Hearing Impairment and Disability

Hearing Impairment and Disability

Edited by Sophie Silva

hayle
medical

New York

Hayle Medical,
750 Third Avenue, 9th Floor,
New York, NY 10017, USA

Visit us on the World Wide Web at:
www.haylemedical.com

ISBN: 978-1-63241-820-3

Cataloging-in-Publication Data

Hearing impairment and disability / edited by Sophie Silva.
p. cm.
Includes bibliographical references and index.
ISBN 978-1-63241-820-3
1. Hearing disorders. 2. Hearing impaired. 3. Deaf. 4. Disabilities. 5. Ear--Diseases. I. Silva, Sophie.
RF290 .H43 2019
617.8--dc23

Table of Contents

Preface

The partial or total inability to hear is referred to as hearing impairment. It may occur in both ears or a single ear. It leads to difficulties in learning a spoken language and social interaction. Some of the factors contributing to hearing loss include aging, infections, genetics, trauma to the ear and birth complications. It can be categorized as mild, moderate, moderate-severe, severe or profound, depending upon the unheard decibels in a particular ear. Otoscopy, tympanometry and auditory function tests such as Weber test, Rinne test, etc. are used to diagnose hearing impairment. Hearing aids are commonly used to assist speech comprehension in such patients. This book provides comprehensive insights into hearing impairment and disability. It elucidates the concepts and innovative models around prospective developments with respect to the diagnosis and treatment of this medical condition. This book will prove to be immensely beneficial to students and researchers in the field of otolaryngology.

This book is a comprehensive compilation of works of different researchers from varied parts of the world. It includes valuable experiences of the researchers with the sole objective of providing the readers (learners) with a proper knowledge of the concerned field. This book will be beneficial in evoking inspiration and enhancing the knowledge of the interested readers.

In the end, I would like to extend my heartiest thanks to the authors who worked with great determination on their chapters. I also appreciate the publisher's support in the course of the book. I would also like to deeply acknowledge my family who stood by me as a source of inspiration during the project.

Editor

Effects of Furosemide on Cochlear Neural Activity, Central Hyperactivity and Behavioural Tinnitus after Cochlear Trauma in Guinea Pig

Wilhelmina H. A. M. Mulders*, Kristin M. Barry, Donald Robertson

The Auditory Laboratory, School of Anatomy, Physiology and Human Biology, The University of Western Australia, Crawley, Western Australia, Australia

Abstract

Cochlear trauma causes increased spontaneous activity (hyperactivity) to develop in central auditory structures, and this has been suggested as a neural substrate for tinnitus. Using a guinea pig model we have previously demonstrated that for some time after cochlear trauma, central hyperactivity is dependent on peripheral afferent drive and only later becomes generated intrinsically within central structures. Furosemide, a loop diuretic, reduces spontaneous firing of auditory afferents. We investigated in our guinea pig model the efficacy of furosemide in reducing 1) spontaneous firing of auditory afferents, using the spectrum of neural noise (SNN) from round window recording, 2) hyperactivity in inferior colliculus, using extracellular single neuron recordings and 3) tinnitus at early time-points after cochlear trauma. Tinnitus was assessed using gap prepulse inhibition of acoustic startle (GPIAS). Intraperitoneal furosemide, but not saline, caused a marked decrease in both SNN and central hyperactivity. Intracochlear perfusion with furosemide similarly reversed central hyperactivity. In animals in which GPIAS measurements suggested the presence of tinnitus (reduced GPIAS), this could be reversed with an intraperitoneal injection with furosemide but not saline. The results are consistent with furosemide reducing central hyperactivity and behavioural signs of tinnitus by acting peripherally to decrease spontaneous firing of auditory afferents. The data support the notion that hyperactivity may be involved in the generation of tinnitus and further suggest that there may be a therapeutic window after cochlear trauma using drug treatments that target peripheral spontaneous activity.

Editor: Berthold Langguth, University of Regensburg, Germany

Funding: Supported by grants from the Royal National Institute for Deaf People (UK) G55, the Medical Health and Research Infrastructure Fund (WA) and The University of Western Australia. The funders had no role in study design, data collection and analysis, decision to publish, or preparation of the manuscript.

Competing Interests: The authors have declared that no competing interests exist.

* E-mail: helmy.mulders@uwa.edu.au

Introduction

A common side-effect of hearing loss is tinnitus, a phantom hearing sensation described as hissing or ringing in the ears [1]. Estimates of the prevalence of chronic tinnitus range from 10 to 15% of the adult population [2–5] but the incidence rises sharply in specific groups such as the elderly, workers in noisy environments and war veterans [6,7]. In about 20% of sufferers, tinnitus significantly affects daily life [8]. A number of previous studies in humans have suggested that the loop diuretic, furosemide may reduce tinnitus in some sufferers [9–11]. The present paper investigates the possible physiological mechanism of such an action.

Although many human studies have described abnormal activity within auditory pathways of tinnitus sufferers [12–15], the exact neural substrate is unknown. Animal models of hearing loss have shown increased spontaneous firing rates in central auditory structures (hyperactivity), alterations in neural synchrony, as well as reorganization [16–21], but exactly how these changes contribute to the development of tinnitus is still debated.

Because primary auditory afferents do not show increased spontaneous firing rates after common types of acoustic trauma [1,18,22], it is often assumed that central hyperactivity is generated intrinsically and is not dependent on peripheral

cochlear activity [1,23,24]. However, using a guinea pig model of acoustic trauma, we have shown that treatments that eliminate or reduce primary auditory nerve firing (cochlear ablation, cochlear cooling or cochlear perfusion with $CoCl_2$), can significantly reduce hyperactivity in inferior colliculus [18,25]. Interestingly, this reduction of hyperactivity could only be fully achieved within the first 6 weeks after trauma, but not at later recovery times [26]. Based on these findings we have hypothesized that there are two distinct stages following cochlear trauma. In the first stage, central hyperactivity is the result of hyperexcitability of central neurons and is still dependent on peripheral afferent drive. This drive comprises the spontaneous firing of surviving primary afferent neurons, which is still present despite the fact that acoustic trauma reduces sensitivity to sound. In the second stage, central neurons become so excitable that they begin to generate their own intrinsic spontaneous firing and hyperactivity therefore becomes relatively independent of peripheral afferent input [27]. If hyperactivity is involved in the development of tinnitus, this suggests there may be a therapeutic window for recent-onset tinnitus in the first stage, using treatments that reduce cochlear afferent firing.

Furosemide is known to reduce primary auditory nerve firing [28]. Therefore in the present study we investigated, in our guinea pig model of cochlear trauma, the effect of furosemide on spontaneous firing of the auditory afferents, on hyperactivity in inferior colliculus and on behavioural measures of tinnitus.

Materials and Methods

Ethics Statement

The experimental protocols were approved by the Animal Ethics Committee of The University of Western Australia (03/100/1007) and were carried out in accordance with the Guidelines from the National Health and Medical Research Council Australia regarding the care and use of animals for experimental procedures. All surgery was performed under anaesthesia and all efforts were made to minimize suffering.

Animals

Thirty-two young adult pigmented guinea pigs of either sex were used. Animals (Tricolor strain) were derived from a local breeding colony at the University of Western Australia. Twenty of these animals were used to assess the therapeutic effects of intraperitoneal injection of furosemide (80 mg/kg) on tinnitus. The remaining twelve animals, weighing between 255 and 395 g at the time of acoustic trauma (10 kHz 124 dB SPL, 2 hours), were used to assess the effect of furosemide on spontaneous activity of the auditory nerve and on central hyperactivity measured in the central nucleus of the inferior colliculus (CNIC) 2 weeks after acoustic trauma. In eight of these animals furosemide (n = 4) or saline (n = 4) was administered intraperitoneally and in the remaining four animals furosemide was administered by intracochlear perfusion (see Fig. 1A).

Behavioural Analysis for Tinnitus: GPIAS and PPI

Behavioural testing for tinnitus consisted of gap prepulse inhibition of acoustic startle (GPIAS) and Prepulse Inhibition (PPI). GPIAS is a variation of PPI. PPI occurs when a weaker prestimulus, or prepulse, inhibits the reaction to a stronger stimulus. GPIAS consists of a comparison between two conditions. Both conditions consist of a background noise and startle pulse which elicits a startle response. However, in one condition, there is a gap within the continuous background noise which precedes the startle pulse. The gap in this case works as a prepulse. In normal animals, this condition results in inhibition of the startle response. It is thought that animals experiencing tinnitus that is qualitatively similar to the background noise, show decreased startle inhibition, i.e. deficits of GPIAS, because the tinnitus "fills in" the gap in the background noise [29,30]. Turner et al. compared GPIAS tests to other behavioural animal models of tinnitus and showed a strong positive correlation between the different methods [30].

A deficit in the GPIAS test could also be due to hearing loss (when an animal does not hear the background noise it cannot detect a gap therein) and therefore a PPI test is performed in parallel to the GPIAS test, using for the prepulse the same parameters as for the background noise in order to establish that the animal can hear the prepulse/background noise. Therefore, animals that fail GPIAS testing but pass PPI testing are thought to have tinnitus [29,30].

Behavioural tests were performed on 20 animals. Seventeen animals, weighing between 332 and 649 g at the time of surgery, were exposed to a unilateral acoustic trauma in order to induce a hearing loss and tinnitus. The remaining 3 animals showed a GPIAS deficit before any cochlear trauma was performed and were therefore discarded from this study.

For behavioural testing, animals were mildly restrained in a clear polycarbonate holder which was placed on a custom-

designed force transducer within a dark soundproof room. Just above the animal's head, two speakers were placed, one to administer the startle stimulus (Radio Shack 401278B; 115 dB SPL, narrowband noise, centre frequency 1 kHz, bandwidth 100 Hz, 20 ms duration, 0.1 ms rise/fall time,) and the other one for continuous background noise (for GPIAS) or a prepulse sound stimulus (for PPI) (Beyer DT 48). Custom-designed software (kindly provided by R. Salvi and D. Stolzberg) and commercial hardware (Tucker-Davis technologies) was used to deliver sound stimuli and record output from the custom-designed startle platform. Acoustic stimuli were calibrated using a ½″ microphone positioned at the location of the animal's external ear canal.

Background noise for GPIAS consisted of a narrowband noise centred at either 8 or 14 kHz (3dB bandwidths = 1 kHz). These two frequency bands were chosen to fall within the centre of peripheral hearing loss (14 kHz) and just below the region of hearing loss (8 kHz). The 14 kHz region is also the region of highest hyperactivity [31] in line with observations in human tinnitus subjects that the tinnitus pitch shows a strong correlation with the frequency region of hearing loss [32]. Intensity could be set at either 60 or 70 dB SPL. For each individual animal the lowest of these two intensity settings for which significant GPIAS ($p < 0.05$, see below: data analysis) would occur was determined and this level was then used throughout further testing for each animal. In the PPI tests the characteristics of the prepulse for PPI were identical to the background noise characteristics for GPIAS. Animals had to pass GPIAS and PPI twice before a cochlear trauma was performed.

A behavioural test consisted of 50 presentations of the startle stimulus with varying intervals (20–30 s) between presentations. Each test consisted of either the 8 or 14 kHz background noise (GPIAS) or pre-pulse stimulus (PPI). During GPIAS testing the startle stimulus was embedded in the continuous background noise and half of the trials contained a 50 ms gap which preceded the startle stimulus by 100 ms (ISI 50 ms). The order of gap (G) and no gap (NG) trials was randomized. During PPI testing the startle stimulus was embedded in silence, and a 50 ms prepulse was presented in half of the trials, but otherwise the PPI test was identical to the GPIAS test. A noise floor test was also performed to obtain a recording of the background level of movement for each animal (20 trials, with no startle or background noise present).

Each testing session contained three behavioural tests. First each animal was allowed to habituate in the soundproof room for 5 min before commencement of testing. Then the first test (50 trials see above) was either a GPIAS or PPI test, using either 8 or 14 kHz background noise or prepulse, respectively. The second test was a noise floor test to ensure that all startle data were above the noise floor in all experiments. Then the third test was again either a GPIAS or PPI test, using the alternate frequency background noise or prepulse, respectively. The order of using 8 and 14 kHz background noise/prepulse was alternated between sessions. There was at least one day between testing sessions. Only one testing session was conducted per day for each animal, with the only exception being the day of treatment. On this day the treatment testing session was conducted 1 hour after the previous session. No animal went through more than three testing sessions in one week in order to reduce the possibility of habituation and acclimatization [29,33,34].

After each test it was determined whether an animal had failed or passed the GPIAS or PPI test. A Mann-Whitney statistical test was applied comparing startle amplitudes with and without GAP or pre-pulse. The animal was deemed to have failed the test when there was no significant difference between the gap/prepulse and

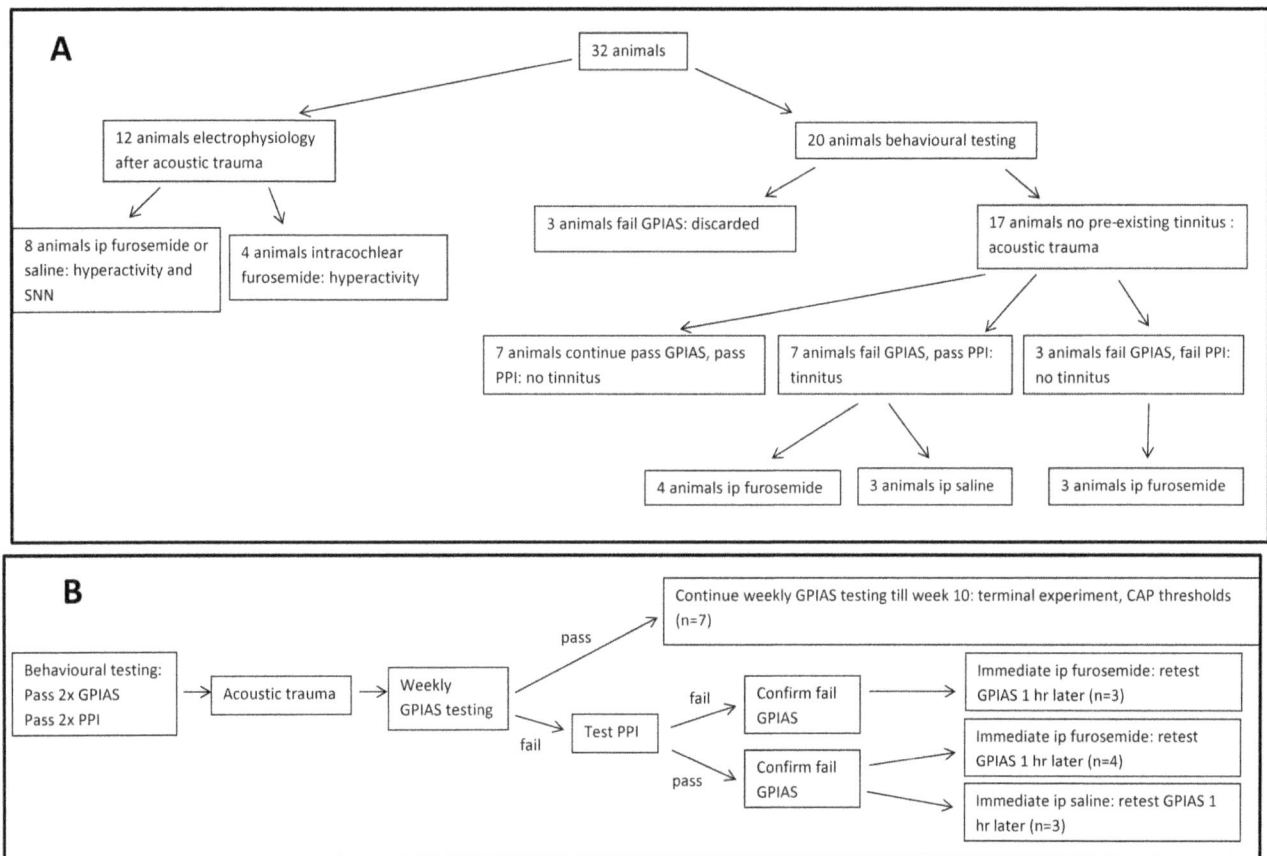

Figure 1. A: Overview of all animals used in the present study as allocated to the different groups. B: Schematic representation of the experimental design of behavioural experiments.

no gap/no prepulse conditions. Passing the test was characterized by a significant difference (significance level $p<0.05$) between the two conditions.

After cochlear trauma, weekly GPIAS testing resumed. When an animal passed the GPIAS test the weekly testing continued. When an animal failed the GPIAS testing (i.e. no significant GPIAS), a PPI test was performed. If the animal passed the PPI test ($p<0.05$) then two days later another GPIAS test was performed. If the animal failed this again and was categorized as a tinnitus animal, it immediately received an i.p. injection of either furosemide (80 mg/kg) or an equivalent amount of saline and was tested again (GPIAS) 1 hour later to assess the effect of treatment on behavioural signs of tinnitus. Three of the animals failed the PPI test as well as the GPIAS test (i.e. no significant pre pulse inhibition) and they also received an immediate i.p. injection of furosemide (80 mg/kg) and were tested again for GPIAS 1 hour later. After the treatment testing, animals underwent a final experiment, at least 3 days later, during which cochlear thresholds on both sides were measured.

Recovery Surgery for Acoustic Trauma

After a subcutaneous injection of 0.1 ml atropine sulphate (0.6 mg/ml), animals received an intraperitoneal injection of Diazepam (5 mg/kg), followed 20 minutes later by an intramuscular injection of Hypnorm (0.315 mg/ml fentanyl citrate and 10 mg/ml fluanisone; 1 ml/kg). When deep anaesthesia was obtained as determined by the absence of the foot withdrawal reflex, the area of incision was shaved and animals were placed on

a heating blanket in a soundproof room and mounted in hollow ear bars. A small opening (approximately 1 mm²) was made in the bulla and an insulated silver wire was placed on the round window. A compound action potential (CAP) audiogram [35] for the frequency range 4–24 kHz was recorded to assess the animals' cochlear sensitivity. All sound stimuli were presented in a closed sound system through a ½″ condenser microphone driven in reverse as a speaker (Bruel and Kjaer, type 4134). The system was calibrated using a 1/8″ condensor microphone in place of the tympanic membrane and an absolute sound calibrator (Bruel and Kjaer type 4231). Pure tone stimuli (10 ms duration, 1 ms rise/fall times) were synthesized by a computer equipped with a DIGI 96 soundcard connected to an analog/digital interface (ADI-9 DS, RME Intelligent Audio Solution). Sample rate was 96 kHz. The interface was driven by a custom-made computer program (Neurosound, MI Lloyd), which was also used to collect single neuron data during the final experiments. CAP signals were amplified (1000x), filtered (100 Hz–3 kHz bandpass) and recorded with a second data acquisition system (Powerlab 4SP, AD Instruments).

When cochlear sensitivity was within the normal range [35], animals received a unilateral acoustic trauma using the closed sound system described above in the left cochlea. For this purpose animals were exposed to a continuous loud tone for 2 h (10 kHz, 124 dB SPL), whilst still anaesthetized. The contralateral ear was blocked with plasticine. Immediately after the acoustic trauma another CAP audiogram was measured, the incision was sutured and buprenorphin (0.05 mg/kg subcutaneously) was given postoperatively as analgesic. Survival time varied between 2 (electro-physiological experiments) and 10 weeks (behavioural experiments).

Surgery for Final Experiments

Animals received a subcutaneous injection with 0.1 ml atropine followed by an intraperitoneal injection of Nembutal (pentobarbitone sodium, 30 mg/kg) and a 0.15 ml intramuscular injection of Hypnorm. Anaesthesia was maintained with full Hypnorm doses every h and half doses of Nembutal every 2 h. When deep anaesthesia was obtained as determined by the absence of the foot withdrawal reflex, the areas of incision were shaved and animals were placed on a heating blanket in a sound proof room and artificially ventilated on carbogen (95% O_2 and 5% CO_2). Paralysis was induced with 0.1 ml pancuronium bromide (2 mg/ml intramuscularly). The electrocardiogram was continuously monitored and heart rate never increased over pre-paralysis levels at any stage of the experiments. After the animals were mounted in hollow ear bars, the left and right cochleae were exposed and CAP audiograms were recorded on both sides with a silver wire placed on the round window as for the recovery procedures. Animals that had been used to assess effects of furosemide on GPIAS were then immediately euthanized with an injection of 0.3 ml Lethabarb (sodium pentobarbitone 325 mg/ml; VIRBAC).

During experiments testing the effects of a single acute intraperitoneal injection of furosemide or saline on central nerve activity, the spontaneous activity of the peripheral auditory nerve fibres was also assessed using the established technique of the spectrum of the neural noise (SNN) recorded from the round window of the noise-damaged cochlea. The latter recording has a prominent peak at approximately 900 Hz which can be used as a measure of the spontaneous activity of the primary afferent fibres [36,37]. To quantify the size of the 900 Hz peak of the SNN, the amplitude of the spectrum between 700 and 1100 Hz was averaged (10 averages/time point).

To obtain extracellular single neuron recordings in the central nucleus of the inferior colliculus (CNIC) a small craniotomy (approximately 4 mm^2) overlying the visual cortex was performed and a glass-insulated tungsten microelectrode [38] was advanced using a stepping motor microdrive along the dorso-ventral axis through the cortex into the CNIC contralateral to the cochlea subjected previously to acoustic trauma. Electrode placement in the CNIC (about 2.5 to 3 mm ventral to the cortical surface) was indicated by the presence of strong sound-driven activity with a short latency (cluster onset latencies <6.5 ms) and a systematic progression from low to high characteristic frequencies (CF) with increasing depth. We have previously confirmed histologically that these response properties correlate with location of the electrode in the CNIC [31]. The craniotomy was covered with 5% agar in saline to improve mechanical stability. When a single neuron was isolated its CF and threshold at CF were determined audio-visually and depth from the cortical surface was recorded using methods described previously [25,39]. In all neurons the spontaneous firing rate was measured for a period of 10 s as previously reported using an identical animal model [18,25,31].

Effects of Furosemide on Central and Peripheral Nerve Activity

To assess the effect of an acute i.p. injection with furosemide (Ilium, Australia, 50 mg/ml furosemide), in 8 animals, spontaneous firing rates of CNIC neurons were collected from the frequency regions between 4 and 24 kHz before (approximately 2 hours of recording) and after an i.p. injection with furosemide (n = 4 animals) or saline (n = 4 animals). These single neuron

recordings were interleaved with measurements of the SNN at regular intervals (every 5 to 15 minutes). After furosemide was injected (80 mg/kg bodyweight i.p.), SNN was monitored until a significant reduction could be observed (between 20 and 30 minutes after injection). We applied the same waiting period (30 minutes) after the saline injections. From that moment single neuron recordings resumed for another 2 hours interleaved with measurements of SNN at regular intervals (every 5 to 15 minutes).

To assess the effect of intracochlear injection of furosemide, a neuron with a high spontaneous firing rate was isolated within the region of the CNIC that showed hyperactivity. Activity from this neuron was then recorded at regular intervals before, during and after the perfusion (recordings of single neurons lasted for up to 130 minutes-see figure 1 D and E). The thresholds to CF tones of the same neurons were also recorded at regular intervals to monitor effects of furosemide on thresholds (see figure 1D and E). For the perfusions, a hole was made in the cochlear apex with the use of a hooked pick and a small hole was made in the scala tympani wall of the basal cochlear turn using a syringe needle. Using a micromanipulator the tip of a glass perfusion pipette was then carefully inserted through the hole in the scala tympani wall. The perfusion pipette contained artificial perilymph (127 mM NaCl, 5 mM KCl, 1 mM MgCl2.6H2O, 1 mM NaH2PO4.H2O, 12 mM NaHCO3, 11 mM glucose and 2 mM CaCl2 at pH 7.4) with furosemide (0.5 mM or 1 mM). Perfusion rate was 2 to 3 µl/min.

Data Analysis

To identify statistically significant differences in spontaneous firing rates before and after intraperitoneal injection with furosemide or saline, a Kruskall-Wallis test was used as the data was not normally distributed, followed by Dunn's multiple comparison tests. The same test was used to assess the effect of furosemide and saline on SNN. We performed statistical analysis at three time points, t = 0 (time of injection) and at t = 20 (between 15–25 min after injection) and t = 120 (between 110 and 125 min after injection). For statistical analysis of the CAP threshold data a one-way ANOVA and Bonferroni's multiple comparison tests were used.

For analysis of each GPIAS and PPI test in each animal, a Mann-Whitney statistical test was used to compare startle amplitudes with and without gap or pre-pulse (significance level p<0.05). For analysis of group data for GPIAS, the percentage suppression in the gap (G) condition compared to the no gap (NG) condition was calculated for each test (% GPIAS = (1-(G/NG))*100). Repeated measures (RM) one-way and two-way ANOVAs were performed comparing the suppression at three different time-points (before acoustic trauma, after acoustic trauma just before drug or control treatment, and after drug or control treatment).

Results

Behavioural Testing Data

Figure 1 shows an overview of all animals and their allocation to the different groups described in detail below (Fig. 1A) as well as a schematic representation of the overall experimental design for the behavioural experiments (Fig. 1B).

Of the 17 animals that showed significant initial GPIAS and PPI and then underwent acoustic trauma, 7 did not develop consistent (twice in one week) GPIAS deficits. Instead, these animals showed robust GPIAS throughout a period of 10 weeks post-acoustic trauma. Their % GPIAS is shown in figure 2A in the presence of both 8 and 14 kHz background noise before the acoustic trauma (black bars) and at 10 weeks post-acoustic trauma (white bars). The fact that these animals continued to pass GPIAS testing suggests they did not develop tinnitus throughout this 10 week period and in addition supports the notion that GPIAS is a robust and consistent phenomenon. The mean audiograms for these animals are shown in figure 2B. The mean cochlear thresholds did not show statistically significant elevations at 10 weeks post-acoustic trauma. This is most likely due to the large variations in the extent of threshold recovery between animals as illustrated in figure 2C, that shows the CAP threshold losses for each individual animal.

Of the 17 animals that showed significant initial GPIAS and PPI and then underwent acoustic trauma, 10 animals did develop GPIAS deficits at time-points between 3 and 6 weeks after acoustic trauma. Nine of these animals developed the GPIAS deficit with 14 kHz background noise and one of them with 8 kHz background noise. They were randomly allocated to a treatment after they were separated on the basis of their PPI data. Seven of these 10 animals showed significant PPI despite the GPIAS deficit, supporting the notion that the GPIAS deficit was due to tinnitus, whereas the other 3 animals also developed a PPI deficit suggesting the GPIAS deficit may not have been due to tinnitus. Four of the 7 animals that showed evidence of tinnitus received an i.p. injection with furosemide and 3 with saline. All 4 animals that received an i.p. injection with furosemide showed individually a return of significant GPIAS, in contrast to the 3 animals that received an i.p. injection with saline. These two groups of animals with intact PPI and different treatments are shown in Figure 3A. Note that only the GPIAS outcomes for the background noise condition (i.e. 8 or 14 kHz centred noise) that revealed the deficit are shown in the group data and this will be done throughout the remainder of this paper. Statistical analysis revealed a significant interaction of time and treatment (F(2, 10) = 10.15, p<0.01). Post-hoc tests revealed that the animals which received furosemide showed significant (p<0.001) improvement in % GPIAS when compared to those animals which received saline. All other comparisons between the two groups were not significant. These findings suggest that furosemide but not saline eliminates the behavioural signs of tinnitus.

Further statistical comparison indicated that within the furosemide treatment group, the % GPIAS before acoustic trauma was significantly higher than after acoustic trauma (p<0.001). Additionally, there was significantly less % GPIAS after acoustic trauma than after treatment with furosemide (p<0.01). No other comparisons within the furosemide group were significant. Within the saline treated group, the % GPIAS before acoustic trauma was significantly higher than both after acoustic trauma (p<0.05) and after treatment with saline (p<0.01). No other comparisons within the saline group were significant. Mean CAP audiograms for these 7 animals that developed tinnitus are shown in figure 3C. Mean thresholds after recovery (varying between 4 and 7 weeks) were elevated compared to before acoustic trauma, but these changes were not statistically significant, most likely due to large inter-animal variation (CAP threshold loss for each individual animal shown in Figure 3D). In addition, there were no statistically significant differences between the threshold loss observed in tinnitus animals compared to the threshold loss observed in non-tinnitus animals.

The remaining 3 acoustic trauma animals that showed GPIAS deficits, also showed PPI deficits, which suggests that their GPIAS deficit may not have been due to tinnitus. These animals also received an i.p. injection with furosemide, but this had no effect on their GPIAS deficits as shown in figure 3B. In this figure the comparison is shown between the results from this group of animals with combined GPIAS deficit and PPI deficit and the

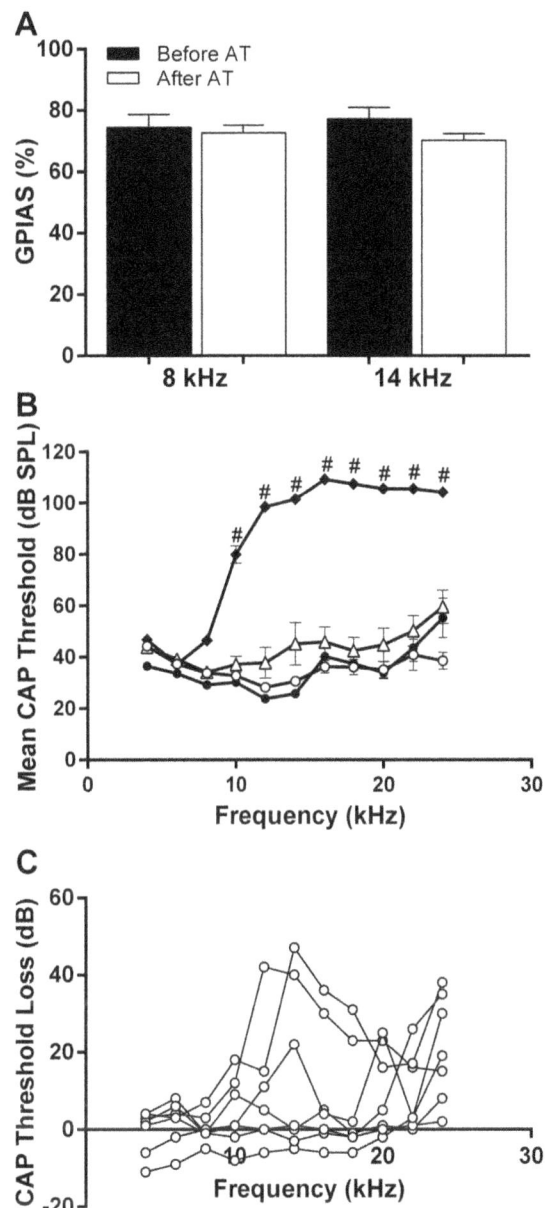

Figure 2. Data from 7 animals that underwent acoustic trauma and that did not develop a GPIAS deficit for a period of 10 weeks A: Histogram showing mean % GPIAS. Shown is % GPIAS measured with 8 and 14 kHz background noise before (black bars) and 10 weeks after trauma (white bars). B: CAP thresholds (mean ± SEM). Left cochlea before acoustic trauma (open circles), immediately after acoustic trauma (black diamonds) and after recovery from acoustic trauma (open triangles). Contralateral control cochlea after recovery (black circles). Statistical significance of differences between pre and post acoustic trauma data: #p<0.001. C: Threshold loss for individual animals at 10 weeks after acoustic trauma.

group of animals described above (GPIAS deficit but no PPI deficit). There was a significant interaction of time and PPI performance (F(2, 10) = 10.15, p<.001). Post-hoc testing showed that after furosemide treatment, animals with impaired PPI showed significantly less % GPIAS than those with intact PPI (p<0.0001). These data show that when reduced GPIAS is associated with reduced PPI, furosemide cannot restore the suppression, unlike the situation when good PPI is still present.

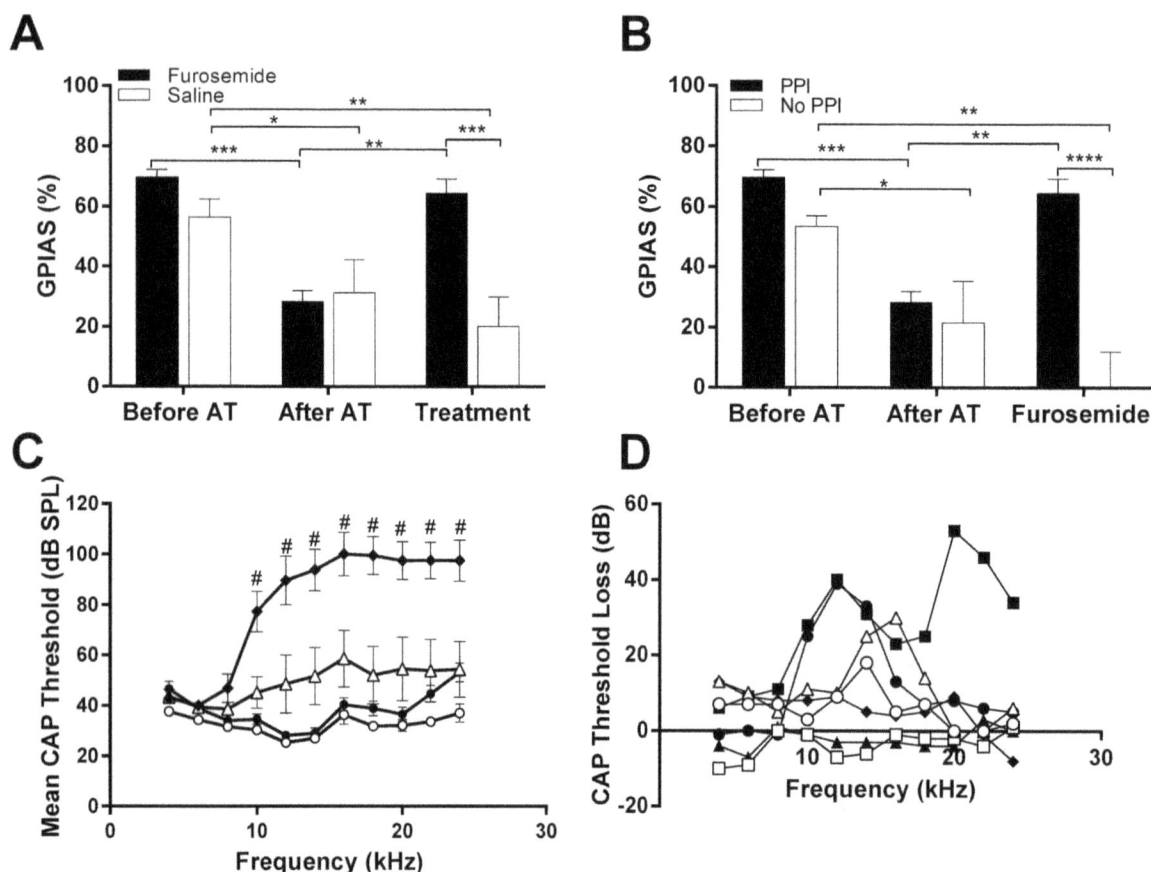

Figure 3. Data from animals that developed GPIAS deficits between 3 and 6 weeks post-trauma Histograms in A and B show % GPIAS before acoustic trauma (AT), after AT and after treatment. A: Data from 4 animals given furosemide (black bars) and 3 animals given saline (white bars). All animals shown in A showed significant PPI. B: Data from 4 animals with significant PPI which were given furosemide (black bars, same animals as in panel A) and 3 animals without significant PPI which were also given furosemide (white bars). Significance is shown from repeated measure two-way ANOVA and post-tests. Statistical significance: *$p<0.05$; **$p<0.01$. ***$p<0.001$. C: CAP thresholds from animals shown in A (mean $\pm$ SEM). Left cochlea before acoustic trauma (open circles), immediately after acoustic trauma (black diamonds) and after recovery from acoustic trauma (open triangles). Contralateral control cochlea after recovery (black circles). Statistical significance of differences between pre and post acoustic trauma data: #$p<0.001$. D: Threshold loss for individual animals shown in A. Black symbols are animals given furosemide and open symbols animals given saline.

This shows that the beneficial action of furosemide is specific to those animals which may have tinnitus and it is therefore unlikely to be having a non-specific effect on startle circuitry *per se*.

Additional statistical comparisons between the intact PPI and impaired PPI animals (Fig. 3B), indicated that within the intact PPI group, the % GPIAS before acoustic trauma was significantly higher than after acoustic trauma ($p<0.01$). Additionally, there was a significantly higher % GPIAS after treatment with furosemide than after acoustic trauma ($p<0.01$). No other comparisons within the intact PPI group were significant. Within the PPI deficit group, the % GPIAS before acoustic trauma was greater than both after acoustic trauma ($p<0.05$) and after treatment with saline ($p<0.01$).

Acute Effects of Furosemide on Peripheral and Central Neural Activity

Figure 4A shows the magnitude of the SNN measured from the round window in 8 different animals before and after i.p. injection with furosemide (n = 4) or saline (n = 4). The SNN can be used as a measure of spontaneous cochlear neural activity [36,37]. In all animals injected with furosemide, the SNN showed a large reduction, which reached a maximum (40 to 70% reduction) 20 to

30 minutes after injection. The SNN remained decreased up to 3 h after injection (the maximum period recorded) in 3 animals but showed recovery to 89% of its initial value in one animal after approximately 2 hours. In contrast, in animals injected with saline, the SNN remained stable. Statistical analysis showed no significant difference between the SNN in the furosemide group and the saline group at time of injection but a significant reduction of SNN after furosemide injection compared to saline injection at t = 20 min and t = 120 min ($p<0.05$). These data show that i.p. administration of furosemide can decrease the spontaneous firing of the primary auditory nerve fibres.

The effects of i.p. injection of furosemide or saline on spontaneous firing rates of single neurons in CNIC, are illustrated in figure 4B. These data were obtained from 8 animals that were exposed to acoustic trauma 2 weeks previously and had therefore developed hyperactivity in CNIC (note that these animals were the same as used for the measurements of SNN described above). The mean spontaneous activity of sampled CNIC neurons before furosemide injection was 8.12 ± 1.1 spikes/sec (ranging from 0 to 74.4 spikes/sec; n = 172 neurons from 4 animals), very similar to the mean spontaneous activity measured in 4 other animals before an injection with saline (8.1 ± 0.8 spikes/sec, ranging from 0 to

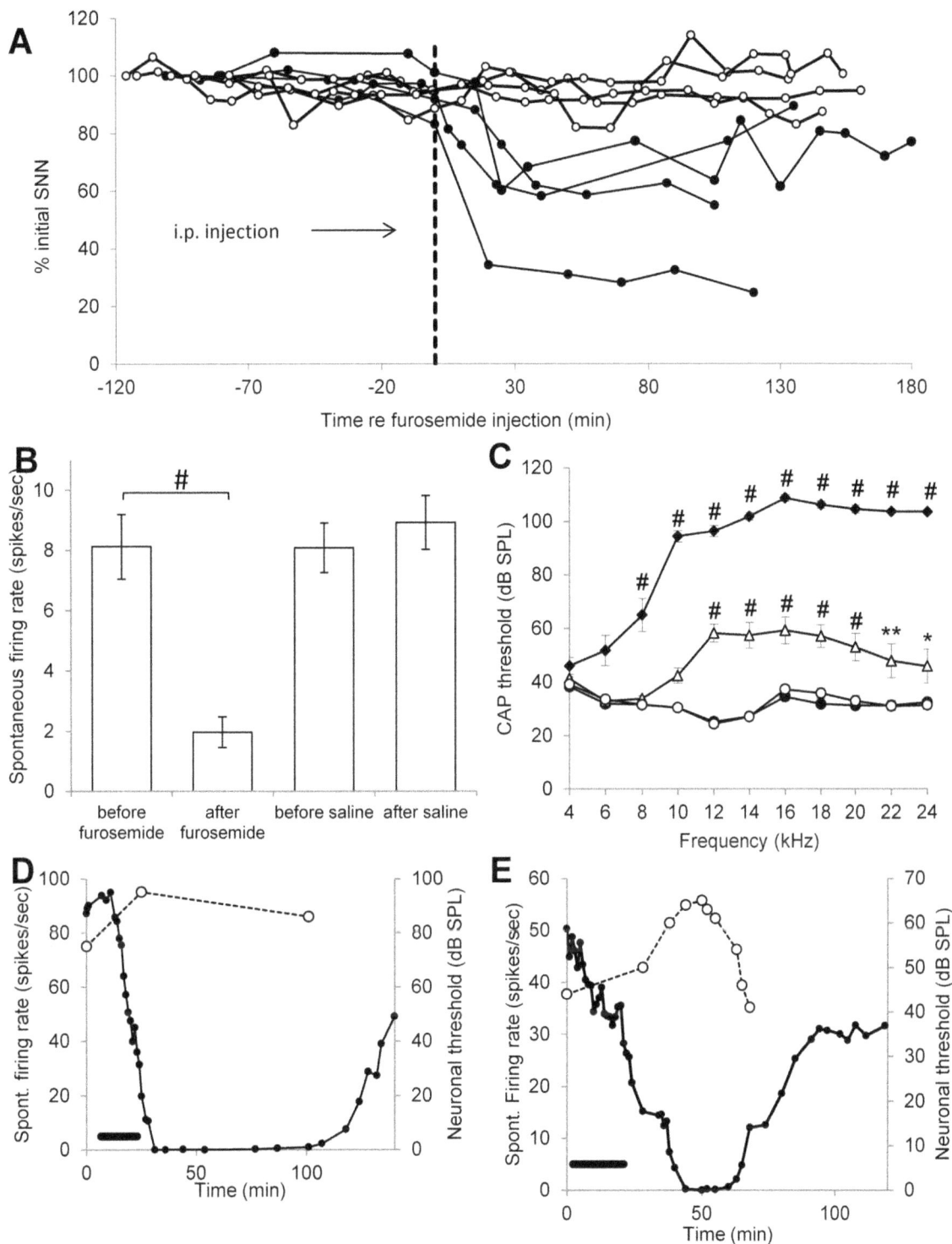

Figure 4. A: Spectrum of neural noise (SNN) recorded from the round window in 8 animals plotted as percentage of original value before and after an i.p. injection with furosemide (black line with filled circles n = 4) or saline (black line with open circle n = 4). Time of injection indicated by dotted line. B: Mean spontaneous firing rate of CNIC neurons recorded before and after i.p. furosemide and before and after saline (n = 4 for each group; mean ± SEM). C: CAP thresholds (mean ± SEM) at different frequencies recorded from the left cochlea before acoustic trauma (open circles), immediately after acoustic trauma (black diamonds) and after recovery from acoustic trauma (open triangles), as well as from the contralateral control cochlea after recovery (black circles). *p<0.05; **p<0.01; #p<0.001 statistical significance as compared to before trauma data. D and E: Spontaneous firing rate of 2 individual neurons from 2 different animals plotted over time before, during and after intracochlear perfusion of furosemide (black circles). Black bar indicates timing of intracochlear perfusion. Open circles indicate measurement of the neuron's threshold to CF tones. Neuronal CF is 10 kHz and 12.4 kHz, in D and E, respectively.

75.9 spikes/sec; n = 235 neurons), indicating levels of neural hyperactivity in good agreement with those previously reported using identical methods [18,26]. After the injection with furosemide (and after a decrease was observed in the averaged SNN as shown in Fig. 4A) the mean spontaneous firing rates in CNIC decreased to 1.97±0.5 spikes/sec (ranging from 0 to 44.8 spikes/sec; n = 179 neurons from 4 animals). This decrease in the spontaneous firing rates after furosemide was statistically significant, both when comparing within each individual animal as well as when using the pooled group data (all p<0.001). In contrast, an injection with saline in the other 4 animals had no effect (8.9±0.9 spikes/sec (ranging from 0 to 77.2 spikes/sec; n = 225 neurons). These data show that an acute i.p. injection with furosemide simultaneously reduced peripheral afferent spontaneous firing (SNN measurements) and lowered the hyperactive spontaneous firing rates seen in IC neurons two weeks after recovery from acoustic trauma.

We were able to record the effect of intracochlear perfusion of furosemide on 6 individual CNIC neurons that showed high spontaneous firing rates varying between 25 to 90 spikes/sec 2 weeks after acoustic trauma. In 5 of these neurons the spontaneous firing rate reduced to 0 spikes/sec and in the remaining neuron spontaneous firing rate reduced by 68.6% (from 34.7 to 10.9 spikes/sec). Four of the neurons were recorded from for long enough to observe partial recovery of spontaneous firing rate. The effect of intracochlear perfusion with furosemide on two of these neurons is illustrated in figures 4D and 4E. In addition, in these figures the thresholds of these neurons to acoustic stimulation are shown (white open circles). These show that furosemide causes a relatively small increase in neuronal thresholds and that these seem to recover at a faster rate than the spontaneous firing rate (note that thresholds for the two neurons shown in Fig. 4D,E are rather high because these neurons emanate from cochlear regions that were subjected to acoustic trauma 2 weeks before recording). These data show that an intracochlear effect of furosemide is sufficient to cause suppression of the hyperactive spontaneous firing rates seen in IC neurons two weeks after recovery from acoustic trauma.

Figure 4C shows the cochlear CAP thresholds after recovery from acoustic trauma in the 8 animals used to describe the i.p. and intracochlear effects of furosemide on neural activity. The effects of acoustic trauma were as described previously [18,31,40]. Immediately after acoustic trauma all CAP thresholds ≥8 kHz were significantly increased compared to before acoustic trauma values, but after 14 to 25 days (our recovery periods) thresholds recovered substantially and were only significantly different from pre-acoustic trauma values at frequencies ≥12 kHz (one-way ANOVA F(32,231) = 89.17, p<0.0001, details from post-hoc analysis shown in figure). No difference was observed between the noise-damaged (before trauma values) and contralateral control cochlear thresholds (measured after recovery from trauma), demonstrating that contralateral control cochlear thresholds remained unaffected by the cochlear trauma on the other side.

Discussion

This paper provides for the first time, direct evidence in a single animal model that a drug treatment that reduces spontaneous firing rates in the auditory nerve, eliminates the hyperactivity in the CNIC caused by acoustic trauma, and also eliminates the behavioural signs of tinnitus.

In agreement with previous studies, acute systemic furosemide caused a reduction of spontaneous firing rates of auditory nerve fibres [28], as demonstrated by decreased SNN [36,37]. This is most likely due to a decreased endocochlear potential, caused by an effect of furosemide on ion transporters in the stria vascularis and subsequent reduction of spontaneous neurotransmitter release from inner hair cells [28,41]. Also in agreement with previous descriptions of the peripheral action of furosemide, the effects on spontaneous cochlear afferent activity were accompanied by relatively minor changes in cochlear neural thresholds that recovered faster than the cochlear spontaneous firing rates. Sewell [28] showed in cats, that primary afferent spontaneous firing is more sensitive than thresholds to falls in endocochlear potential induced by furosemide. This suggests that furosemide, or related drugs, could be used to selectively reduce primary afferent spontaneous firing without major effects on hearing sensitivity, which could be beneficial for any future therapeutic application.

A major finding was that acute administration of furosemide also caused a marked reduction in the spontaneous hyperactivity that developed in the CNIC after acoustic trauma. These findings are in agreement with our previous studies showing an elimination of central hyperactivity after other treatments directly reducing cochlear neural output [18,25].

Finally, in animals with unequivocal behavioural evidence of tinnitus (reduced GPIAS and intact PPI), an i.p. injection with furosemide, but not saline, dramatically altered the result of GPIAS testing, showing a return of significant GPIAS, suggesting that furosemide reduced the level of tinnitus in these animals. The effect was robust in that all animals in this group showed a return of GPIAS after furosemide, whereas none did so after saline. Similar observations of the effectiveness of furosemide were made in 3 other animals in our laboratory that developed failures in GPIAS after mechanical lesion of the cochlea or that had pre-existing GPIAS deficits before a trauma to the cochlea (data not shown). We have previously shown that mechanical lesions also results in hyperactivity in IC neurons [42]. A specific therapeutic effect of furosemide on tinnitus is further supported by the fact that 3 animals that showed a GPIAS deficit but also a PPI deficit, did not respond positively to furosemide administration, since in these animals the GPIAS deficit was most likely due to factors other than tinnitus (see below). This suggests that furosemide does not exert its effects via a general effect on acoustic startle.

Approximately 60% of animals subjected to acoustic trauma (10 out of 17 animals) developed repeatable deficits of GPIAS. A deficit of GPIAS can be an indication of tinnitus as GPIAS testing strongly correlates with other behavioural testing paradigms for tinnitus [30]. However, a deficit in GPIAS could also be a result of hearing loss, habituation or unknown startle circuitry deficits [29,30,43] and we included the PPI test in our experiments in order to screen for these possibilities. Indeed, when also tested for PPI, 30% of these animals with GPIAS deficits (17% of total), also showed a PPI deficit. The remaining animals with GPIAS deficits showed significant PPI and these latter animals (41% of total numbers receiving acoustic trauma) could therefore be categorized as fulfilling criteria consistent with their experiencing tinnitus. Because the pre-pulse stimulus had the same acoustic characteristics as the background noise used in the GPIAS test, this provided valuable confirmation that the animals could still detect the background noise and that their startle circuitry was functioning normally. The percentage of animals showing tinnitus shows large variations between studies, i.e. in guinea pigs (57%; 4 out of 7 animals) [29], in mice (50%) [44] or in rats (between 30 and 75%) [45–48]. This could be due to species differences or to the different parameters of cochlear trauma between different studies. The fact that not all animals develop signs of tinnitus is in agreement with human population data showing that not all individuals with a hearing loss develop tinnitus [2,4].

Taken together, our results seem to provide a mechanism for the possible therapeutic effect of furosemide in treating tinnitus, which has in fact been reported in human patients [9,11,49]. However, there are several important qualifications that must be placed on this conclusion.

First, the dose of furosemide (80 mg/kg) that we used for i.p injection is more than 10 times the usual hourly intravenous dose recommended in humans for treatment of severe renal and cardiovascular conditions, and it is higher than the oral dose used in the past for treatment of human tinnitus. However, direct comparison between human and guinea pig is not possible (for example different metabolic rates [50] might mean a lower dose could be used in human to produce therapeutic effects on tinnitus) and clearly more work is needed to elucidate whether lower doses that are suitable for human application can produce the physiological and behavioural effects we report here.

Second, the present study used only a single dose of furosemide and involved a single session of behavioural testing immediately after. Hence it is not known if the behavioural effects seen are long lasting or whether chronic administration of furosemide would be required to permanently suppress central hyperactivity and tinnitus.

Third, furosemide might affect CNIC hyperactivity via direct central actions, since the Na-K-2Cl co-transporter found in the inner ear is also expressed centrally [51] and a central effect cannot be ruled out by the present experiments. However, the fact that we saw changes in peripheral neural activity after i.p furosemide and also observed complete elimination of spontaneous hyperactivity in CNIC neurons after local intracochlear injection, is compatible with the notion that an intracochlear action of furosemide is sufficient to induce the central effects.

Fourth, we have only investigated the effects of furosemide between 3–8 weeks after cochlear trauma. Our previous work showed that the peripheral dependence of central hyperactivity is temporary [18], and that the central-intrinsic phase emerges at

around 8 to 12 weeks post–trauma [27]. At this latter stage, both hyperactivity and tinnitus should become resistant to furosemide treatment and further animal studies are needed to test this hypothesis. Nonetheless, our present data could provide a physiological explanation for the partial success of furosemide treatment in human tinnitus patients [9,11,49]. Risey et al. [11] reported that 50% of patients experienced alleviation of tinnitus after furosemide administration and we suggest that patients who did not respond to furosemide, had tinnitus that was in the second, central-intrinsic, phase. Cesarani et al. [9] showed acute positive effects of furosemide in 74% of patients, with increased effectiveness when treatment was given during the first 3 months after tinnitus onset. Others also showed greater beneficial effects of furosemide treatment in patients with fresh cases of deafness than old cases of deafness, again supporting our hypothesis [10].

Finally, although the major finding of this paper strengthens the notion of a link between central neural hyperactivity and tinnitus, this relationship is by no means clear. Hyperactivity in CNIC develops rapidly (within hours after cochlear trauma) [52], as does auditory cortex hyperactivity [19,53], but tinnitus in our animals was only observed a minimum of 3 weeks after cochlear trauma. This suggests that tinnitus development requires the involvement of other brain regions. Other brain regions that have been suggested to be involved include the limbic system and recently, the paraflocculus of the cerebellum [54,55].

Acknowledgments

The authors thank R. Salvi and D. Stolzberg for generous sharing of software and advice.

Author Contributions

Conceived and designed the experiments: WHAMM KMB DR. Performed the experiments: WHAMM KMB DR. Analyzed the data: WHAMM KMB DR. Contributed reagents/materials/analysis tools: WHAMM DR. Wrote the paper: WHAMM KMB DR.

References

1. Eggermont JJ, Roberts LE (2004) The neuroscience of tinnitus. TRENDS in neuroscience 27: 676–682.
2. Shargorodsky J, Curhan GC, Farwell WR (2010) Prevalence and characteristics of tinnitus among US adults. Am J Med 123: 711–718.
3. Vio MM, Holme RH (2005) Hearing loss and tinnitus: 250 million people and a US$10 billion potential market. Drug Discov Today 10: 1263–1265.
4. Axelsson A, Ringdahl A (1989) Tinnitus–a study of its prevalence and characteristics. Br J Audiol 23: 53–62.
5. Salvi R, Lobarinas E, Sun W (2009) Pharmacological treatments for tinnitus: new and old. Drugs Fut 34: 381–400.
6. Yankaskas K (2013) Prelude: noise-induced tinnitus and hearing loss in the military. Hear Res 295: 3–8.
7. Mrena R, Savolainen S, Kiukaanniemi H, Ylikoski J, Makitie AA (2009) The effect of tightened hearing protection regulations on military noise-induced tinnitus. Int J Audiol 48: 394–400.
8. Andersson G, Kaldo V (2004) Internet-based cognitive behavioral therapy for tinnitus. J Clin Psychol 60: 171–178.
9. Cesarani A, Capobianco S, Soi D, Giuliano DA, Alpini D (2002) Intratympanic dexamethasone treatment for control of subjective idiopathic tinnitus: our clinical experience. Int Tinnitus J 8: 111–114.
10. Nakai Y, Yamane H, Minowa Y, Go K, Fukumaru M, et al. (1982) Application of loop diuretics for treatment of sensorineural hearing impairment. Experimental and clinical study. Acta Otolaryngol 94: 37–43.
11. Risey JA, Guth PS, Amedee RG (1995) Furosemide Distinguishes Central and Peripheral Tinnitus. Int Tinnitus J 1: 99–103.
12. Lockwood AH, Salvi RJ, Burkard RF, Galantowicz PJ, Coad ML, et al. (1999) Neuroanatomy of tinnitus. Scand Audiol Suppl 51: 47–52.
13. Melcher JR, Sigalovsky IS, Guinan JJ, Jr., Levine RA (2000) Lateralized tinnitus studied with functional magnetic resonance imaging: abnormal inferior colliculus activation. J Neurophysiol 83: 1058–1072.
14. Lanting CP, de Kleine E, van Dijk P (2009) Neural activity underlying tinnitus generation: results from PET and fMRI. Hear Res 255: 1–13.
15. Gu JW, Halpin CF, Nam EC, Levine RA, Melcher JR (2010) Tinnitus, diminished sound-level tolerance, and elevated auditory activity in humans with clinically normal hearing sensitivity. J Neurophysiol 104: 3361–3370.
16. Eggermont JJ, Komiya H (2000) Moderate noise trauma in juvenile cats results in profound cortical topographic map changes in adulthood. Hear Res 142: 89–101.
17. Finlayson PG, Kaltenbach JA (2009) Alterations in the spontaneous discharge patterns of single units in the dorsal cochlear nucleus following intense sound exposure. Hear Res 256: 104–117.
18. Mulders WH, Robertson D (2009) Hyperactivity in the auditory midbrain after acoustic trauma: dependence on cochlear activity. Neuroscience 164: 733–746.
19. Norena AJ, Eggermont JJ (2003) Changes in spontaneous neural activity immediately after an acoustic trauma: implications for neural correlates of tinnitus. Hear Res 183: 137–153.
20. Vogler DP, Robertson D, Mulders WH (2011) Hyperactivity in the ventral cochlear nucleus after cochlear trauma. J Neurosci 31: 6639–6645.
21. Robertson D, Irvine DR (1989) Plasticity of frequency organization in auditory cortex of guinea pigs with partial unilateral deafness. J Comp Neurol 282: 456–471.
22. Liberman MC, Dodds LW (1984) Single-neuron labeling and chronic cochlear pathology. II. Stereocilia damage and alterations of spontaneous discharge rates. Hear Res 16: 43–53.
23. Brozoski TJ, Bauer CA (2005) The effect of dorsal cochlear nucleus ablation on tinnitus in rats. Hear Res 206: 227–236.
24. Zacharek MA, Kaltenbach JA, Mathog TA, Zhang J (2002) Effects of cochlear ablation on noise induced hyperactivity in the hamster dorsal cochlear nucleus: implications for the origin of noise induced tinnitus. Hear Res 172: 137–143.
25. Mulders WH, Seluakumaran K, Robertson D (2010) Efferent pathways modulate hyperactivity in inferior colliculus. J Neurosci 30: 9578–9587.
26. Mulders WH, Robertson D (2011) Progressive centralization of midbrain hyperactivity after acoustic trauma. Neuroscience 192: 753–760.

27. Robertson D, Bester C, Vogler D, Mulders WH (2013) Spontaneous hyperactivity in the auditory midbrain: relationship to afferent input. Hear Res 295: 124–129.
28. Sewell WF (1984) The relation between the endocochlear potential and spontaneous activity in auditory nerve fibres of the cat. J Physiol 347: 685–696.
29. Dehmel S, Eisinger D, Shore SE (2012) Gap prepulse inhibition and auditory brainstem-evoked potentials as objective measures for tinnitus in guinea pigs. Front Syst Neurosci 6: 42.
30. Turner JG, Brozoski TJ, Bauer CA, Parrish JL, Myers K, et al. (2006) Gap detection deficits in rats with tinnitus: a potential novel screening tool. Behav Neurosci 120: 188–195.
31. Mulders WH, Ding D, Salvi R, Robertson D (2011) Relationship between auditory thresholds, central spontaneous activity, and hair cell loss after acoustic trauma. J Comp Neurol 519: 2637–2647.
32. Norena A, Micheyl C, Chery-Croze S, Collet L (2002) Psychoacoustic characterization of the tinnitus spectrum: implications for the underlying mechanisms of tinnitus. Audiol Neurootol 7: 358–369.
33. Davis M (1974) Sensitization of the rat startle response by noise. J Comp Physiol Psychol 87: 571–581.
34. Faraday MM, Grunberg NE (2000) The importance of acclimation in acoustic startle amplitude and pre-pulse inhibition testing of male and female rats. Pharmacol Biochem Behav 66: 375–381.
35. Johnstone JR, Alder VA, Johnstone BM, Robertson D, Yates GK (1979) Cochlear action potential threshold and single unit thresholds. J Acoust Soc Am 65: 254–257.
36. McMahon CM, Patuzzi RB (2002) The origin of the 900 Hz spectral peak in spontaneous and sound-evoked round-window electrical activity. Hear Res 173: 134–152.
37. Patuzzi RB, Brown DJ, McMahon CM, Halliday AF (2004) Determinants of the spectrum of the neural electrical activity at the round window: transmitter release and neural depolarisation. Hear Res 190: 87–108.
38. Merrill EG, Ainsworth A (1972) Glass-coated platinum-plated tungsten microelectrodes. Med Biol Eng 10: 662–672.
39. Ingham NJ, Bleeck S, Winter IM (2006) Contralateral inhibitory and excitatory frequency response maps in the mammalian cochlear nucleus. Eur J Neurosci 24: 2515–2529.
40. Dong S, Mulders WH, Rodger J, Woo S, Robertson D (2010) Acoustic trauma evokes hyperactivity and changes in gene expression in guinea-pig auditory brainstem. Eur J Neurosci 31: 1616–1628.
41. Rybak LP, Morizono T (1982) Effect of furosemide upon endolymph potassium concentration. Hear Res 7: 223–231.
42. Dong S, Mulders WH, Rodger J, Robertson D (2009) Changes in neuronal activity and gene expression in guinea-pig auditory brainstem after unilateral partial hearing loss. Neuroscience 159: 1164–1174.
43. Lobarinas E, Hayes SH, Allman BL (2013) The gap-startle paradigm for tinnitus screening in animal models: limitations and optimization. Hear Res 295: 150–160.
44. Middleton JW, Kiritani T, Pedersen C, Turner JG, Shepherd GM, et al. (2011) Mice with behavioral evidence of tinnitus exhibit dorsal cochlear nucleus hyperactivity because of decreased GABAergic inhibition. Proc Natl Acad Sci U S A 108: 7601–7606.
45. Zhang J, Zhang Y, Zhang X (2011) Auditory cortex electrical stimulation suppresses tinnitus in rats. J Assoc Res Otolaryngol 12: 185–201.
46. Wang H, Brozoski TJ, Turner JG, Ling L, Parrish JL, et al. (2009) Plasticity at glycinergic synapses in dorsal cochlear nucleus of rats with behavioral evidence of tinnitus. Neuroscience 164: 747–759.
47. Kraus KS, Mitra S, Jimenez Z, Hinduja S, Ding D, et al. (2010) Noise trauma impairs neurogenesis in the rat hippocampus. Neuroscience 167: 1216–1226.
48. Ruttiger L, Singer W, Panford-Walsh R, Matsumoto M, Lee SC, et al. (2013) The reduced cochlear output and the failure to adapt the central auditory response causes tinnitus in noise exposed rats. PLoS One 8: e57247.
49. Alpini D, Cesarani A, Giuliano DA, Capobianco S (2004) Tinnitus: pharmacological topodiagnosis. Int Tinnitus J 10: 91–93.
50. Gillooly JF, Brown JH, West GB, Savage VM, Charnov EL (2001) Effects of size and temperature on metabolic rate. Science 293: 2248–2251.
51. Blaesse P, Airaksinen MS, Rivera C, Kaila K (2009) Cation-chloride cotransporters and neuronal function. Neuron 61: 820–838.
52. Mulders WH, Robertson D (2013) Development of hyperactivity after acoustic trauma in the guinea pig inferior colliculus. Hear Res 298: 104–108.
53. Seki S, Eggermont JJ (2003) Changes in spontaneous firing rate and neural synchrony in cat primary auditory cortex after localized tone-induced hearing loss. Hear Res 180: 28–38.
54. Bauer CA, Kurt W, Sybert LT, Brozoski TJ (2013) The cerebellum as a novel tinnitus generator. Hear Res 295: 130–139.
55. De Ridder D, Elgoyhen AB, Romo R, Langguth B (2011) Phantom percepts: tinnitus and pain as persisting aversive memory networks. Proc Natl Acad Sci U S A 108: 8075–8080.

2

Disrupted Bone Remodeling Leads to Cochlear Overgrowth and Hearing Loss in a Mouse Model of Fibrous Dysplasia

Omar Akil[1,9], Faith Hall-Glenn[2,9], Jolie Chang[1], Alfred Li[3], Wenhan Chang[3], Lawrence R. Lustig[1]*, Tamara Alliston[2]*, Edward C. Hsiao[4]*

1 Department of Otolaryngology, Head & Neck Surgery, University of California San Francisco, San Francisco, California, United States of America, 2 Department of Orthopaedic Surgery, University of California San Francisco, San Francisco, California, United States of America, 3 Endocrine Unit and Bone Imaging Core, San Francisco VA Medical Center, San Francisco, California, United States of America, 4 Division of Endocrinology and Metabolism, and the Institute for Human Genetics, Department of Medicine, University of California San Francisco, San Francisco, California, United States of America

Abstract

Normal hearing requires exquisite cooperation between bony and sensorineural structures within the cochlea. For example, the inner ear secretes proteins such as osteoprotegrin (OPG) that can prevent cochlear bone remodeling. Accordingly, diseases that affect bone regulation can also result in hearing loss. Patients with fibrous dysplasia develop trabecular bone overgrowth resulting in hearing loss if the lesions affect the temporal bones. Unfortunately, the mechanisms responsible for this hearing loss, which could be sensorineural and/or conductive, remain unclear. In this study, we used a unique transgenic mouse model of increased G_s G-protein coupled receptor (GPCR) signaling induced by expression of an engineered receptor, Rs1, in osteoblastic cells. These ColI(2.3)$^+$/Rs1$^+$ mice showed dramatic bone lesions that histologically and radiologically resembled fibrous dysplasia. We found that ColI(2.3)$^+$/Rs1$^+$ mice showed progressive and severe conductive hearing loss. Ossicular chain impingement increased with the size and number of dysplastic lesions. While sensorineural structures were unaffected, ColI(2.3)$^+$/Rs1$^+$ cochleae had abnormally high osteoclast activity, together with elevated tartrate resistant acid phosphatase (TRAP) activity and receptor activator of nuclear factor kappa-B ligand (Rankl) mRNA expression. ColI(2.3)$^+$/Rs1$^+$ cochleae also showed decreased expression of Sclerostin (Sost), an antagonist of the Wnt signaling pathway that normally increases bone formation. The osteocyte canalicular networks of ColI(2.3)$^+$/Rs1$^+$ cochleae were disrupted and showed abnormal osteocyte morphology. The osteocytes in the ColI(2.3)$^+$/Rs1$^+$ cochleae showed increased expression of matrix metalloproteinase 13 (MMP-13) and TRAP, both of which can support osteocyte-mediated peri-lacunar remodeling. Thus, while the ossicular chain impingement is sufficient to account for the progressive hearing loss in fibrous dysplasia, the deregulation of bone remodeling extends to the cochlea as well. Our findings suggest that factors regulating bone remodeling, including peri-lacunar remodeling by osteocytes, may be useful targets for treating the bony overgrowths and hearing changes of fibrous dysplasia and other bony pathologies.

Editor: Dominique Heymann, Faculté de médecine de Nantes, France

Funding: This work was supported by Hearing Research Inc (TA, LL), NIH R01 DE019284 (TA), and NIH K08 AR056299 (ECH). The funders had no role in study design, data collection/analysis, decision to publish, or preparation of the manuscript.

Competing Interests: The authors have declared that no competing interests exist.

* E-mail: Edward.Hsiao@ucsf.edu (ECH); llustig@ohns.ucsf.edu (LL); tamara.alliston@ucsf.edu (TA)

9 These authors contributed equally to this work.

Background

Bone remodeling, a critical process in the maintenance of skeletal homeostasis, integrates bone formation and bone resorption [1]. Abnormalities in bone remodeling cause significant morbidity, including deformity and disability associated with inherited diseases of abnormal bone formation and bone fragility associated with aging and osteoporosis. Not surprisingly, diseases that severely change bone remodeling can also affect hearing since the auditory transduction mechanism is embedded within bone [2–6].

Interactions between the structures of the cochlea, such as the bony otic capsule and the organ of Corti, are essential for hearing. In the embryo, the cochleae form through bidirectional signaling between the sensorineural structures and developing bone [7]. In adults, cells within the organ of Corti normally secrete soluble factors to suppress remodeling of cochlear bone by osteoclasts and osteoblasts [8,9]. The importance of this crosstalk is evident in bone syndromes where these pathways are disrupted. For example, otosclerosis and osteogenesis imperfecta tarda are characterized by sensorineural, conductive, and mixed forms of hearing loss [10–12].

Patients with fibrous dysplasia (FD; OMIM #174800) of bone have lesions containing dense fibro-cellular infiltrate and increased trabecular bone formation. FD is caused by activating mutations in the G_s G-protein coupled receptor (GPCR) signaling pathway, which increases cyclic adenosine monophosphate (cAMP) levels [13–15]. As many as 20% of FD patients have hearing loss [16–

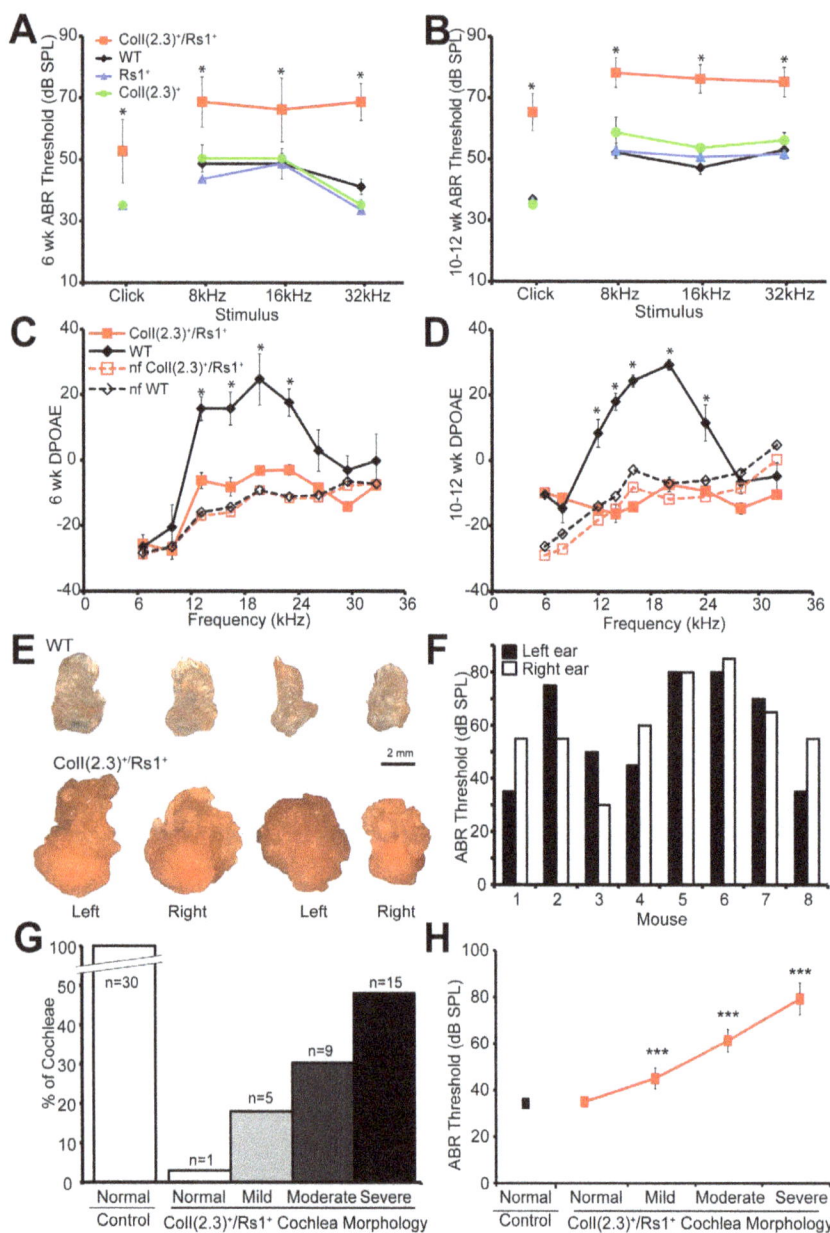

Figure 1. Progressive hearing loss observed in Coll(2.3)$^+$/Rs1$^+$ mice with fibrous dysplasia-like lesions correlates to the severity of dysplastic cochlear lesions. (A, B) ABR thresholds (decibels of sound pressure level, dBSPL) were measured in 6-week-old and 10–12-week-old Coll(2.3)$^+$/Rs1$^+$ (mutant), WT, and Coll(2.3)$^-$/Rs1$^+$ and Coll(2.3)$^+$/Rs1$^-$ (single transgenic) mice. Coll(2.3)$^+$/Rs1$^+$ mice showed higher ABR thresholds at. Click stimulus and at 8, 16, and 32 kHz stimuli when compared to WT and single transgenic mice at both 6- and 10–12-week-old time points. Male and female mice were analyzed together. **(C)** DPOAEs were also measured at 6-weeks and 10–12-weeks. WT and Coll(2.3)$^+$/Rs1$^+$ mice and compared to WT and Coll(2.3)$^+$/Rs1$^+$ background noise floor (nf) measurements of all experimental noise sources used. Coll(2.3)$^+$/Rs1$^+$ mutant DPOAEs at 6, 12, 18, 24, 32 kHz frequencies showed levels similar to nf controls compared to normal WT DPOAEs at 6 weeks of age. Male and female mice were analyzed together. **(D)** Increased differences between WT and Coll(2.3)$^+$/Rs1$^+$ DPOAE recordings were observed in 10–12 week-old mice. *, p<0.05. **(E)** Images of dissected cochleae from two representative sets of Coll(2.3)$^+$/Rs1$^+$ and WT 12-week-old mice showed gross abnormalities caused by fibrous lesion growth compared to WT cochlea. Scale bar = 2 mm. **(F)** Click ABR thresholds were measured in the left and right ears of 12-week mice (n = 8), with highly variable differences observed in the same mouse. Male and female mice were analyzed together. **(G)** A rank-order histological grading system (see methods for criteria) was used to group the severity of Coll(2.3)$^+$/Rs1$^+$ cochlear lesions into normal, mild, moderate, and severe lesions from 30 Coll(2.3)$^+$/Rs1$^+$ cochleae. When compared to 30 normal WT cochleae which all had normal morphology, chi-squared analysis showed p<0.0001. **(H)** The categorized lesions from 15 control (30 cochleae) and 15 Coll(2.3)$^+$/Rs1$^+$ mice (30 cochleae) were compared to measured ABR thresholds. N = 1 cochlea that appeared normal; 5 cochleae with mild lesions; 9 cochleae with moderate lesions; and 15 cochlea with severe lesions, as in (G). Male and female mice were analyzed together. ***, p<0.0001 when compared to control ABR threshold.

22]. Disrupted bone remodeling leading to the overgrowth of temporal bones is thought to contribute to this progressive hearing loss in FD patients, which also can be either conductive, sensorineural, or both [18,19]. However, the traditional methods of discriminating conductive *vs.* sensorineural hearing loss require intact bone physical properties to make that distinction. Thus our goal was to elucidate the mechanisms responsible for hearing loss in fibrous dysplasia.

In this study, we used a transgenic mouse model of increased G_s-GPCR signaling to better define the mechanisms by which FD causes hearing loss. The complexity of the *GNAS* locus and embryonic lethality of constitutively-active $G_s\alpha$ signaling [23] preclude direct genetic modifications to introduce the classical *GNAS* mutations that cause fibrous dysplasia. Since GPCRs signal through a limited number of canonical pathways including G_s and G_i that ultimately regulate intracellular cAMP levels, we developed a method of inducing regulated G_s signaling in cells by engineered receptors such as RASSLs (receptors activated solely by synthetic ligands). RASSLs are powerful tools for studying GPCR signaling as they no longer respond to endogenous hormones but can be activated by synthetic small-molecule ligands [24]. In addition, RASSLs are small genes easily expressed in constructs and transgenes allowing precise spatial and temporal regulation. RASSLs have proven to be useful for dissecting GPCR signaling in complex tissues including bone, brain, and heart [24–27].

Mice expressing the engineered G_s-GPCR Rs1 in osteoblastic cells using the Collagen I 2.3 kb promoter fragment [ColI(2.3)+/Rs1+ mice] develop bone phenotypes that strongly resemble fibrous dysplasia of the bone, including increased trabecular bone formation, cortical erosions, and disorganized bone formation with rapid turnover and remodeling [26]. We used this dramatic phenotype to determine how FD-like lesions may affect the otic capsule and cochlea and elucidate the mechanisms that contribute to FD-induced hearing loss.

Materials and Methods

Mouse Strains

ColI(2.3)+/Rs1+ mice were generated as previously described [26] by mating mice with a collagen type 1α 2.3 kb promoter fragment driving the tTA ("TEToff" system) driver transgene [FVB/NJ-Tg(Col1a1-tTA)139Niss/Mmucd; MMRRC accession 030758-MU] with mice carrying the TetO-Rs1 responder transgene [FVB/N-Tg(tetO-HTR4*D100A)2Niss/Mmmh; MMRRC accession 029993-MU]. Double-transgenic mice [abbreviated here as ColI(2.3)+/Rs1+ mice] maintained off of doxycycline showed strong activation of G_s-GPCR signaling in osteoblastic cells [26] and developed their fibrous dysplastic bone phenotype postnatally [28]. These mice were maintained on an FVBN background, a strain with minimal auditory defects [29]. Wild type [WT; ColI(2.3)−/Rs1−] or single-transgenic [ColI(2.3)+/Rs1− and ColI(2.3)−/Rs1+] mice showed no identifiable bone phenotype and were collectively used as controls. Prior studies showed no sexual dimorphism in the bone phenotype [26,28,30] including differences in body length or weight. Our study combined the results from male and female mice for the morphological analyses and auditory testing. Only male mice were used for the gene expression and immunohistochemistry studies to minimize any potential effects of sex on bone formation and remodeling. This study was carried out in strict accordance with the recommendations in the Guide for the Care and Use of Laboratory Animals of the National Institutes of Health. All procedures and protocols were approved by the University of California, San Francisco Institutional Animal Care and Use

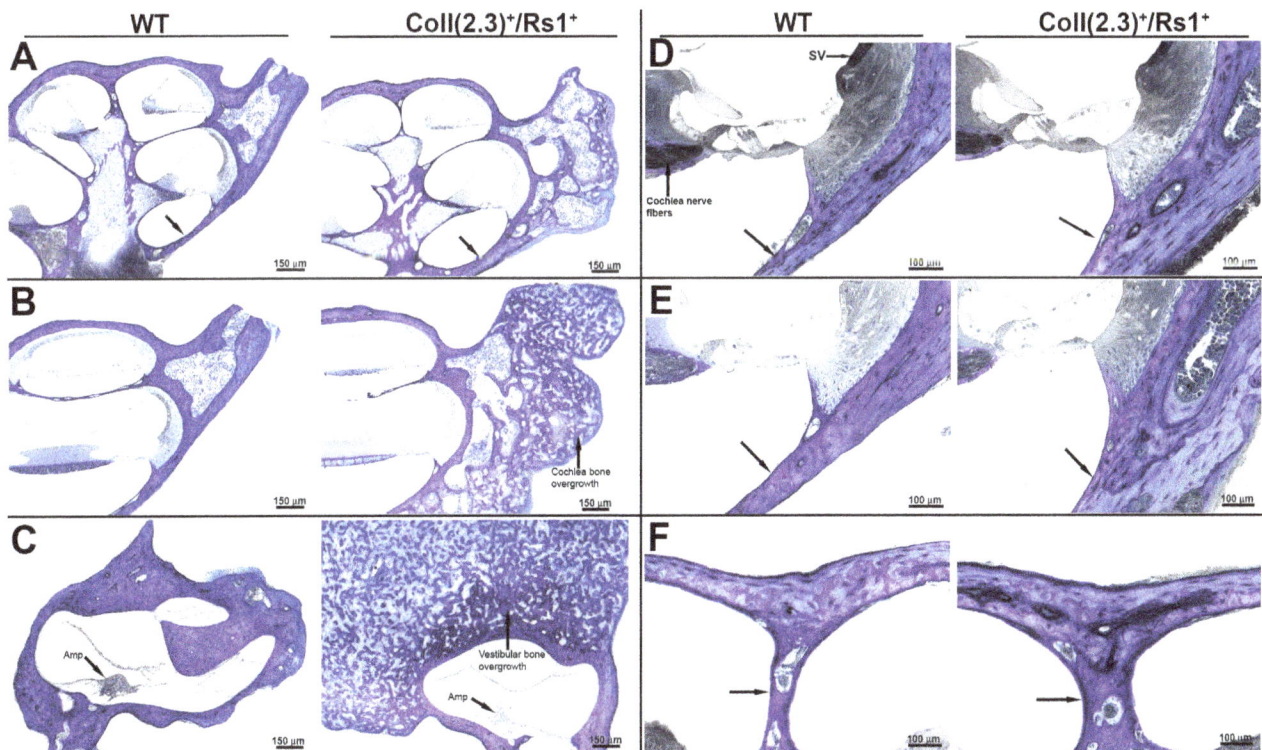

Figure 2. Irregular lesions in ColI(2.3)+/Rs1+ cochlea involve the apex and the labyrinth causing thickening of the otic capsule. (A–C) Cochlea from 12-week-old WT and ColI(2.3)+/Rs1+ mice were stained for toluidine blue and examined histologically. Mixed boney fibrous lesions were often observed surrounding ColI(2.3)+/Rs1+ cochlea compared to WT controls. ColI(2.3)+/Rs1+ cochlea had multiple fibrous boney overgrowths of the vestibular bone compared to normal WT morphology. Scale bar, 150 μm. **(D–F)** The walls of ColI(2.3)+/Rs1+ cochleae showed significant thickening in comparison to WT cochleae, possibly due to the overall thickening of the surrounding otic capsule. The stria vascularis (SV) in the ColI(2.3)+/Rs1+ mice appear normal. Scale bar, 100 μm.

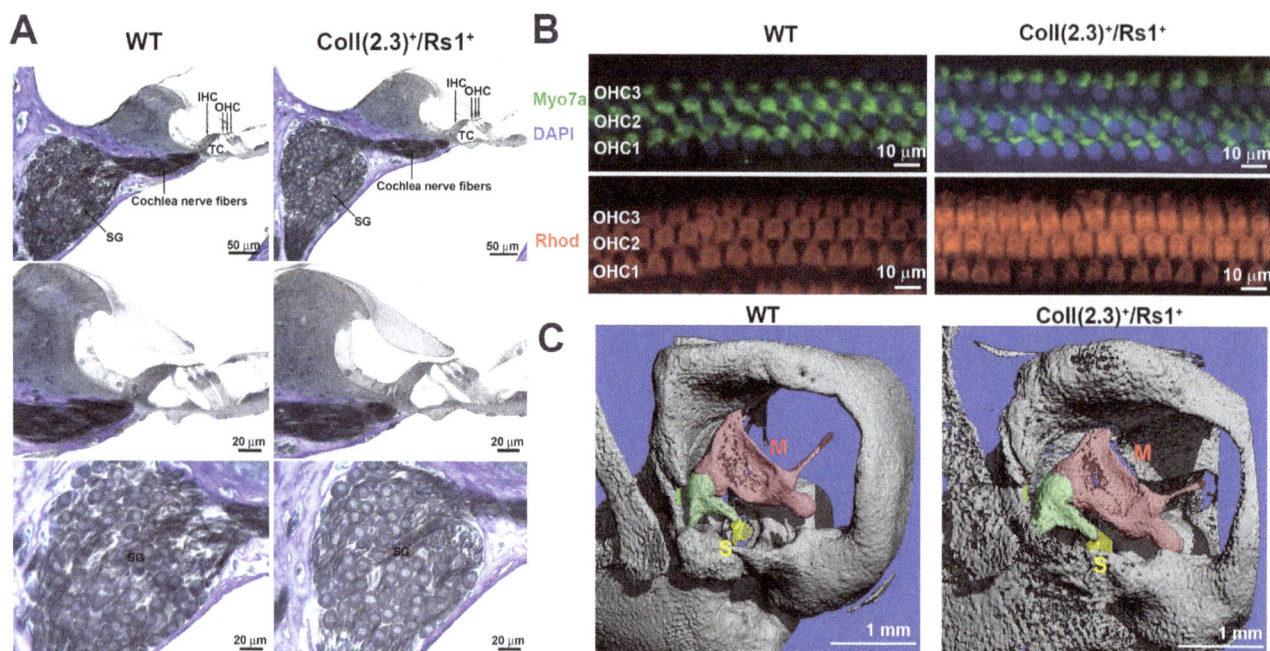

Figure 3. Sensorineural structures of CollI(2.3)⁺/Rs1⁺ mice are normal despite the bony overgrowth affecting the ossicular chain. (A) Histological analysis of the sensorineural structures of 12-week-old WT and CollI(2.3)⁺/Rs1⁺ revealed no gross abnormalities in the organ of Corti (OC), tunnel of Corti (TC), inner hair cells (IHC), or outer hair cells (OHC). **(B)** Whole mount immunofluorescence preparations of the outer hair cells revealed no visible differences in hair cell structure or number in CollI(2.3)⁺/Rs1⁺ in comparison to WT structures. **(C)** Micro computed x-ray tomography of the temporal bones was examined. A region of interest including the middle ear was selected in WT and CollI(2.3)⁺/Rs1⁺ at 12-week-old mice. CollI(2.3)⁺/Rs1⁺ temporal bones showed significant bony overgrowth of the middle ear compared to WT. The ossicles are structurally identifiable and are affected in the CollI(2.3)⁺/Rs1⁺ mice [malleus (M), incus (I), and stapes (S)].

Committee (#AN086974 and #AN098643). All procedures were performed under anesthesia, and all efforts were made to minimize suffering.

Cochlear Morphology Assessments

A rank-order grading system was used to rate the condition and the severity of CollI(2.3)⁺/Rs1⁺ cochlear bone lesions based on the amount of bone overgrowth at 12 weeks observed by a single experimenter who was blinded to the hearing results at the time of scoring. Control cochleae categorized as a "cochlea with no abnormal bone overgrowth," and correlated with evoked acoustic brainstem response (ABR) thresholds of 30 to 35 dB. Mild bony lesions were grouped based on the presence of small cochlear lesions, whereas moderate bony lesions were categorized as large growths on the cochlea and the labyrinth area. Severe bony lesions were grouped based on very large bone overgrowths involving the bulla and overgrowth on the labyrinth area.

Auditory Assessments

Hearing tests were performed on control and CollI(2.3)⁺/Rs1⁺ littermates at 6 and 10–12 weeks of age in a soundproof chamber as described [31–33]. Briefly, mice were anesthetized by intraperitoneal injection of a mixture of ketamine hydrochloride (Ketaset, 100 mg/kg) and xylazine hydrochloride (Xyla-ject, 10 mg/kg). Body temperature was maintained with a heating pad and monitored throughout the hearing testing.

The evoked ABR thresholds were differentially recorded from the scalp of control and CollI(2.3)⁺/Rs1⁺ mice using subdermal needle electrodes at the vertex, below the pinna of the left ear (reference probe), and below the contralateral ear (ground probe). The sound stimuli included clicks (5 ms duration; 31 Hz) and tone pips at 8, 16, and 32 kHz (10 ms duration; cos2 shaping; 21 Hz). Measurements were recorded using the TDT BioSig III system (Tucker Davis Technologies). For each stimulus, electroencephalographic (EEG) activity was recorded for 20 ms at a sampling rate of 25 kHz and filtered (0.3–3 kHz). Waveforms from 512 stimuli were averaged for click responses, and 1000 stimuli for frequency specific stimuli (8, 16, and 32 kHz). ABR waveforms were recorded in 5 dB sound pressure level (SPL) intervals down from the maximum amplitude. The threshold was defined as the lowest stimulus level at which response peaks for waves I-V were clearly and repetitively present upon visual inspection. These threshold judgments were confirmed by analysis of stored waveforms. One-way ANOVA with Bonferroni post-hoc testing was used to determine statistical significance, defined as $p < 0.05$.

Distortion product oto-acoustic emissions (DPOAE) were measured using an acoustic probe placed in the left external auditory canal. Stimuli consisted of two primary tones delivered simultaneously with a frequency ratio of $f1/f2 = 1.25$. Tones were digitally synthesized at 100 kHz using SigGen software. The primary tones with geometric mean (GM) frequencies ranging from 6 to 36 kHz and equal levels (L1 = L2 = 60 dB SPL) were presented *via* two separate speakers (EC1; Tucker Davis Technologies) to the acoustic probe. DPOAE responses (2f1–f2) were recorded using an ER10B microphone assembly (Etymotics Research) within the acoustic probe and the TDT BioSig III system (Tucker Davis Technologies). Responses were amplified, digitally sampled at 100 kHz, and averaged over 50 discrete spectra. Fast Fourier transforms were computed from averaged responses. For each stimulus set, the DPOAE amplitude level at 2f1–f2 was extracted, and sound pressure levels for data points 100 Hz above and below the DPOAE frequency were averaged

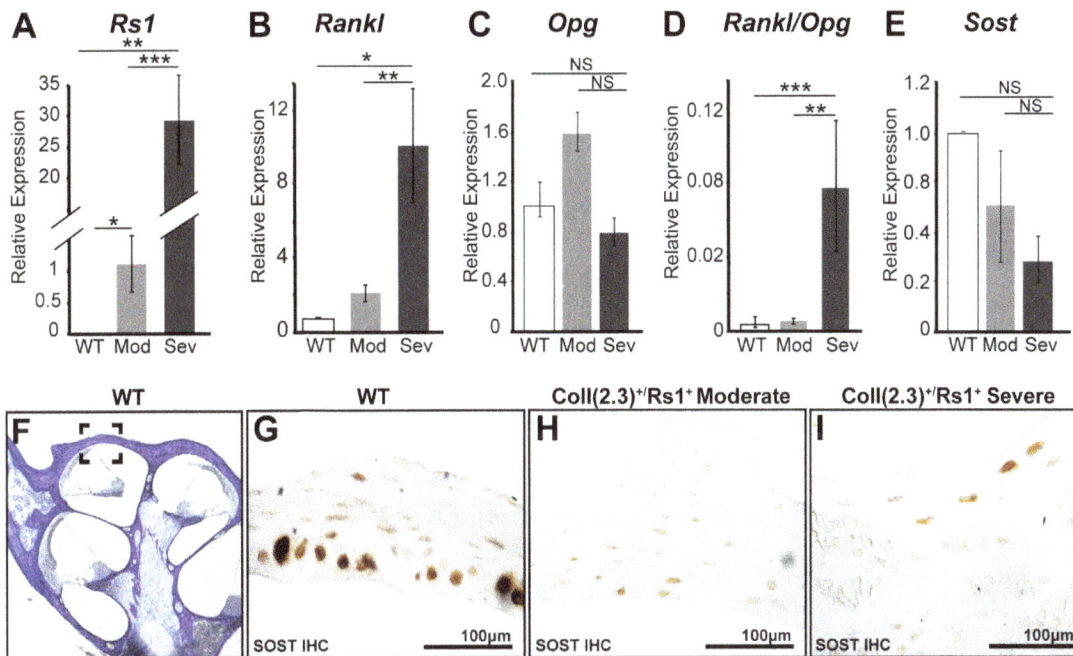

Figure 4. Markers of osteoclast-mediated bone remodeling is reactivated in CoII(2.3)$^+$/Rs1$^+$ cochlea. Markers of bone remodeling were assessed by immunohistochemistry on dissected 12-week-old male WT and CoII(2.3)$^+$/Rs1$^+$ cochlea with moderate (Mod) and severe (Sev) fibrous lesions using quantitative PCR. (**A**) Rs1 transgene expression was absent in WT controls and elevated in moderate (**, p = 0.01) and elevated 30-fold in severe CoII(2.3)$^+$/Rs1$^+$ cochlea (***, p<0.001). (**B**) *Rankl*, a marker for osteoclast differentiation and activity was significantly increased in CoII(2.3)$^+$/Rs1$^+$ severe cochlea when compared to WT and moderate CoII(2.3)$^+$/Rs1$^+$ cochlea (*, p<0.05; **, p<0.01). No statistically significant differences were observed in moderate CoII(2.3)$^+$/Rs1$^+$ cochlea compared to WT (p=0.63). (**C**) There were also no statistically significant changes observed in *Osteoprotegrin* expression in moderate and severe CoII(2.3) $^+$/Rs1$^+$ cochlea compared to WT cochlea (p=0.29, and p=0.645 respectively). (**D**) The ratios of *Rankl* and osteoclast inhibitory factor *osteoprotegrin* (*Opg*) were significantly increased in CoII(2.3)$^+$/Rs1$^+$ severe cochlea compared to moderate CoII(2.3)$^+$/Rs1$^+$ (**, p<0.01) and WT cochlea (***, p<0.005) indicating that osteoclast mediated remodeling is increased in CoII(2.3)$^+$/Rs1$^+$ severe cochlea. (**E**) No statistically significant changes were observed in *Sost* expression in CoII(2.3)$^+$/Rs1$^+$ moderate and severe cochlea compared to WT expression (p=0.73 and p=0.43 respectively). Error bars are mean +/− SEM of triplicate measurements, n=5 WT and 5 each of CoII(2.3)$^+$/Rs1$^+$ moderate and severe cochleae. (**F**) A specific area of the otic capsule (indicated by box) was examined immunohistochemical analysis. (**G–I**) Immunohistochemistry for SOST showed visibly significant decreases in expression in moderate and severe CoII(2.3)$^+$/Rs1$^+$ cochlea compared to WT cochlea.

for the noise floor measurements. DPOAE levels were plotted as a function of primary tone GM frequency. Statistical analysis was performed using ANOVA with Bonferroni post-hoc tests with significance defined as p<0.05.

Histological Analysis

Histological analyses were performed as previously described for plastic [31–33] and paraffin embedded sections [34]. To histologically preserve the sensorineural structures in plastic sections, freshly-dissected cochleae were perfused through the round and oval windows with a solution of 2.5% paraformaldehyde and 1.5% glutaraldehyde in 0.1 M phosphate buffered solution (PBS) at pH 7.4. Cochleae were incubated in the same fixative overnight at 4°C, rinsed with 0.1 M PBS, and post-fixed in 1% osmium tetroxide for two hours prior to embedding in Araldite 502 resin (Electron Microscopy Sciences). 5 μm sections were stained with toluidine blue for histological analysis.

For paraffin sections, dissected cochleae were fixed in 4% paraformaldehyde in PBS overnight. Cochleae were decalcified by incubation at 4°C in 10% ethylenediaminetetraacetic acid (EDTA) for 2–4 days, followed by serial ethanol dehydration and embedding in paraffin. 6 μm thick sections were permeabilized in 0.3% Triton X-100 in PBS, processed for antigen retrieval with Ficin (Invitrogen), and blocked for intrinsic peroxidase activity with 3% hydrogen peroxide. Sections were rinsed in PBS/0.2%

Tween (PBST) and blocked with 10% normal horse serum (Vector labs) for 2 h at room temperature. Sections were then incubated with the following primary antibodies overnight at 4°C: anti-MMP-13 (1:50 dilution; Abcam, ab-39012) and anti-Sclerostin (1:50 dilution; R&D systems, AF1589). Sections were rinsed with PBST and incubated with biotinylated secondary anti-goat and -rabbit antibodies (Vector labs), followed by PBST rinses and incubation with the ABC Elite avidin/biotin blocking kit (Vector labs). 3, 3′-diaminobenzidine (DAB) substrate peroxidase substrate antigen labeling kit (Vector labs) was used to visualize protein expression. Tartrate resistant acid phosphatase (TRAP) staining to assess osteoclast and osteocyte mediated bone remodeling in WT and FD cochleae was performed using the TRAP stained system (Sigma) as previously described [34].

Whole-mount Immunofluorescence Hair Cell Analysis

Immunofluorescence studies were conducted on whole-mount cochleae of the CoII(2.3)$^+$/Rs1$^+$ and control mice as described [32,33]. Cochleae were perfused with 4% PFA in 0.1 M PBS at pH 7.4 and kept in the fixative overnight at 4°C. Cochleae were then decalcified with 5% EDTA in 0.1 M PBS for 2–3 days. Following decalcification, the otic capsule and outer membranes were removed. The remaining organ of Corti was incubated with the anti-myosin VIIa antibody (a hair-cell specific marker; 1:50 dilution in PBS; Proteus Biosciences, Cat# 25-6790) and

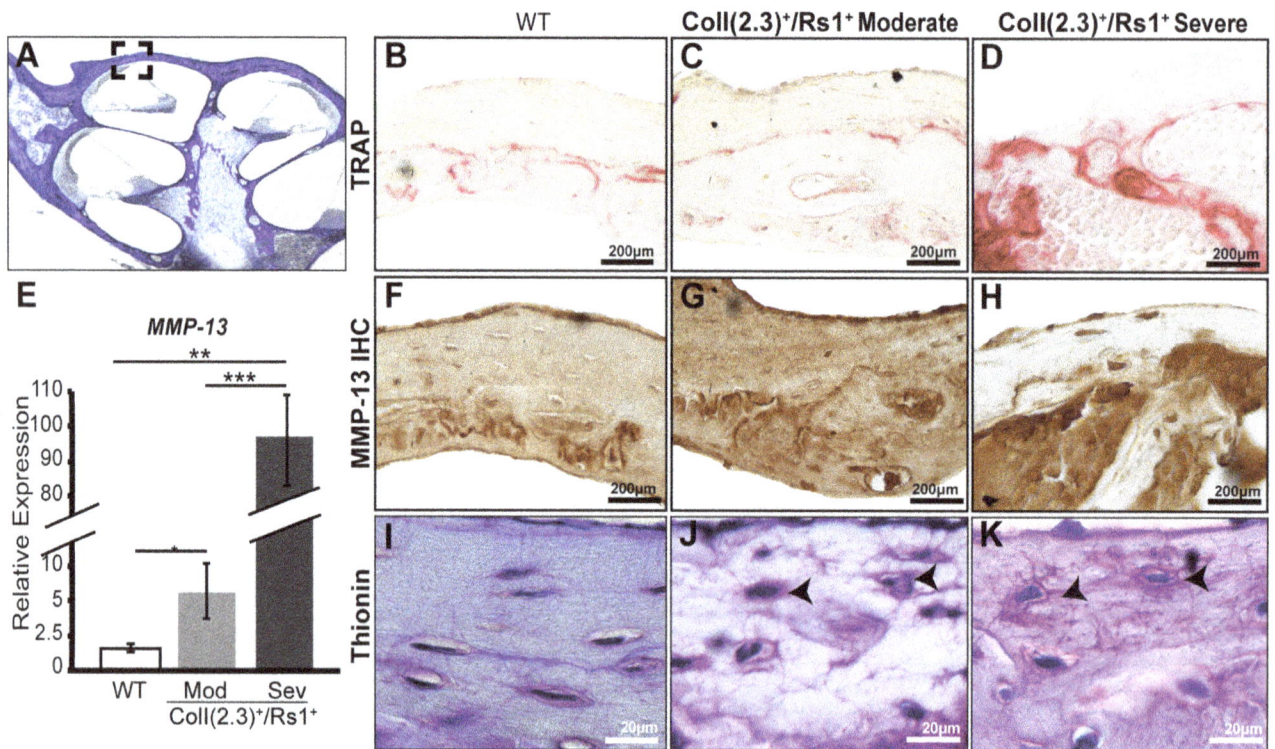

Figure 5. Abnormal peri-lacunar remodeling in cochlear fibrous dysplasia. (A) 12-week-old cochlea from male WT and ColI(2.3)$^+$/Rs1$^+$ cochleae were examined for markers of peri-lacunar remodeling in a specific area of the otic capsule. **(B–D)** TRAP, a marker for osteoclast activity, was elevated in moderate and severe ColI(2.3)$^+$/Rs1$^+$ otic capsules compared to the low levels observed in WT controls. **(E)** The expression of osteocyte secreted remodeling factor, MMP-13 was significantly increased 7-fold in moderate (**, $p < 0.005$) and 100 fold in severe ColI(2.3)$^+$/Rs1$^+$ cochleae (***, $p < 1 \times 10^{-05}$) compared to WT cochleae. (n = 6 male WT, n = 5 male ColI(2.3)$^+$/Rs1$^+$ moderate, and n = 5 male ColI(2.3)$^+$/Rs1$^+$ severe cochlea). Error bars are mean +/− SEM of triplicate measurements. **(F–H)** Immunohistochemistry showed that MMP-13 expression was confined to the otic capsule in WT cochleae, but the domain of expression is increased in ColI(2.3)$^+$/Rs1$^+$ moderate and severe cochlea. **(I–K)** Thionin staining of the canalicular network was examined in WT and ColI(2.3)$^+$/Rs1$^+$ moderate and severe cochleae. The canalicular network in WT cochlea shows normal elliptical osteocyte morphology and connectivity. ColI(2.3)$^+$/Rs1$^+$ moderate and severe cochleae show an abnormal rounded osteocyte morphologies with disrupted and disorganized canalicular networks of varying severity (n = 5 males per genotype).

incubated overnight at 4°C. Whole-mount cochleae were rinsed twice for 10 min with PBS and then incubated for 2 h with a goat anti-rabbit IgG antibody conjugated to Cy3 (1:2000 dilution in PBS, Jackson ImmunoResearch, 111-165-003). The whole mounts were rinsed in PBS twice for 15 min and incubated with rhodamine–phalloidin (stock solution of 200 U/ml methanol, diluted 1:100 in PBS for working solution) for one hour. Whole mounts were then rinsed with PBS, further microdissected into individual turns for surface preparation, and then exposed for 15 min at room temperature to the fluorescent dye 4,6-diamidino-2-phenylindole (DAPI, Sigma-Aldrich; 1.5 µg/ml in PBS) to mark nuclei. The cochlear whole mounts were rinsed in PBS and mounted on glass slides in anti-fade FluorSave reagent (Calbiochem, 34589). Hair cells in the organ of Corti were visualized by epifluorescence.

Micro-computed Tomography (µCT)

The temporal bones and ossicles of WT and ColI(2.3)$^+$/Rs1$^+$12-week mice were imaged *in situ* by micro-computed tomography (µCT-50; Scanco Medical AG, Bassersdorf, Switzerland) as described [35]. The scanning region was determined by the anterior end of the sphenoid bone and extended through the posterior region of the occipital bone. The desired region was scanned at a voxel size of 4.8 µm, using an energy potential of 55 kVp and intensity of 109 µA. The region of interest was then

analyzed using µCT evaluation software (version 6.0; Scanco Medical AG). The evaluation script was set at Gaussian sigma of 0.8, support of two, and lower threshold of 280 grayscale units, which corresponds to a bone density of 490 mg HA/cm^3. Three-dimensional renderings were created using µCT 3D visualization software (version 3.8; Scanco Medical AG). False coloring of the ossicles was added using Adobe Photoshop CS.

RNA Extraction and Quantitative Reverse Transcriptase PCR (qRT-PCR)

RNA was isolated from whole cochleae from 12-week WT and ColI(2.3)$^+$/Rs1$^+$ mice. Tissues were frozen in liquid nitrogen and crushed with a mortar and pestle in TRIZOL RNA isolation reagent (Invitrogen). Chloroform extraction was performed and samples were prepared for RNA purification and on-column DNase I digestion using a Qiagen RNeasy column, following the manufacturer's instructions. RNA was reverse transcribed into cDNA using Superscript (Biorad) as recommended by the manufacturer. Quantitative PCR was performed using a ViiA 7 Real time PCR System (Life Technologies). Gene expression was assessed using Taqman probes (Life Technologies) for the Rs1 transgene (Human HTR4, Hs00168380_m1); *Mmp-13* (Mm00439491); Sclerostin (*Sost*) (Mm00470479); and *Rankl* (Mm00441906). All expression values were normalized to *Gapdh* (Mm 99999915_g1). All graphs represent fold changes of

ColI(2.3)$^+$/Rs1$^+$ mice relative to wild type control littermates. Statistical analysis was performed using Student's t-test with p< 0.05 considered statistically significant.

Results

Cochlear Bone Overgrowth and Conductive Hearing Loss is Evident in a Mouse Model with Fibrous Dysplasia-like Bone Formation

As previously described, ColI(2.3)$^+$/Rs1$^+$ mice show severe trabecular overgrowth in all bones, including those of the skull [26]. As expected, the ABR threshold of the single-transgenic mice did not differ from WT littermates at 6 or 10–12 weeks of age (Figure 1A,B). However, ColI(2.3)$^+$/Rs1$^+$ mice consistently showed significant ABR threshold elevations in response to click- and frequency-specific tone-burst stimuli (8, 16, and 32 kHz) (Figure 1A,B). This increase in ABR threshold was higher in the 10–12-week-old ColI(2.3)$^+$/Rs1$^+$ mice than in 6-week-old mice, demonstrating a progressive decline in hearing as the mice aged over this timeframe.

We next performed distortion product otoacoustic emission (DPOAE) testing to assess outer hair cell and efferent auditory function since reduced DPOAE levels can indicate outer hair cell (OHC) contractility defects or the presence of a conductive hearing deficit. Although the DPOAE responses were intact in the control mice, the DPOAE responses in ColI(2.3)$^+$/Rs1$^+$ mice were significantly reduced to a level close to or below the background noise level (Figure 1C,D). This loss of DPOAE in ColI(2.3)$^+$/Rs1$^+$ mice is thus due to either the presence of a conductive hearing loss or abnormal outer hair cell motility.

Morphological examination of the cochleae showed that most, but not all, of the cochleae from the ColI(2.3)$^+$/Rs1$^+$ mice had multiple spongy, bony overgrowths involving the bulla (not shown), cochlear apex, and labyrinth (Figure 1E). The phenotypic variability of the lesions was reflected in the greater standard deviations of ABRs in ColI(2.3)$^+$/Rs1$^+$ mice (Figure 1A), both between individual mice and between ears in the same ColI(2.3)$^+$/ Rs1$^+$ mouse (Figure 1F). These lesions often obscured many of the traditional landmarks including the oval and round window niche. In some cases, the ossicles also appeared to be enmeshed in the bony lesions though the ossicles themselves appeared to have normal morphology. To quantify this change, we applied rank-ordered morphology scoring (Figure 1G) to the cochlea. We found that the degree of bone lesion severity correlated with the amount of hearing loss (Figure 1H), suggesting that the bony overgrowth contributed to the hearing loss observed in the ColI(2.3)$^+$/Rs1$^+$ mice.

Taken together, these data suggest that the hearing loss in ColI(2.3)$^+$/Rs1$^+$ mice was potentially conductive, possibly due to ossicular fixation. Furthermore, the variability seen in the bony overgrowth likely accounted for the variability in the ABR and DPOAE values, even between left and right cochlea in the same mouse.

Fibrodysplastic-like Lesions Result in Thicker Otic Capsule Wall and Involve the Apex and the Labyrinthe Area of the Cochlea

We next used detailed histological analysis to better understand the microscopic changes occurring within the cochlea in ColI(2.3)$^+$/Rs1$^+$ mice. The ColI(2.3)$^+$/Rs1$^+$ mice showed aggressive bony and fibrous overgrowths that surrounded the otic capsule and the adjacent vestibular labyrinth as compared to WT controls (Figure 2A–C). The most severely affected areas were in

bone adjacent to the cochlea and the labyrinth. Although the FD lesions often increased the thickness of the outer wall of the cochlea (Figure 2A, 2D–E, black arrows) as well as the mid-modiolar bone separating the apical scala (Fig. 2F black arrows), no lesions were observed involving the inner cortex of the otic capsule or centrally in the bony spiral modiolus (Figure 2A). The stria vascularis (SV), organ of Corti (OC) and tunnel of Corti (TC) (Figure 2A–B, 2D–E) were also normal. Thus, although the otic capsule bone showed some histologic defects, whether the hearing loss in ColI(2.3)$^+$/Rs1$^+$ mice is sensorineural or conductive remained unclear.

Intact Sensorineural Structures of ColI(2.3)$^+$/Rs1$^+$ Cochlea

We next examined the integrity of the organ of Corti, spiral ganglion (SG), inner hair cells (IHCs), outer hair cells (OHCs), and cochlear nerve fibers to assess if the observed hearing loss could be caused by sensory or neuronal defects (Figure 3A). Cells in the organ of Corti and spiral ganglia had normal size and morphology. Cochlear mid-turn surface preparations stained with Myosin 7a, a marker for hair cells [32,33], demonstrated normal numbers of OHCs. Additional labeling with rhodamine, a stain for actin, also revealed that OHC steriocillia and cuticular plates were present in both the WT and ColI(2.3)$^+$/Rs1$^+$ cochlea (Figure 3B). These results showed no significant histological differences between WT and ColI(2.3)$^+$/Rs1$^+$ cochlear sensorineural structures.

To more fully examine the integrity of bony structures in the ear, we performed microCT analysis of the temporal bones. In some cochlea, the ossicles were directly affected with malformations and increased bone, as well as impingement by FD lesions originating from surrounding bone (Figure 3C). In contrast, WT cochlea showed normal morphology.

These morphometric and histologic analyses demonstrate that the observed hearing loss in the ColI(2.3)$^+$/Rs1$^+$ mice was predominantly due to conductive loss from the FD lesions impinging upon the ossicular chain and sound conduction mechanism, with no objective evidence of a sensory or neural component to the hearing loss.

Defective Regulation of Bone Remodeling in ColI(2.3)$^+$/ Rs1$^+$ Cochlea

We next sought to understand the molecular mechanisms that led to the striking bony overgrowth in the cochlea in the ColI(2.3)$^+$/Rs1$^+$ mice. In long bones of ColI(2.3)$^+$/Rs1$^+$ mice, high levels of G$_s$ activation resulted in significantly increased bone remodeling and increased markers of bone turnover [26]. However, normal cochlear bone does not undergo classical osteoblast- and osteoclast-mediated remodeling [3], making it unclear what cellular mechanisms induce temporal bone fibrous dysplasia formation.

To determine if variable expression of key bone cell regulatory factors were responsible for severity of the FD lesions seen in the transgenic mice, we compared the gene expression in the WT cochleae $vs.$ moderate and severely affected ColI(2.3)$^+$/Rs1$^+$ cochleae. As expected, Rs1 expression in the total cochleae was higher in the severely affected samples (Figure 4A). $Rankl$, a secreted factor produced by osteoblasts and osteocytes that increases osteoclast recruitment, differentiation, activity, and survival [36], showed significantly higher expression in the ColI(2.3)$^+$/Rs1$^+$ cochlea, and was more dramatically elevated in severe ColI(2.3)$^+$/Rs1$^+$ lesions surrounding the cochlea (Figures 4B and 5D). Interestingly, no changes were observed in the mRNA levels of the osteoblast secreted RANKL antagonist, $osteoprotegrin$ (Opg), in moderate and severe ColI(2.3)$^+$/Rs1$^+$ cochlea compared to WT (Figure 4C). *Rankl/Opg* ratios [37] used as a measure of osteolytic balance [38] were significantly increased in the severely-affected ColI(2.3)$^+$/Rs1$^+$ cochleae as compared to ColI(2.3)$^+$/Rs1$^+$ moderate and WT cochlea (Figure 4D).

We next examined the expression of sclerostin, a protein encoded by the gene *Sost*, to assess osteocyte activity. Sclerostin is an osteocyte-derived antagonist of the osteoinductive Wnt signaling pathway [39,40]. Normally, Sclerostin suppresses new bone formation [40]. Loss-of-function mutations in sclerostin result in progressive bone overgrowth in diseases, such as sclerosteosis [41] and van Buchem's disease [42], which are also associated with hearing loss. To determine if this regulatory mechanism was also impaired in the FD-like lesions in the cochlea of ColI(2.3)$^+$/Rs1$^+$ mice, we assessed sclerostin protein and *Sost* gene expression by immunohistochemistry and quantitative PCR. We observed no statistically significant decreases in *Sost* mRNA expression in moderate or severe ColI(2.3)$^+$/Rs1$^+$ cochlea compared to WT cochlea (Figure 4E). However, immunohisto-chemistry revealed that Sclerostin protein expression was qualita-tively decreased in moderate and severe ColI(2.3)$^+$/Rs1$^+$ lesions compared to WT (Figure 4F–I). Taken together, these data suggest that ColI(2.3)$^+$/Rs1$^+$ cochlea may exhibit increased bone remod-eling due in part to decreased sclerostin expression by osteocytes, which may activate osteoblast mediated bone remodeling [43].

Perilacunar Remodeling is Disrupted in FD Cochlea

Perilacunar remodeling (PLR) is mediated by osteocytes in the canalicular network that remodel the local bone matrix to maintain bone quality and systemic mineral homeostasis [40,44–47]. In PLR, osteocytes, in addition to osteoclasts, secrete tartrate resistant acid phosphatase (TRAP) [47] and matrix metallopro-teinases (MMPs) [34,48,49] to drive bone resorption and remodeling.

We thus focused on *Rankl* and *MMP-13* to investigate the role of PLR in normal and ColI(2.3)$^+$/Rs1$^+$ cochlear bone. *Rankl* mRNA expression was elevated in the ColI(2.3)$^+$/Rs1$^+$ cochlear bone (Figure 4B), as was TRAP staining of histological sections (Figures 5A–D). We found that *Mmp-13* mRNA expression was low in WT cochleae; in contrast, *Mmp-13* mRNA expression was significantly increased in both moderate and severe double mutant cochleae (Figure 5E). In the WT cochlea, MMP-13 protein was highly localized within the otic capsule (Figure 5F), in the same areas where Sclerostin and TRAP are maximally expressed (Figures 4G and 5B). In the ColI(2.3)$^+$/Rs1$^+$ cochlea not only are *Mmp-13* mRNA and protein levels increased (Figure 5E), but the normal distinctive localization is also disrupted (Figure 5G, H) with increased expression in both osteocytes and in cochlear bone matrix. Thus, in the severe FD-like lesions, the level and localization of TRAP and MMP-13 expression is greatly expanded beyond the narrow zones in which they are normally expressed (Figures 5D, H and 5B, F, respectively).

Integrity of the canalicular network is normally required to maintain osteocyte viability and function, which directly influences bone quality [50] as demonstrated in MMP-13 deficient mice, which show defective PLR and a disrupted canalicular network [34]. To identify if a similar disruption occurs in the ColI(2.3)$^+$/Rs1$^+$ mice, we used thionin staining to visualize the canalicular network of 12-week moderately and severely affected ColI(2.3)$^+$/Rs1$^+$ cochleae. The thionin staining revealed highly disorganized dendritic processes and abnormal osteocyte morphology relative to the aligned canalicular organization observed in WT cochlear bone (Figure 5J, K, and I respectively).

Taken together, these results demonstrate that the normally limited bone remodeling and turnover in the cochlea is

hyperactivated in moderate and severe ColI(2.3)$^+$/Rs1$^+$ cochleae, and is accompanied by decreased levels of sclerostin and increased markers of osteoclast and perilacunar bone remodeling (TRAP, RANKL, and MMP-13).

Discussion

Many fibrous dyplasia patients develop progressive hearing loss through mechanisms that remain unclear. In this study, we investigated the cause of fibrous dysplasia-associated hearing loss using the ColI(2.3)$^+$/Rs1$^+$ mouse model that develops invasive FD-like lesions [26]. We found that ColI(2.3)$^+$/Rs1$^+$ mice developed progressive hearing loss due to FD-like lesions that often surrounded the ossicular chain and obstructed the oval and round window regions of the cochlea. These bony defects prohibited sound propagation into the cochlea, resulting in elevations in ABR and loss of DPOAEs. Further, the elevation of ABR thresholds significantly correlated with the severity of FD lesions in the cochlea. Histological and immunofluorescent analysis of the organ of Corti revealed no abnormalities, decreasing the likelihood that a sensorineural deficit caused the hearing loss.

We found that the severity of hearing loss and bony lesions in the ColI(2.3)$^+$/Rs1$^+$ mice correlated with deregulation of factors implicated in the control of bone remodeling, including RANKL, SOST, TRAP, and MMP-13. Relative to WT littermates, ColI(2.3)$^+$/Rs1$^+$ cochleae had lower levels of factors that suppress bone remodeling, but higher levels of factors that promote it. Specifically, we found that the expression of SOST, an osteocyte-specific negative regulator of bone remodeling [40], was signifi-cantly reduced in the ColI(2.3)$^+$/Rs1$^+$ cochleae and correlated to the severity of graded FD lesions. In contrast, TRAP, a marker for active bone remodeling by osteoclasts and osteocytes [47], was increased in moderate and severely affected ColI(2.3)$^+$/Rs1$^+$ cochleae. This area of TRAP overexpression was most pro-nounced in the otic capsule.

We and other groups previously showed that PLR is essential for maintaining the osteocyte canalicular network [34,47]. MMP-13 is a key PLR enzyme, and its deficiency causes disruption of the canalicular network [34]. Here, we observed increased MMP-13 expression in moderate and severe ColI(2.3)$^+$/Rs1$^+$ cochlear lesions compared to WT cochleae. Elevated MMP-13 expression was also associated with canalicular disorganization, often with enlarged canalicular channels around osteocytes and with altered morphology. In addition, we consistently observed MMP-13 staining in the pericellular matrix and intracellular space, in addition to the bone matrix staining that is typically observed. This altered MMP-13 localization in the severe FD mice may indicate that Rs1 expression is associated with a protein processing defect or change in the localization of bone matrix proteins, and may account for a decrease in bone matrix maturation we observed previously in long bones [51]. Collectively, these results suggest that elevated G$_s$ signaling in ColI(2.3)$^+$/Rs1$^+$ mice, and possibly also in FD patients, may cause hyper-activation of osteocyte-mediated PLR as well as bone remodeling by osteoclasts and osteoblasts, ultimately leading to hearing loss by bony overgrowths that affect the conductive mechanisms of the ear.

Surprisingly, while the FD-like lesions were easily identified in the bony structures surrounding the cochlea, the most severe lesions largely spared the cochlea itself. We speculate that this protection may result from the unique regulation of bone remodeling in the cochlea – which is very limited relative to bone remodeling in the rest of the skeleton [8]. A key inhibitor of osteoclast activity, osteoprotegrin (OPG), is normally enriched in the cochlea relative to other sites in the body [52]. In mice, OPG is produced at high levels by fibrocytes within the spiral ligament and secreted in the perilymph [52,53]. Mice deficient in OPG show excessive remodeling throughout the middle and inner ear resulting in severe hearing loss [3]. Similar pathology is also found in human patients with Juvenile Paget's disease [54]. We found that the high level of *Opg* expression in the cochlea was maintained in the ColI(2.3)$^+$/Rs1$^+$ cochleae. Therefore, even though osteoblastic-cell-specific activation of G$_s$-GPCR signaling in our ColI(2.3)$^+$/Rs1$^+$ mouse model increases the *Rankl/Opg* ratios, the elevated cochlear OPG may be sufficient to spare cochlear bone from the most severe FD lesions. These findings in the cochlea motivate further study on the possible role for OPG in suppressing the progression of FD lesions in the ear or at other sites.

While there are cases of FD causing sensorineural hearing loss in humans, it has been hypothesized that this is due to auditory neural compression from the FD bone changes [18]. The results in our mouse model with FD like lesions would support that mechanism, as well as possibly physical changes to the ossicular chain, as opposed to pathologic changes of sensory structures as seen in such lesions as cochlear otosclerosis [10]. These results point to a role for peri-lacunar remodeling in the cochlea that may be disrupted in FD.

In conclusion, our results show that the cochlea is a unique bony structure characterized by limited bone turnover that confers protection from proliferative and metabolically active FD bony lesions. The invasive fibro-osseous lesions seen in this mouse model cause conductive hearing loss through involvement of the ossicular chain, in a manner very similar to that seen in humans. These mechanisms could be new pharmacologic targets to treat the skeletal or hearing manifestations of FD or other skeletal diseases.

Acknowledgments

We thank Corey Cain, Hannah Kim, and the San Francisco VA Medical Center Bone Imaging Core for their technical assistance and discussions.

Author Contributions

Conceived and designed the experiments: OA FHG ECH JC TA LL. Performed the experiments: OA JC FHG AL WC ECH. Analyzed the data: OA FHG JC AL WC LL TA ECH. Wrote the paper: OA FHG LL TA ECH. Performed the hearing tests and subsequent data analysis (Figure 1): OA JC. Performed the histology and immunofluorescence experiments and subsequent data analysis (Figures 2, 3A, and 3B): OA. Performed the histological, immunohistological, and quantitative PCR studies, and the data analysis (Figures 4 and 5): FHG. Performed the microCT imaging and performed the data analysis with ECH (Figure 3C): AL WC. Analyzed the results together and prepared the manuscript: OA FHG LL TA ECH.

References

1. Raggatt LJ, Partridge NC (2010) Cellular and molecular mechanisms of bone remodeling. The Journal of biological chemistry 285: 25103–25108.
2. Feng X, McDonald JM (2011) Disorders of bone remodeling. Annual review of pathology 6: 121–145.
3. Zehnder AF, Kristiansen AG, Adams JC, Kujawa SG, Merchant SN, et al. (2006) Osteoprotegrin knockout mice demonstrate abnormal remodeling of the otic capsule and progressive hearing loss. The Laryngoscope 116: 201–206.
4. Lyford-Pike S, Hoover-Fong J, Tunkel DE (2012) Otolaryngologic manifestations of skeletal dysplasias in children. Otolaryngologic clinics of North America 45: 579–598, vii.
5. Chang JL, Brauer DS, Johnson J, Chen CG, Akil O, et al. (2010) Tissue-specific calibration of extracellular matrix material properties by transforming growth factor-beta and Runx2 in bone is required for hearing. EMBO reports 11: 765–771.
6. Clayton AE, Mikulec AA, Mikulec KH, Merchant SN, McKenna MJ (2004) Association between osteoporosis and otosclerosis in women. The Journal of laryngology and otology 118: 617–621.
7. Driver EC, Kelley MW (2009) Specification of cell fate in the mammalian cochlea. Birth defects research Part C, Embryo today : reviews 87: 212–221.
8. Sorensen MS (1994) Temporal bone dynamics, the hard way. Formation, growth, modeling, repair and quantum type bone remodeling in the otic capsule. Acta oto-laryngologica Supplementum 512: 1–22.
9. Kao SY, Kempfle JS, Jensen JB, Perez-Fernandez D, Lysaght AC, et al. (2013) Loss of osteoprotegerin expression in the inner ear causes degeneration of the cochlear nerve and sensorineural hearing loss. Neurobiology of disease 56: 25–33.
10. Cureoglu S, Baylan MY, Paparella MM (2010) Cochlear otosclerosis. Current opinion in otolaryngology & head and neck surgery 18: 357–362.
11. Cureoglu S, Schachern PA, Ferlito A, Rinaldo A, Tsuprun V, et al. (2006) Otosclerosis: etiopathogenesis and histopathology. Am J Otolaryngol 27: 334–340.
12. Santos F, McCall AA, Chien W, Merchant S (2012) Otopathology in Osteogenesis Imperfecta. Otol Neurotol 33: 1562–1566.
13. Kobilka BK (2007) G protein coupled receptor structure and activation. Biochimica et biophysica acta 1768: 794–807.
14. Spiegel AM, Weinstein LS (2004) Inherited diseases involving g proteins and g protein-coupled receptors. Annual review of medicine 55: 27–39.
15. Pollandt K, Engels C, Kaiser E, Werner M, Delling G (2001) Gsalpha gene mutations in monostotic fibrous dysplasia of bone and fibrous dysplasia-like low-grade central osteosarcoma. Virchows Archiv : an international journal of pathology 439: 170–175.
16. Cole DE, Fraser FC, Glorieux FH, Jequier S, Marie PJ, et al. (1983) Panostotic fibrous dysplasia: a congenital disorder of bone with unusual facial appearance, bone fragility, hyperphosphatasemia, and hypophosphatemia. American journal of medical genetics 14: 725–735.
17. DiCaprio MR, Enneking WF (2005) Fibrous dysplasia. Pathophysiology, evaluation, and treatment. The Journal of bone and joint surgery American volume 87: 1848–1864.
18. Megerian CA, Sofferman RA, McKenna MJ, Eavey RD, Nadol JB, Jr. (1995) Fibrous dysplasia of the temporal bone: ten new cases demonstrating the spectrum of otologic sequelae. The American journal of otology 16: 408–419.
19. Morrissey DD, Talbot JM, Schleuning AJ, 2nd (1997) Fibrous dysplasia of the temporal bone: reversal of sensorineural hearing loss after decompression of the internal auditory canal. The Laryngoscope 107: 1336–1340.
20. Papadakis CE, Skoulakis CE, Prokopakis EP, Nikolidakis AA, Bizakis JG, et al. (2000) Fibrous dysplasia of the temporal bone: report of a case and a review of its characteristics. Ear, nose, & throat journal 79: 52–57.
21. Riddle ND, Bui MM (2013) Fibrous dysplasia. Archives of pathology & laboratory medicine 137: 134–138.
22. Lietman SA, Levine MA (2013) Fibrous dysplasia. Pediatric endocrinology reviews : PER 10 Suppl 2: 389–396.
23. Weinstein LS (2006) G(s)alpha Mutations in Fibrous Dysplasia and McCune-Albright Syndrome. J Bone Miner Res 21 Suppl 2: P120–124.
24. Conklin BR, Hsiao EC, Claeysen S, Dumuis A, Srinivasan S, et al. (2008) Engineering GPCR signaling pathways with RASSLs. Nature methods 5: 673–678.
25. Coward P, Wada HG, Falk MS, Chan SD, Meng F, et al. (1998) Controlling signaling with a specifically designed Gi-coupled receptor. Proc Natl Acad Sci U S A 95: 352–357.
26. Hsiao EC, Boudignon BM, Chang WC, Bencsik M, Peng J, et al. (2008) Osteoblast expression of an engineered Gs-coupled receptor dramatically increases bone mass. Proceedings of the National Academy of Sciences of the United States of America 105: 1209–1214.
27. Redfern CH, Degtyarev MY, Kwa AT, Salomonis N, Cotte N, et al. (2000) Conditional expression of a Gi-coupled receptor causes ventricular conduction delay and a lethal cardiomyopathy. Proc Natl Acad Sci U S A 97: 4826–4831.
28. Hsiao EC, Boudignon BM, Halloran BP, Nissenson RA, Conklin BR (2010) Gs G protein-coupled receptor signaling in osteoblasts elicits age-dependent effects on bone formation. Journal of bone and mineral research : the official journal of the American Society for Bone and Mineral Research 25: 584–593.
29. Zheng QY, Johnson KR, Erway LC (1999) Assessment of hearing in 80 inbred strains of mice by ABR threshold analyses. Hearing research 130: 94–107.
30. Hsiao EC, Millard SM, Louie A, Huang Y, Conklin BR, et al. (2010) Ligand-mediated activation of an engineered gs g protein-coupled receptor in osteoblasts increases trabecular bone formation. Mol Endocrinol 24: 621–631.
31. Akil O, Chang J, Hiel H, Kong JH, Yi E, et al. (2006) Progressive deafness and altered cochlear innervation in knock-out mice lacking prosaposin. The Journal of neuroscience : the official journal of the Society for Neuroscience 26: 13076–13088.
32. Akil O, Lustig LR (2012) Severe vestibular dysfunction and altered vestibular innervation in mice lacking prosaposin. Neuroscience research 72: 296–305.
33. Akil O, Seal RP, Burke K, Wang C, Alemi A, et al. (2012) Restoration of hearing in the VGLUT3 knockout mouse using virally mediated gene therapy. Neuron 75: 283–293.
34. Tang S, Herber RP, Ho S, Alliston T (2012) Matrix metalloproteinase-13 is required for osteocytic perilacunar remodeling and maintains bone fracture

resistance. Journal of bone and mineral research : the official journal of the American Society for Bone and Mineral Research.

35. Dvorak-Ewell MM, Chen TH, Liang N, Garvey C, Liu B, et al. (2011) Osteoblast extracellular Ca2+ -sensing receptor regulates bone development, mineralization, and turnover. Journal of bone and mineral research : the official journal of the American Society for Bone and Mineral Research 26: 2935–2947.

36. Wada T, Nakashima T, Hiroshi N, Penninger JM (2006) RANKL-RANK signaling in osteoclastogenesis and bone disease. Trends in molecular medicine 12: 17–25.

37. Boyce BF, Xing L (2007) Biology of RANK, RANKL, and osteoprotegerin. Arthritis research & therapy 9 Suppl 1: S1.

38. Grimaud E, Soubigou L, Couillaud S, Coipeau P, Moreau A, et al. (2003) Receptor activator of nuclear factor kappaB ligand (RANKL)/osteoprotegerin (OPG) ratio is increased in severe osteolysis. The American journal of pathology 163: 2021–2031.

39. Tu X, Rhee Y, Condon KW, Bivi N, Allen MR, et al. (2012) Sost downregulation and local Wnt signaling are required for the osteogenic response to mechanical loading. Bone 50: 209–217.

40. van Bezooijen RL, Roelen BA, Visser A, van der Wee-Pals L, de Wilt E, et al. (2004) Sclerostin is an osteocyte-expressed negative regulator of bone formation, but not a classical BMP antagonist. The Journal of experimental medicine 199: 805–814.

41. Balemans W, Ebeling M, Patel N, Van Hul E, Olson P, et al. (2001) Increased bone density in sclerosteosis is due to the deficiency of a novel secreted protein (SOST). Human molecular genetics 10: 537–543.

42. van Lierop AH, Hamdy NA, van Egmond ME, Bakker E, Dikkers FG, et al. (2013) Van Buchem disease: clinical, biochemical, and densitometric features of patients and disease carriers. Journal of bone and mineral research : the official journal of the American Society for Bone and Mineral Research 28: 848–854.

43. Cullinane DM (2002) The role of osteocytes in bone regulation: mineral homeostasis versus mechanoreception. Journal of musculoskeletal & neuronal interactions 2: 242–244.

44. Belanger LF (1969) Osteocytic osteolysis. Calcified tissue research 4: 1–12.

45. Bonewald LF (2011) The amazing osteocyte. Journal of bone and mineral research : the official journal of the American Society for Bone and Mineral Research 26: 229–238.

46. Qing H, Bonewald LF (2009) Osteocyte remodeling of the perilacunar and pericanalicular matrix. International journal of oral science 1: 59–65.

47. Qing H, Ardeshirpour L, Pajevic PD, Dusevich V, Jahn K, et al. (2012) Demonstration of osteocytic perilacunar/canalicular remodeling in mice during lactation. Journal of bone and mineral research : the official journal of the American Society for Bone and Mineral Research 27: 1018–1029.

48. Holmbeck K, Bianco P, Pidoux I, Inoue S, Billinghurst RC, et al. (2005) The metalloproteinase MT1-MMP is required for normal development and maintenance of osteocyte processes in bone. Journal of cell science 118: 147–156.

49. Inoue K, Mikuni-Takagaki Y, Oikawa K, Itoh T, Inada M, et al. (2006) A crucial role for matrix metalloproteinase 2 in osteocytic canalicular formation and bone metabolism. The Journal of biological chemistry 281: 33814–33824.

50. Milovanovic P, Zimmermann EA, Hahn M, Djonic D, Puschel K, et al. (2013) Osteocytic Canalicular Networks: Morphological Implications for Altered Mechanosensitivity. ACS nano.

51. Kazakia GJ, Speer D, Shanbhag S, Majumdar S, Conklin BR, et al. (2011) Mineral Composition is Altered by Osteoblast Expression of an Engineered G(s)-Coupled Receptor. Calcified tissue international 89: 10–20.

52. Zehnder AF, Kristiansen AG, Adams JC, Merchant SN, McKenna MJ (2005) Osteoprotegerin in the inner ear may inhibit bone remodeling in the otic capsule. The Laryngoscope 115: 172–177.

53. Lacey DL, Timms E, Tan HL, Kelley MJ, Dunstan CR, et al. (1998) Osteoprotegerin ligand is a cytokine that regulates osteoclast differentiation and activation. Cell 93: 165–176.

54. Whyte MP, Obrecht SE, Finnegan PM, Jones JL, Podgornik MN, et al. (2002) Osteoprotegerin deficiency and juvenile Paget's disease. N Engl J Med 347: 175–184.

3

Disruption of Ion-Trafficking System in the Cochlear Spiral Ligament Prior to Permanent Hearing Loss Induced by Exposure to Intense Noise: Possible Involvement of 4-Hydroxy-2-Nonenal as a Mediator of Oxidative Stress

Taro Yamaguchi, Reiko Nagashima, Masanori Yoneyama, Tatsuo Shiba, Kiyokazu Ogita*

Laboratory of Pharmacology, Faculty of Pharmaceutical Sciences, Setsunan University, Hirakata, Osaka, Japan

Abstract

Noise-induced hearing loss is at least in part due to disruption of endocochlear potential, which is maintained by various K^+ transport apparatuses including Na^+, K^+-ATPase and gap junction-mediated intercellular communication in the lateral wall structures. In this study, we examined the changes in the ion-trafficking-related proteins in the spiral ligament fibrocytes (SLFs) following *in vivo* acoustic overstimulation or *in vitro* exposure of cultured SLFs to 4-hydroxy-2-nonenal, which is a mediator of oxidative stress. Connexin (Cx)26 and Cx30 were ubiquitously expressed throughout the spiral ligament, whereas Na^+, K^+-ATPase α1 was predominantly detected in the stria vascularis and spiral prominence (type 2 SLFs). One-hour exposure of mice to 8 kHz octave band noise at a 110 dB sound pressure level produced an immediate and prolonged decrease in the Cx26 expression level and in Na^+, K^+-ATPase activity, as well as a delayed decrease in Cx30 expression in the SLFs. The noise-induced hearing loss and decrease in the Cx26 protein level and Na^+, K^+-ATPase activity were abolished by a systemic treatment with a free radical-scavenging agent, 4-hydroxy-2,2,6,6-tetramethylpiperidine 1-oxyl, or with a nitric oxide synthase inhibitor, $N^ω$-nitro-L-arginine methyl ester hydrochloride. *In vitro* exposure of SLFs in primary culture to 4-hydroxy-2-nonenal produced a decrease in the protein levels of Cx26 and Na^+, K^+-ATPase α1, as well as Na^+, K^+-ATPase activity, and also resulted in dysfunction of the intercellular communication between the SLFs. Taken together, our data suggest that disruption of the ion-trafficking system in the cochlear SLFs is caused by the decrease in Cxs level and Na^+, K^+-ATPase activity, and at least in part involved in permanent hearing loss induced by intense noise. Oxidative stress-mediated products might contribute to the decrease in Cxs content and Na^+, K^+-ATPase activity in the cochlear lateral wall structures.

Editor: Utpal Sen, University of Louisville, United States of America

Funding: This work was supported in part by grants-in-aid for scientific research to K.O.(project# 4042) from the Ministry of Education, Culture, Sports, Science, and Technology, Japan. Additional funding was received from Setsunan University for this study. The funders had no role in study design, data collection and analysis, decision to publish, or preparation of the manuscript.

Competing Interests: The authors have declared that no competing interests exist.

* Email: ogita@pharm.setsunan.ac.jp

Introduction

Mammalian cochlear spiral ligament (SL) fibrocytes (SLFs) of the mesenchymal non-sensory regions play important roles in the cochlear physiology of hearing. Their role includes the transport of K^+ from the endolymph into the hair cells to generate the endocochlear potential (EP), which is essential for the transduction of sound by hair cells [1–3]. Once hair cells are activated by sound, the EP generated through the flow of K^+ from the endolymph into the hair cells. It has been postulated that a K^+-recycling pathway toward the stria vascularis (SV) via the SLFs in the cochlear lateral wall structures is critical for proper hearing, although the exact mechanism operating in this pathway has not been definitively determined [2]. Previous reports demonstrated that acoustic overstimulation produces alteration of the EP, as well as hearing loss [4,5]. These findings suggest that acoustic injury is at least in part attributable to the abnormal EP induced by

dysfunction of the SV and SL in the cochlear lateral wall structures. However, the mechanism underlying the acoustic overstimulation-induced dysfunction of the lateral wall structures is not fully understood.

Accumulating evidence indicates that gap junction (GJ)-mediated intercellular communication (GJ-IC) plays an important role in maintaining the unique ionic composition of the endolymph and intracellular ion content, both of which are crucial to cochlear functions. GJs are intercellular membrane channels that possess the unique feature of directly connecting the cytoplasm of neighboring cells. The GJ is formed by the juxtaposition of 2 hexameric structures (termed hemichannels or connexons) composed of connexins (Cxs) at the GJ plaques, where a large number of GJs cluster at the cell-cell contact points. Non-sensory cells in the cochlea are connected extensively by GJs that facilitate intercellular ionic and biochemical coupling for GJ-IC. The cochlear GJs are assembled with 2 subtypes of Cx family proteins, i.e., Cx26 and Cx30, which are widely distributed in the basal and intermediate cells of the SV, the supporting cells, the spiral limbus, and the spiral prominence [6,7]. Evidence for involvement of Cxs in hearing ability comes from the finding that mutations in the Cx26-encoding gene (GJB2) cause at substantial portion (20–50%) of the cases of human non-syndromic hereditary deafness, which is one of the most common human birth defects. A large number of reports on human GJB2 mutations linked to prelingual deafness indicated loss-of-function mutations that effectively null the utility of Cx26 in the cochlea [8]. Disturbance of the GJ complex of Cx26 would be expected to disrupt the recycling of K^+ from the synapses at the base of the hair cells through the supporting cells and SLFs in the cochlea. The disruption of K^+ recycling is known to decrease sound-induced cochlear responses, resulting in sensorineural hearing loss [9]. In the present study, therefore, we evaluated whether Cx-related GJ-IC in the cochlear lateral wall structures is involved in the mechanism underlying noise-induced hearing loss.

Na^+, K^+-ATPase is a well-known enzyme that participates in the active transport of Na^+ and K^+, and plays important roles in maintaining cochlear function of the inner ear [10–12]. Cytochemical studies showed that strong activity of Na^+, K^+-ATPase is detectable in the SV and spiral prominence of the cochlear lateral wall structures, with the highest level of activity in the marginal cells of the SV [10,13,14]. However, little expression of Na^+, K^+-ATPase is found in the organ of Corti.

To the best of our knowledge, there have been very few reports regarding the functional role of Cxs in acquired sensorineural hearing loss. Although previous studies showed changes in the EP and K^+ concentration in the endolymph after exposure to noise [4,15], there has been no direct evidence for the involvement of a decrease in cochlear Na^+, K^+-ATPase activity in noise-induced hearing loss. In the present study, we investigated changes in Cx26 and Cx30 expression levels as well as Na^+, K^+-ATPase activity in the cochlear lateral wall structures following exposure to noise in vivo. Based on our previous study showing that exposure to noise in vivo produces 4-hydroxy-2-nonenal (4-HNE) in the lateral wall structures of the cochlea [16], we further investigated the in vitro effect of 4-HNE on the expression level of Cxs and on Na^+, K^+-ATPase activity in primary cultures of the SLFs.

Materials and Methods

Materials

Carbenoxolone, 4-hydroxy-2,2,6,6-tetramethylpiperidine-N-oxyl (tempol), and N^ω-nitro-L-arginine methyl ester (L-NAME) were purchased from Sigma-Aldrich Co. (St. Louis, MO, U.S.A.). 4-HNE was supplied from Cayman Chemical (Ann Arbor, MI. USA). Mouse monoclonal antibodies against Cx26 and Na^+, K^+-ATPase α1 were obtained from Zymed Laboratories, Inc. (South San Francisco, CA, USA) and Santa Cruz Biotechnology, Inc. (Santa Cruz, CA, USA), respectively. Rabbit polyclonal antibodies against Cx30, S100β, and glyceraldehyde-3-phosphate dehydrogenase (GAPDH) were obtained from Zymed Laboratories, Inc. (South San Francisco, CA, USA), FabGennix Inc. (Frisco, TX, USA), and Santa Cruz Biotechnology, Inc. (Santa Cruz, CA, USA), respectively. Alexa-Fluor 598-conjugated anti-rabbit IgG (H+L) antibody, Alexa-Fluor 488-conjugated anti-mouse IgG (H+L) antibody, Calcein-AM, and 1,1-dioctadecyl-3,3,3′,3′-tetramethylindocarbocyanine perchloric acid (DiI) were purchased from Life Technology Co. (Carlsbad, CA, USA). Diaminobenzidine/hydrogen peroxide solution (Histofine) came from Nitirei Co. (Tokyo, Japan). Streptavidin-biotin complex peroxidase kit, poly-L-lysine hydrobromide, and trypsin solution were from Nacalai

Tesque, Inc. (Kyoto, Japan). Polyvinylidene fluoride membranes (Immobilon-P) were obtained from Millipore (Bedford, MA, USA). Western Lightning Chemoluminescence Reagent Plus was purchased from PerkinElmer Life Science Products, Inc. (Boston, MA, U.S.A.). All other chemicals used were of the highest purity commercially available.

Animal treatment

The protocol used here met the guidelines of the Japanese Society for Pharmacology and was approved by the Committee for Ethical Use of Experimental Animals at Setsunan University. All efforts were made to minimize animal suffering, to reduce the number of animals used, and to utilize alternatives to in vivo techniques. Adult male Std-ddY mice weighing 26–28 g, which we routinely use for neuroscience studies, were housed in metallic breeding cages in a room with a light-dark cycle of 12 h–12 h and a humidity of 55% at 23°C and given free access to food and water. To remove animals with natural auditory impairment, we measured their auditory brainstem response (ABR) before use and selected those animals with normal acoustic sense in the present study.

Intense noise exposure

The mice were anesthetized with chloral hydrate (500 mg/kg, i.p.) and exposed to 110-dB sound-pressure level (SPL) of octave-band noise, centered at 8 kHz, for 1 h within a sound chamber [17]. Each animal was placed in a cage. The sound chamber was fitted with a speaker (300HT; FOSTEX, Tokyo, Japan) driven by a noise generator (SF-06; RION, Tokyo, Japan) and power amplifier (DAD-M100proHT; FLYING MOLE, Shizuoka, Japan). To ensure uniformity of the stimulus, we calibrated and measured the sound levels with a sound-level meter (NL-26; RION, Tokyo, Japan), which was positioned at the level of the animal's head. As a control, naïve animals were placed in the same cage without noise.

ABR recording

For ABR measurements, stainless steel-needle electrodes were placed at the vertex and ventro-lateral to the left and right ears. Electroencephalogram recording was performed with an extracellular amplifier Digital Bioamp system (BAL-1; Tucker-Davis Technologies, FL, USA), and waveform storing and stimulus control were performed by using Scope software of the Power Lab system (Power Lab 2/20; AD Instruments, Castle Hill, Australia). Sound stimuli were produced by a coupler-type speaker (ES1spc; Bioresearch Center, Nagoya, Japan) inserted into the external auditory canal of the mouse. Tone-burst stimuli, 0.1 ms rise/fall time (cosine gate) and 1-ms flat segment, were generated by using a Real-Time Processor (RP2.1; Tucker-Davis Technologies, FL, USA); and the amplitudes were specified by use of a Programmable Attenuator (PA5; Tucker-Davis Technologies, FL, USA). Sound levels were calibrated with a sound-level meter (TYPE 6224; ACO CO., LTD.). ABR waveforms were recorded for 12.8 ms at a sampling rate of 40,000 Hz by using 50–5000 Hz bandpass-filter settings. Waveforms from 500 stimuli were averaged. For recording, animals were anesthetized (500 mg/kg chloral hydrate, i.p.). The thresholds of ABR were determined before noise exposure and immediately (0) and on day 7 afterward at 12 kHz, by using a 5-dB SPL minimum step size down from the maximum amplitude. The hearing threshold was defined as the lowest stimulus intensity that produced a reliable wave I of the ABR. Because the constraining test tones at 4, 12, and 20 kHz were set to SPLs of less than 90 dB, the respective thresholds were recorded as 100 dB for the calculation of the threshold shift value when there was no response due to profound hearing impairment.

Histological assessment

The mice were anesthetized deeply with chloral hydrate (500 mg/kg, i.p.) and intracardially perfused with saline and subsequently with 4% (wt/vol) paraformaldehyde in 0.1 M sodium phosphate buffer (pH 7.4). Their cochleae were removed quickly. The round and oval windows and the apex of the cochlea were opened and then perfused with Bouin's solution (picric acid: 37% (vol/vol) formaldehyde: acetic acid = 15:5:1). The tissues were subsequently kept at room temperature overnight. The post-fixed cochlea was embedded in paraffin, and then sections at 5 μm thickness were prepared by using a microtome. The sections were deparaffinized with xylene and then rehydrated by passage through ethanol at graded concentrations of 50 to 100% (vol/vol) and then immersion in water. Immunoreactivity was determined by the avidin-biotin-peroxidase method. For the immunostaining of Cx26 and Cx30, the sections were washed with Tris-buffered saline (pH 7.5) containing 0.03% (wt/vol) Tween 20 (TBST) and then incubated with 0.03% (vol/vol) H_2O_2 in methanol for 5 min. After having been blocked with 10% (vol/vol) normal goat serum in TBST for 1 h at room temperature, serial sections were incubated with mouse monoclonal antibody against Cx26 (1:200) or rabbit polyclonal antibody against Cx30 (1:200) at 4°C overnight, followed by biotinylated anti-mouse IgG antibody or biotinylated anti-rabbit IgG antibody for 30 min at room temperature, and then with ABC solution for 1 h at room temperature. The peroxidase reaction was visualized by use of diaminobenzidine/hydrogen peroxide solution.

For double labeling with antibodies against Cx26 and Cx30 or S100β, sections covered with 10 mM sodium citrate buffer (pH 7.0) were first microwaved in a microwave oven for 10 min. After having been blocked with 10% (vol/vol) normal goat serum in TBST for 1 h at room temperature, the sections were incubated with primary antibodies against Cx26 and Cx30 or S100β at 4°C overnight. After having been washed with TBST, the sections were then reacted for 2 h at room temperature with secondary antibodies (Alexa Fluor 488-conjugated anti-mouse IgG for Cx26 and Alexa Fluor 598-conjugated anti-rabbit IgG for Cx30 or S100β). For double labeling with antibodies against Na^+, K^+-ATPase α1 and S100β, the sections were first microwaved as above and then blocked with 10% (vol/vol) normal goat serum in TBST for 1 h at room temperature, after which they were if the sections were first incubated with one primary antibody and then incubated with the other one, then "sequentially" would apply. But I assume that you would have used a mixture of both primary antibodies as the first step incubated with primary antibodies at 4°C overnight. After having been washed with TBST, the sections were next reacted for 2 h at room temperature with secondary antibodies (Alexa Fluor 488-conjugated anti-mouse IgG for Na^+, K^+-ATPase α1 and Alexa Fluor 598-conjugated anti-rabbit IgG for S100β). Finally, the sections were incubated with Hoechst 33342 (5 mg/mL) for 20 min at room temperature; and positive cells were determined by viewing with an Olympus U-LH100HG fluorescence microscope.

Semi-quantitative RT-PCR and real-time PCR

For RT-PCR assays, total RNA was isolated from cortical neurons with Trizol by following the manufacturer's instructions (Invitrogen Co., California, USA). One microgram of total RNA was reverse transcribed to prepare cDNA by using Oligo(dT)$_{15}$ primer in accordance with Ready-To-Go You-Prime First-Stranded Beads (GE Healthcare UK Ltd, Buckinghamshire, England). Aliquots of cDNA were then amplified with a 0.4 μM concentration of each primer set: 5'-AAATGTCTGCTATGA-CAAGTCCTTC-3'(forward) and 5'-CTTTGAGCTCCTCTT-CTTTCTTGTT-3'(reverse) for the Cx43-encoding gene (GJA1); 5'-CCGTCTTCATGTACGTCTTTTACAT-3' (forward) and 5'-ATACCTAACGAACAAATAGCACAGC-3'(reverse) for the Cx26-encoding gene (GJB2); 5'-AGTTTATACGTGGGGGA-GAAGAGAAA-3' (forward) and 5'-TGGTACCCATTGTA-GAGGAAGTAGA-3'(reverse) for the Cx30-encoding gene (GJB6); and 5'-GCCAAGTATGATGACATCAAGAAG-3' (forward) and 5'-TCCAGGGGTTTCTTACTCCTTGGA-3'(reverse) for GAPDH in 25 μL of reaction mixture containing 0.2 mM concentration of each dNTP, 0.625 units Taq DNA polymerase, 10 mM Tris–HCl (pH 8.3), 50 mM KCl, 1.5 mM $MgCl_2$, and 0.001% gelatin. Reactions were carried out for a total of 25–30 cycles with the use of a Thermal cycler, and then the PCR products were analyzed by performing 1% agarose gel electrophoresis. For real-time PCR assays, an aliquot of cDNA was amplified by using a 0.2 μM concentration of each primer set for GJA1, GJB2, GJB6, and GAPDH genes in 12.5 μL of STBR Premix Ex Taq (Takara Bio Inc, Shiga, Japan).

Immunoblot analysis

Cochlear SL structures were quickly removed and immersed in ice-cold homogenizing buffer consisting of 10 mM Tris-HCl buffer (pH 7.5), 0.32 M sucrose, 1 mM EDTA, 1 mM EGTA, 5 mM dithiothreitol, phosphatase inhibitors (10 mM sodium β-glycerophosphate and 1 mM sodium orthovanadate), and 1 μg/mL each of protease inhibitors [(p-amidinophenyl)methanesulfonyl fluoride, benzamidine, leupeptin, and antipain], homogenized in 30 μL of the homogenizing buffer, and then immediately boiled for 10 min in a solution comprising 2% (wt/vol) SDS, 5% (vol/vol) 2-mercaptoethanol, 10% (vol/vol) glycerol, and 0.01% (wt/vol) bromophenol blue. The samples were stored at −80°C until used for immunoblot analysis.

The immunoblot analysis was carried out as described previously [18]. Briefly, an aliquot (10 μg) of sample was loaded onto a 10% (wt/vol) polyacrylamide gel for detection of Cx26, Cx30, and GAPDH. The proteins were transferred to a polyvinylidene fluoride membrane and blocked with 5% (wt/vol) skim milk dissolved in washing buffer [Tris-buffered saline containing 0.05% (wt/vol) Tween 20]. The membranes were incubated with the desired primary antibody for 2 h at room temperature, then washed with the above washing buffer for 3 cycles of 5 min each, and subsequently incubated with horseradish peroxidase-conjugated antibodies against mouse IgG and rabbit IgG for 1 h at room temperature. Proteins reactive with the antibody were detected with the aid of Western Lightning Chemoluminescence Reagent Plus, which procedure was followed by exposure to X-ray films.

Na^+, K^+-ATPase activity

Na^+, K^+-ATPase activity was determined by colormetrically measuring the amount of inorganic phosphate released from the substrate ATP [14]. Cochlear lateral wall structures were quickly removed and homogenized in ice-cold HEPES buffer (pH 7.5). An aliquot (6 μg protein) of the homogenate was incubated 10 min at 37°C in reaction buffer consisting of 40 mM Tris-HCl buffer (pH 7.5), 150 mM KCl, and 1.2 M NaCl in the absence or presence of 100 μM ouabain and then further incubated 30 min at 37°C in the reaction buffer containing 10 mM ATP and 30 mM $MgSO_4$. The reaction was terminated by the addition of 12% perchloric acid and 0.84% ammonium molybdate to measure the released inorganic phosphate. The specific activity was calculated from the values obtained in the absence and presence of ouabain and expressed as $\mu mol \cdot min^{-1} \cdot mg \ protein^{-1}$.

Primary cultures of SLFs

Mouse cochleae were removed from 5 animals under sterile conditions, and transferred to ice-cold Dulbecco's phosphate-buffered saline containing 100 U/mL penicillin, 0.1 mg/mL streptomycin, and 33 mM glucose. Following opening of the cochlear bone, the SL tissues were dissected with fine forceps. The SL tissues were cut into small longitudinal segments and then placed into type 1 collagen-coated Petri dishes (35 mm) containing 0.3 mL of culture medium consisting of DMEM supplemented with 10% fetal bovine serum (FBS), 100 U/mL penicillin, and 0.1 mg/mL streptomycin. At 3 and 4 days *in vitro* (DIV), 0.7 mL and 1 mL of fresh culture medium, respectively, was added to each Petri dish. The tissue segments were further cultured for 6 days with a change of the culture medium every 3 days. During the culture period, the cells migrated from the tissue segments and reached confluence at 10 DIV. The cells were then rinsed with phosphate-buffered saline and incubated with 0.25% trypsin solution for 5 min at 37°C to induce cell detachment. Culture medium was then added and gently triturated to suspend the cells. After centrifugation at $900 \times g$ for 5 min, the cells were washed twice with culture medium by gentle trituration and centrifugation. The cells were seeded at a density of 1,000 cells/0.5 mL in 4-well dishes (Nunc, Denmark) that had been previously coated with poly-L-lysine hydrobromide and then cultured for the desired periods with a change of culture medium every 3 days. Usually at 12 DIV, the cells were used for experiments. The cultures were always maintained at 37°C in 95% (vol/vol) air -5% (vol/vol) CO_2.

Fluorescent dye-transfer assay

Cultures of SLFs were labeled simultaneously with calcein-AM and DiI as donor cells. Calcein-AM is cleaved by cytosolic esterases and then becomes able to permeate GJs. DiI associates with cell membranes and fails to be transferred to unlabeled cells [19]. The labeled cells (donor cells) were harvested with a 0.25% trypsin solution for 5 min, rinsed, and seeded onto unlabeled cells, which had been cultured as acceptor cells. These cells were then cultured for 4.5 h to allow the donor cells to establish GJ-IC with the acceptor cells (Figure 1). The number of cells receiving calcein from the donor cells provides an index of GJ-IC. The transfer of calcein to the acceptor cells from the donor cells was completely blocked by pretreatment for 4 h with 200 μM carbenoxolone, which completely and reversibly blocks the GJ-IC under certain experimental conditions [19].

Data analysis

The area under the curve was calculated by analyzing the densitometric data by the software Lane Analyzer ver. 3 (Copyright Rise Co., Ltd. & Atto Corp. 1999–2001). Each result was expressed as the mean ± S.E.M., and the statistical significance of differences was determined by one-way ANOVA with the Bonferroni/Dunnett *post hoc* test or the Mann-Whitney *U*-test.

Results

Localization of Cx26, Cx30, and Na⁺, K⁺-ATPase α1 in the lateral wall structures

Multiple isoforms of 3 subunits (α, β, and γ) comprise the Na⁺, K⁺-ATPase oligomer. Of these subunits, the α subunit has the binding sites for ATP and cations (Na⁺ and K⁺). The cochlear GJs

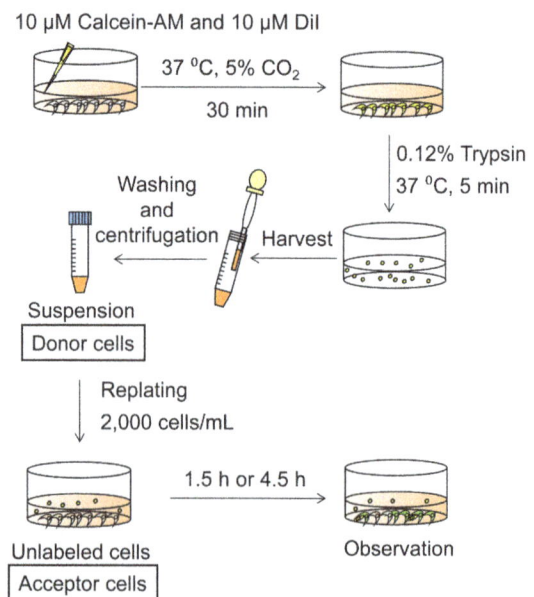

Figure 1. Procedure for fluorescent dye-transfer assay. Cultures of the SLFs prepared from the cochlea of naïve animals were labeled with both DiI (*red*) and calcein-AM (*green*) as donor cells (*yellow*). The donor cells were then seeded onto unlabeled cells (acceptor cells), and the cultures were incubated for 1.5 or 4.5 h.

are assembled with Cx26 and Cx30 [6,7]. Thus, we examined the expression of ion-transport proteins including Cx26, Cx30, and the α1 subunit of Na⁺, K⁺-ATPase in the lateral wall structures of naïve adult mouse. Histological assessment by immunostaining revealed that Na⁺, K⁺-ATPase α1 was located predominantly in the type 2/4 SLFs and in the entire SV (Figure 2b; see Figure 2a for locations of these cells or structure). Cx26 was expressed mainly in the type 1 cells and in the basal cells of the SV with weak expression in the type 2/4 cells; whereas Cx30 was found in all SLFs and in the basal cells of the SV (Figure 2c). Co-localization of Cx26 and Cx30 was observed in the adhesion sites of the SLFs (Figure 2c at high magnification).

Developmental changes in the expression of Cx26, S100β, and Na⁺, K⁺-ATPase α1 in the lateral wall structures

A previous report demonstrated that the various types of SLFs in the postnatal rat have different processes of proliferation and differentiation [20]. Using immunostaining, thus, we determined the expression levels of Na⁺, K⁺-ATPase α1 and Cx26 in the lateral wall structures at the postnatal ages of day 7 (P7), P10, P14, and P35 (Figure 3). S100β is a family protein of S100, which is known to express in the type 1/2 cells of the SLFs [21]. Na⁺, K⁺-ATPase α1 appeared in the type 2/4 SLFs and in the SV even at P7. The level of Na⁺, K⁺-ATPase α1 was very weak at P7 and gradually increased up to the adult age (P35, Figure 3a). Cx26 was found mainly in the basal cells of the SV, but not in the SLFs, even at P7. At P10, Cx26 started to appear in the type 1 cells with the level increasing up to P35 (Figure 3b).

Effect of noise exposure on mRNA level of GJ genes in the SL

To determine hearing loss and hair-cell damage following noise exposure, we measured the ABR immediately and on day 7 after a

(a)

(b)

(c)

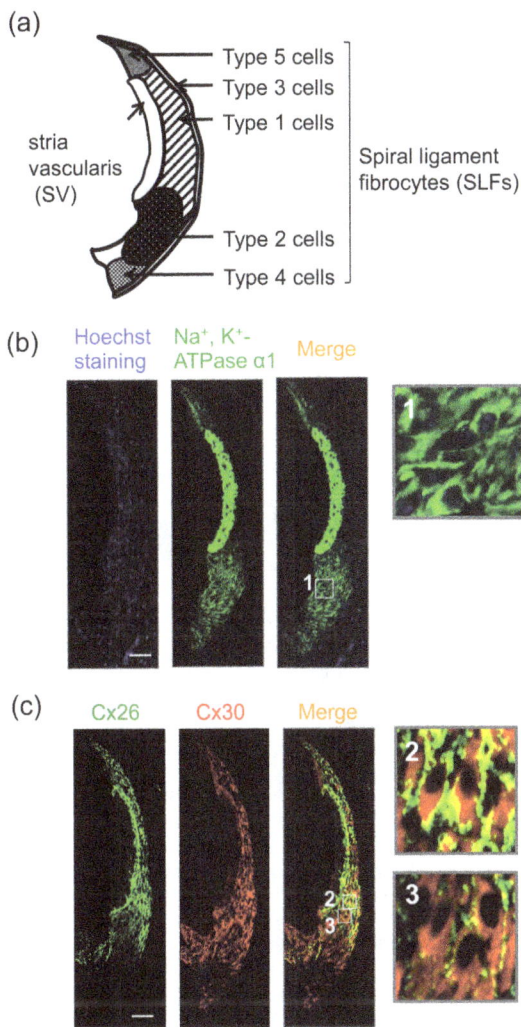

Figure 2. Localization of Cx26, Cx30, and Na⁺, K⁺-ATPase α1 in the lateral wall structures. Mice at the postnatal age of 5 weeks were fixed for preparation of cochlear slices, which were then stained with Hoechst 33342 and immunostained for Cx26, Cx30, and Na⁺, K⁺-ATPase α1 in the lateral wall structures. (**a**) Diagram of various types (types 1–5) of fibrocytes in the lateral wall structures. (**b**) Typical images of Hoechst 33342 staining (*blue*) and Na⁺, K⁺-ATPase α1 immunostaining (*green*) in the lateral wall structures of mice. The rightmost panel is a higher magnification image of the framed squares "1" in the adjacent image. (**c**) Typical images of immunostaining for Cx26 (*green*) and Cx30 (*red*) in the lateral wall structures of mice at the postnatal age of 5 weeks. The rightmost panels are higher magnification images of the framed squares "2" and "3" in the adjacent merged image. Yellow color denotes co-localization of Cx26 and Cx30. These experiments were carried out at least 4 times under the same experimental conditions, with similar results. Scale bar = 50 μm.

(a) Na⁺, K⁺-ATPase α1/S100β

(b) Cx26/S100β

Figure 3. Developmental changes in Cx26, S100β, and Na⁺, K⁺-ATPase α1 in the lateral wall structures. Mice of various postnatal ages were fixed for preparation of cochlear slices, which were then stained with Hoechst 33342 and immunostained for Cx26, Na⁺, K⁺-ATPase α1, and S100β in the lateral wall structures. (**a**) Typical images of immunostaining for Na⁺, K⁺-ATPase α1 (*green*) and S100β (*red*) in the lateral wall structures of mice at P7 to P35. (**b**) Typical images of immunostaining for Cx26 (*green*) and S100β (*red*) in the lateral wall structures of mice at P7 to P35. These experiments were carried out at least 4 times under the same experimental conditions, with similar results. Scale bar = 50 μm.

Semi-quantitative RT-PCR (Figure 4a) and real-time PCR (Figure 4b) both revealed a decrease in the mRNA level of GJB2 in the SL at 2-h post-noise exposure. However, no significant change was seen in the mRNA levels of GJA1 and GJB6 there under the same experimental conditions.

Effect of noise exposure on the protein levels of Cx26 and Cx30 in the SL

We next determined the protein levels of Cx26 and Cx30 in the SL of naïve and noise-exposed animals. Figure 5 shows the Cx26 level at various time points following noise exposure. Immunoblot analysis revealed that noise exposure produced a dramatic decrease in the Cx26 level at 4 h, 24 h, and on day 7 post-exposure (Figure 5a). In addition to immunoblot analysis, immunostaining revealed this noise-induced decrease in the Cx26 level in the type 1 cells of the SL and in basal cells of the SV from at least 2 h to 24 h (day 1) post-exposure (Figure 5b). The decrease in Cx26 in the SV remained even later on day 7, although the Cx26 level in the basal cells returned until the naïve one from days 2 to 7 post-exposure.

Figure 6 shows the Cx30 level at various time points following noise exposure. Immunoblot analysis using the protein samples prepared from the SV revealed that Cx30 expression markedly decreased at least on day 7 post-exposure (Figure 6a). This noise-

1-h exposure to noise at 110 dB SPL. Noise was effective in shifting the ABR threshold at the frequencies of 4, 12, and 20 kHz immediately after exposure. Immediately post-exposure, the ABR threshold shifts were from 40 to 80 dB at all frequencies. The ABR threshold shifts induced by noise remained more than 20 dB even on day 7 post-exposure (data not shown). These results suggest that noise at 110 dB SPL produced a permanent threshold shift. Under these experimental conditions, we examined the effect of noise exposure on the mRNA level of GJA1, GJB2, and GJB6, which are the coding genes for Cx43, Cx26, and Cx30, respectively.

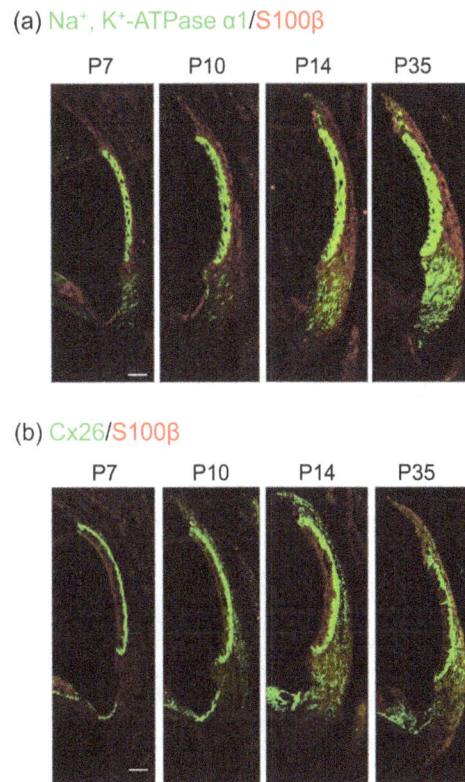

(a)

(b)

2 h after noise exposure

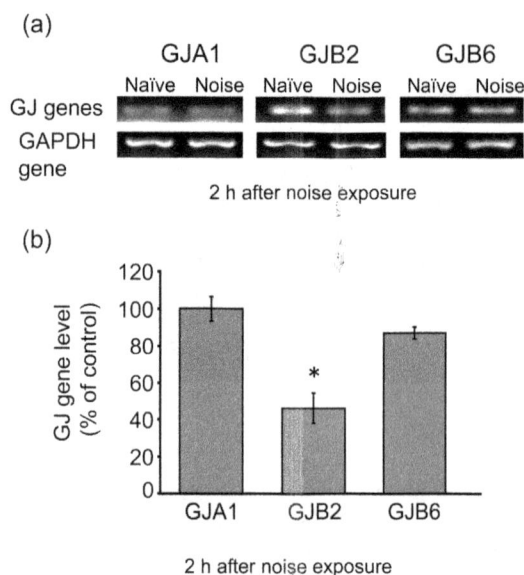

Figure 4. Effect of noise exposure on the mRNA level of Cxs in the SL. Animals were exposed to noise at 110 dB SPL for 1 h. At 2-h post-exposure, total RNA was isolated from the SL and subjected to semi-quantitative RT-PCR (**a**) and real-time PCR (**b**) analyses for determination of the mRNA level of GJA1 (Cx43), GJB2 (Cx26), GJB6 (Cx30), and GAPDH. Values are the mean ± S.E. from 5 separate animals per each group. *$P<0.05$, significantly different from control value obtained for naïve animals.

(a)

Time after noise exposure

(b)

Figure 5. Effect of noise exposure on the protein level of Cx26 in the SL. Animals were exposed to noise at 110 dB SPL for 1 h. (**a**) Tissue lysates were prepared from the SL of the cochlear at the various time points indicated post-noise exposure as well as from that of naïve animals for determination of Cx26 levels by immunoblot analysis. Values are the means ± S.E. from 4–7 separate animals per each group. *$P<0.05$, significantly different from control value obtained for naïve animals. (**b**) At the various time points indicated post-exposure, animals were fixed for preparation of the cochlear slices, which were then immunostained for Cx26 in the lateral wall structures of the cochlea. These experiments were carried out at least 6 times under the same experimental conditions, with similar results. 0 h, immediately after noise exposure.

induced decrease in the level of Cx30 protein was found in the type 2/4 cells on day 2 and afterwards, followed by that in the type 1 cells on day 7 post-exposure (Figure 6b).

Effect of noise exposure on Na⁺, K⁺-ATPase activity in the SL

To evaluate whether Na⁺, K⁺-ATPase changed as a noise-induced event in the lateral wall structures, we determined the mRNA level of Na⁺, K⁺-ATPase α1 and Na⁺, K⁺-ATPase activity in tissue lysates prepared from the SL of naïve and noise-exposed animals (Figure 7). Noise exposure dramatically decreased both the mRNA level of Na⁺, K⁺-ATPase α1 and Na⁺, K⁺-ATPase activity at least 2 h post-exposure. Importantly, this noise-induced decrease was maintained at least up to day 7 post-exposure.

Effect of tempol and L-NAME on noise-induced permanent hearing loss and noise-induced events in the SL

Evidence for involvement of oxidative stress in noise-induced hearing loss comes from our previous findings that noise-induced hearing loss is prevented by treatment with tempol and L-NAME, which are a reactive oxygen species scavenger and nitric oxide synthase inhibitor, respectively [16]. To evaluate if oxidative stress was involved in the noise-induced decreases in the Cx26 level and Na⁺, K⁺-ATPase activity, we examined the effect of tempol and L-NAME applied separately on the noise-induced decreases in Cx26 level and Na⁺, K⁺-ATPase activity in the SL, as well as on the noise-induced shift in the ABR threshold, under the same experimental conditions. Noise exposure produced a significant decrease in the Cx26 level and a remarkable shift in the ABR threshold (Table 1). As expected, tempol and L-NAME had the ability to abolish both events induced by noise exposure. In addition to Cx26, the noise-induced decrease in Na⁺, K⁺-ATPase

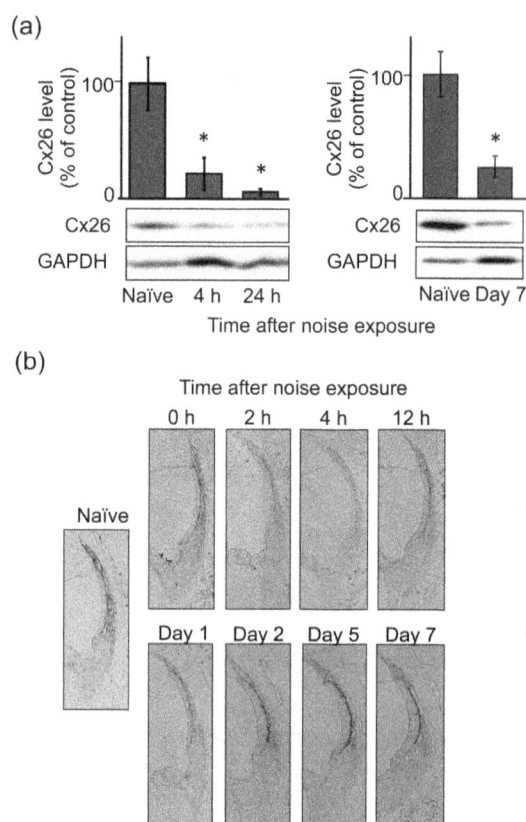

activity was prevented by tempol or L-NAME at the same doses as effective in abolishing the threshold shift (Figure 8).

Effect of 4-HNE on the GJ-IC and Cx26 level in SLF cultures

Our previous report demonstrated that 4-HNE-protein adducts, the 4-HNE of which is the major aldehydic product of lipid peroxidation and believed to be largely responsible for the cytopathological effects observed during oxidative stress [22], are produced in the lateral wall structures following noise exposure under the same experimental conditions as used in the present study [16]. To elucidate the effect of 4-HNE on GJ-IC in the SLFs of the cochlea, we used a fluorescent dye-transfer assay to determine whether an exposure to 4-HNE would affect GJ-IC in cultures of SLFs. Figure 9a shows fluorescence micrographs taken at 1.5- and 4.5-h incubation in the absence of 4-HNE. Both DiI (*red*) and calcein-AM (*green*) were observed in the donor cells, but almost not in the acceptor cells, at 1.5-h incubation. At 4.5-h incubation, expectedly, calcein-AM spread from the donor cells to the adjacent acceptor cells, indicating establishment of GJ-IC in the cultures. Under the same experimental conditions, an

(a)

(b)

Time after noise exposure

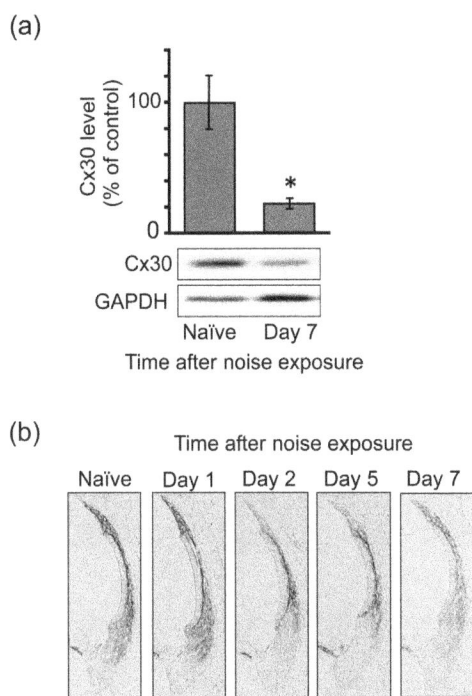

Figure 6. Effect of noise exposure on the protein level of Cx30 in the SL. Animals were exposed to noise at 110 dB SPL for 1 h. (a) Tissue lysates were prepared from the SL of the cochlea on day 7 post-noise exposure as well as from that of naïve animals for determination of Cx30 levels by immunoblot analysis. Values are the means ± S.E. from 4 separate animals per each group. *$P<0.05$, significantly different from control value obtained for naïve animals. (b) At the various time points indicated post-exposure, animals were fixed for preparation of cochlear slices, which were then immunostained for Cx30 in the lateral wall structures of the cochlea. These experiments were carried out at least 6 times under the same experimental conditions, with similar results.

(a)

(b)

Figure 7. Effect of noise exposure on the mRNA level and activity of Na$^+$, K$^+$-ATPase in the SL. (a) Animals were exposed to noise at 110 dB SPL for 1 h. At 2 h post-exposure, total RNA was isolated from the cochlear SL and subjected to real-time PCR analyses for determination of the mRNA level of Na$^+$, K$^+$-ATPase α1 and GAPDH. (b) Tissue lysates were prepared from the cochlear SL at the various time points indicated post-noise exposure as well as from that of naïve animals for determination of Na$^+$, K$^+$-ATPase activity. Values are the mean ± S.E. from 5–10 separate animals per each group. *$P<0.05$, significantly different from control value obtained for naïve animals.

exposure to 4-HNE at the concentration of 1 to 20 μM dramatically decreased the spread of calcein-AM to the acceptor cells in a concentration-dependent manner (Figure 9b). The level of Cx26 was gradually decreased by the exposure to 4-HNE almost in an exposure time-dependent manner (Figure 9c). 4-HNE failed to show any signs of cytotoxicity toward the SLFs under the same experimental conditions (data not shown).

Effect of 4-HNE on Na$^+$, K$^+$-ATPase in SLF cultures

To elucidate the involvement of 4-HNE in the noise-induced decrease in Na$^+$, K$^+$-ATPase activity in the SL, we assessed the change in Na$^+$, K$^+$-ATPase activity and protein levels of Na$^+$, K$^+$-ATPase subunits in the cultured SLFs during the culture in the absence or presence of 4-HNE. Exposure to 4-HNE at the concentration of 1 μM significantly decreased Na$^+$, K$^+$-ATPase activity by a 10-min exposure or longer (Figure 10a). Under the same experimental conditions, the protein level of the Na$^+$, K$^+$-ATPase α1 subunit was significantly decreased by exposure to 4-HNE in a exposure time-dependent manner (Figure 10b). However, no significant change by exposure to 4-HNE, at least when used at 1 μM, was seen in the protein level of the Na$^+$, K$^+$-ATPase β1 subunit.

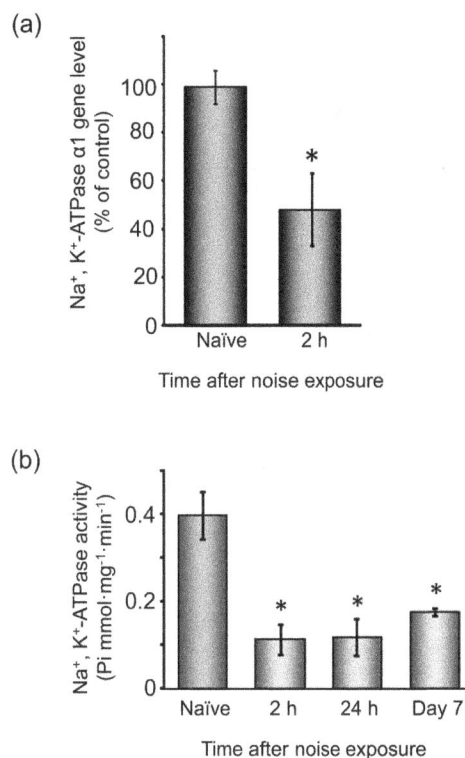

Discussion

The primary aim of the present study was to determine whether disruption of the ion- trafficking system such as GJ-IC and Na$^+$, K$^+$-ATPase activity in the lateral wall structures of the cochlea would be involved in the process producing hearing loss. To this end, we used an *in vivo* model of hearing loss induced by the exposure to intense noise, as well as the primary cultures of SLFs as an *in vitro* system. In the *in vivo* model, previously established by us, noise at different SPLs produced hearing loss with a temporary or permanent threshold shift of the ABR in an SPL-dependent manner [16]. Noise at lower SPL (90 and 100 dB) or higher SPL (110 and 120 dB) produced hearing loss with a temporary or permanent threshold shift, respectively. Indeed, our current data showing that noise at 110 dB SPL produced permanent hearing loss strongly supports our previous findings. In the present study, we demonstrated at the first time that a prolonged decrease in the levels of GJ-comprising proteins, Cx26 and Cx30, and Na$^+$, K$^+$-ATPase activity occurred in the lateral wall structures prior to hearing loss induced by acoustic overstimulation. These events prior to the hearing loss were abolished by tempol, a free radical-scavenging agent, which ameliorated the hearing loss under the same experimental conditions. These results allow us to propose that disruption of ion-trafficking including GJ-IC and active transport of Na$^+$ and K$^+$ in the lateral wall structures contributed

Table 1. Effect of treatment with tempol or L-NAME on ABR threshold shift and the decrease in Cx26 level in noise-exposed mice.

Treatment	Cx26 level (% of control)	ABR threshold shift (dB)			
		Time point of measurement	4 kHz	12 kHz	20 kHz
None	21.9±13.9**	Immediately	50.3±5.5	63.8±5.0	63.8±5.2
		Day 7	20.2±1.5	33.0±2.6	33.0±2.6
Tempol	53.8±17.9#	Immediately	41.7±4.4#	41.7±1.7#	43.3±1.7##
		Day 7	1.7±1.7##	5.0±0.1##	10.0±2.9##
L-NAME	45.2±4.2##	Immediately	38.3±1.7#	45.0±2.9##	43.3±1.7##
		Day 7	3.3±.7##	10.0±0.1##	8.3±1.7##

Mice were exposed to noise at 110 dB SPL for 1 h. At 30 min before the onset of noise exposure, the animals were given tempol (30 mg/kg, i.p.) or L-NAME (1 mg/kg, i.p.). The ABR threshold was assessed at the frequencies of 4, 12, and 20 kHz on immediately and day 7 post-noise exposure. Values are the mean ± S.E. from 3–12 separate animals per each group. For determination of the Cx26 level by immunoblot analysis, tissue lysates were prepared from the SL at 4 h post-noise exposure. Values are the mean ± S.E. from 4 separate animals per each group.
**$P<0.01$, significantly different from control value obtained for naïve animals.
#$P<0.05$,
##$P<0.01$, significantly different from the value obtained for noise-exposed animals without drug treatment.

to the permanent hearing loss induced by acoustic overstimulation. In addition to the findings from the *in vivo* model, those from the *in vitro* system using SLFs in primary culture demonstrated at the first time that one of the main mediators of oxidative stress, 4-HNE, had the ability to cause dysfunction of GJ-IC and attenuation of Na$^+$, K$^+$-ATPase activity effected by down-regulation of the Na$^+$, K$^+$-ATPase α1 level. Based on our previous findings that 4-HNE is produced in the lateral wall structures prior to hearing loss induced by intense noise [16], it is possible that 4-HNE produced by noise expose contributed to hearing loss through disruption of the ion-trafficking system in the lateral wall structures of the cochlea. However, other oxidants may be involved in noise-induced disruption of the ion-trafficking system in the lateral wall structures of the cochlea. Further studies may elucidate any oxidants involved in these events induced by acoustic overstimulation.

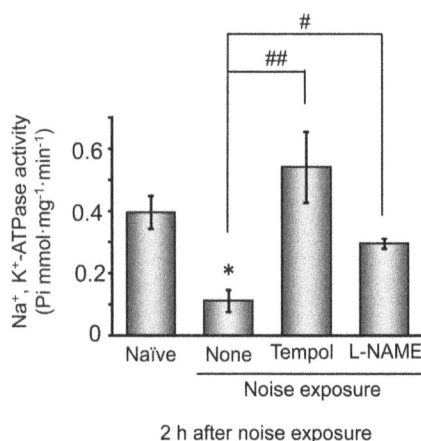

Figure 8. Effect of tempol and L-NAME on Na$^+$, K$^+$-ATPase activity in the SL. Mice were exposed to noise at 110 dB SPL for 1 h. At 30 min before the onset of noise exposure, the animals were given tempol (30 mg/kg, i.p.) or L-NAME (1 mg/kg, i.p.). Tissue lysates were prepared from the SL for determination of Na$^+$, K$^+$-ATPase activity. Values are the mean ± S.E. from 3–10 separate animals per each group. *$P<0.05$, significantly different from control value obtained for naïve animals. #$P<0.05$, ##$P<0.01$, significantly different from the value obtained for noise-exposed animals without drug treatment.

Ion-trafficking system in the lateral wall structures and hearing ability

Endolymph contains 150 mM K$^+$, 2 mM Na$^+$, and 20 μM Ca^{2+} and maintains the EP at +80 mV, which is crucial for maintenance of hearing ability [23]. The EP enhances the sensitivity of hair cells by increasing the driving force for K$^+$ influx and Ca^{2+} permeation, which amplify the motility of hair bundles [24,25]. It is proposed that noise exposure-induced hearing loss is at least in part due to a reduction in the EP [12,26,27]. After K$^+$ enters into the hair cells in the organ of Corti by acoustic stimulation, K$^+$ must cycle back to the endolymph through the pathway comprising perilymph, supporting cells, and lateral wall structures [1,28,29]. In the lateral wall structures, the ion-trafficking system comprising Na$^+$, K$^+$-ATPase, ion transporters, and GJs contributes to the K$^+$ transport and is essential for generation of the EP. The current data showed that Na$^+$, K$^+$-ATPase and Cx26 reached high levels in the lateral wall structures at P14 (Figure 3a and 3b). Considering that the onset of hearing ability in rodents occurs at postnatal days 13–14 (P13–14), our current data support the proposition that Na$^+$, K$^+$-ATPase and GJs play an important role for establishing and maintaining the EP and hearing ability. Thus, our present proposition that the decreases in Cx contents and Na$^+$, K$^+$-ATPase activity in the lateral wall structures, indicating disruption of the ion-trafficking system, induced hearing loss through would be feasible.

Cxs and noise-induced hearing loss

Non-sensory cells in the cochlea are connected extensively by GJs that facilitate intercellular ionic and biochemical coupling. Several different Cx proteins have been reported to be expressed in the mammalian inner ear. These include Cx26, Cx30, Cx31, and Cx43 [6,30,31,32]. Cx26 and Cx30 are the prominent members co-assembled in most of the cochlear GJs [6]. In the lateral wall structures of mice at adult age (P35), co-expression of Cx26 and Cx30 was observed in the type 1 SLFs and basal cells of the SV (Figure 2c). However, the type 2 SLFs had Cx30 but little Cx26. Therefore, the type 1 and type 2 SLFs expressed hetero-GJs composed of Cx26/Cx30 and homo-GJs of Cx30, respectively. Mutations in the genes encoding Cx26 and Cx30 are also known to cause a substantial portion of the cases of human non-syndromic hereditary deafness, which is one of the most common human birth defects [33]. The current data indicated that

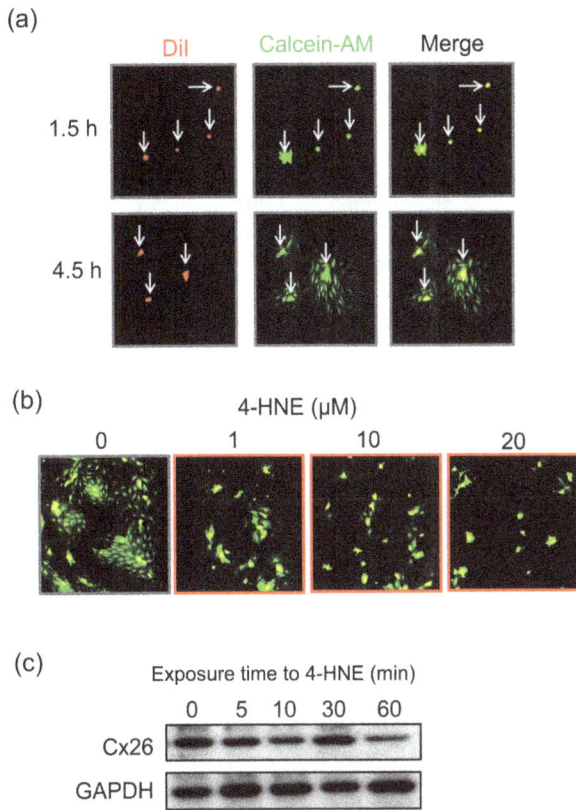

Figure 9. Effect of 4-HNE on GJ-IC and Cx26 level in SLF cultures. Cultures of the SLFs prepared from the cochlea of naïve animals were subjected to fluorescent dye-transfer assay for determination of GJ-IC. The SLFs were labeled with both DiI (*red*) and calcein-AM (*green*) as donor cells. The donor cells were then seeded onto unlabeled cells (acceptor cells), and the cultures were incubated for 1.5 or 4.5 h in the absence or presence of 4-HNE. (**a**) Time-dependent intercellular trafficking of calcein AM in the SLFs without treatment with 4-HNE. White arrows denote the donor cells. (**b**) The cells were incubated for 4.5 h in the presence of either vehicle or 4-HNE at the different concentrations indicated. (**c**) The level of Cx26 in the SLFs was determined by immunoblot analysis at the various time points indicated after the addition of 4-HNE at 10 μM. These experiments were carried out at least 4 times under the same experimental conditions, with similar results.

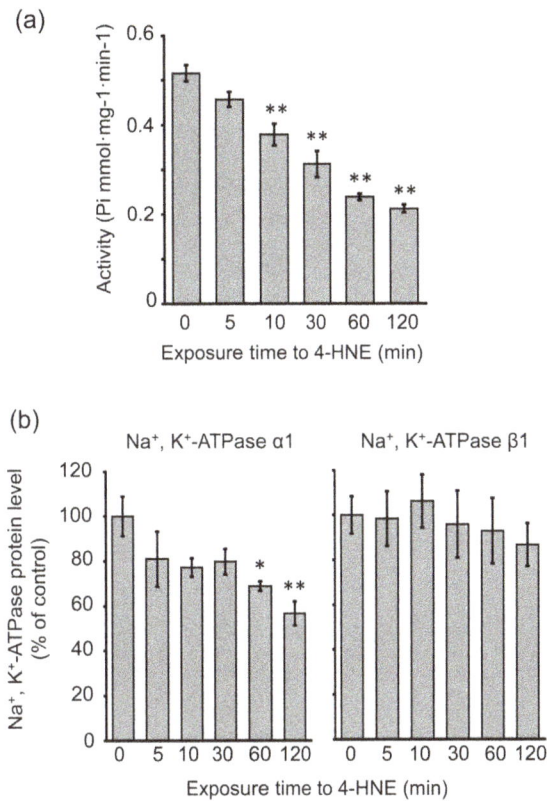

Figure 10. Effect of 4-HNE on Na$^+$, K$^+$-ATPase in SLF cultures. Cultures of the SLFs prepared from the cochlea of naïve animals were incubated for the indicated times in the presence of 4-HNE at 0.1 μM and then examined for Na$^+$, K$^+$-ATPase activity (**a**) and the protein level of Na$^+$, K$^+$-ATPase α1 and β1 subunits (**b**). Values are the mean ± S.E. from 4 independent experiments. *$P<0.05$, significantly different from control value obtained for untreated cells.

exposure to noise produced an immediate and prolonged decrease in the level of Cx26 in the type 1 SLFs and basal cell of the SV. In addition, the results of the RT-PCR analysis allows us to propose that such exposure decreased the gene expression of Cx26, but not that of Cx43 or Cx30, at least immediately post exposure. The noise-induced decrease in Cx26 was prevented by the free radical-scavenging agent and the nitric oxide synthase inhibitor, which use improved the noise-induced hearing loss. These findings suggest that the immediate and prolonged decrease in Cx26 was crucial for noise-induced hearing loss through dysfunction of GJ-IC in the lateral wall structures.

To elucidate the involvement of oxidative stress in GJ-IC in the SL, we used primary cultures of the SLFs derived from adult mice. Our previous data indicated that exposure to noise causes marked expression of 4-HNE-adduct proteins in the SL [16]. 4-HNE is known to form Michael adducts with focal adhesion kinase, β-catenin, paxillin, VE-cadherin, ZO-1, and the actin cytoskeleton in endothelial cells [34], indicating that these junction proteins and cytoskeleton are involved in 4-HNE-induced alterations of cell-cell

adhesion in endothelial cells. It is also known that 4-HNE directly binds to insulin receptor substrate-1/-2 proteins and degrades it in adipocytes [35]. In addition, our preliminary data using the cultures of the SLFs showed that 4-HNE was co-localized with Cx43, the level of which decreased after 4-HNE exposure (data not shown). In the present study, we demonstrated that 4-HNE has the ability to decrease Cx26 level and to disrupt the GJ-IC, but not to damage, in the SLFs. These results suggest that 4-HNE directly contributes to the disruption of the GJ-IC through the decrease in Cxs in the SLFs. Furthermore, these *in vitro* data allow us to propose the idea that exposure to noise *in vivo* disrupted the GJ-IC in cells of the lateral wall structures by causing a decrease in contents of Cxs induced at least in part by the formation of 4-HNE. However, the mechanism underlying this 4-HNE-induced decrease remains to be explored in the future.

Na$^+$, K$^+$-ATPase and noise-induced hearing loss

Multiple isoforms of 3 subunits, α, β, and γ, comprise the Na$^+$, K$^+$-ATPase oligomer. The α subunit contains the binding sites for ATP and the cations, whereas the glycosylated β subunit ensures correct folding and membrane insertion of the α subunits. The small γ subunit co-localizes with the α subunit in nephron segments, where it increases the affinity of Na$^+$, K$^+$-ATPase for ATP. The β subunit, but not the γ subunit, is essential for normal activity of Na$^+$, K$^+$-ATPase. The α subunit is subject to being phosphorylated at select serine residues. Na$^+$, K$^+$-ATPase also is well known to participate in the active ion transport in the inner ear and to play an important role in maintaining cochlear function [10–12]. In the present study, we demonstrated that exposure to noise *in vivo* decreased the activity of Na$^+$, K$^+$-ATPase in the SL. The current data that both the free radical-scavenging agent and nitric oxide synthase inhibitor abolished the noise-induced decrease in Na$^+$, K$^+$-ATPase activity allows us to propose that this noise-induced event was due to excess oxidative stress and/or nitric oxide generation. Indeed, the *in vitro* exposure of the SLF cultures to 4-HNE decreased the activity and α1 subunit protein level of Na$^+$, K$^+$-ATPase. Thus, it seems likely that this 4-HNE-induced decrease in Na$^+$, K$^+$-ATPase activity was due to the decrease in the α1 subunit level. However, we currently have no idea regarding the mechanism underlying the 4-HNE-induced decrease in the α1 subunit level, although 4-HNE is known to bind to Na$^+$, K$^+$-ATPase in striatal synaptosomes [36]

Conclusions

In the present study, we demonstrated at first time that noise-induced hearing loss was at least in part due to the disruption of the ion-trafficking system, involving a decrease in the levels of Cxs and in Na$^+$, K$^+$-ATPase activity in the lateral wall structures. Formation of 4-HNE by excessive oxidative stress was considered to be operative in the disruption of GJ-IC in the SL. However, it would be required for future studies to validate the hypothesis that 4-HNE is involve in noise-induced hearing loss. In addition, further evaluation of the mechanism underlying the disruption of GJ-IC should contribute to the development of therapeutics for noise-induced hearing loss.

Author Contributions

Conceived and designed the experiments: TY RN KO. Performed the experiments: TY RN. Analyzed the data: TY RN KO. Contributed reagents/materials/analysis tools: MY TS. Wrote the paper: TY RN KO.

References

1. Wangemann P (2002) K$^+$ cycling and the endocochlear potential. Hear Res 165: 1–9.
2. Weber PC, Cunningham CD 3rd, Schulte BA (2001) Potassium recycling pathways in the human cochlea. Laryngoscope 111: 1156–1165.
3. Delprat B, Ruel J, Guitton MJ, Hamard G, Lenoir M, et al. (2005) Deafness and cochlear fibrocyte alterations in mice deficient for the inner ear protein otospiralin. Mol Cell Biol 25: 847–853.
4. Konishi T, Salt AN, Hamrick PE (1979) Effects of exposure to noise on ion movement in guinea pig cochlea. Hear Res 1: 325–342.
5. Melichar I, Syka J, Ulehlová L (1980) Recovery of the endocochlear potential and the K$^+$ concentrations in the cochlear fluids after acoustic trauma. Hear Res 2: 55–63.
6. Forge A, Becker D, Casalotti S, Edwards J, Marziano N, et al. (2003) Gap junctions in the inner ear: comparison of distribution patterns in different vertebrates and assessment of connexin composition in mammals. J Comp Neurol 467: 207–731.
7. Ahmad S, Chen S, Sun J, Lin X (2003) Connexins 26 and 30 are co-assembled to form gap junctions in the cochlea of mice. Biochem Biophys Res Commun 307: 362–368.
8. Hoang Dinh E, Ahmad S, Chang Q, Tang W, Stong B, et al. (2009) Diverse deafness mechanisms of connexin mutations revealed by studies using in vitro approaches and mouse models. Brain Res 1277: 52–69.
9. Lefebvre PP, Malgrange B, Lallemend F, Staecker H, Moonen G, et al. (2002) Mechanisms of cell death in the injured auditory system: otoprotective strategies. Audiol Neurootol 7: 165–170.
10. Kerr TP, Ross MD, Ernst SA (1982) Cellular localization of Na$^+$, K$^+$-ATPase in the mammalian cochlear duct: significance for cochlear fluid balance. Am J Otolaryngol 3: 332–338.
11. Schulte BA, Adams JC (1989) Distribution of immunoreactive Na$^+$, K$^+$-ATPase in gerbil cochlea. J Histochem Cytochem 37: 127–134.
12. Wangemann P (1995) Comparison of ion transport mechanisms between vestibular dark cells and strial marginal cells. Hear Res 90: 149–157.
13. Hsu CJ (1992) Changes in activity of cytochrome oxidase in the cochleae of guinea pigs with experimental endolymphatic hydrops. J Formos Med Assoc 91: 258–262.
14. Gratton MA, Smyth BJ, Schulte BA, Vincent DA Jr (1995) Na,K-ATPase activity decreases in the cochlear lateral wall of quiet-aged gerbils. Hear Res 83: 43–50.
15. Li W, Zhao L, Jiang S, Gu R (1997) Effects of high intensity impulse noise on ionic concentrations in cochlear endolymph of the guinea pig. Chin Med J (Engl) 110: 883–886.
16. Nagashima R, Yamaguchi T, Tanaka H, Ogita K (2010) Mechanism underlying the protective effect of tempol and N$^\omega$-nitro-L-arginine methyl ester on acoustic injury: possible involvement of c-Jun N-terminal kinase pathway and connexin26 in the cochlear spiral ligament. J Pharmacol Sci 114: 50–62.
17. Nagashima R, Sugiyama C, Yoneyama M, Kuramoto N, Kawada K, et al. (2007) Acoustic overstimulation facilitates the expression of glutamate-cysteine ligase catalytic subunit probably through enhanced DNA binding of activator protein-1 and/or NF-kB in the murine cochlea. Neurochem Int. 51: 209–215.
18. Nagashima R, Ogita K (2006) Enhanced biosynthesis of glutathione in the spiral ganglion of the cochlea after in vivo treatment with dexamethasone in mice. Brain Res 1117: 101–108.
19. Goldberg GS, Bechberger JF, Naus CC (1995) A pre-loading method of gap junctional communication by fluorescent dye transfer. Biotechniques 18: 490–497.
20. Mutai H, Nagashima R, Fujii M, Matsunaga T (2009) Mitotic activity and specification of fibrocyte subtypes in the developing rat cochlear lateral wall. Neuroscience 163: 255–1263.
21. Suko T, Ichimiya I, Yoshida K, Suzuki M, Mogi G (2000) Classification and culture of spiral ligament fibrocytes from mice. Hearing Res 140: 137–144.
22. Mercer RW, Biemesderfer D, Bliss DP Jr, Collins JH, Forbush B 3rd (1993) Molecular cloning and immunological characterization of the gamma polypeptide, a small protein associated with the Na,K-ATPase. J Cell Biol 121: 579–586.
23. Von Bekesy G (1952) Resting potentials inside the cochlear partition. Nature 169: 241–242.
24. Vassout P (1984) Effects of pure tone on endocochlear potential and potassium ion concentration in the guinea pig cochlea. Acta Otolaryngol 98: 199–203.
25. Ide M, Morimitsu T (1990) Long term effects of intense sound on endocochlear DC potential. Auris Nasus Larynx 17: 1–10.
26. Hibino H, Kurachi Y (2006) Molecular and physiological bases of K$^+$ circulation in the mammalian inner ear. Physiology 21: 336–345.
27. Chan DK, Hudspeth AJ (2005) Ca^{2+} current-driven nonlinear amplification by the mammalian cochlea in vitro. Nat Neurosci 8: 149–155.
28. Kikuchi T, Adams JC, Miyabe Y, So E, Kobayashi T (2000) Potassium ion recycling pathway via gap junction systems in the mammalian cochlea and its interruption in hereditary nonsyndromic deafness. Med Electron Microsc 33: 51–56.
29. Spicer SS, Schulte BA (1998) Evidence for a medial K$^+$ recycling pathway from inner hair cells. Hear Res 118: 1–12.
30. Kikuchi T, Kimura RS, Paul DL, Adams JC (1995) Gap junctions in the rat cochlea: immunohistochemical and ultrastructural analysis. Anat Embryol 191: 101–118.
31. Lautermann J, ten Cate WJ, Altenhoff P, Grümmer R, Traub O, et al. (1998) Expression of the gap-junction connexins 26 and 30 in the rat cochlea. Cell Tissue Res 294: 415–420.
32. Zhao HB (2005) Connexin26 is responsible for anionic molecule permeability in the cochlea for intercellular signalling and metabolic communications. Eur J Neurosci 21: 1859–1868.
33. Rabionet R, Gasparini P, Estivill X (2000) Molecular genetics of hearing impairment due to mutations in gap junction genes encoding beta connexins. Hum Mutat 16: 190–202.
34. Usatyuk PV, Parinandi NL, Natarajan V (2006) Redox regulation of 4-hydroxy-2-nonenal-mediated endothelial barrier dysfunction by focal adhesion, adherens, and tight junction proteins. J Biol Chem 281: 35554–35566.
35. Demazay D, Mas JC, Rocchi S, Van Obberghen E (2008) FALDH reverses the deleterious action of oxidative stress induced by lipid peroxidation product 4-hydroxynonenal on insulin signaling in 3T3L1 adipocytes. Diabetes 57: 1216–1226.
36. Fleuranceau-Morel P, Barrier L, Fauconneau B, Piriou A, Huguet F (1999) Origin of 4-hydroxynonenal incubation-induced inhibition of dopamine transporter and Na+/K+ adenosine triphosphate in rat striatal synaptosomes. Neurosci Lett 277: 91–94.

4

Gene Expression Changes for Antioxidants Pathways in the Mouse Cochlea: Relations to Age-related Hearing Deficits

Sherif F. Tadros[1,2¤a], **Mary D'Souza**[1,2¤b], **Xiaoxia Zhu**[1,2,3], **Robert D. Frisina**[1,2,3]*

1 International Center for Hearing & Speech Research, National Technical Institute for the Deaf, Rochester Institute of Technology, Rochester, New York, United States of America, **2** Otolaryngology Dept., University of Rochester Medical School, Rochester, New York, United States of America, **3** Depts. Chemical & Biomedical Engineering, Communication Sciences & Disorders, and Global Center for Hearing & Speech Research, University of South Florida, Tampa, Florida, United States of America

Abstract

Age-related hearing loss – presbycusis – is the number one neurodegenerative disorder and top communication deficit of our aged population. Like many aging disorders of the nervous system, damage from free radicals linked to production of reactive oxygen and/or nitrogen species (ROS and RNS, respectively) may play key roles in disease progression. The efficacy of the antioxidant systems, e.g., glutathione and thioredoxin, is an important factor in pathophysiology of the aging nervous system. In this investigation, relations between the expression of antioxidant-related genes in the auditory portion of the inner ear – cochlea, and age-related hearing loss was explored for CBA/CaJ mice. Forty mice were classified into four groups according to age and degree of hearing loss. Cochlear mRNA samples were collected and cDNA generated. Using Affymetrix® GeneChip, the expressions of 56 antioxidant-related gene probes were analyzed to estimate the differences in gene expression between the four subject groups. The expression of Glutathione peroxidase 6, Gpx6; Thioredoxin reductase 1, Txnrd1; Isocitrate dehydrogenase 1, Idh1; and Heat shock protein 1, Hspb1; were significantly different, or showed large fold-change differences between subject groups. The Gpx6, Txnrd1 and Hspb1 gene expression changes were validated using qPCR. The Gpx6 gene was upregulated while the Txnrd1 gene was downregulated with age/hearing loss. The Hspb1 gene was found to be downregulated in middle-aged animals as well as those with mild presbycusis, whereas it was upregulated in those with severe presbycusis. These results facilitate development of future interventions to predict, prevent or slow down the progression of presbycusis.

Editor: Luis Eduardo Soares Netto, Instituto de Biociencias - Universidade de São Paulo, Brazil

Funding: Research was supported by National Institutes of Health Grants P01 AG009524 from the National Institute on Aging, P30 DC005409 from the National Institute on Deafness & Communication Disorders, USA. The funders had no role in study design, data collection and analysis, decision to publish, or preparation of the manuscript.

Competing Interests: The authors have declared that no competing interests exist.

* E-mail: Rfrisina@usf.edu

¤a Current address: Macquarie University, Little Bay, NSW, Australia
¤b Current address: Rochester, New York, United States of America

Introduction

Oxidative stress has a definite role in cell aging. The multifactorial approach of explaining the processes of aging in the ear and brain results in different theories. Some of these theories explain aging as an evolutionary effect (e.g. mutation accumulation theory, particularly for the mitochondrial genome), others explain it as a molecular effect (e.g., gene regulation theory), a cellular effect (e.g., telomere length theory), or a systemic effect (e.g., neuroendocrine and immunological theories).

One of the main cellular theories of aging is the free radical theory. According to this, aging is the result of accumulative effects of oxidative insults throughout the life span [1] caused by reactive oxygen and/or nitrogen species (ROS and RNS, respectively) [2–5]. The main source of ROS in the cell is the mitochondrial leakage of electrons, followed by production of superoxides, and hydrogen peroxide (H_2O_2) [6–7]. The lack of ability to scavenge all of these oxidants from the cell leads to DNA, lipids and protein damage [8–11]. Lipid damage, in turn, can lead to calcium (Ca++)

influx and pathological changes in the cells [12–13]. DNA damage can be more permanent, cumulative and have more devastating consequences than lipid or protein damage. The fact that mitochondria continue to replicate, and that the mitochondrial genome almost entirely codes for proteins, makes mitochondrial DNA (mtDNA) oxidative damage very important and potentially dangerous to cellular health, even relative to nuclear DNA damage [1,14–15].

Thiol-reducing systems, glutathione (GSH) and thioredoxin (Trx) are two major cellular antioxidant systems that play an important role in maintaining the proper intracellular redox concentration. Other redox compounds, such as nicotinamide adenine dinucleotides (NADPH, NADH), ascorbic acid (Vitamin C), tocopherols (Vitamin E), lipoic acid, and ubiquinone (Q10), in addition to antioxidant enzymes like dimutate superoxide (SOD-1 and SOD-2), catalases and peroxidases also play roles in cell protection [16]. The balance between these systems and ROS/RNS production is vital for cell survival. Decreases in levels of antioxidants along with overwhelming exposure to oxidative stress can accelerate the process of cellular age-related damage [17–19]. Due to its high intracellular concentration, *GSH* is thought to be largely responsible for antioxidant protective effects inside cells and organelles. In addition to its action as a major antioxidant defense, Trx may play an important role in the redox regulation of protein thiols involved in signal transduction, gene regulation and cell growth [16,20–21].

Age-related hearing loss is the number one neurodegenerative disorder and top communication deficit of our growing aged population; and along with arthritis and cardiovascular disease, one of the top three chronic medical conditions of the elderly. The CBA mouse strain has been one of the most useful in terms of understanding the behavioral, neural and molecular bases of age-related hearing loss at both sensory end-organ (inner ear: cochlear) and brain (central auditory system) levels [22–25]. In the present study, age- and function-related changes in antioxidant-related cochlear gene expression in different age groups of CBA mice were investigated. Utilizing gene microarrays, candidate genes that may participate in presbycusis – age-related hearing loss - at the cochlear level were identified.

Methods

The present investigation utilized methodologies similar to Tadros, Frisina and colleagues [26–28].

Animal Model

CBA/CaJ mice were bred in-house and housed according to institutional protocol, with original breeding pairs obtained from Jackson Laboratories. All animals had similar environmental and non-ototoxic history. The CBA mouse is a model organism for human presbycusis because it loses its hearing progressively over its lifespan. The young adult group was used as the baseline group for gene expression data analyses (e.g., calculation of fold changes). Functional hearing measurements were obtained prior to sacrifice similar to our previous investigations of the biological bases of presbycusis [29–31]. Before data acquisition, individual mice were microscopically examined for evidence of external ear canal and middle ear obstruction. Mice with clearly visualized, healthy tympanic membranes were included. This study was carried out in strict accordance with the recommendations in the Guide for the Care and Use of Laboratory Animals of the National Institutes of Health, and all procedures were fully approved by the University of Rochester Vivarium Committee on Animal Resources.

Functional Hearing Assessment
Distortion Product Otoacoustic Emissions (DPOAEs). Ipsilateral acoustic stimulation and simultaneous measurement of DPOAEs were accomplished with the Tucker Davis Tech. (TDT) BioSig III system. Stimuli were digitally synthesized at 200 kHz

using SigGen software applications with the ratio of frequency 2 (F2) to frequency 1 (F1) constant at 1.25; L1 was equal to 65 dB sound pressure level (SPL) and L2 was equal to 50 dB SPL as calibrated in a 0.1-mL coupler simulating the mouse ear canal. After synthesis, F1, F2, were each passed through an RP2.1 D/A converter to PA5 programmable attenuators. Following attenuation, the signals went to ED1 speaker drivers which fed into the EC1 electrostatic loudspeakers coupled to the ear canal through short, flexible tubes with rigid plastic tapering tips. For DPOAE measurements, resultant ear canal sound pressure was recorded with an ER10B+ low-noise microphone and probe (Etymotic) housed in the same coupler as the F1 and F2 speakers. The output of the ER10B+ amplifier was put into an MA3 microphone amplifier, whose output went to an RP2.1 A/D converter for sampling at 200 kHz. A fast Fourier transform (FFT) was performed with TDT BioSig software on the resultant waveform. The magnitude of F1, F2, the 2f1-f2 distortion product, and the noise floor of the frequency bins surrounding the 2f1-f2 components were measured from the FFT. The procedure was repeated for geometric mean frequencies ranging from 5.6 to 44.8 kHz (eight frequencies per octave) to adequately assess the neuroethologically functional range of mouse hearing.

Mice were anesthetized with a mixture of ketamine and xylazine (120 and 10 mg/kg body weight, respectively) by intraperitoneal injection before all experimental sessions. All recording sessions were completed in a soundproof acoustic chamber (lined with Sonex) with body temperature maintained with a heating pad. Before recording, the operating microscope (Zeiss) was used to place the stimulus probe and microphone in the test ear, and the coupler for the speaker for the contralateral noise source was placed into the opposite ear canal. Both couplers were placed close to the tympanic membrane. The recording session duration was limited by depth of anesthesia, and lasted approximately 1 hour per animal.

Auditory Brainstem Responses (ABRs). During this procedure, 5.0 mg/10.0 gm body weight general anesthetic, Avertin (Tribromoethanol, delivered IP), was used to anaesthetize the mice. Normal body temperature was maintained at 38°C with a Servo heating pad. Auditory brainstem responses were measured in response to tone pips of 3, 6, 12, 24, 32, and 48 kHz presented at a rate of 11 bursts/sec. Auditory brainstem responses were recorded with subcutaneous platinum needle electrodes placed at the vertex (noninverting input), right-side mastoid prominence (inverted input), and tail (indifferent site). Electroencephalographic (EEG) activity was differentially amplified (50 or 100 X) (Grass Model P511 EEG amplifier), then put into an analogue-to-digital converter (AD1, TDT) and digitized at 50 kHz. Each averaged response was based on 300–500 stimulus repetitions recorded over 10-millisec epochs. Contamination by muscle and cardiac activities was prevented by rejecting data epochs in which the

Table 1. ANOVA results of genechip signal log ratios between groups and average fold changes of validated genes.

Gene ID	Gene Name	ANOVA (Sig. Log. Ratio)	GeneChip Average Fold Change		
			Middle Age	Old Mild	Old Severe
1425964_x_at	Hspb1	P = 0.0598, F = 3.11, df = 2,29	−0.7729	−1.245	0.5188
1452135_at	Gpx6	P = 0.0681, F = 2.95, df = 2,29	0.9848	1.550	1.310
1421529_a_at	Txnrd1	P = *0.0219, F = 4.37, df = 2,29	−0.1404	−1.138	−1.485
1419821_s_at	Idh1 (NADP+)	P = *0.0131, F = 5.05, df = 2,29	−0.2129	−1.032	−1.612

* denotes statistical significance at 0.05 level.

single-trace electroencephalogram contained peak-to-peak amplitudes exceeding 50 μV. The ABR was recorded in a small sound-attenuating chamber.

Sample Isolation

Upon completion of the physiological recording sessions, the mice were sacrificed by cervical dislocation. The brains were immediately dissected using a Zeiss stereomicroscope and placed in ice-cold saline. The soft tissues of forty CBA mice cochleae were dissected. The two cochleae of each mouse were pooled together to form one sample per mouse. All samples were placed in cold Trizol (Invitrogen, CA) and stored at −80°C for gene microarray and real time PCR processing.

Microarray gene expression processing

Gene Chip. One Affymetrix M430A high-density oligonucleotide array set (A) (Affymetrix Inc., Santa Clara, CA) was used for each cochlea sample. Each array contains 22,600 probe sets analyzing the expression of over 14,000 mouse genes. Eleven pairs of 25-mer oligonucleotides that span the coding region of the genes represent each gene. Each probe pair consists of a perfect match sequence that is complementary to the mRNA target and a mismatch sequence that has a single base pair mutation in a region critical for target hybridization; this sequence serves as a control for non-specific hybridization. Sequences used in the design of the array were selected from GenBank, dbEST, and RefSeq.

Sample Preparation

RNA Extraction. These procedures are described in detail in our previous microarray articles [26–28].

cDNA Synthesis. For gene array analysis, cDNA synthesis was performed with 20 μg of total RNA using the Superscript Choice cDNA Synthesis Kit (Invitrogen). For qPCR, nuGen cDNA reagents kit was used to generate a high fidelity cDNA, which was modified at the 3′ end to contain an initiation site for T7 RNA polymerase. Detailed protocol is found in www.nugeninc.com.

***In-vitro* Transcription (IVT) and Fragmentation.** Clean up of double-stranded cDNA was done according to the Affymetrix GeneChip Expression analysis protocol. Synthesis of Biotin-labeled cRNA was performed by adding 1 μg of cDNA to 10X IVT labeling buffer, IVT labeling NTP mix, IVT labeling enzyme mix and RNase-free water, then incubated at 37°C for 16 hours. The Biotin-labeled cRNA was cleaned up according to the Affymetrix GeneChip expression analysis protocol and a 20 μg of full-length cRNA from each sample was fragmented by adding 5X fragmentation buffer and RNase-free water, followed by incubation at 94°C for 35 min. The standard fragmentation procedure produces a distribution of RNA fragment sizes from approximately 35 to 200 bases. After the fragmentation, cDNA, full-length cRNA and fragmented cRNA were analyzed by electrophoresis using the Agilent Bioanalyzer 2100 to assess the appropriate size distribution prior to microarray hybridization.

Target Hybridization, Washing, Staining and Scanning. GeneChip M430A probe arrays (Affymetrix) were hybridized, washed and stained according to the manufacturer's instructions in a fluidics station. The arrays were scanned using a Hewlett Packard confocal laser scanner and visualized using GeneChip 5.1 software. Three data files were created, namely image data (.dat), cell intensity data (.cel) and expression probe analysis data (.chp) files. Detailed protocols for sample preparation and target labeling assays for expression analysis can be found at http://www.Affymetrix.com.

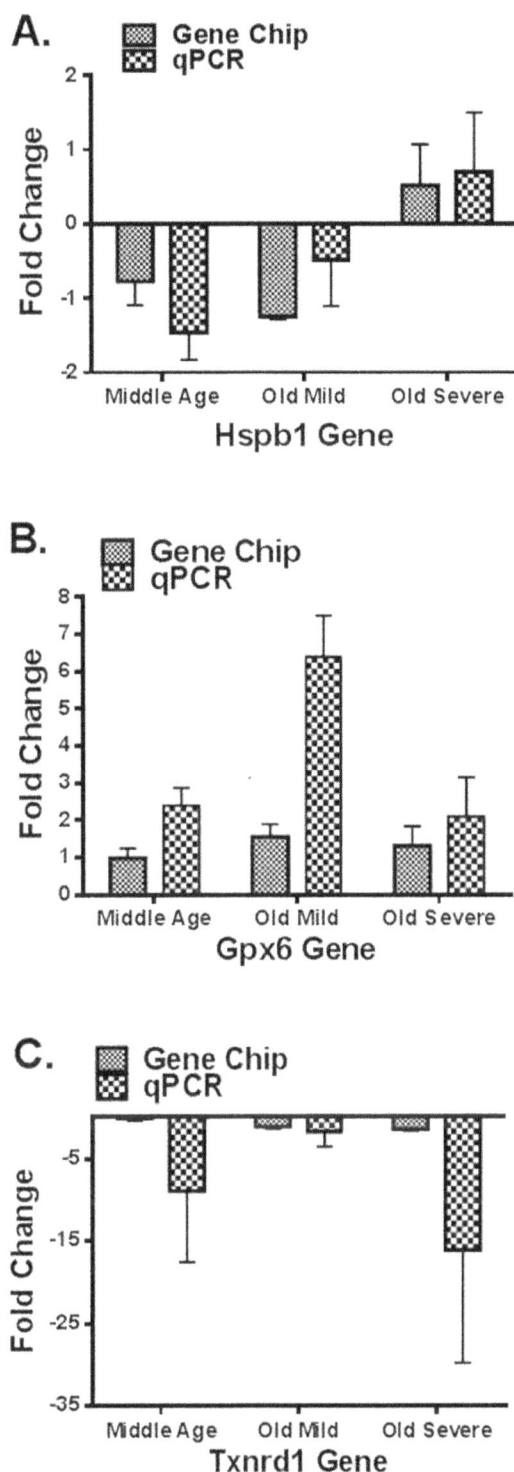

Figure 1. A): **For both GeneChip and real-time PCR, fold changes of *Hspb1* gene expression in the cochleae of middle age, old mild hearing loss, and old severe hearing loss groups showed upregulation with age and hearing loss.** B): For both GeneChip and real-time PCR, fold changes of *Gpx6* gene expression in cochlea samples showed upregulation in all age groups compared to the young group. C): For both GeneChip and real-time PCR, fold changes of *Txnrd1* gene expression in the cochleae of middle age, old mild hearing loss, and old severe hearing loss groups showed downregulation with age and hearing loss.

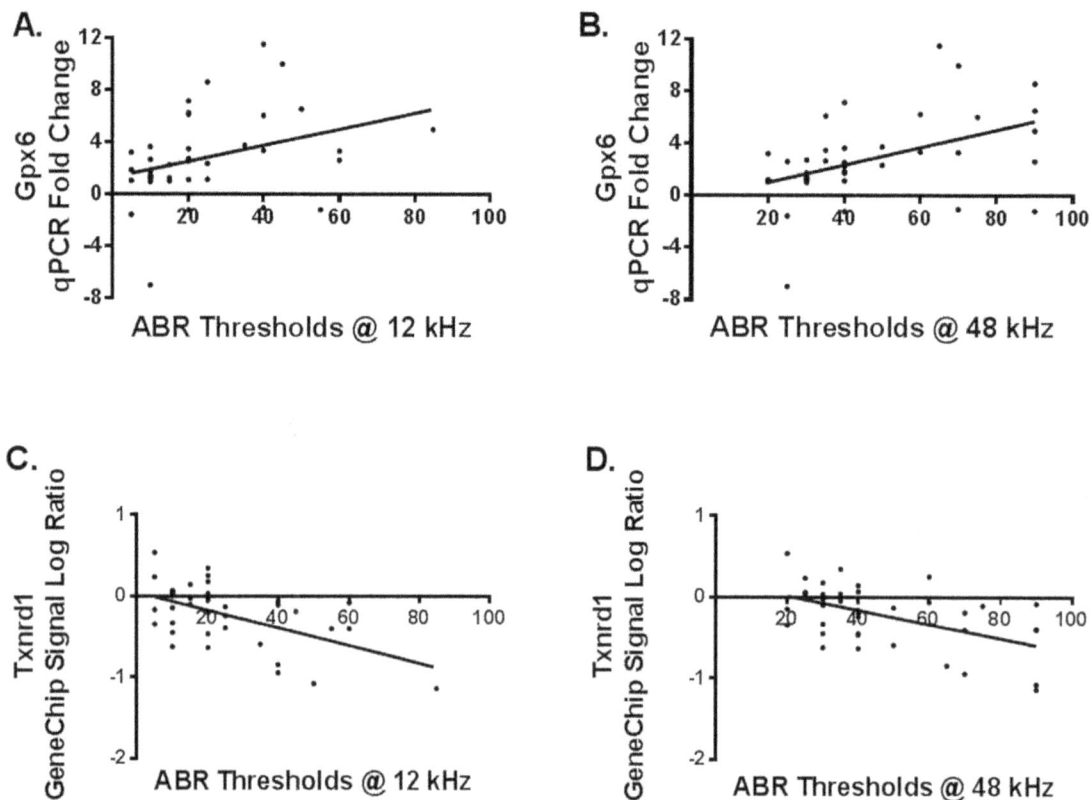

Figure 2. ABR thresholds correlation with gene expression A) and B): The correlations between *Gxp6* **qPCR fold changes and ABR thresholds at 12 kHz and 48 kHz are two examples of the significant correlations of gene expression changes with ABR test results.** C) and D): The correlations between *Txnrd1* signal log ratio and ABR thresholds at 12 kHz and 48 kHz were significant.

GeneChip Data Access

The entire microarray probe-set from each GeneChip 430A and individual CBA mouse phenotypic (hearing measures) data have been submitted to the GEO-NCBI database, and have been approved with the following Series reference #: GSE GSE49543. These GeneChip data can be accessed via, http://www.ncbi.nlm.nih.gov/geo/query/acc.cgi?acc = GSE49543. The probe-sets used in the current article were derived from the above GEO-NCBI accession number GSE49543. All steps were conducted according to the MIAME (Minimum Information About a Microarray Experiment) checklist [61].

Real-time PCR (qPCR)

The primer/probe used in quantification of gene expression was acquired from TaqMan® Gene Expression Assays-on-Demand products (AOD) from Applied Biosystems, Inc. (Foster City, CA, USA).

Detailed information about the PCR protocols is found in www.appliedbiosystems.com, and in our previous microarray articles [26–28].

Statistical Analyses

GeneChip Expression Analysis. After assessing chip quality, the Affymetrix GeneChip Operating Software (GCOS) automatically generates the (.cel) image file from the (.dat) data file. The signal log ratio of each sample determined the difference in expression of the studied gene in that sample from the mean expression of that gene in all samples from the young adult mice. A signal log ratio of 1.0 indicates an increase of the transcript level by

2 fold and −1.0 indicates a decrease by 2 fold. A signal log ratio of zero indicates no change.

For the fifty-six antioxidant-related genechip probes, one-way Analysis of Variance (ANOVA) (95% confidence limit) was used to compare between the signal log ratio values of the different subject groups. In addition, fold changes of all samples were calculated from signal log ratios using the following equations:

$$Fold\ Change = 2^{signal\ log\ ratio} \text{if signal log ratio} \geq 0 \text{ or}$$

$$(-1)x2^{(-SignalLogRatio)} \text{if signal log ratio} < 0$$

Real Time PCR Analysis

The threshold cycle (C_T) values were measured to detect the threshold of each of four significant genes of interest and *GAPDH* gene in all samples [32–33]. Each sample was measured in triplicate and normalized to the reference *GAPDH* gene expression. The C_T value of each well was determined and the average of the three wells of each sample was calculated. For samples that showed no expression of the test gene, the value of minimum expression was used for statistical analysis.

Delta $C_T(\Delta C_T)$ for test gene of each sample was calculated using the equation:

$$\Delta C_T = C_T \text{ Test Gene}_T\ GAPDH$$

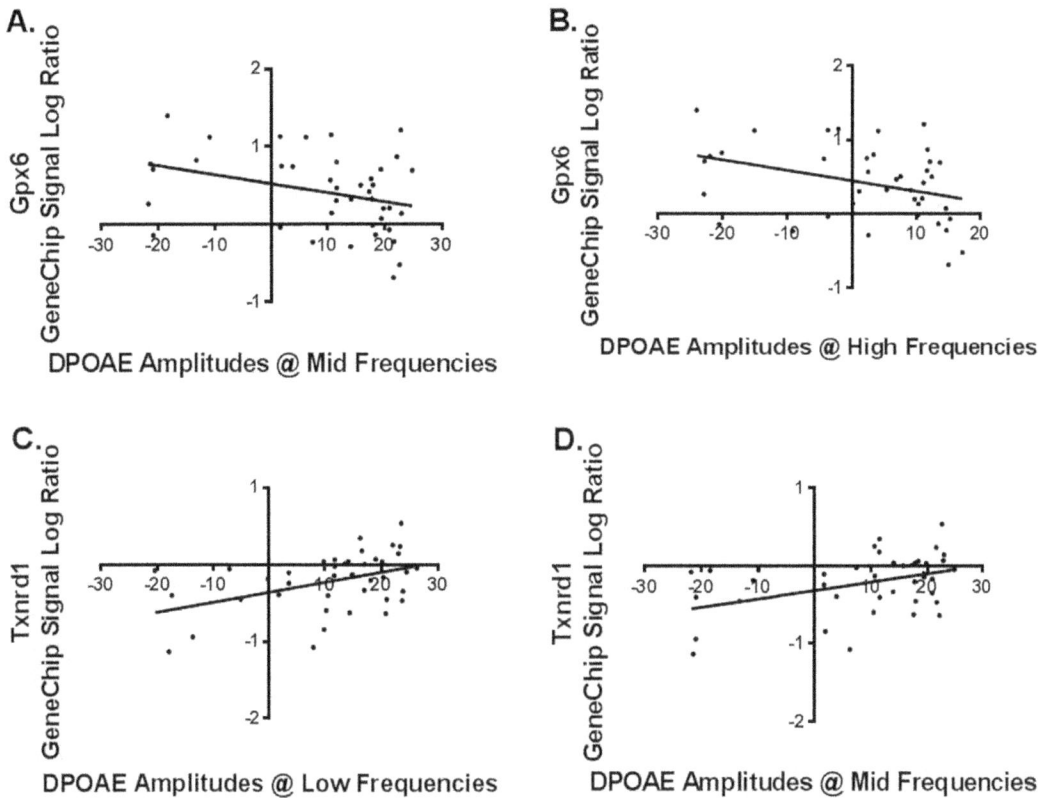

Figure 3. DPOAE amplitudes correlation with gene expression A) and B): The correlations between *Gxp6* signal log ratio and DPOAE amplitudes at mid and high frequencies, are two examples of the significant correlations of gene expression changes with DPOAE test results. C) and D): The correlations between *Txnrd1* signal log ratio and DPOAE amplitudes at low and mid frequencies were significant.

Delta delta $C_T(\Delta\Delta C_T)$ was calculated using the following equation:

$$\Delta\Delta C_T = \Delta C_T \text{ Sample Average } \Delta C_T \text{ young group}$$

The fold change in the test gene expression was finally calculated from the formula:

Fold change $2^{(-\Delta\Delta C_T)}$ if $\Delta\Delta C_T \leq 0$ or $(-1)\big/2^{(-\Delta\Delta C_T)}$ if $\Delta\Delta C > 0$

A statistical evaluation of real time PCR results was performed using one-way ANOVA to compare between ΔC_T for test gene expression in young age, middle age, old age mild presbycusis, and old age severe presbycusis groups.

For the three significantly different genes on genechip and/or qPCR, linear regression analyses were employed to find correlations between the signal log ratio values or fold change and the functional hearing measurements. These measurements were the distortion product otoacoustic emission (DPOAE) amplitudes at low frequencies (5.6 kHz to 14.5 kHz), mid frequencies (15.8 kHz to 29.0 kHz) and high frequencies (31.6 kHz to 44.8 kHz), in addition to auditory brainstem response thresholds (ABR) at 3, 6, 12, 24, 32 and 48 kHz. The GraphPad Prism 4 software was used to perform the one-way ANOVA and the linear regression statistics.

Results

Subject Groups: Age and Hearing Functionality

The sample set segregated into 4 groups based upon age, DPOAE levels and ABR thresholds: young adult control with good hearing (N = 8, 4 males, 4 females, age = 3.5+/−0.4 mon), middle-aged with good hearing (N = 17, 8 males, 9 females, age = 12.3+/−1.3 mon), old with mild presbycusis (N = 9, 4 males, 5 females, age = 27.7+/−3.4 mon) and old with severe presbycusis (N = 6, 2 males, 4 females, age = 30.6+/−1.9 mon). Detailed audiological data were presented in Tadros et al. [26–27].

Microarray gene expression

Fifty-six antioxidant-related gene probes were present on the microarray, and these were selected for further analysis. Statistical computations comparing the *signal log ratios* (Table 1) and *fold changes* of middle age, old mild hearing loss, and old severe hearing loss subject groups showed significant differences in expression or large fold-changes for four genes: *Gpx6*, *Txnrd1*, *Idh1*, and *Hspb1*. These gene expression changes were selected for validation by using real-time PCR (qPCR). In our selection of the genes to validate with real-time PCR, we relied on either a significant statistical difference of gene expression between groups (e.g., in the case of Txnrd1 and Idh1) or a large numerical difference in the microarray average fold change of the young adult group compared to the middle and old groups (e.g., in the case of Hspb1 and Gpx6). For Hspb1 and Gpx6, although the signal log ratio differences were not statistically significant, notice that there is a strong trend for gene expression group differences.

Table 2. Correlation between Gpx6 gene expression and audiological measurements.

	Sig. Log Ratio (GeneChip)	Fold Change (GeneChip)	Fold Change (qPCR)
ABR 3 kHz	$p = 0.187$, $r^2 = 0.045$, $F = 1.803$	$p = 0.239$, $r^2 = 0.0362$, $F = 1.426$	$p = 0.186$, $r^2 = 0.046$, $F = 1.815$
ABR 6 kHz	$p = 0.065$, $r^2 = 0.087$, $F = 3.618$	$p = 0.113$, $r^2 = 0.0648$, $F = 2.632$	$p = 0.075$, $r^2 = 0.081$, $F = 3.352$
ABR 12 kHz	$p =$ *$\mathbf{0.019}$, $r^2 = 0.137$, $F = 6.028$	$p =$ *$\mathbf{0.047}$, $r^2 = 0.100$, $F = 4.237$	$p =$ *$\mathbf{0.029}$, $r^2 = 0.119$, $F = 5.170$
ABR 24 kHz	$p =$ *$\mathbf{0.014}$, $r^2 = 0.149$, $F = 6.658$	$p = 0.051$, $r^2 = 0.0963$, $F = 4.050$	$p =$ *$\mathbf{0.048}$, $r^2 = 0.0989$, $F = 4.175$
ABR 32 kHz	$p =$ *$\mathbf{0.019}$, $r^2 = 0.136$, $F = 5.984$	$p = 0.052$, $r^2 = 0.0959$, $F = 4.031$	$p =$ *$\mathbf{0.022}$, $r^2 = 0.130$, $F = 5.699$
ABR 48 kHz	$p =$ **$\mathbf{0.002}$, $r^2 = 0.222$, $F = 10.84$	$p =$ *$\mathbf{0.011}$, $r^2 = 0.159$, $F = 7.186$	$p =$ **$\mathbf{0.004}$, $r^2 = 0.204$, $F = 9.721$
DPOAE Low Freq.	$p = 0.117$, $r^2 = 0.0634$, $F = 2.572$	$p = 0.269$, $r^2 = 0.0319$, $F = 1.255$	$p = 0.579$, $r^2 = 0.008$, $F = 0.312$
DPOAE Mid Freq.	$p =$ *$\mathbf{0.037}$, $r^2 = 0.109$, $F = 4.652$	$p = 0.159$, $r^2 = 0.0515$, $F = 2.064$	$p = 0.237$, $r^2 = 0.037$, $F = 1.44$
DPOAE High Freq.	$p =$ *$\mathbf{0.027}$, $r^2 = 0.123$, $F = 5.305$	$p = 0.119$, $r^2 = 0.0625$, $F = 2.535$	$p = 0.217$, $r^2 = 0.039$, $F = 1.576$

* denotes statistical significance at 0.05 level;
** at the 0.01 level.

Real-time PCR (qPCR)

Three genes out of the four validated microarray genes showed comparable results for both the genechip and the qPCR. These three genes were: *Hspb1* ($p =$ *0.0345, $F = 3.79$, $df = 2,29$) and *Gpx6* ($p =$ **0.0011, $F = 8.644$, $df = 2,29$) that showed significant up-regulation and *Txnrd1* ($p = 0.6575$, $F = 0.4254$, $df = 2,29$) that showed down-regulation with age and hearing loss. For *Idh1* gene, the qPCR results did not show consistency with the genechip data. Figures 1A–1C show quantitative comparisons between fold changes for the genechip microarray expression changes and those for the qPCR.

Correlation between gene expression and hearing measurements

Linear regression tests were used to analyze the correlations between hearing measurements (ABR thresholds and DPOAE amplitudes) and gene expression for both the genechip and qPCR expression levels. For *Gpx6* expression upregulation, genechip and q-PCR data showed significant correlations with both ABR thresholds and DPOAE amplitudes (Table 2) (Figs. 2A–B, 3A–B). For *Txnrd1* gene expression down-regulation, genechip signal log ratios and fold changes showed statistically significant correlations with ABR thresholds and DPOAE amplitudes (Table 3) (Fig. 2C–D, 3C–D). No significant correlations were found between *Hspb1* gene expressions as measured by qPCR and audiological tests. This may be, because the qPCR method is overall more sensitive than the genechip, for individual gene analyses. When the qPCR results are used to calculate fold changes, the results can have more variability than the genechip fold changes, sometimes reducing the statistical power of the correlations.

Discussion

Antioxidant Systems

The antioxidant systems, thiol-reducing Glutathione (GSH) and thioredoxin (Trx), are the main cellular defense mechanisms against free radicals. Catalyzed by the glutathione and thioredoxin peroxidases, GSH and Trx can scavenge free radicals and reduce peroxides producing glutathione disulfide (GSSG) and thioredoxin disulfide, respectively. This oxidized form of glutathione and thioredoxine can be converted back to the reduced form by glutathione and thioredoxine reductases in a reaction requiring NADPH. Since glutathione is the most abundant intracellular

redox, in addition to its major role as an antioxidant, the GSH/GSSG ratio is considered as an indicator of the cellular redox environment and has a major influence on cell proliferation and differentiation [20,34]. Thioredoxin system has an equally important role as an antioxidant and redox regulating system. In addition it plays a key role in DNA synthesis and activation of transcription factors that regulate cell growth [21]. In cases of oxidative stress, these two antioxidant systems act, both in parallel and interactive ways, to reduce ROS/RNS concentration and regulate redox cellular environment [17,35].

Glutathione peroxidase (Gpx) isoforms are a family of enzymes that slightly vary in properties [36]. The classic intracellular *Gpx1* is expressed in varies types of tissues and *Gpx3* is found intensively in plasma, kidney, adrenal gland, and weakly in heart, lung and cerebellum [37–38]. *Gpx6* has been identified based on its close homology with *Gpx3* [39] and expressed in embryos and adult olfactory epithelium. The expression of Gpx isoforms differs depending on tissue type.

Thioredoxin reductase (Txnrd) is a selenoprotein. It has three isoforms *Txnrd1* (cytosolic), *Txnrd2* (mitochondrial) and *Txnrd3* (TGR or thioredoxin and glutathione reductase) [40–45]. The inhibition of thioredoxine reductase enzyme may have a devastating effect on the cell due to the inhibition of the whole thioredoxin system [46]. In addition to its antioxidant effect, it has been reported that *Txnrd1* plays an important role in the control of basal p53 activity [47].

Heat shock proteins (Hsps) are a multi-functional family of proteins. Under stressful conditions, as infection, inflammation, exposure to toxins, elevated temperature or other stress conditions, Hsps have a cytoprotective function through working as a molecular chaperon to repair or remove denatured proteins and inhibit apoptosis [48–49].

Antioxidants and Cochlea

Different tissues in the cochlea may respond differently to the damaging ROS but the effects of oxidative stress and antioxidant systems on aging cochlea are well known [50–52]. Some reports showed a significant lower activity of glutathione-related antioxidant enzymes with noise exposure and drugs [53–55]. Mutation of the gene of *Gpx1* was reported to increase the vulnerability to noise-induced and age-related hearing loss in mice [56]. Ebselen, a Gpx mimic seleno-organic compound, was found to have a protective effect on cochlea against acoustic trauma, gentamicin and cisplatin [57–58]. Though the role of thioredoxin system in

Table 3. Correlation between *Txnrd1* gene expression and audiological measurements.

	Sig. Log Ratio (GeneChip)	Fold Change (GeneChip)	Fold Change (qPCR)
ABR 3 kHz	$p=0.083$, $r^2=0.0768$, $F=3.161$	$p=0.077$, $r^2=0.079$, $F=3.304$	$p=0.516$, $r^2=0.011$, $F=0.429$
ABR 6 kHz	$P=$ **0.004**, $r^2=0.195$, $F=9.189$	$p=$ **0.006**, $r^2=0.180$, $F=8.339$	$p=0.561$, $r^2=0.009$, $F=0.345$
ABR 12 kHz	$p=$ ***0.0003**, $r^2=0.293$, $F=15.75$	$p=$ ***0.0009**, $r^2=0.255$, $F=13.00$	$p=0.833$, $r^2=0.0012$, $F=0.045$
ABR 24 kHz	$p=$ **0.002**, $r^2=0.222$, $F=10.87$	$p=$ **0.006**, $r^2=0.181$, $F=8.395$	$p=0.849$, $r^2=0.0009$, 0.037
ABR 32 kHz	$p=$ **0.0066**, $r^2=0.179$, $F=8.272$	$p=$ **0.0079**, $r^2=0.172$, $F=7.875$	$p=0.746$, $r^2=0.0028$, $F=0.107$
ABR 48 kHz	$p=$ ***0.0006**, $r^2=0.269$, $F=13.96$	$p=$ **0.0012**, $r^2=0.245$, $F=12.36$	$p=0.909$, $r^2=0.0003$, $F=0.013$
DPOAE Low Freq.	$p=$ **0.005**, $r^2=0.188$, $F=8.822$	$p=$ **0.0065**, $r^2=0.179$, $F=8.283$	$p=0.355$, $r^2=0.0226$, $F=0.877$
DPOAE Mid Freq.	$p=$ **0.008**, $r^2=0.171$, $F=7.818$	$p=$ **0.004**, $r^2=0.195$, $F=9.213$	$p=0.478$, $r^2=0.013$, $F=0.515$
DPOAE High Freq.	$p=$ *0.034**, $r^2=0.113$, $F=4.823$	$p=$ **0.0075**, $r^2=0.174$, $F=7.981$	$p=0.598$, $r^2=0.007$, $F=0.282$

* denotes statistical significance at 0.05 level;
** at the 0.01 level;
*** at the 0.001 level.

the central nervous system has been established [16], its protective effect in the cochlea is still needed to be explored. It was reported that *Txnrd* activation in strial melanocytes by low level acoustic stimulation (LLAS) might be the cause of reduced susceptibility to temporary noise-induced threshold shift [59]. *Hsps* are divided into families according to their molecular weight. Heat shock protein b1 (*Hspb1*), also called Hsp27, has been found in the outer hair cells of rat cochlea and may provide a protection to these cells against auditory trauma or oxidative stress. In addition, the presence of high levels of Hsp27 in the cuticular plate and lateral wall of outer hair cells may help the regulation of the actin cytoskeleton against mechanical strain [60]. A limitation of the present study is that we cannot be sure about the importance of the up-regulation of Hspb1 expression in old age with severe hearing loss. It could be explained as an attempt to protect the cochlear hair cells from age-linked acoustic trauma and stress, which requires further investigation.

In the present investigation, *Txnrd1* was found to be downregulated while both *Gpx6* and *Hspb1* were upregulated in the CBA mouse cochlea with age and hearing loss. These findings may be explained as an exhaustion of the thioredoxin system with oxidative stress, and a compensatory mechanism by both the glutathione system and heat shock proteins in cochlear cells to scavenge the excess free radicals. *Hspb1* changes showed upregulation only in the old severe hearing loss group that may indicate its main relation with hearing loss. Though further studies may be needed to provide the functional and histological proof of the protective effect of antioxidants on age related hearing loss, the strong correlations between both *Txnrd1* or *Gpx6* expression on one hand and ABR thresholds and DPOAE amplitudes on the other hand, point to direct relations of the expression of these genes in the cochlea with age and hearing loss. The downregulation of *Txnrd1* expression may have a special therapeutic significance for future efforts at prevention and/or treatment of presbycusis through gene therapy techniques.

Recently, Tanaka et al. [62] studied the expression pattern of 84 oxidative stress and antioxidant defense-related genes in F344/NHsd male albino rats, dividing their subject groups *solely* according to age. In the present study, we used CBA/CaJ mice, both males and females, to study 56 oxidative stress-related genes and divided the animals into four groups according to two criteria, *both* their age and audiological test (ABR and DPOAEs) results.

This categorization helped us to more clearly differentiate between the effects of age and degree of hearing loss in the old age groups, on the oxidative stress gene expression. Tanaka and colleagues reported a statistically significant difference in expression between age groups in thirteen genes (one was down-regulated and twelve were up-regulated with age). Five genes were glutathione- and thioredoxin-related (Gpx6, Gpx3, Gstk1, Txnip, and Gsr). The expression of these genes was correlated to age but not to hearing loss. Note that Tanaka et al. grouped their data for multiple sound frequencies, whereas correlations were made with individual sound frequencies in the present study. Many of the genes that were correlated to both age and hearing loss have cytoprotective functions or have both survival and apoptotic function (Scd1, Cygb, Duo2, Aass, Slc38a5, Nqo1, Vim, and Dhcr24). In terms of similarities, Tanaka et al. reported changes in the Txnip gene, and we observed the down-regulation of a related gene: thioredoxin reductase 1 (Txnrd1). Note that Tanaka et al. did not find a correlation between the expression of Gpx6 and the degree of hearing loss, but both studies confirm the importance of this gene that is upregulated with age in both the mouse and rat cochlea, presumably to help preserve hearing in old age. The differences in findings for other genes may relate to the different species employed, the type of microarray utilized, or differences in the analysis of the microarray and qPCR results carried out in both studies. Lastly, notice also that the individual effects of age and of hearing loss in the expression patterns could not be clearly addressed in Tanaka et al.'s study, and this issue will be interesting to address in subsequent investigations.

Acknowledgments

We thank John Housel for collecting the ABR recordings, and Enza Daugherty and Shannon Salvog for project support. Supported by NIH Grants P01 AG009524 from the National Institute on Aging, and P30 DC005409 from the National Institute on Deafness & Communication Disorders, USA.

Author Contributions

Conceived and designed the experiments: SFT MD XZ RDF. Performed the experiments: SFT MD XZ. Analyzed the data: SFT MD XZ RDF. Contributed reagents/materials/analysis tools: SFT MD XZ. Wrote the paper: SFT MD XZ RDF.

References

1. Harman D (2003) The free radical theory of aging. Antiox Redox Signal 5:557–561.
2. Quiles JL, Ochoa JJ, Ramirez-Tortosa MC, Huertas JR, Mataix J (2006) Age-related mitochondrial DNA deletion in rat liver depends on dietary fat unsaturation. J Gerontol 61A(2): 107–114.
3. Lopez-Diazguerrero NE, Luna-Lopez A, Gutierrez-Ruiz MC, Zentella A, Konigsberg M (2005) Susceptibility of DNA to oxidative stressors in young and aging mice. Life Sci 77: 2840–2854.
4. Mariani E, Polidori MC, Cherubini A, Mecocci P (2005) Oxidative stress in brain aging, neurodegenerative and vascular diseases: An overview. J Chrom Biol 827:65–75.
5. Weinert BT, Timiras PS (2003) Theories Aging J Appl Physiol 95:1706–1716.
6. Linford NJ, Schriner SE, Rabinovitch PS (2006) Oxidative damage and aging: Spotlight on mitochondria. Cancer Res 66(5):2497–2499.
7. Lanaz G (1988) Role of mitochondria in oxidative stress and ageing. Biochem Biophys Acta. 1366: 63–67.
8. Dalle-Donne I, Rossi R, Colombo R, Giustarini D, Milzani A (2006) Biomarkers of oxidative damage in human disease. Clin Chem 52(4):601–623.
9. Joseph JA, Shukitt-Hale B, Casadesus G, Fisher D (2005) Oxidative stress and inflammation in brain aging: Nutritional considerations. Neurochem Res 30: 927–935.
10. Joseph JA, Denisova NA, Fisher D, Bickford P, Prior R, et al. (1998) Age-related neuro-degeneration and oxidative stress: Putative nutritional intervention. Neurol Clin 16:747–755.
11. Joseph JA, Denisova NA, Fisher D, Shukitt-Hale B, Bickford P, et al. (1998) Membrane and receptor modifications of oxidative stress vulnerability in aging: Nutritional considerations. Ann NY Acad Sci 854:268–276.
12. Ikeda K, Sunose H, Takasaka T (1993) Effects of free radicals on the intracellular calcium concentration in the isolated outer hair cell of the guinea pig cochlea. Acta Otolaryngol 13:137–141.
13. Clerici WJ, DiMartino DL, Prasad MR (1995) Direct effects of reactive oxygen species on cochlear outer hair cell shape in vitro. Hear Res 84:30–40.
14. Van Remmen H, Richardson A (2001) Oxidative damage to mitochondria and aging. Exp Gerontol 36:957–968.
15. Seidman MD (2000) Effects of dietary restriction and antioxidants on presbyacusis. Laryngoscope 110:727–738.
16. Patenaude A, Murthy MRV, Mirault ME (2005) Emerging roles of thioredoxin cycle enzymes in the central nervous system. Cell Mol Life Sci 62:1063–1080.
17. Yamawaki H, Berk BC (2005) Thioredoxin: a multifunctional antioxidant enzyme in kidney, heart and vessels. Curr Opin Nephrol Hypertens 14:149–153.
18. Lynch ED, Kil J (2005) Compounds for the prevention and treatment of noise-induced hearing loss. Drug Discovery Today 10(19):1291–1298.
19. Sohal RS, Weindruch R (1996) Oxidative stress, caloric restriction, and aging. Science 273:59–63.
20. Schafer FQ, Buettner GR (2001) Redox environment of the cell as viewed through the redox state of the glutathione disulfide/glutathione couple. Free Radical Biol Med 30:1191–1212.
21. Gan L, Yang XL, Lui Q, Xu HB (2005) Inhibitory effects of thioredoxin reductase antisense RNA on the growth of human hepatocellular carcinoma cells. J Cell Biochem 96:653–664.
22. Zhu X, Vasilyeva ON, Kim S-H, Jacobson M, Romney J, et al. (2007) Auditory efferent system declines precede age-related hearing loss: Contralateral suppression of otoacoustic emissions in mice. J Comp Neurol 503:593–604.
23. Frisina RD (2010) Aging Changes in the Central Auditory System. In: Adrian Rees, Alan Palmer Handbook of Auditory Science: The Auditory Brain. Oxford: Oxford Univ. Press, Ch. 17, pp 415–436.
24. Frisina RD, Newman SR, Zhu X (2007) Auditory efferent activation in CBA mice exceeds that of C57s for varying levels of noise. J Acoust Soc Am 121: EL-29–34.
25. Frisina RD, Singh A, Bak M, Bozorg S, Seth R, et al. (2011) F1 (CBA x C57) mice show superior hearing in old age relative to their parental strains: Hybrid vigor or a new animal model for "Golden Ears"? Neurobiol Aging 32:1716–1724.
26. Tadros SF, D'Souza M, Zettel ML, Zhu X, Lynch-Erhardt M, et al. (2007) Serotonin 2B receptor: Upregulated with age and hearing loss in mouse auditory system. Neurobiol Aging 28:1112–1123.
27. Tadros SF, D'Souza M, Zettel ML, Zhu X, Frisina RD (2007) Glutamate-related gene expression changes with age in the mouse auditory midbrain. Brain Res 1127:1–9.
28. Christensen N, D'Souza M, Zhu X, Frisina RD (2009) Age-related hearing loss: Aquaporin 4 gene expression changes in the mouse cochlea and auditory midbrain. Brain Res 1253:27–34.
29. Jacobson M, Kim S, Romney J, Zhu X, Frisina RD (2003) Contralateral suppression of distortion-product otoacoustic emissions declines with age: A comparison of findings in CBA mice with human listeners. Laryngoscope 113(10):1707–1713.
30. Guimaraes P, Zhu X, Cannon T, Kim S, Frisina RD (2004) Sex differences in distortion product otoacoustic emissions as a function of age in CBA mice. Hear Res 192(1–2):83–89.
31. Varghese GI, Zhu X, Frisina RD (2005) Age-related declines in distortion product otoacoustic emissions utilizing pure tone contralateral stimulation in CBA/CaJ mice. Hear Res 209:60–67.
32. Giulietti A, Overbergh L, Valckx D, Decallonne B, Bouillon R, et al. (2001) An overview of real-time quantitative PCR: Applications to quantify cytokine gene expression. Methods 25:386–401.
33. Baik SY, Jung KH, Choi MR, Yang BH, Kim SH, et al. (2005) Fluoxetine-induced up-regulation of 14-3-3zeta and tryptophan hydroxylase levels in RBL-2H3 cells. Neurosci Lett 374:53–57.
34. Maher P (2005) The effects of stress and aging on glutathione metabolism. Ageing Res Rev 4:288–314.
35. Casagrande S, Bonetto V, Fratelli M, Gianazza E, Eberini I, et al. (2002) Glutathionylation of human thioredoxin: a possible crosstalk between the glutathione and thioredoxin systems. Proc Natl Acad Sci USA 99:9745–9749.
36. Meseguer M, Garrido N, Simon C, Pellicer A, Remohi J (2004) Concentration of glutathione and expression of glutathione peroxidases 1 and 4 in fresh sperm provide a forecast of the outcome of cryopreservation of human spermatozoa. J Androl 25(5):773–780.
37. Drew JE, Farquharson AJ, Arthur JR, Morrice PC, Duthie GC (2005) Novel sites of cytosolic glutathione peroxidase expression in colon. FEBS Lett 579:6135–6139.
38. Fukuhara R, Kageyama T (2005) Structure, gene expression, and evolution of primate glutathione peroxidases. Comp Biochem Phys 141(4):428–436.
39. Kryukov GV, Castellano S, Novoselov SV, Lobanov AV, Zehtab O, et al. (2003) Characterization of mammalian selenoproteomes. Science 300:1439–1443.
40. Madeja Z, Sroka J, Nystrom C, Bjorkhem-Bergman L, Nordman T, et al. (2005) The role of thioredoxin reductase activity in selenium-induced cytotoxicity. Biochem Pharmacol 69:1765–1772.
41. Sun QA, Su D, Novoselov SV, Carlson BA, Hatfield DL, et al. (2005) Reaction mechanism and regulation of mammalian thioredoxin/glutathione reductase. Biochem 44:14528–14537.
42. Sun QA, Kirnarsky L, Sherman S, Gladyshev VN (2001) Selenoprotein oxidoreductase with specificity for thioredoxin and glutathione systems. Proc Nat Acad Sc USA 98:3673–3678.
43. Sun QA, Wu Y, Zappacosta F, Jeang KT, Lee BJ, et al. (1999) Redox regulation of cell signaling by selenocysteine in mammalian thioredoxin reductases. J Biol Chem 274:24522–24530.
44. Lee SR, Kim JR, Kwon KS, Yoon HW, Levine RL, et al. (1999) Molecular cloning and characterization of a mitochondrial selenocysteine-containing thioredoxin reductase from rat liver. J Biol Chem 274:4722–4734.
45. Miranda-Vizuete A, Damdimopoulos AE, Pedrajas JR, Gustafsson JA, Spyrou G (1999) Human mitochondrial thioredoxin reductase cDNA cloning, expression and genomic organization. Eur J Biochem 261:405–412.
46. Witte AB, Anestal K, Jerremalm E, Ehrsson H, Arner ESJ (2005) Inhibition of thioredoxin reductase but not of glutathione reductase by the major classes of alkylating and platinum-containing anticancer compounds. Free Radical Biol Med 39:696–703.
47. Seemann S, Hainaut P (2005) Roles of thioredoxin reductase 1 and APE/Ref-1 in the control of basal p53 stability and activity. Oncogene 24:3853–3863.
48. Mikuriya T, Sugahara K, Takemoto T, Tanaka K, Takeno K, et al. (2005) Geranylgeranylacetone, a heat shock protein inducer, prevents acoustic injury in the guinea pig. Brain Res 1065:107–114.
49. Bruey JM, Ducasse C, Bonniaud P, Ravagnan L, Susin SA, et al. (2000) Hsp 27 negatively regulates cell death by interacting with cytochrome C. Nat Cell Biol 2:645–652.
50. Staecker H, Zheng QY, Van De Water TR (2001) Oxidative stress in aging in the C57B16/J mouse cochlea. Acta Otolaryngol 121:666–672.
51. Rabinowitz PM, Wise JP, Mobo BH, Antonucci PG, Powell C, et al. (2002) Antioxidant status and hearing function in noise-exposed workers. Hear Res 173:164–171.
52. Kawamoto K, Sha SH, Minoda R, Izumikawa M, Kuriyama H, et al. (2003) Antioxidant gene therapy can protect hearing and hair cells from ototoxicity. Mol Ther 9(2):173–181.
53. Klemens JJ, Meech RP, Hughes LF, Somani S, Campbell KC (2003) Antioxidant enzyme levels inversely covary with hearing loss after amikacin treatment. J Am Acad Audiol 14(3):134–143.
54. Rybak LP, Husain K, Evenson L, Morris C, Whitworth C, et al. (1997) Protection by 4-methylthiobenzoic acid against cisplatin-induced ototoxicity: antioxidant system. Pharmacol Toxicol 81(4):173–179.
55. Ravi R, Somani SM, Rybak LP (1995) Mechanism of cisplatin ototoxicity: antioxidant system. Pharmacol Toxicol 76:386–394.
56. Ohlemiller KK, McFadden SL, Ding DL, Lear PM, Ho YS (2000) Targeted mutation of the gene for cellular glutathione peroxidase (Gpx1) increases noise-induced hearing loss in mice. J Assoc Res Otolaryngol 1(3):243–254.
57. Pourbakht A, Yamasoba T (2003) Ebselen attenuates cochlear damage caused by acoustic trauma. Hear Res 181:100–108.
58. Lynch ED, Gu R, Pierce C, Kil J (2005) Reduction of acute cisplatin ototoxicity and nephrotoxicity in rats by oral administration of allopurinol and ebselen. Hear Res 201:81–89.

59. Barrenas ML, Hellstrom PA (1996) The effect of low level acoustic stimulation on susceptibility to noise in blue- and brown-eyed young human subjects. Ear Hear 17(1):63–68.

60. Leonova EV, Fairfield DA, Lomax MI, Altschuler RA (2002) Constitutive expression of Hsp27 in the rat cochlea. Hear Res 163:61–70.

61. Brazma A, Hingamp P, Quackenbush J, Sherlock G, Spellman P, et al. (2001) Minimum information about a microarray experiment (MIAME)-toward standards for microarray data. Nature Genetics 29(4): 365–371.

62. Tanaka C, Coling DE, Manohar S, Chen GD, Hu BH, et al. (2012) Expression pattern of oxidative stress and antioxidant defense-related genes in the aging Fischer 344/NHsd rat cochlea. Neurobiol Aging 33(8):1842.e1–1842.e14.

5

Gap43 Transcription Modulation in the Adult Brain Depends on Sensory Activity and Synaptic Cooperation

Nicole Rosskothen-Kuhl*, Robert-Benjamin Illing

Neurobiological Research Laboratory, Department of Otorhinolaryngology, University of Freiburg, Freiburg, Germany

Abstract

Brain development and learning is accompanied by morphological and molecular changes in neurons. The growth associated protein 43 (Gap43), indicator of neurite elongation and synapse formation, is highly expressed during early stages of development. Upon maturation of the brain, Gap43 is down-regulated by most neurons with the exception of subdivisions such as the CA3 region of hippocampus, the lateral superior olive (LSO) and the central inferior colliculus (CIC). Little is known about the regulation of this mRNA in adult brains. We found that the expression of Gap43 mRNA in specific neurons can be modulated by changing sensory activity of the adult brain. Using the central auditory system of rats as a model, Gap43 protein and mRNA levels were determined in LSO and CIC of hearing-experienced rats unilaterally or bilaterally deafened or unilaterally stimulated by a cochlear implant (CI). Our data indicate that Gap43 is a marker useful beyond monitoring neuronal growth and synaptogenesis, reflecting also specific patterns of synaptic activities on specific neurons. Thus, unilateral loss of input to an adult auditory system directly causes asymmetrical expression of Gap43 mRNA between LSOs or CICs on both sides of the brainstem. This consequence can be prevented by simple-patterned stimulation of a dysfunctional ear by way of a CI. We suggest that as a function of input balance and activity pattern, Gap43 mRNA expression changes as cells associate converging afferent signals.

Editor: Berta Alsina, Universitat Pompeu Fabra, Spain

Funding: The authors have no support or funding to report.

Competing Interests: The authors declare that no competing interests exist.

* E-mail: nicole.rosskothen@uniklinik-freiburg.de

Introduction

In the auditory system of the adult mammalian brain, FBJ osteosarcoma oncogene *fos* (also known as *c-fos*) is one of the first genes activated by sensory activity evoked either by acoustical or electrical intracochlear stimulation (EIS) [1,2]. Its protein is a monomer of the heterodimeric Fos-Jun activator protein-1 (AP-1) transcription factor [3]. AP-1 triggers the expression of many genes, among them the growth associated protein Gap43 [4]. This phosphoprotein is neuron-specific and expressed in neuronal somata, axons, and growth cones during pre- and early postnatal development [5,6]. Gap43 plays a key role during neurite outgrowth in ontogeny and regeneration as well as in early stages of synaptogenesis [7].

In transgenic mice overexpressing *gap43*, aberrant neuronal connections develop [8]. By contrast, complete *gap43* knock-down in mice is lethal in 90% of all cases during the first three weeks of postnatal life [9]. Rekart et al. [10] observed significant memory impairments when Gap43 levels were reduced by 50%. Using Gap43 gene silencing in the olivo-cerebellar system, Gap43 is shown to be essential for maintenance of climbing fiber structure and to promote sprouting after lesion of the inferior olive [11,12]. Overall, these studies provide evidence that Gap43 is crucial for neuronal network formation.

During postnatal maturation, Gap43 is down-regulated by most neurons and only specific regions of the mammalian brain maintain high levels of Gap43 mRNA [13,14]. The adult hippocampal CA3 region known to be involved in life-long neuronal plasticity and learning [15,16] and the lateral superior olive (LSO) as well as the central inferior colliculus (CIC) are notable examples. This suggests that they maintain a responsiveness to reshape their neuronal affiliations upon varying patterns of neuronal activity into adulthood [17,18]. However, little is known about the factors regulating Gap43 expression in the adult brain.

It has been shown that re-expression of Gap43 protein can be induced by cochlear ablation in the mature auditory brainstem, involving an early phase of low Gap43 levels up to 3 days, and a Gap43 re-expression phase starting after 3 days of deafness with a local maximum of Gap43 protein after 7 days of cochlear ablation [19].

The auditory brainstem nuclei LSO and CIC are indispensable for the binaural computation of sound localization. In order to fulfill this function, LSO neurons receive sensory-driven signals originating from both ears to evaluate interaural level differences (ILD) of acoustic stimuli. Encoding of ILDs depends on excitatory (glutamatergic) input from the cochlear nucleus (CN) and inhibitory (glycinergic) input from the medial nucleus of the trapezoid body (MNTB) of the same side [20–25]. Frequency-specific signals arriving from both ears remain tonotopically ordered [26].

The central and major region of the tripartite inferior colliculus (IC) receives tonotopically ordered bilaterally ascending afferents from LSO, lateral lemniscus, CN, and medial superior olive (MSO) [27], and descending input from the auditory cortex and other forebrain regions [28]. Whilst the uncrossed pathways from

LSO to CIC are mainly inhibitory, the dominating projection is crossed and excitatory [29].

The utilization of binaural signal processing for spatially directed behavior requires a fine-tuning of neuronal activity depending on converging synaptic inputs. This fine-tuning takes place in postnatal development and needs to be continually readjusted throughout life. Considering the crucial roles of LSO and CIC in binaural signal processing [30,31], we investigated the effect of experimentally induced deviations in binaural input on *gap43* transcription in their neurons. Gap43 was chosen as an indicator for a neuron's readiness for activity-dependent structural readjustment of nerve net circuitry. Our hypothesis was that the transcription of *gap43* should change depending on level or pattern of neuronal activity.

Materials and Methods

Animals

Twenty nine adult female Wistar rats aged 6 to 16 weeks were used. Care and use of the animals as reported here were approved by the appropriate agency (Regierungspräsidium Freiburg, permission number G-10/83). Rats were anesthetized by an intraperitoneal (i.p.) injection of a mixture of ketamine (50 mg/kg body weight; cp-Pharm Handelsgesellschaft mbH, Burgdorf, Germany) and xylazine (5 mg/kg body weight; Rompun, Bayer-Leverkusen, Germany) before ear bone removal or cochlear opening with electrode insertion. For pain reduction, rats received an intramuscular injection of carprofen (4–5 mg/kg body weight, RIMADYL, Pfizer GmbH, Berlin, Germany). Preceding transcardial perfusion, rats were given a lethal dose of sodium-thiopental (i.p., 250 mg/kg body weight of Trapanal, Nycomed, Konstanz, Germany).

Experimental Groups

Animals were divided into four experimental groups (Table 1). Guided by previous results [19,32], we distinguished an 'early' phase covering 1 and 3 days after deafness or EIS from a 'midterm' phase including 5 and 7 days following deafness or EIS. We investigated an additional 'late' phase at 70 days for selected cases (Table 1).

Group one constitutes age matched controls (Co) without cochlear implant (CI) insertion. To ensure that these control rats had normal hearing, we first tested the motor response to a handclap (Preyer's reflex [33]) three days before sacrifice (Fig. 1). We then checked tympanic membrane and middle ear under a microscope to verify that hearing is not impaired due to damage of the tympanic membrane or an inflammation of the middle ear. Eventually, we measured the auditory brainstem responses (ABRs) (Fig. 1). For the ABR recording, steel needle electrodes were placed subcutaneously at vertex and mastoids and a 20 Hz train of click stimuli was presented to one side through a brass pipe inserted into the outer ear canal, while the other ear was masked by white noise at the same sound pressure level (SPL). The SPL was stepwise increased, attempting to elicit an ABR at hearing threshold visualized by an averager (Multiliner E; Evolution 1.70c; Toennies & Jäger GmbH, Höchberg, Germany). The ABR mean amplitudes were set after 300 sweeps recorded in a frequency band of 0.1 to 3 kHz (Fig. 2A).

In order to estimate the impact of naturally occurring sound intensities on the transcription of *gap43*, we removed the malleus unilaterally or bilaterally three days before perfusion in five rats leading to a rise of hearing threshold by 50 dB [34]. No statistically significant difference was found against the animals without any intervention by any histochemical measure.

Table 1. Experimental Groups.

Group	1 (Co)	2 (bd)		3 (ud)			4 (us)	
treatment	none/malleus removal	bilateral CI implantation		unilateral CI implantation			unilateral CI implantation+EIS	
duration of experiments	–	early (1+3 days implanted)	midterm (5+7 days implanted)	early (1+3 days implanted)	midterm (5+7 days implanted)	late (70 days implanted)	early (1+3 days EIS)	midterm (5+7 days EIS)
no. of LSOs	16	4	4	4i/4c	4i/4c	3i/3c	3i/3c	3i/3c
no. of CICs	16	4	4	4i/4c	4i/4c	3i/3c	3i/3c	3i/3c

c: contralateral; i: ipsilateral; Co: control; *bd*: bilateral deaf; *ud*: unilateral deaf; *us*: unilateral stimulation; EIS: electrical intracochlear stimulation.

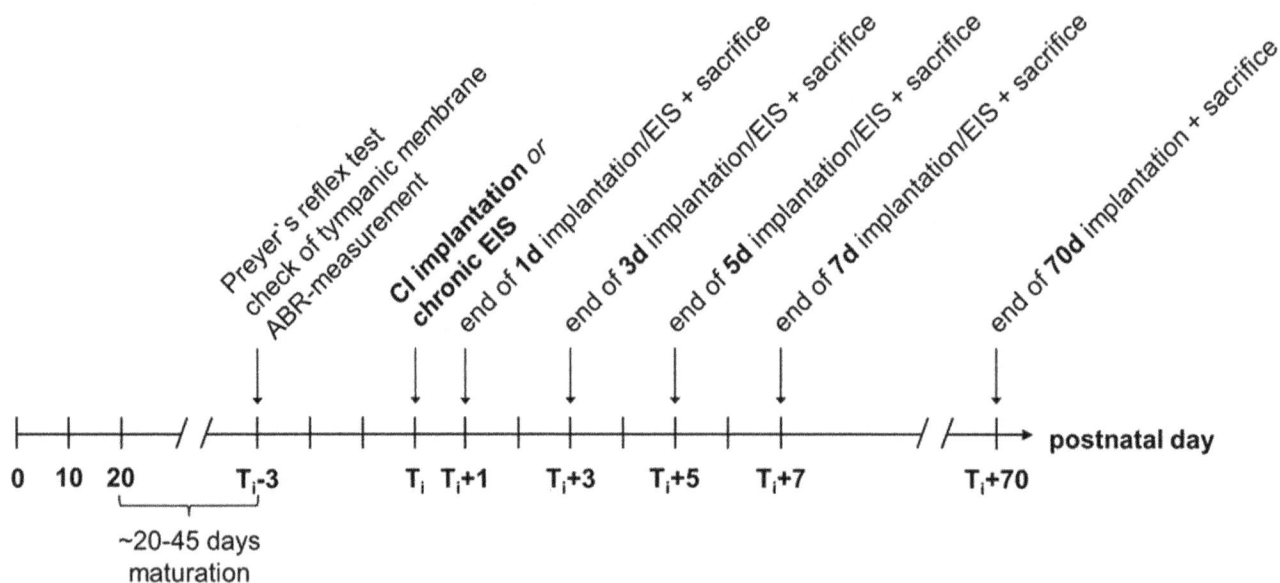

Figure 1. Experimental Design. T_i: time of implantation of a passive electrode dummy or onset of electrical intracochlear stimulation (EIS); d: day(s).

The second experimental group included bilaterally deafened (*bd*) rats (Table 1). Normal hearing was verified by ABR measurement before rats were deafened by bilateral insertion of a CI into the cochlea (Fig. 1). The operation consisted of exposing the cochlea by a retroauricular surgical approach. Preserving the facial nerve, tympanic membrane and malleus were removed and the opening in the bulla tympani was widened to provide good visibility of the cochlea. A 0.6 mm wide hole was made with a diamond drill in the bony wall of the medial turn of the cochlea and two rings of an electrode carrier dummy were inserted without being activated. One and 3 days (early group) as well as 5 and 7 days (midterm group) after electrode insertion, rats were anesthetized for electrode explantation immediately followed by transcardial perfusion (Fig. 1).

The third experimental group consisted of unilaterally deafened (*ud*) rats (Table 1). Unilateral deafness was again induced by CI insertion into the left cochlea, while the right cochlea remained intact. The electrode carrier remained in place for 1 and 3 days, 5 and 7 days, or 70 days. To verify total deafness by CI insertion in experimental groups two and three, we measured the ABRs due to click presentation 1, 3, 5 and/or 7 days after implantation (Fig. 2B).

Finally, experimental group four consisted of unilaterally CI stimulated (*us*) rats (Table 1) as early or midterm group members. Normal hearing capacity was checked before CI stimulation as described for the control group (Fig. 1). The surgical procedure included approach and opening of the cochlea as described above. Before bipolar electrode insertion into the medial turn of the cochlea, the electrode connection device was fixed on the skull with small threaded screws. The electrode carrier was then pulled through under the skin and inserted into the cochlea following the retroauricular surgical approach. To stabilize electrode position, the bulla was filled with 4% lukewarm agar. After hardening, the wound was surgically closed.

Chronic EIS

The implanted device was connected to the external stimulator (CI in a box) by way of a swivel (Fig. 3). The stimulator was connected to a communicator, both kindly provided by Cochlear

Germany GmbH & Co. KG. The swivel, directly placed over a centered hole in the cage lid, guaranteed unhindered mobility of the rat during stimulation. Still under anesthesia, the CI was activated to record the electrically evoked auditory brainstem response (EABR; Fig. 2C) with steel needle electrodes placed subcutaneously at vertex and mastoids, respectively. EABR measurement was performed to corroborate correct placement of stimulation electrodes and to determine an appropriate current level. The EABR was visualized using an averager (Multiliner E, Evolution 1.70c, Toennies), calculating mean amplitudes of 500 sweeps in a frequency band of 0.1 to 10 kHz. We aimed to obtain maximal EABR amplitudes of 9 μV±10% by adjusting the current level of EIS to match acoustic stimuli of 90 dB above hearing threshold, causing specific tonotopic activation of central auditory neurons (Figs. 2A, C and 8). After recovering from anesthesia, the CI was activated for causing local activation of the spiral ganglion. Bipolar stimulation consisted of 50 pulses per second biphasic stimuli with a phase width of 50 μs [35]. During chronic stimulation, a companion rat resided in the right part of the cage to avoid detrimental effects of social deprivation (Fig. 3).

Immunohistochemistry (IHC)

Following completion of postoperative survival time or stimulation period, animals received a lethal dose of sodium-thiopental and were transcardially perfused with a fixative containing 4% paraformaldehyde in 0.1 M phosphate buffer at pH 7.4. After the brain was removed from the skull and soaked in 20% RNase/DNase-free sucrose buffer overnight, parts containing CN, LSO, and CIC were cryo-cut into 30 μm thick frontal sections. Following incubation with 0.045% H_2O_2, 1% sodium-borohydride (only for Fos staining) and 1% milk powder, each in 0.02 M sodium phosphate buffer at pH 7.4 for 30 min, sections were exposed to a primary antibody raised in goat against Fos protein (SC-52-G, 1:2000, lot. no. A2810, Santa Cruz Biotechnology Inc., Santa Cruz, USA), or raised in mouse against Gap43 protein (MAB347, 1:5000, lot. no. LV178643/NG1894354, Millipore Biosciences, Temecula, USA). After incubation for 48 h at 4°C, a biotinylated secondary anti-goat (BA-5000, 1:200, Vector Labo-

A

ABR, hearing ear

B

ABR, deaf ear

C

EABR, hearing-experienced rat

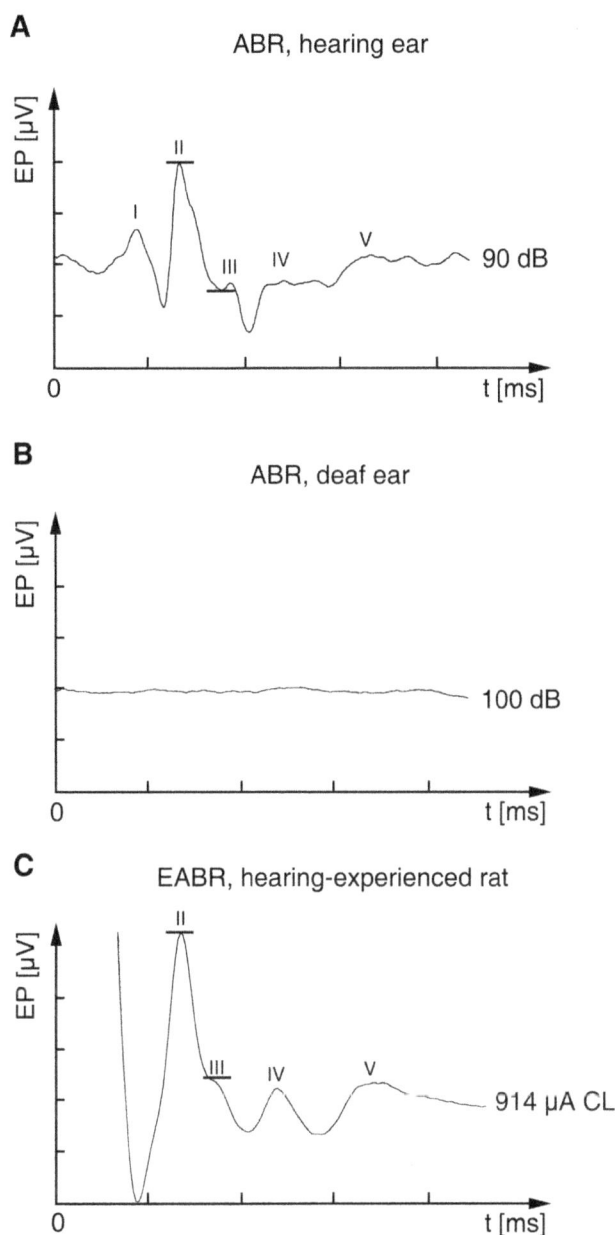

Figure 2. Acoustically and electrically evoked brain-stem responses (ABR/EABR). (A, B) Hearing ear stimulated at 90 dB (A) and an ear deafened by electrode insertion stimulated at 100 dB (B). (C) Representative EABR response of a hearing-experienced rat at a current level (CL) of 914 μA. Typically, the ABR of a hearing rat showed five distinguishable peaks (I–V), four of them (II–V) recognizable in the EABR. The black horizontal lines indicate the range of amplitude measurement. x-axis: 2 ms per unit; y-axis: 4 μV per unit; EP: evoked potential.

ratories, Inc., Burlingame, USA) or anti-mouse antibody (BA-2001, 1:200, Vector Laboratories) was added. Visualization of anti-Fos (goat) and anti-Gap43 (mouse)-binding sites was based on intensification by the avidin-biotin-technique (Vector Laboratories), followed by 3,3′ diaminobenzidine tetrahydrochloride (Sigma, Taufkirchen, Germany). Controls omitting primary antibodies were run to verify their specificity and lack of unspecific binding by the secondary antibody. Neuronal nuclei of the parabrachial region always containing Fos immunoreactivity served as positive staining controls [36].

Synthesis of Fos and Gap43 Fragment for in-situ Hybridization (ISH)

Gap43 mRNA was isolated (PAXgene RNA Kit 762174 preAnalytiX, QIAGEN, Hilden, Germany) from rat CN at postnatal day 10, while for Fos fragment synthesis mRNA was isolated from adult rat CN after 2 h EIS. Afterwards, subsequent complementary DNA (cDNA) synthesis was performed using standard techniques (Omniscript RT Kit 205111, QIAGEN).

Gap43 DNA fragment amplification. Based on the cDNA, a specific DNA fragment (191 bp) of the Gap43 gene [NCBI: NM_017195.3, GI: 166091453] flanked with the T3 and T7 promoters was amplified with the following primers: Gap43 F4 (T3)

(5′-ATTAACCCTCACTAAAGGGATGCAGAAAGCAGC-CAAGCTGAGGA-3′), and Gap43 R3 (T7)

(5′-GGGCAACGTGGAAAGCCGTTTCTTGGGATAT-CACTCAGCATAAT-3′).

Fos DNA fragment amplification. Based on the cDNA, a specific DNA fragment (313 bp) of the Fos gene [NCBI: NM_022197, GI: 148298807] was amplified with the following primers: F1-FBJ/Fos (5′-AGCTCCCACCAGTGTCTACC-3′), and R1-JB/Fos 5′-CCACGGAGGAGACCAGAGTG-3′.).

Riboprobe construction. The Fos fragment was subcloned into pCR4-TOPO (K4595-01, Invitrogen, Carlsbad, USA) to construct subclone pCR4 Fos. From this construct a linearized Fos fragment was amplified, which is flanked by the T3 and T7 promoters. For both fragments, digoxigenin-labeled antisense riboprobes were generated, from the 191 bp rat Gap43 cDNA and the 313 bp rat Fos cDNA after transcription with T7 (for Gap43) or T3 (for Fos) RNA polymerase (for Gap43: Cat. No. 10881767001; for Fos: Cat. No. 11031163001, Roche Applied Science, Mannheim, Germany). Sense riboprobes were made after transcription with T3 (for Gap43) or T7 (for Fos) RNA polymerase (for Gap43: Cat. No. 11031163001, for Fos: Cat. No. 10881767001, Roche Applied Science). These sense probes served as control to verify that the complementary transcript failed to generate any staining in the entire CN, LSO (cp. Fig. 4, inset in A, B), and CIC, (cp. Fig. 5, inset in E, F).

In-situ Hybridization (ISH)

Thirty micrometer thick cryo-cut frontal brain sections were collected in 2× standard saline citrate (SSC) buffer (Invitrogen, Life Technologies GmbH, Darmstadt, Germany). Sections were washed in 2× SSC buffer for 15 min. Before pre-hybridization, they were pretreated in a 1:1 dilution of 2× SSC and a hybridization buffer consisting of 50% formamide (Carl Roth GmbH, Karlsruhe, Germany), 4× SSC (Invitrogen), 10% dextransulfate (Sigma), 1× Denhardt's solution (AMRESCO Inc., Solon, USA), 250 μg/ml heat-denatured cod and herring sperm DNA (Roche Diagnostics GmbH, Mannheim, Germany), and 625 μg/ml tRNA from E. coli MRE 600 (Roche) for 15 min. Pre-hybridization in hybridization buffer at 55°C lasted for 60 min. Hybridization was done overnight at 55°C in the same solution with the addition of 100 ng/ml digoxigenin (DIG)-labeled Fos and 1000 ng/ml DIG-labeled Gap43 antisense or sense complementary RNA, respectively. After hybridization, sections were washed twice in 2× SSC for 15 min at room temperature, 2× SSC and 50% formamide (MERCK KGAA, Darmstadt, Germany) for 15 min, 0.1× SSC and 50% formamide for 15 min, and twice in 0.1× SSC for 15 min at 65°C each. For immunological detection of DIG-labeled hybrids, brain sections

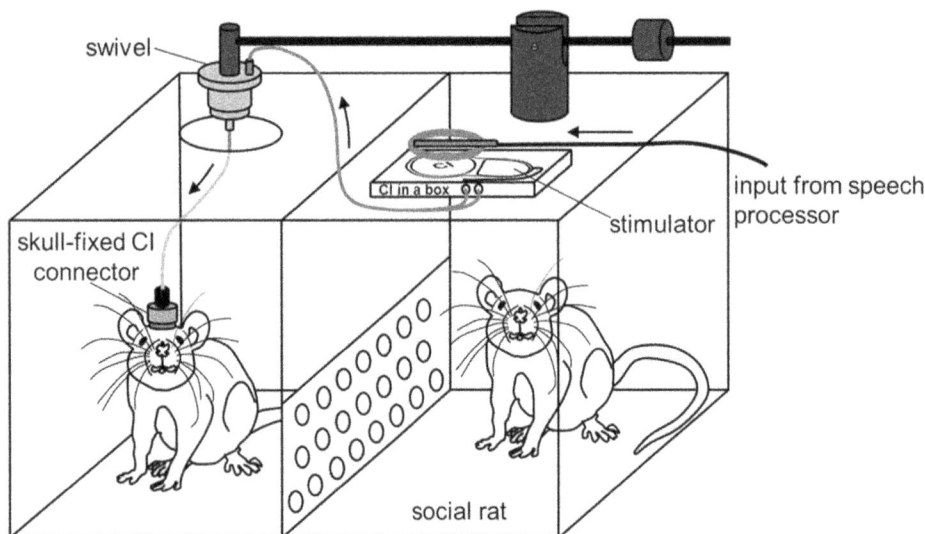

Figure 3. In-house designed setup for chronic electrical intracochlear stimulation (EIS). The rat in the left part of the cage is stimulated using a skull-fixed cochlear-implant (CI) connector. The implanted device was connected to the external stimulator 'CI in a box' by way of a swivel. The input for the CI delivers the speech processor. During chronic stimulation, a companion rat resided in the right part of the cage to avoid detrimental effects of social deprivation.

were treated twice in buffer 1 (100 mM Tris/HCl, pH 7.5; 150 mM NaCl) for 10 min each, blocked in buffer 2 (1% blocking reagent [Roche] in buffer 1) for 60 min at room temperature, and incubated overnight at 4°C with the anti-DIG Fab fragment from sheep tagged with alkaline phosphatase (1:1500, Roche) in buffer 2. For the preparation of color reaction, sections were equilibrated in buffer 1 for 2× 10 min each and in buffer 3 (100 mM Tris/HCl, pH 9.5; 100 mM NaCl; 50 mM MgCl$_2$) for 10 min. Afterwards, nitroblue tetrazolium (0.34 mg/ml, Roche) and 5-bromo-4-chloro-3-indolyl-phosphate, 4-toluidine salt (0.17 mg/ml, Roche) were added to buffer 3. Development of the color reaction was performed in the dark at room temperature, eight hours for Gap43 mRNA staining, and 9 h for Fos mRNA staining. The color reaction was stopped by transfer sections into distilled water. Finally, sections were mounted on glass slides, dehydrated in increasing grades of alcohol, cleared in xylene, and coverslipped with DPX (Sigma-Aldrich, Steinheim, Germany).

Detection and Quantification of Gap43 mRNA Staining Intensity

To quantify changes in Gap43 mRNA expression, the mean of staining intensities for Gap43 mRNA were detected throughout LSO and CIC on both sides of the brainstem. Color photographs were taken from sections of the left (l)/ipsilateral (i) and right (r)/contralateral (c) side of mRNA stained LSOs and CICs through a x10 (for LSO) or a x5 (for CIC) objective with a digital camera (AxioCam, Zeiss, Jena, Germany) at 8 bit conversion. Under graphics software (Adobe Photoshop CS, Adobe Systems Inc., San Jose, USA) global variations in staining intensity of sections from different animals were compensated by setting the median of each photograph to 217 (for LSO) or 185 (for CIC). We then extracted the red channel of each photograph. Selection of a region of interest (ROI) was done using the lasso tool (Figs. 4A, 5A, dashed lines). For LSO, the ROI was defined by tracing the histologically visible border of each LSO, whereas the same defined ROI was always used for CIC of different rats. Detection of the mean staining intensity of Gap43 mRNA positive neurons in LSO and CIC was performed inside ROIs by using the filling tool at

tolerance 10 (for LSO) or 11 (for CIC). Due to this definition of staining intensity, LSO and CIC lacking Gap43 mRNA positive neurons had a mean value of 0, whereas a maximally stained single neuron has a staining intensity of around140 (for LSO) or 170 (for CIC). Due to the looser packing of neurons and the restriction of positive neurons to only a part of the ROI, mean values of staining intensity per ROI detected in this study varied between 2 and 14 for LSO, and between 0.5 and 1.7 for CIC, across all types of experiments.

Statistical Analysis

Statistical analysis was done with Prism (GraphPad Software, La Jolla, USA) and Microsoft Office Excel 2003 (Microsoft Germany GmbH, Unterschleißheim, Germany). Mean staining intensities and their standard error (SEM) for Gap43 mRNA were determined for LSO and CIC in twenty nine brains of three to seven pairs of sections (Figs. 4A, 5A, dashed line). Across the respective auditory area on each side, ratios of left-to-right (controls and *bd* rats) or ipsilateral-to-contralateral (*ud* and *us* rats) sides were calculated for subsequent statistical analysis (Figs. 6, 7).

Differences of means were identified by one-way analysis of variance (ANOVA) with significance level set to p<0.05. The F-values of each ANOVA test with their degrees of freedom (DF) are specified in the legends of Figs. 6 and 7. Supplemented by Dunnett post-hoc test, significant differences of means of experimental groups with the single control group were determined. To determine means that are significantly different from each other within a defined subset, Tukey post-hoc test was added. Significant differences of means for selected pairings of groups were calculated by combining one-way ANOVA with Sidak post-hoc test. Again, the significance level was set to p<0.05. Significance levels were distinguished as (***/###) for p<0.001, (**) for p<0.01, (*/#) for p<0.05. To detect differences between left and right brainstem side of controls, a two-tailed unpaired t-test was used with confidence interval set to p<0.05.

Preparatory statistics of three different control groups: non-operated control rats (I) as well as rats with unilateral (II) or bilateral (III) malleus removal, revealed that Gap43 mRNA

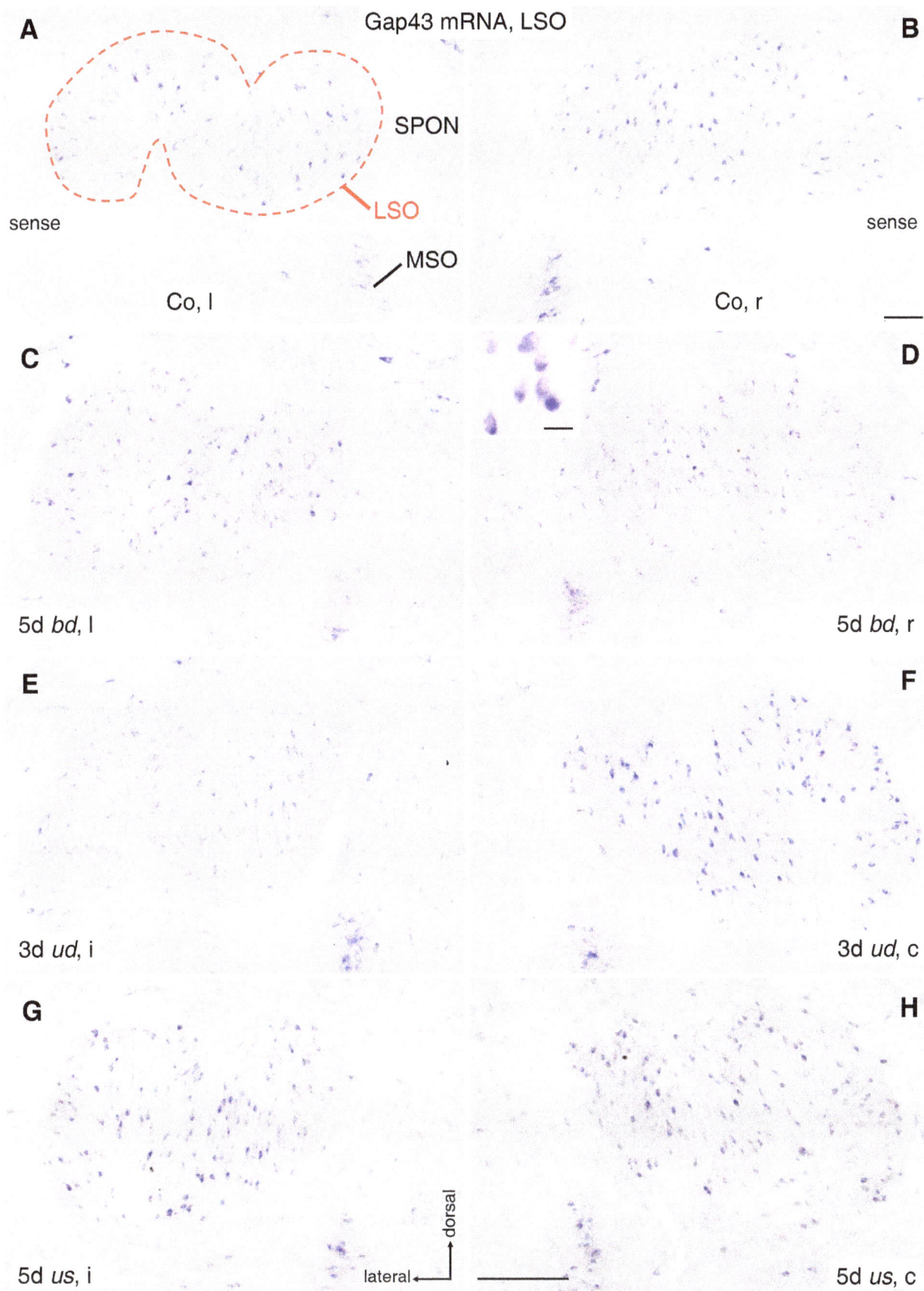

Figure 4. Gap43 mRNA staining in lateral superior olive (LSO). (A, B) A basal level of Gap43 mRNA was seen in neuronal cell bodies (purple dots) of the entire left (A) and right (B) LSO (dashed outline) of untreated control rats (Co). The insets show lack of staining in corresponding sections

after use of Gap43 sense probe. Scale bar for insets: 0.2 mm. (C, D) Gap43 mRNA expression in left (C) and right (D) LSO after 5 days (d) of bilaterally deaf (*bd*) rats is equivalent to control level. Inset in D shows Gap43 mRNA positive neurons at higher magnification. Scale bar of inset: 20 μm. (E) Following 3d of unilateral deafness (*ud*), Gap43 mRNA expression decreased in neurons of LSOi compared to controls. (F) Simultaneously, the expression increased contralaterally. (G, H) After 5d of unilateral stimulation (*us*), high bilaterally balanced Gap43 mRNA levels were observed. Scale bar for A to H: 0.2 mm. SPON: superior paraolivary nucleus; MSO: medial superior olive; l: left; r: right; i: ipsilateral; c: contralateral.

expression was indistinguishable among them. Specifically, no statistical differences were detected between ipsilateral-to-contralateral ratios of *gap43* transcription of the three different groups (n = 8/30 rats/slices; for LSO: (I): 1.02±0.028, mean ± SEM; (II): 0.99±0.06; (III): 0.89±0.06; for CIC: (I): 0.99±0.032; (II): 1.14±0.03; (III): 1.01±0.06; p>0.05 for all), leading to a pooling of all control rats to one group (see 'Experimental groups') for the following statistic of this study.

Gap43 staining levels were evaluated for bilaterally deafened (*bd*) rats. Staining levels were indistinguishable between both sides of LSO and of CIC, respectively, as well as between the two time windows studied (LSO: 4/25 rats/slices; early *bd* l: 2.94±0.34; early *bd* r: 3.32±0.37; midterm *bd* l: 3.63±0.40; midterm *bd* r: 3.49±0.53; CIC: 4/24 rats/slices; early *bd* l: 0.59±0.042; early *bd* r: 0.62±0.04; midterm *bd* l: 0.62±0.045; midterm *bd* r: 0.63±0.05; p>0.05 for all). Consequently, we combined the Gap43 mRNA staining intensities of LSOs or CICs to one group for further statistical analysis.

Results

Intracochlear Electrode Insertion Induces Total Deafness

Bilaterally opening the cochleae and inserting electrodes into their medial turn consistently disabled implanted rats to show a motor response to a handclap (Preyer's reflex). This indicates a rise of ABR threshold beyond 81 dB SPL [33]. Audiometry revealed a rise of hearing threshold by 100 dB (Fig. 2B) against normal hearing controls (Fig. 2A), implying total deafness. Correspondingly, unilateral electrode implantation caused unilateral deafness.

Neurons of the Mature Auditory Brainstem Maintain *gap43* Transcription

Under control conditions, neurons throughout LSO (Fig. 4A, B) and in the ventral part of CIC (Fig. 5A, B) possessed a notable level of Gap43 mRNA in their cytoplasm (Figs. 4D, 5D inset), showing a mean staining intensity of 4.56±0.42 for LSO (Fig. 6B) and 0.66±0.041 for CIC (Fig. 6D), both against 0 for the mean staining level obtained by using the sense probe (Figs. 4A, B, 5E, F insets). Because of a staining ratio close to 1 (for LSO: 0.96±0.03; for CIC: 1.03±0.03; p>0.05 for left vs. right by t-test; Fig. 6A, C), brains were proved to be symmetrical and control data were pooled from both sides of the brainstem.

Our experiments demonstrated that even if sensory-evoked activity fails due to bilateral hearing loss, the basal transcription of *gap43* was unaffected in neurons of LSO and CIC (cp. 4C, D). Statistical evaluation of the mean Gap43 mRNA staining intensity of LSO and CIC revealed no significant difference compared to the staining intensity of control rats (for LSO: *bd*: 3.32±0.2; Co: 4.56±0.42; for CIC: *bd*: 0.62±0.66; Co: 0.66±0.04; p>0.05 for both; Fig. 6B, D).

Asymmetric Sensory Activity Results in Imbalanced *gap43* Transcription. LSO

Already by 1 day after *ud*, a significant imbalance of Gap43 mRNA staining intensity was found between ipsilateral (i) and contralateral (c) LSO (Fig. 4E, F), with an ipsilateral-to-contralateral ratio of staining intensity significantly smaller than under

control conditions (n = 19/92 rats/slices; *ud*: 0.39±0.02; Co: 0.96±0.03; p<0.001; cp. Fig. 6A). For the generation of Fig. 6, data of early, midterm, and late *ud* rats were pooled (cp. Fig. 7). This imbalance resulted from an increase of Gap43 mRNA staining intensity on the contralateral side (*ud* c: 10.51±0.46; p<0.001; Fig. 6B), while the ipsilateral side remained at control level (*ud* i: 4.17±0.32; Co: 4.56±0.42; p>0.05; Figs. 6B, 7B). A quantitative evaluation of randomly selected sets of LSOs from Co, *ud* and *us* rats revealed that these changes in staining levels were not due to varying numbers of stained neurons (n = 9/34 rats/slices; F = 1.712, DFn = 2, DFd = 31; p>0.05; Fig. 4).

In order to see if a once unbalanced auditory system has the potential to re-balance itself after a longer period of deafness, Gap43 mRNA staining intensity was studied after 70 days of *ud*. Still, we detected a significant imbalance of Gap43 mRNA staining between both sides of LSO indicated by a ratio significantly smaller than for controls (late *ud*: 0.50±0.03; Co: 0.96±0.03; p<0.001; Fig. 7A).

CIC

Within 1 day of *ud*, a sustained imbalance of Gap43 mRNA staining intensity developed between ipsilateral and contralateral CIC (Fig. 5C, D). The ipsilateral-to-contralateral ratio of staining intensity was significantly larger than for controls (n = 19/89 rats/slices; Co: 1.03±0.03; *ud*: 1.82±0.08; p<0.001; Figs. 6C, 7C). Unlike the situation in LSO, this imbalance resulted from a significant increase of Gap43 mRNA staining intensity on the ipsilateral side (*ud* i: 1.09±0.06; p<0.001; Fig. 6D), while the contralateral side remained at control level (*ud* c: 0.62±0.03; Co: 0.66±0.04; p>0.05; Figs. 6D, 7D).

As described for LSO, CIC was still out of balance after 70 days of *ud* (Fig. 5E, F). By this time, an ipsilateral-to-contralateral staining ratio indistinguishable from early and midterm *ud* rats (early: 1.87±0.15; midterm: 1.81±0.13; late *ud*: 1.77±0.08; p>0.05; Fig. 7C) was seen. This led *us* to pool all three groups for statistical evaluation as shown in Fig. 6C, D.

Unilateral EIS Results in Balanced *gap43* Transcription in Auditory Brainstem Regions. LSO

Within the group of *us* rats, neurons throughout both LSOs expressed balanced levels of Gap43 mRNA independent of stimulation duration (Fig. 4G, H). As a result, the ipsilateral-to-contralateral staining ratio for Gap43 mRNA was found to be close to 1 and thus indistinguishable from controls (n = 14/55 rats/slices; *us*: 1.03±0.03; Co: 0.96±0.03; p>0.05; Figs. 6A, 7A). Compared to the corresponding ratio in *ud* rats, a significant difference was detected (n = 17/91 rats/slices; *us*: 1.03±0.03; *ud*: 0.39±0.02; p<0.001; Figs. 6A, 7A). Unlike controls and LSOi of *ud* rats, the mean staining intensity of Gap43 mRNA positive neurons was bilaterally increased for all stimulation times (n = 25/117 rats/slices; *us* i: 8.91±0.66; *us* c: 8.72±0.62; *ud* i: 4.17±0.32; Co: 4.56±0.42; p<0.001 for all; Figs. 6B, 7B).

CIC

As described for LSO, stimulation of one ear by a CI resulted in a bilaterally balanced transcription of *gap43* within the cytoplasm of neurons located ventrally in CIC (Fig. 5G, H). Evaluation of the

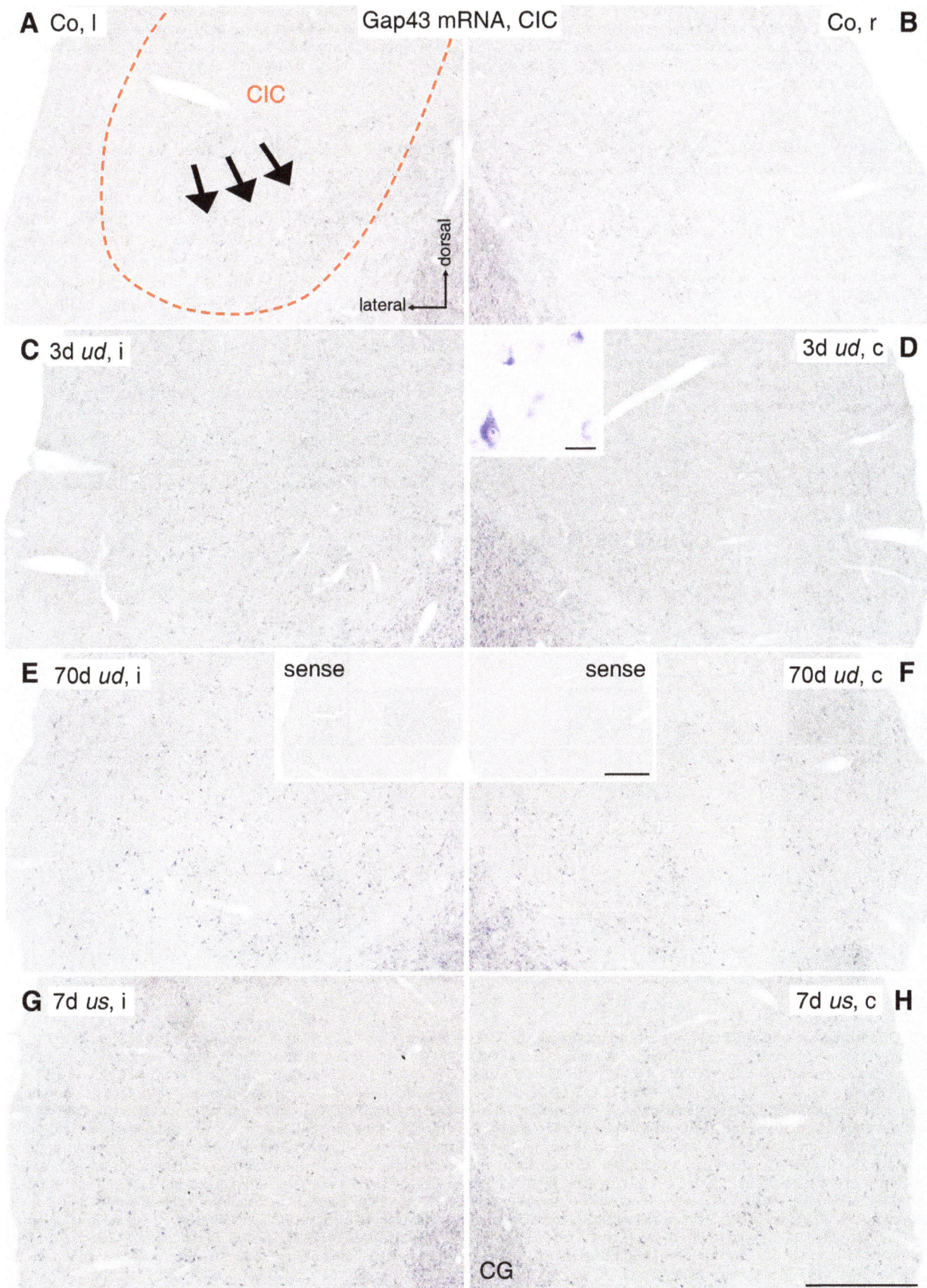

Figure 5. Gap43 mRNA staining in central inferior colliculus (CIC). (A, B) In the untreated control group (Co), Gap43 mRNA positive neurons (purple dots) in CIC (dashed outline) were mainly localized ventrally (arrows). (C, D) 3 days (d) after unilateral deafness (ud), Gap43 mRNA level

increased in CICi (C), while expression was decreased in CICc (D). The inset shows a higher magnification of stained CIC neurons. Scale bar in inset: 20 μm. (E, F) After 70d of *ud*, Gap43 mRNA expression rose bilaterally in CIC, with a significantly higher level on the ipsilateral side (E) compared to the contralateral side (F). Insets show control staining after incubation with Gap43 sense probe. Scale bar for insets: 0.2 mm. (G, H) Unilateral stimulation (*us*) for 7d resulted in an increase of Gap43 mRNA levels in ventral CIC on ipsilateral (G) and contralateral (H) side. Scale bar for A to H: 0.2 mm. l: left; r: right; i: ipsilateral; c: contralateral; CG: central gray.

ipsilateral-to-contralateral staining intensity revealed a ratio close to 1 for all different stimulation periods (Figs. 6C, 7C) and similar to controls (n = 14/60 rats/slices; *us*: 1.06±0.03; Co: 1.03±0.03; p>0.05), but significantly different from *ud* rats (n = 17/89 rats/slices; *us*: 1.06±0.03; *ud*: 1.82±0.08; p<0.001; Fig. 6C). However, the mean Gap43 mRNA staining intensities in *us* rats were bilaterally increased compared to controls as well as to CICc of *ud* rats (n = 25/121 rats/slices; *us* i: 0.93±0.07; *us* c: 0.89±0.07; *ud* c: 0.62±0.03; Co: 0.66±0.04; p = 0.0385 for Co vs. *us* c; p = 0.0085 for Co vs. *us* i; p = 0.0049 for *ud* c vs. *us* c; p = 0.0007 for *ud* c vs. *us* i; Fig. 6D). By contrast to the increase in Gap43 staining intensities in LSO, the increase in CIC was mainly based on a substantial rise of *gap43* transcription after the early period of *us* (Fig. 7D).

Adult *gap43* Transcription in Other Auditory Brainstem Regions

The ventral cochlear nucleus (VCN) of rats remained virtually free of any hybridization under all conditions (cp. Fig. 8A). Apart from LSO and CIC, Gap43 mRNA staining was prominent in neurons of MSO and still noticeable in shell neurons of LSO and in neurons of various other subnuclei of the superior olivary complex. As staining in all of these regions remained unaffected by any experimental condition (Fig. 4), they were not considered any further in this study.

Gap43 Protein Expression in the Adult Auditory Brainstem

Immunohistochemistry for Gap43 protein in VCN of normal adult rats revealed faintly labeled immunopositive boutons previously shown to be presynaptic endings [37] across the entire

Gap43 mRNA staining intensity

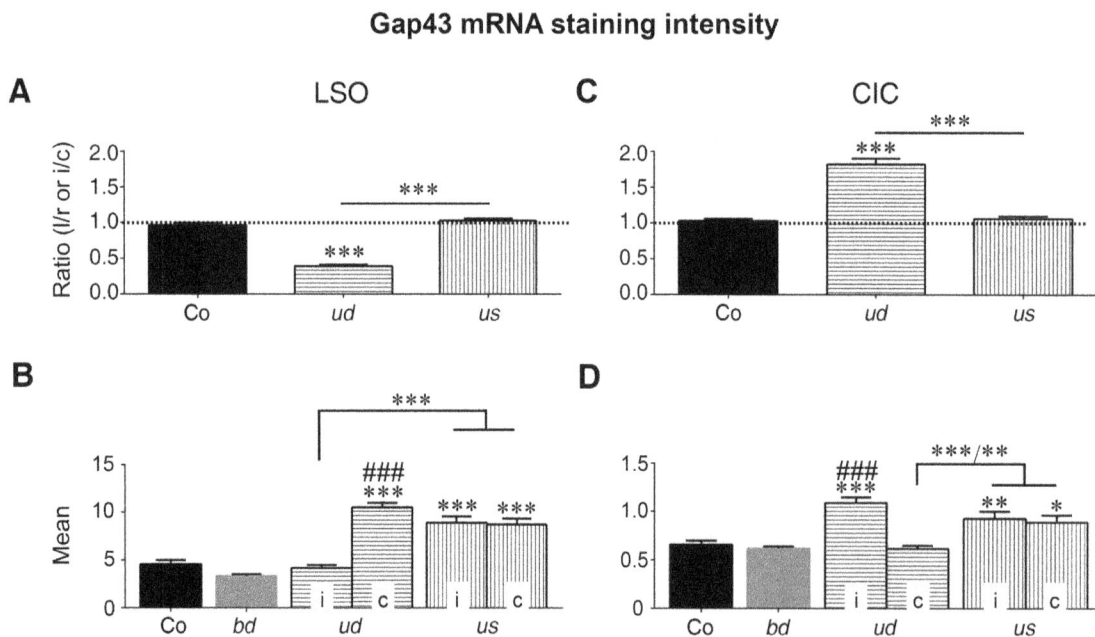

Figure 6. Quantification of Gap43 mRNA staining intensities in LSO (A, B) and CIC (C, D). Bilateral comparison of left-to-right or ipsilateral-to-contralateral staining intensities in LSO (A) and CIC (C) indicates that Gap43 mRNA was different between both sides of the brainstem if sensory stimulation was reduced on one side only (LSO: n = 19/92 rats/slices; F = 45.48, DFn = 2, DFd = 118; *ud*: 0.39±0.02; Co: 0.96±0.03; CIC: n = 19/89 rats/slices; F = 201.5, DFn = 2, DFd = 116; *ud*: 1.82±0.08; Co: 1.03±0.03; p<0.001 for both). EIS in the ear of one side with the other ear continuing transduction of acoustically signals maintained ipsilateral-to-contralateral balance as in controls (LSO: n = 6/29 rats/slices; *us*: 1.03±0.03; CIC: n = 6/30 rats/slices, *us*: 1.06±0.03; p>0.05 for both). Dotted line indicates bilateral symmetry (1.0). Significant differences against control level are indicated by asterisks above bars. Significant divergences between *ud* and *us* rats are indicated by lines with associated asterisks. (B) Staining results of *gap43* transcription in LSO (n = 29/142 rats/slices; F = 53.89, DFn = 5, DFd = 278) indicates that the staining intensity increased significantly against controls (Co) in LSOc due to unilateral deafness (*ud*; n = 19/89 rats/slices; p<0.001), and in bilateral LSO after unilateral stimulation (*us*; n = 14/55 rats/slices; p< 0.001 for both). Additionally, staining intensity in *ud* rats on the contralateral side was significantly higher than for bilaterally deafened (*bd*) rats (n = 15/87 rats/slices; ###: p<0.001). Staining intensities of both LSOs of *us* rats were higher than the ipsilateral intensity of *ud* rats (n = 17/90 rats/slices; p<0.001 for both). (D) Staining results of *gap43* transcription in CIC (n = 29/145 rats/slices; F = 18.71, DFn = 5, DFd = 284) revealed that the level increased against controls in CICi due to *ud* (n = 19/91 rats/slices; p<0.001), and in bilateral CIC after *us* (n = 14/56 rats/slices; p = 0.0085 for Co vs. *us* i; p = 0.0385 for Co vs. *us* c). Mean staining intensity of CIC of *bd* rats was significantly different from CICi of *ud* rats (n = 15/89 rats/slices; ###: p< 0.001), whereas both sides of *us* rats rose against CICc of *ud* rats (n = 17/95 rats/slices; p = 0.0007 for *us* i vs. *ud* c; p = 0.0049 for *us* c vs. *ud* c). Significance levels: (***/###) for p<0.001, (**) for p<0.01, (*) for p<0.05. LSO: lateral superior olive; CIC: central inferior colliculus; i: ipsilateral; c: contralateral.

Gap43 mRNA staining intensity

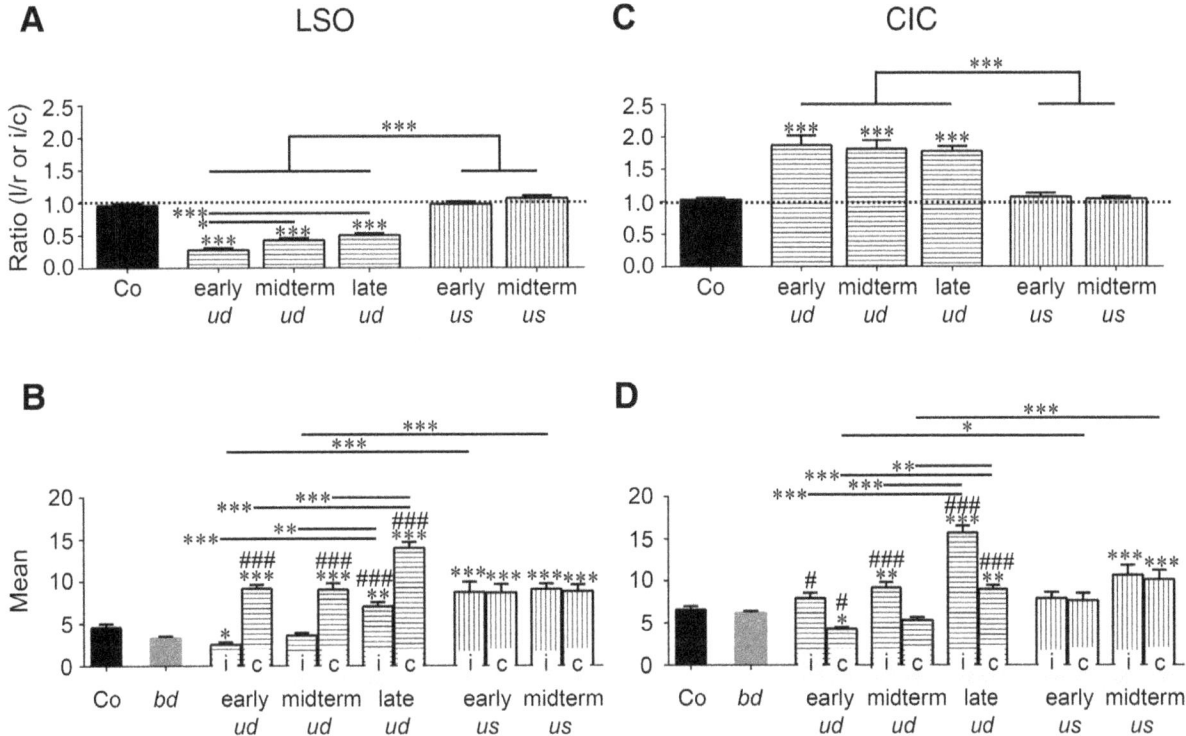

Figure 7. Quantification of Gap43 mRNA staining intensities in LSO (A, B) and CIC (C, D) in experimental subgroups. (A, C) Bilateral comparison of left-to-right or ipsilateral-to-contralateral staining intensity of LSO (A) and CIC (C) indicates that Gap43 mRNA was significantly different between both sides of the brainstem if sensory stimulation was reduced on one side only (*ud*) compared to control (LSO: n = 19/92 rats/slices; F = 102.5, DFn = 5, DFd = 115; early *ud*: 0.28±0.03; midterm *ud*: 0.42±0.04; late *ud*: 0.50±0.03; Co: 0.96±0.03; CIC: n = 19/89 rats/slices; F = 19.34, DFn = 5, DFd = 119; early *ud*: 1.87±0.15; midterm *ud*: 1.81±0.13; late *ud*: 1.77±0.08; Co: 1.03±0.03; p<0.001 for all). Comparison of the ratios of the three subgroups of *ud* rats showed significant differences among temporal groups only for LSO (p = 0.0208 for early *ud* vs. midterm *ud*; p<0.001 for early *ud* vs. late *ud*). Activating a cochlear implant on one ear (*us*) with the other ear hearing acoustically maintained an ipsilateral-to-contralateral balance (LSO: n = 6/29 rats/slices; early *us*: 0.98±0.04; midterm *us*: 1.07±0.04; CIC: n = 6/30 rats/slices, early *us*: 1.07±0.06; midterm *us*: 1.05±0.03; p> 0.05 for all). For both LSO and CIC, significant differences were detected between the subgroups of *ud* and *us* rats (p<0.001 for all). Dotted line indicated bilateral symmetry (1.0). Significant differences against control level were indicated by asterisks above bars. (B) Results for *gap43* transcription in LSO (n = 29/142 rats/slices) indicated that staining intensity increased significantly against controls (Co) in LSOc of *ud* rats independent of the duration of deafness (n = 19/89 rats/slices; F = 37.55, DFn = 11, DFd = 272; p<0.001). By contrast, the mean staining intensity decreased after early *ud* in LSOi (p = 0.0158), while it increased significantly after late *ud*, compared to controls (p = 0.0069). Additionally, the staining intensity of all *ud* rats on the contralateral side was significantly higher as compared to bilaterally deafened (*bd*) rats (n = 15/87 rats/slices; F = 86.54, DFn = 6, DFd = 167; ###: p<0.001). On the ipsilateral side, a significant rise against the staining intensity of *bd* was verified only following a longer duration of *ud* (###: p<0.001). A comparison of late *ud* rats with early and midterm *ud* rats showed a bilateral increase of mean Gap43 mRNA staining intensity with sustained duration of deafness (F = 27.52, DFn = 9, DFd = 170; p = 0.002 for midterm *ud* i vs. late *ud* i; p<0.001 for all other). After *us*, neurons in both LSOs increased their *gap43* transcription level independent of stimulation duration against controls (F = 37.55, DFn = 11, DFd = 272; p<0.001 for all). Staining intensities of LSOi of both subgroups of *us* rats were higher than the ipsilateral intensities of isochronously *ud* rats (n = 17/90 rats/slices; F = 27.52, DFn = 9, DFd = 170; p<0.001 for both). (D) Results for *gap43* transcription in CIC (n = 29/145 rats/slices) showed that staining intensity increased against controls in CICi of *ud* rats after a midterm and late period of deafness (n = 19/91 rats/slices; F = 25.16, DFn = 11, DFd = 278; p = 0.0028 for midterm ud i vs. Co; p<0.001 for late *ud* i vs. Co). By contrast, the mean staining intensity decreased after early *ud* in CICc (p = 0.0094), while it increased significantly after late *ud* compared to controls (p = 0.0094). Staining intensities of all *ud* rats on the ipsilateral side were significantly higher than for bilaterally deafened (*bd*) rats (n = 15/89 rats/slices; F = 57.93, DFn = 6, DFd = 171; #: p = 0.03 for early *ud* i vs. *bd*; ###: p<0.001 for other both). Contralaterally, a significant rise against the staining intensity of *bd* was seen only following longer lasting *ud* (###: p<0.001), while it significantly decreased after early *ud* (#: p = 0.01). A comparison of late *ud* rats with early and midterm *ud* rats showed a bilateral increase of mean Gap43 mRNA staining intensities with duration of deafness (F = 22.22, DFn = 9, DFd = 180; p = 0.001 for midterm *ud* c vs. late *ud* c; p<0.001 for all other). After *us*, both CICs increased their *gap43* transcription level significantly only after a midterm duration of *us* compared to control (25.16, DFn = 11, DFd = 278; p<0.001 for both). Staining intensities of CICc of both subgroups of *us* rats were higher than the contralateral intensities of isochronously *ud* rats (n = 17/95 rats/slices; F = 22.22, DFn = 9, DFd = 180; p = 0.0155 for early *us* c vs. early *ud* c; p<0.001 for midterm *us* c vs. midterm *ud* c). Significance levels: (***/###) for p<0.001, (**) for p<0.01, (*/#) for p<0.05. LSO: lateral superior olive; CIC: central inferior colliculus; i: ipsilateral; c: contralateral.

nucleus (cp. Fig. 8B and arrowheads in inset). This basal level of specific staining persisted independent of experimental treatment (cp. Fig. 8B) and was generally more prominent than we reported in our earlier work [19,37], for which tissue fixation including glutaraldehyde was used.

In LSO, no obvious changes in Gap43 protein expression were observed despite prominent changes in Gap43 mRNA level in the

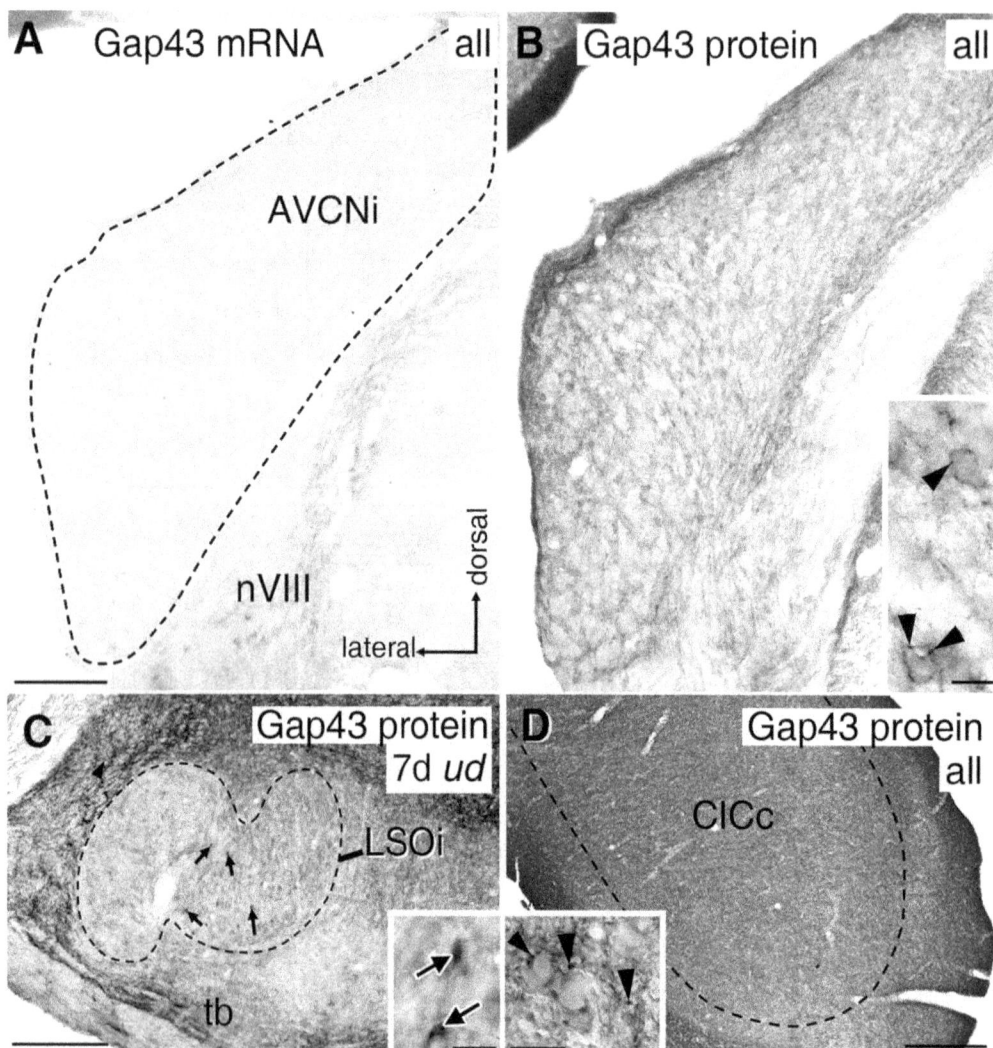

Figure 8. Gap43 mRNA and protein expression in auditory brainstem. (A) Anteroventral cochlear nucleus (AVCN, dashed line) was devoid of Gap43 mRNA staining on both sides under any experimental condition. (B) Faintly stained Gap43 protein-positive axonal boutons were present throughout AVCN in controls and all experimental conditions. Inset: higher magnification of immuno-positive presynaptic endings (arrowheads). (C) Gap43 protein expression in lateral olivocochlear neurons (arrows) within LSOi (dashed line) required at least 5 days (d) of electrode implantation independent of its activation. Inset: close-up of Gap43 protein-positive neurons (arrows) and boutons following 7d of *ud*. (D) Throughout CIC (dashed line), Gap43 immunoreactivity was always present. Inset: close-up of immuno-positive presynaptic endings (arrowheads). Scale bars for A to D: 0.2 mm. Scale bars of insets B to D: 20 μm. LSO: lateral superior olive; CIC: central inferior colliculus; nVIII: 8th cranial nerve; tb: trapezoid body; i: ipsilateral; c: contralateral; *ud*: unilateral deafness.

cytoplasm of neurons. Only isolated cells contained Gap43 protein on the deaf or stimulated side (Fig. 8C, arrows and inset). However, development of Gap43 protein within these neuronal somata, likely to be LOC neurons [38], required at least 5 days of deafness or chronic EIS. A basal level of immunopositive fibers and presynaptic endings was observed in LSO, with the highest density consistently found in its medial region. These Gap43 immunoreactive endings appeared to remain unaltered on both sides of LSO in all four experimental groups (cp. Fig. 8C).

On the level of CIC, Gap43 immunoreactivity was notable in an area-wide network of stained thin fibers and small boutons which we identified as presynaptic endings in an ultrastructural investigation (unpublished results) (Fig. 8D, and arrowheads in inset). As described for LSO, immunoreactivity was found to be unaffected by experimental treatment on both sides of the brainstem.

Expression of Fos mRNA and Protein Decreases with Increasing Stimulation Time

Fos mRNA and protein staining served as a marker for the effectiveness of tonotopic activation of auditory brainstem neurons. In controls, only a negligible number of Fos mRNA and protein positive neurons was seen anywhere in the auditory brainstem (cp. Fig. 9A, B, inset). Activated by chronic EIS showing four identifiable positive peaks in the EABR (Fig. 2C), neurons in the ipsilateral anteroventral cochlear nucleus (AVCNi) contained Fos mRNA and protein in a regionally restricted area. This region corresponded tonotopically to the intracochlear stimulation site (Fig. 9). A correspondingly restricted population of Fos positive neurons was seen in LSOi and CICc [39]. Following one day of sustained EIS, only a sparse level of Fos mRNA positive neurons was observed, while a slightly reduced but still recognizable number of neurons expressing Fos protein existed in these auditory

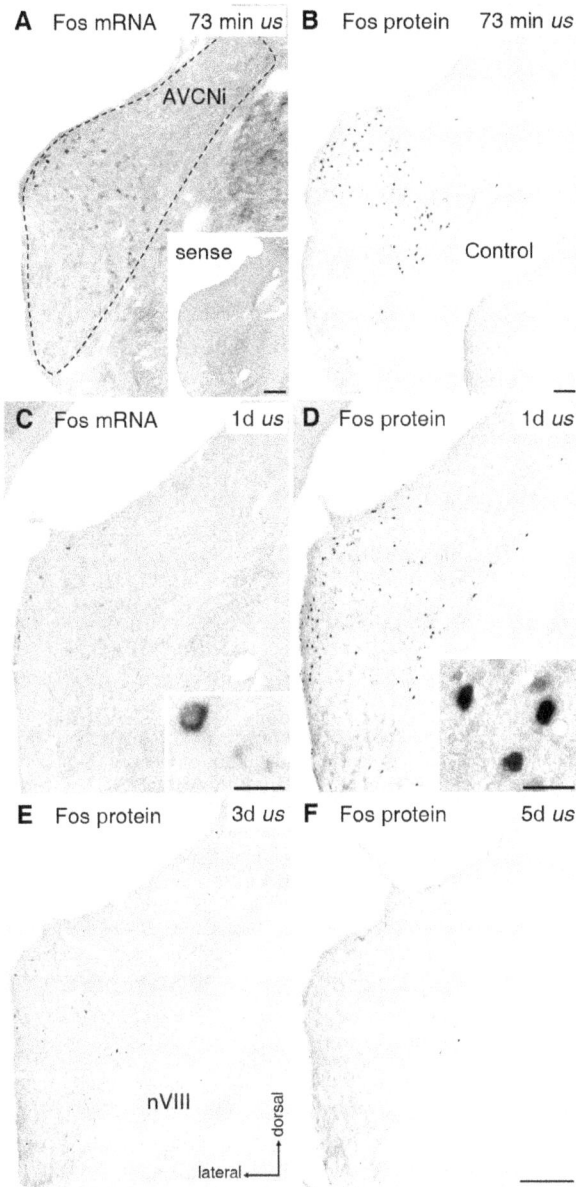

Figure 9. The effectiveness of electrical intracochlear stimulation (EIS) on neurons of the anteroventral cochlear nucleus (AVCN). Fos mRNA (A) and Fos protein (B) closely corresponded locally after EIS for under 2 h duration. (A, C) Fos mRNA expression (black dots) in neurons of ipsilateral (i) AVCN after 73 min (A; cp. Illing and Rosskothen-Kuhl, 2012) and 1 day (d) (C) of unilateral stimulation (us). Fos-positive neurons were spatially limited to regions tonotopically corresponding to frequencies processed at the site of intracochlear electrode position. The number of labeled neurons was higher after 73 min than after 1d of us. Inset A: AVCNi was devoid of staining after incubation with Fos sense probe. Inset C: higher magnification of mRNA-positive neurons, showing strongest staining in cytoplasm. (B, D) Fos protein staining (black dots) in AVCNi after 73 min (B; cp. Illing and Rosskothen-Kuhl, 2012) and 1d (D) of us. Protein expression was spatially limited to a band tonotopically corresponding to intracochlear stimulation position. Inset B: AVCNi of control. Scale bars in insets A and B: 0.2 mm. Inset D: higher magnification of Fos protein positive nuclei in AVCNi. Scale bars in insets C and D: 20 μm. (E) Three days after sustained EIS a strong decrease in the number of Fos protein positive nuclei was observable. (F) Following 5d of us, no further protein positive nuclei were detectable. Scale bar for A to E: 0.2 mm. nVIII: 8th cranial nerve.

regions (cp. Fig. 9C, D). By 3 days of chronic EIS, the number of neurons stained for Fos protein has even more decreased in the activated area (Fig. 9E). Following EIS for longer than 3 days, no mRNA and protein positive neurons were detected in VCN, LSO, and CIC (cp. Fig. 9F).

Discussion

This study is the first to demonstrate that *gap43* transcription may be modulated by the level and pattern of sensory activity in an intact adult mammalian brain. Studies involving transgenic mice overexpressing *gap43*, *gap43* knock-down, or *gap43* gene silencing have collected an impressive body of evidence suggesting the protein Gap43 to be involved in axonal growth and the formation and plasticity of synaptic contacts [8–12]. Specifically, the neuronal transcription of *gap43* is changed asymmetrically in the central auditory brainstem as soon as sensory evoked activity is unilaterally lost. However, the formation of such asymmetry between both sides of the brainstem can be prevented. A simple-patterned stimulation of the auditory nerve on the side of a deaf ear is sufficient to maintain the bilateral balance of Gap43 mRNA on the levels of LSO and CIC (Fig. 10).

Asymmetric Activation of the Adult Auditory System Triggers Imbalanced *gap43* Transcription

In a normally functioning adult rat brain and in brains of unilaterally or bilaterally hearing impaired rats, neurons of LSO and CIC maintain the same ipsilateral-to-contralateral ratios of *gap43* transcription close to 1. Based on this result, we pooled these groups as our statistical reference (Co; Figs. 6, 7). The lack of massive molecular changes by a rise of hearing threshold of 50 dB suggests that even a notably dampened auditory environment is sufficient to maintain a qualitatively normal pattern of neuronal activity due to aural and interaural stimulation. The level of this transcription remains unchanged by a bilateral loss of sensory input. However, total deafness of only one ear quickly results in an asymmetric change of *gap43* transcription when comparing both sides of the brainstem. One cause for this molecular imbalance must be the changed ratio of excitatory-to-inhibitory inputs of LSO and CIC neurons. While neurons in LSOi and CICc are released from their ascending excitatory input, neurons in LSOc and CICi lost their ascending inhibitory input [20,29] (Fig. 10C).

However, despite a changed excitatory-to-inhibitory ratio in LSO and CIC under ud, Gap43 mRNA levels rose only on the side where stimulation-dependent inhibition was silenced. If LSOi of ud rats receives glycinergic inhibition from MNTBi but no longer excitation from VCNi, neurons maintain a basal level of *gap43* transcription. The same applies when CICc is no longer excited by a crossed innervation from VCNi and LSOi, but inhibitory afferents from LSOc [40,41] are still active (Fig. 10C). By contrast, if LSOc lost its stimulation-dependent inhibition by way of MNTBc, an increase of Gap43 mRNA results (Fig. 10C). The same applies if CICi is excited by the sensory activated VCNc across the midline, but now misses inhibition from silenced LSOi and VCNi as a consequence of deafness [29,42]. Remarkably, this deafness-dependent induction of bilaterally asymmetric expression of Gap43 mRNA appeared to be stable. Even an auditory system unilaterally deafened for a longer time failed to recover the initial Gap43 mRNA symmetry by an intrinsic regime (cp. Fig. 5E, F), a finding matching earlier observations made after unilateral cochlear ablation [18].

It is important to note that spiking activity cannot be the sole cause for *gap43* transcription or its modulation. If it were, we should have seen some change in Gap43 mRNA expression of

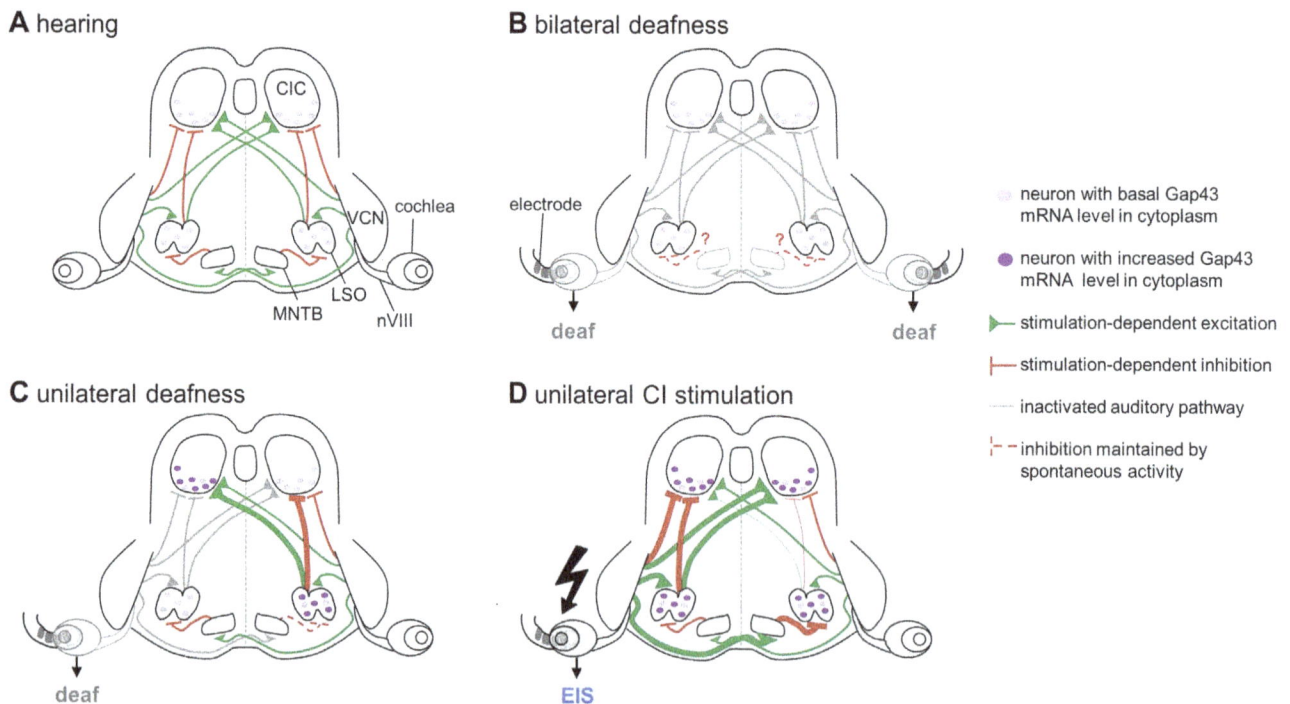

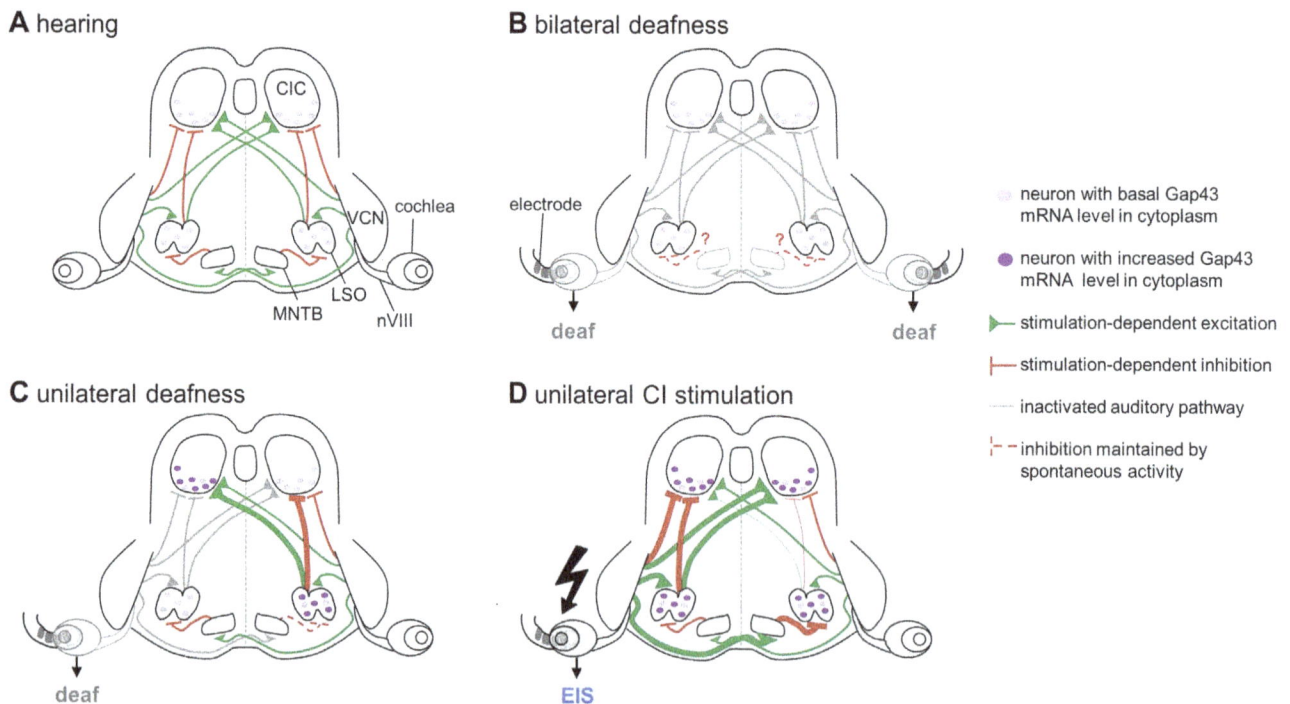

Figure 10. Expression level of Gap43 mRNA depends on synaptic cooperation in auditory brainstem nuclei. (A) Under control conditions, neurons in LSO and CIC of both sides of the brainstem receive stimulation-dependent excitatory (green) and inhibitory (red) inputs defining a functional balance with respect to metabotropic receptor activation to generate a basal level of Gap43 mRNA expression (light purple dots). (B) Induction of bilateral deafness silences all stimulation-dependent inputs (gray), leaving Gap43 mRNA levels unchanged. Question marks indicate a possible influence of spontaneous activity in MNTB neurons of unknown significance. (C) Unilateral deafness causes an imbalance of excitation and inhibition on neurons. Loss of excitation (gray) remained ineffective in modulating Gap43 mRNA levels in LSOi and CICc, whereas loss of stimulation-dependent inhibition for LSO via MNTB induces a significant increase of Gap43 mRNA staining level (dark purple dots) in LSOc and CICi. (D) Following unilateral EIS, excitatory afferents of neurons in LSOi and CICc as well as inhibitory afferents on neurons in LSOc and CICi were kept active even if the CI induced input is stronger-than-normal (thick lines). This resulted in a deviation from the normal excitatory-to-inhibitory input ratio and led to a rise of *gap43* transcription in neurons of these auditory regions (dark purple dots). nVII: 8th cranial nerve; MNTB: medial nucleus of the trapezoid body; LSO: lateral superior olive; CI: cochlear implant; CIC: central inferior colliculus; EIS: electrical intracochlear stimulation; VCN: ventral cochlear nucleus.

VCN neurons which we never did. This evidence is the first to suggest that neuronal activity plays upon *gap43* transcription in a fundamentally different way than upon *fos* transcription.

Unilateral EIS Prevents Asymmetric *gap43* Transcription in the Auditory Brainstem

When one ear of hearing-experienced adult rats was supplied with a CI and electrically stimulated while the other continued transduction of acoustic signals, a tonotopic expression of neurons containing Fos mRNA or protein was seen only in auditory regions of the electrically activated pathway (Fig. 9 [39]). This observation implies that both sides of the auditory brainstem received different strengths and patterns of sensory-evoked input. Remarkably, the same tonotopically restricted simple-patterned CI stimulation maintained the symmetry of *gap43* transcription in LSO and CIC on both sides of the brainstem rather than letting it drift into bilateral imbalance (Fig. 10D). Apparently, CI stimulation can remedy molecular consequences of a failing ear by giving auditory brainstem circuits an input sufficient to maintain synaptic cooperation on both sides of the brainstem. However, the expression level of Gap43 mRNA is significantly increased on both sides of the brainstem under this specific condition of mixed bilateral activation. An increase of Gap43 mRNA expression can also be induced by nerve crush of the facial nerve followed by

retrograde electrical stimulation of its nucleus in the adult mammalian brain [43].

Given the presence of Gap43 mRNA and the moldability of its quantity, we propose that the molecular machinery for neural circuit adaptation and reorganization is maintained in the adult auditory brainstem waiting to be unlocked. Our study shows that variations in strength and pattern of sensory input have significant impact on the expression of plasticity-related genes, such as that encoding for Gap43. We demonstrated that levels of Gap43 mRNA expression reflect altered sensory activity in conjunction with a shifted ratio between excitation and inhibition on neurons of the auditory brainstem.

Rules Governing the Modulation of *gap43* Transcription

Considering the modulation of the basal level of *gap43* transcription under various experimental conditions, we propose the following rule: Gap43 mRNA expression rises above baseline level in neurons whenever the ratio of their excitatory-to-inhibitory input changes, but only as long as both types of synapses are active (Fig. 10).

In case of bilateral hearing loss (*bd*), neurons of LSO and CIC lost both excitatory and inhibitory synaptic inputs, failing to detect a deviation from their standard ratio. As a result, neurons maintained *gap43* transcription as normal (Fig. 10A, B).

When sensory input failed on one side only (*ud*), a sustained basal *gap43* transcription persisted in neurons of LSOi and CICc, since they lost their excitatory input (Fig. 10C). By contrast, neurons in LSOc increased *gap43* transcription since stimulation-dependent inhibition by MNTBc failed due to inactivation of driving neurons in VCNi, while excitation from VCNc remained effective. As neurons of MNTB maintain a moderate spontaneous activity [44,45], glycinergic presynaptic endings on LSOc neurons are still effective in supporting second messenger systems. It is unknown if this spontaneous activity is maintained in a totally deaf brain (Fig. 10B, question marks). Thus, LSOc neurons are more strongly excited than normally but are still affected by glycinergic synapses so that second messenger cascades triggered from both glutamatergic and glycinergic receptors can interact intracellularly and increase Gap43 mRNA expression.

This dependence of *gap43* transcription on synaptic cooperation marks a sharp contrast to the regulation of *fos* expression apparently characterizing neurons exclusively or predominantly affected by excitatory input. From all 16 sites investigated for their Gap43 mRNA expression (LSO and CIC bilaterally under 4 experimental conditions, cp. Fig. 10), CICi under *ud* is the one not readily explained by the rule suggested above. As CICi under *ud* should lose inhibition by LSOi and VCNi but maintain strong excitation supplied by LSOc and VCNc, we need to additionally postulate that a disinhibition of its neurons may be sufficient to directly increase the *gap43* transcription (Fig. 10C).

Compensating a dysfunctional ear by EIS (*us*) increased sensory activity in an otherwise deaf ear. As a consequence, LSOi and CICc received a stronger-than-normal excitatory synaptic input, and inhibition is increased for LSOc and CICi at the same time. This resulted in a deviation from the normal excitatory-to-inhibitory input ratio and led to a rise of *gap43* transcription in neurons of these auditory regions (Fig. 10D).

Comparison of Gap43 mRNA and Protein Levels in the Auditory Brainstem

An important question concerns the unlocking of a neuron's potential to grow as indicated by the intracellular presence of Gap43 mRNA. Translation into protein does not trivially follow from mRNA expression. In our study, basal levels of Gap43 protein known to be quickly transported from the neuronal soma to its nerve terminals [46] were observed independent of experimental treatment (Fig. 8B–D).

VCN

By postnatal day 28, *gap43* transcription almost completely disappears from the rat VCN [18]. Correspondingly, we detected no Gap43 mRNA positive neurons in VCN of adult rats (Fig. 8A). Since this remained unchanged under any experimental condition, we suggest that VCN neurons lack the competence for initiating growth responses in adulthood. However, a basal level of Gap43 protein always existed in presynaptic endings throughout VCN (Fig. 8B, and arrowheads in inset). Since Gap43 mRNA was absent from VCN, the source of the Gap43 protein has to be elsewhere. A plausible candidate is the superior olivary complex. Cholinergic medial olivocochlear neurons of the ventral nucleus of the trapezoid body are known to be a major source for Gap43 protein in VCN [37,38,47]. Additionally, small neurons of the LSO of which some were calbindin positive [48,49], and shell neurons of the periolivary region around the LSO maintain axons heading for VCN and are potential parent cell bodies of presynaptic endings found there [48].

LSO

While the deviation of Gap43 mRNA expression from baseline level followed from changes of the ratio of excitatory-to-inhibitory synaptic input driven from both ears in LSO (Fig. 6A, B), levels of Gap43 protein failed to do so. Instead, only selected LSO neurons expressed this protein on the side of deafness-inducing electrode implantation by 5 days, independent of EIS (Fig. 8C, arrows and inset). Following cochlear ablation in adult rats, such neurons emerge throughout LSOi by 5 to 7 days and were identified as lateral olivocochlear cells [19]. We demonstrated before [38] that these neurons do not have the ability to sprout into VCN after cochlear ablation.

CIC

Ventral neurons within CIC changed their *gap43* transcription as a function of balance and strength of binaural activity. Simultaneously, numerous presynaptic endings positive for Gap43 protein were found throughout CIC and remained unaltered under different experimental conditions (Fig. 8D, and inset). Complying with physiological studies investigating interactions of bilateral acoustic stimulation in IC [31], our observations reinforce the concept of IC neurons maintaining a potential for experience-dependent adjustments even at adult age.

Overall, in the system studied here, no obvious quantitative relationship between the presence of Gap43 mRNA and protein was detected. It seems plausible, though, to suspect some functional reason behind energy and logistics expenses required for maintaining Gap43 mRNA expression in specific neuronal populations of the adult auditory brainstem. Neurons containing Gap43 mRNA in LSO and CIC may be waiting and ready for neuroplastic growth that might require another yet unidentified 'go' signal. It would be extremely important to identify the nature of this signal for understanding adult brain plasticity in general, and to put it to use for therapeutic approaches of CI patients in particular.

Gap43 Transcription does not Trivially Depend on Fos Expression

Looking for the upstream regulation of *gap43* expression, the transcription factor AP-1 and Fos as one of its monomers are obvious candidates [4,50]. The results of the present study unequivocally indicate that the transcription of *gap43* does not trivially depend on the availability of Fos. Stimulating the auditory system by unilateral EIS, Fos mRNA and protein expression increased in VCNi, LSOi, or CICc [34,39,51–53] (Fig. 9), among others. In *ud* rats, no increase of Fos expression was detectable in regions of the auditory pathway on the opposite side, but neurons of LSOc and CICi significantly increased their Gap43 mRNA transcription.

Looking closer, a local activation of the medial turn of the cochlea by EIS resulted in a tonotopically restricted Fos expression within most central auditory regions [2,39] (Fig. 9). However, a matching local restriction was not recognizable in the *gap43* transcription pattern of LSO or CIC under identical stimulation conditions. As mentioned above, VCN prominently expressing Fos after 1 or 3 days of chronic EIS never showed Gap43 mRNA positive neurons. For these reasons, no evidence can be cited to assume a dominant role of Fos in the regulation of *gap43* transcription. Apparently, then, regulation of *gap43* expression must be under the control of additional or other intracellular signaling pathways.

Clinical Relevance

In adult humans, monaural deafness can be a result of acute hearing loss, cochlear ossification, or acoustic neuroma surgery. Different medical response modalities exist for these patients, ranging from 'no treatment' up to providing the deaf ear with one of various types of hearing aids [54]. Recent studies demonstrate that EIS by way of a CI improves hearing abilities in patients with single-sided deafness and is superior to alternative treatment options mostly relying on monaural hearing alone [54,55]. Binaural hearing is more demanding on network functions and must have cellular and molecular correlates. We propose that our findings of molecular changes in auditory neurons due to variations in the strength and pattern of sensory input provide important details about these network dynamics. A major outcome of our study is that even a simple-patterned CI stimulation may remedy molecular consequences of a failing ear in central auditory neurons.

Conclusion

As suggested by Moore and Shannon [56], a deeper understanding of central auditory plasticity responses is required to further improve the effectiveness of CI-brain-interactions in patients. Proceeding in this direction, our study identifies a regulating mechanism including the transcription of the plasticity and growth associated gene *gap43* within the adult auditory brainstem. From these data we derive the hypothesis that the level of *gap43* transcription rises when two conditions are met: (1) the ratio of excitation to inhibition must deviate from normal, and (2) both types of synapses, excitatory and inhibitory, must be active to invoke second messenger cascades to interact intracellularly. In our series of experiments, these conditions are met if one ear is completely deafened or else permanently activated by EIS. With this study we provide new insights into the readiness of neurons in the adult brainstem to initiate axonal growth. The next step must be to find out how to unlock this potential.

Acknowledgments

We thank H. Hildebrandt, E. Michalk, A. Rauch, P. Janz, H. Kunert, and A. Perera for helpful discussions and proof reading the article, A. Reisch for co-development of the chronic CI setup, P. Pedersen and J. John for expert technical help, M. Kuhl for technical assistance, R. Birkenhäger and S. Weis for synthesis of in-situ hybridization probes, S. Hoff for technical assistance with probe synthesis, and R. Laszig for continuous support. Stimulation electrodes, programming software, and hardware components were kindly provided by Cochlear Germany GmbH and Co. KG, Germany.

Author Contributions

Conceived and designed the experiments: NRK RBI. Performed the experiments: NRK. Analyzed the data: NRK RBI. Wrote the paper: NRK RBI.

References

1. Ehret G, Fischer R (1991) Neuronal activity and tonotopy in the auditory system visualized by c-fos gene expression. Brain Res 567: 350–354.
2. Rosskothen N, Hirschmüller-Ohmes I, Illing RB (2008) AP-1 activity rises by stimulation-dependent c-Fos expression in auditory neurons. Neuroreport 19: 1091–1093.
3. Sheng M, Greenberg ME (1990) The regulation and function of c-fos and other immediate early genes in the nervous system. Neuron 4: 477–85.
4. de Groen PC, Eggen BJ, Gispen WH, Schotman P, Schrama LH (1995) Cloning and promoter analysis of the human B-50/GAP-43 gene. J Mol Neurosci 6: 109–119.
5. Meiri KF, Pfenninger KH, Willard MB (1986) Growth associated protein GAP-43, a polypeptide that is induced when neurons extend axons, is a component of growth cones and corresponds to pp46, a major polypeptide of a subcellular fraction enriched in growth cones. Proc Natl Acad Sci U S A 83: 3537–3541.
6. Gerin CG, Madueke IC, Perkins T, Hill S, Smith K, et al. (2011) Combination strategies for repair, plasticity, and regeneration using regulation of gene expression during the chronic phase after spinal cord injury. Synapse 65: 1255–1281.
7. Benowitz LI, Routtenberg A (1997) GAP-43: an intrinsic determinant of neuronal development and plasticity. Trends Neurosci 20: 84–91.
8. Aigner L, Arber S, Kapfhammer JP, Laux T, Schneider C, et al. (1995) Overexpression of the neural growth-associated protein GAP-43 induces nerve sprouting in the adult nervous system of transgenic mice. Cell 83: 269–278.
9. Strittmatter SM, Fankhauser C, Huang PL, Mashimo H, Fishman MC (1995) Neuronal pathfinding is abnormal in mice lacking the neuronal growth cone protein GAP-43. Cell 80: 445–452.
10. Rekart JL, Meiri K, Routtenberg A (2005) Hippocampal-dependent memory is impaired in heterozygous GAP-43 knockout mice. Hippocampus 15: 1–7.
11. Grasselli G, Mandolesi G, Strata P, Cesare P (2011) Impaired sprouting and axonal atrophy in cerebellar climbing fibres following in vivo silencing of the growth-associated protein GAP-43. PLoS One 6: e20791.
12. Grasselli G, Strata P (2013) Structural plasticity of climbing fibers and the growth-associated protein GAP-43. Front Neural Circuits 7: 25.
13. Bendotti C, Servadio A, Samanin R (1991) Distribution of GAP-43 mRNA in the brain stem of adult rats as evidenced by in situ hybridization: localization within monoaminergic neurons. J Neurosci 11: 600–607.
14. Benowitz LI, Perrone-Bizzozero NI (1991) The expression of GAP-43 in relation to neuronal growth and plasticity: When, where, how, and why? Prog Brain Res 89: 69–87.
15. Kruger L, Bendotti C, Rivolta R, Samanin R (1993) Distribution of GAP-43 mRNA in the adult rat brain. J Comp Neurol 333: 417–34.
16. Casoli T, Stefano GD, Fattoretti P, Solazzi M, Delfino A, et al. (2003) GAP-43 mRNA detection by in situ hybridization, direct and indirect in situ RT-PCR in hippocampal and cerebellar tissue sections of adult rat brain. Micron 34: 415–22.
17. Yao GL, Kiyama H, Tohyama M (1993) Distribution of GAP-43 (B50/F1) mRNA in the adult rat brain by in situ hybridization using an alkaline phosphatase labeled probe. Mol Brain Res 18: 1–6.
18. Illing RB, Cao QL, Förster CR, Laszig R (1999) Auditory brainstem: development and plasticity of GAP-43 mRNA expression in the rat. J Comp Neurol 412: 353–372.
19. Illing RB, Horváth M, Laszig R (1997) Plasticity of the auditory brainstem: effects of cochlear lesions on GAP-43 immunoreactivity in the rat. J Comp Neurol 382: 116–138.
20. Moore MJ, Caspary DM (1983) Strychnine block binaural inhibition in lateral superior olivary neurons. J Neurosci 3: 237–242.
21. Sanes DH, Rubel EW (1988) The ontogeny of inhibition and excitation in the Gerbil lateral superior olive. J Neurosci 8: 682–700.
22. Tollin DJ (2003) The lateral superior olive: A functional role in sound source localization. Neuroscientist 9: 127–143.
23. Caspary DM, Finlayson PG (1991) Superior olivary complex: Functional neuropharmacology of the principal cell types. In: Altschuler RA, Bobbin RP, Clopton BM, Hoffman DW, editors, Neurobiology of Hearing: the Central Auditory System. Raven Press, New York, NY. 141–161.
24. Schwartz IR (1992) The superior olivary complex and lateral lemniscal nuclei. In: Webster B, Popper AN, Fay RR, editors, The Mammalian Auditory Pathways: Neuroanatomy. Springer-Verlag, New York, NY. 117–167.
25. Kullmann PH, Ene FA, Kandler K (2002) Glycinergic and GABAergic calcium responses in the developing lateral superior olive. Eur J Neurosci 15: 1093–104.
26. Kandler K, Clause A, Noh J (2009) Tonotopic reorganization of developing auditory brainstem circuits. Nat Neurosci 12: 711–717.
27. Malmierca MS (2003) The structure and physiology of the rat auditory system: an overview. Int Rev Neurobiol 58: 147–211.
28. Winer JA, Larue DT, Diehl JJ, Hefti BJ (1998) Auditory cortical projections to the cat inferior colliculus. J Comp Neurol 400: 147–174.
29. Saint Marie RL, Ostapoff EM, Morest DK, Wenthold RJ (1989) Glycine-immunoreactive projection of the cat lateral superior olive: possible role in midbrain ear dominance. J Comp Neurol 279: 382–396.
30. Kelly JB, Glenn SL, Beaver CJ (1991) Sound frequency and binaural response properties of single neurons in rat IC. Hear Res 56: 273–280.
31. Mei HX, Cheng L, Tang J, Fu ZY, Wang X, et al. (2012) Bilateral collicular interaction: modulation of auditory signal processing in amplitude domain. PLoS One 7, e41311.
32. Hildebrandt H, Hoffmann NA, Illing RB (2011) Synaptic reorganization in the adult rat's ventral cochlear nucleus following its total sensory deafferentation. PLoS One 6, e23686.
33. Jero J, Coling DE, Lalwani AK (2001) The use of Preyer's reflex in evaluation of hearing in mice. Acta Otolaryngol 121: 585–589.
34. Illing RB, Michler SA (2001) Modulation of P-CREB and expression of c-Fos in cochlear nucleus and superior olive following electrical intracochlear stimulation. Neuroreport 12: 875–878.

35. Jakob T, Illing RB (2008) Laterality, intensity, and frequency of electrical intracochlear stimulation are differentially mapped into specific patterns of gene expression in the rat auditory brainstem. Audiol Med 6: 215–227.

36. Illing RB, Michler SA, Kraus KS, Laszig R (2002) Transcription factor modulation and expression in the rat auditory brainstem following electrical intracochlear stimulation. Exp Neurol 175: 226–244.

37. Meidinger MA, Hildebrandt-Schoenfeld H, Illing RB (2006) Cochlear damage induces GAP-43 expression in cholinergic synapses of the rat cochlear nucleus in the adult rat: A light and electron microscopical study. Eur J Neurosci 23: 3187–3199.

38. Kraus KS, Illing RB (2004) Superior olivary contributions to auditory system plasticity: medial but not lateral olivocochlear neurons are the source of cochleotomy-induced GAP-43 expression in the ventral cochlear nucleus. J Comp Neurol 475: 374–390.

39. Rosskothen-Kuhl N, Illing RB (2010) Nonlinear development of the populations of neurons expressing c-Fos under sustained electrical intracochlear stimulation in the rat auditory brainstem. Brain Res 1347: 33–41.

40. Kelly JB, Li L (1997) Two sources of inhibition affecting binaural evoked responses in the rat's inferior colliculus: the dorsal nucleus of the lateral lemniscus and the superior olivary complex. Hear Res 104: 112–126.

41. Saint Marie RL, Baker RA (1990) Neurotransmitter-specific uptake and retrograde transport of [3H] glycine from the inferior colliculus by ipsilateral projections of the superior olivary complex and nuclei of the lateral lemniscus. Brain Res 524: 244–253.

42. Thompson AM, Schofield BR (2000) Afferent projections of the superior olivary complex. Microsc Res Tech 51: 330–354.

43. Sharma N, Marzo SJ, Jones KJ, Foecking EM (2010) Electrical stimulation and testosterone differentially enhance expression of regeneration-associated genes. Exp Neurol. 223: 183–191.

44. Smith PH, Joris PX, Yin TC (1998) Anatomy and physiology of principal cells of the medial nucleus of the trapezoid body (MNTB) of the cat. J Neurophysiol 79: 3127–3142.

45. Sommer I, Lingenhöhl K, Friauf E (1993) Principal cells of the rat medial nucleus of the trapezoid body: an intracellular in vivo study of their physiology and morphology. Exp Brain Res 95: 223–39.

46. Skene JH, Willard M (1981) Characteristics of growth-associated polypeptides in regenerating toad retinal ganglion cell axons. J Neurosci 1: 419–426.

47. Fredrich M, Zeber AC, Hildebrandt H, Illing RB (2013) Differential molecular profiles of astrocytes in degeneration and re-innervation after sensory deafferentation of the adult rat cochlear nucleus. Eur J Neurosci 38: 2041–56.

48. Horváth M, Kraus KS, Illing RB (2000) Olivocochlear neurons sending axon collaterals into the ventral cochlear nucleus of the rat. J Comp Neurol 422: 95–105.

49. Illing RB, Rosskothen-Kuhl N, Fredrich M, Hildebrandt H, Zeber AC (2010) Imaging the plasticity of the central auditory system on the cellular and molecular level. Audiol Med 8: 63–76.

50. Diolaiti D, Bernardoni R, Trazzi S, Papa A, Porro A, et al. (2007) Functional cooperation between TrkA and p75(NTR) accelerates neuronal differentiation by increased transcription of GAP-43 and p21(CIP/WAF) genes via ERK1/2 and AP-1 activities. Exp Cell Res 14: 2980–2992.

51. Rosskothen-Kuhl N, Illing RB (2012) The impact of hearing experience on signal integration in the auditory brainstem: A c-Fos study of the rat. Brain Res 1435: 40–55.

52. Bischoff P, Rosskothen-Kuhl N, Illing RB (2013) Systemically antagonizing L-type calcium channels modifies intensity and pattern of Fos expression evoked by electrical intracochlear stimulation in the adult rat auditory brainstem. Otolarygology S3: 005. doi:10.4172/2161-119X. S3-005.

53. Illing RB, Rosskothen-Kuhl N (2012) The Cochlear Implant in Action: Molecular Changes Induced in the Rat Central Auditory System. In: Umat C, Tange RA, editors. Cochlear Implant Research Updates. ISBN: 978-953-51-0582-4, InTech, DOI: 10.5772/34440. 137–166.

54. Arndt S, Aschendorff A, Laszig R, Beck R, Schild C, et al. (2011) Comparison of pseudobinaural hearing to real binaural hearing rehabilitation after cochlear implantation in patients with unilateral deafness and tinnitus. Otol Neurotol 32: 39–47.

55. Firszt JB, Holden LK, Reeder RM, Waltzman SB, Arndt S (2012) Auditory abilities after cochlear implantation in adults with unilateral deafness: A pilot study. Otol Neurotol 33: 1339–1346.

56. Moore DR, Shannon RV (2009) Beyond cochlear implants: awakening the deafened brain. Nat Neurosci 12: 686–691.

6

Contribution of Auditory Working Memory to Speech Understanding in Mandarin-Speaking Cochlear Implant Users

Duoduo Tao[1,2], Rui Deng[1], Ye Jiang[1], John J. Galvin III[2,3], Qian-Jie Fu[1,2,3], Bing Chen[1]*

1 Department of Otology and Skull Base Surgery, Eye Ear Nose and Throat Hospital, Fudan University, Shanghai, China, 2 Division of Communication and Auditory Neuroscience, House Research Institute, Los Angeles, California, United States of America, 3 Department of Head and Neck Surgery, David Geffen School of Medicine, UCLA, Los Angeles, California, United States of America

Abstract

Purpose: To investigate how auditory working memory relates to speech perception performance by Mandarin-speaking cochlear implant (CI) users.

Method: Auditory working memory and speech perception was measured in Mandarin-speaking CI and normal-hearing (NH) participants. Working memory capacity was measured using forward digit span and backward digit span; working memory efficiency was measured using articulation rate. Speech perception was assessed with: (a) word-in-sentence recognition in quiet, (b) word-in-sentence recognition in speech-shaped steady noise at +5 dB signal-to-noise ratio, (c) Chinese disyllable recognition in quiet, (d) Chinese lexical tone recognition in quiet. Self-reported school rank was also collected regarding performance in schoolwork.

Results: There was large inter-subject variability in auditory working memory and speech performance for CI participants. Working memory and speech performance were significantly poorer for CI than for NH participants. All three working memory measures were strongly correlated with each other for both CI and NH participants. Partial correlation analyses were performed on the CI data while controlling for demographic variables. Working memory efficiency was significantly correlated only with sentence recognition in quiet when working memory capacity was partialled out. Working memory capacity was correlated with disyllable recognition and school rank when efficiency was partialled out. There was no correlation between working memory and lexical tone recognition in the present CI participants.

Conclusions: Mandarin-speaking CI users experience significant deficits in auditory working memory and speech performance compared with NH listeners. The present data suggest that auditory working memory may contribute to CI users' difficulties in speech understanding. The present pattern of results with Mandarin-speaking CI users is consistent with previous auditory working memory studies with English-speaking CI users, suggesting that the lexical importance of voice pitch cues (albeit poorly coded by the CI) did not influence the relationship between working memory and speech perception.

Editor: Howard Nusbaum, The University of Chicago, United States of America

Funding: This work was funded in part by the Special Fund for Projects of Ministry of Health of China (#201202005), the National Nature Science Foundation of China (#81371087), Shanghai Science and Technology Commission Medical Guide Project (#134119a1800), and by National Institutes of Health (NIH) grant R01-DC004993. The funders had no role in study design, data collection and analysis, decision to publish, or preparation of the manuscript.

Competing Interests: The authors have declared that no competing interests exist.

* E-mail: entdtao@gmail.com

Introduction

The cochlear implant (CI) has been very successful in restoring hearing and communication to many adult and pediatric patients with severe hearing loss. Despite this success, CI speech performance remains much poorer than that of normal hearing (NH) listeners, and there is much variability in CI outcomes [1–6]. Previous studies have used demographic information (e.g., age at implantation, duration of deafness, etc.), etiology of deafness, CI device type and speech processing strategy, educational and family background to explain the variability in CI outcomes, but with limited success [7,8]. Other factors may also contribute to the variability in CI outcomes, such as CI users' perceptual, cognitive and linguistic capabilities. Pisoni and colleagues [9–11] have investigated some of these "higher-level" measures to explain individual differences in information processing that may underlie speech performance and language development.

One such higher-level process is working memory, which can be defined as a temporary storage mechanism for awareness, sensory perception or information retrieved from long-term memory [12]. Short-term memory may be considered to be a subset of working memory. In speech, short-term working memory is used to encode, store, maintain, and retrieve phonological and lexical representations of words for both speech perception and production [13]. Short-term working memory bridges the sensory input and a listener's long-term pattern representations. One way to assess short-term working memory is to measure the number of familiar items that can be recalled in correct serial order. Digit span recall is commonly used to measure verbal working memory capacity. Forward digit span requires a listener to repeat a sequence of digits in the correct order; backward digit span requires a listener to repeat a sequence of digits in reverse order [9,10,14–18]. Forward digit span is considered to be a measure of rapid phonological coding skill, with relatively little cognitive processing demand, while backward digit span requires greater cognitive load [19,20]. Forward and backward digit span can be used to estimate the capacity of short-term working memory [10].

Verbal rehearsal speed (i.e., articulation rate) can be used to measure the efficiency of short-term working memory [10]. Articulation rate is measured by asking listeners to repeat words in meaningful or non-meaningful sentences, which typically contains approximately seven syllables [21]. Different from digit span tasks, articulation rate may reflect listeners' ability to keep and retrieve information in short-term memory for more complex linguistic processes, such as word recognition, sentence recognition and speech production. Articulation rate, a measure of working memory efficiency, has been correlated with working memory capacity [9,10,22,23].

Previous studies have shown that short-term working memory is linked to NH children's ability to recognize and learn new words [24,25]. NH children's ability to mimic the sound of nonsense words has also been correlated with vocabulary and novel word learning [24,26]. Other research [27] has suggested that speech and language development are closely associated with verbal working memory. Speech perception and language processing are closely correlated, and both depend on rapid and efficient phonological coding of speech in short-term memory [13,25,28].

When the auditory periphery is impaired, listeners may experience a greater cognitive load that may be due to limited capacity and/or efficiency of short-term working memory. Stiles et al. [29] compared performance of six- to nine-year-olds with mild to moderate hearing loss to that of NH peers for phonological and visuospatial tasks that targeted short-term memory. Although articulation rate and vocabulary were lower in hearing-impaired (HI) children than in NH peers, there was no significant difference in speech performance between NH and HI children. This result is in contrast to those for children who use a CI. Watson et al [30] found significantly lower digit span and articulation rate (using nonsense words) performance for CI children than for NH peers. Pisoni et al. [22] reported similar results for digit span performance in older CI children. Watson et al [30] compared cortical recordings and working memory performance in age-matched NH and CI listeners. Results showed a significant correlation between the mismatch negativity activation (pre-attentive) and auditory working memory in NH children, but not in CI children. The authors suggested that severe hearing impairment may have disrupted or limited language development in CI children. Taken together, these studies also suggest that severe hearing loss, as experienced by pediatric CI users, may also impair normal development of short-term working memory.

Pisoni and Geers [9] found significant correlations between auditory digit span and speech performance in 43 pediatric CI participants with a relatively homogeneous demographic background, even after several years of CI experience [22]. Pisoni and Cleary [10] measured forward and backward digit span, articulation rate and spoken word recognition in 176 pediatric CI participants. Correlation analyses showed that 20% of the variance in word recognition scores could be explained by

articulation rate (i.e., working memory efficiency), with 7% of the variance explained by digit span performance (i.e., working memory capacity). Nittrouer et al. [31] measured serial recall of non-rhyming nouns, rhyming nouns and non-rhyming adjectives in NH adults and children, as well as CI children. Results showed that CI children were less accurate in serial recall than NH children. However, the rate of recall did not significantly differ between CI and NH children, suggesting that working memory capacity, rather than working memory efficiency (as suggested by the Pisoni studies), may explain the variance in speech performance among CI children.

Given these somewhat inconsistent findings regarding the effects of short-term working memory on CI users' speech performance, we compared working memory and speech in young Mandarin-speaking CI listeners. In this study, we investigated the relationship between working memory and understanding of lexical tones (single syllables), disyllables, and sentences in Mandarin-speaking listeners. We hypothesized that, consistent with previous studies with English-speaking listeners, Mandarin-speaking CI listeners would exhibit deficits in both working memory capacity and efficiency, compared with NH listeners. We also hypothesized that the different linguistic processing demands of a tonal language such as Mandarin Chinese might affect the relationship between working memory and speech performance, compared to previous studies with English-speaking listeners. Similar to previous studies by Pisoni and colleagues, working memory capacity was assessed using forward and backward digit span recall, and working memory efficiency was estimated using articulation rate.

Materials and Methods

Ethics Statement

This study was approved by the Institutional Review Board protocol of Shanghai Eye Ear Nose and Throat Hospital, Fudan University, China. Written informed consent was obtained from each participant prior to enrollment in this study.

Participants

Thirty-two CI users (21 pre-lingually deafened and 11 post-lingually deafened) participated in the experiment and completed all tests. All CI subjects were unilaterally implanted. CI participants all used the same device (Nucleus-24; Cochlear Corp.) and speech-processing strategy (Advanced Combination Encoder, or ACE). CI participants' mean age at testing was 13.0 years (SD = 4.0, range: 6.0–26.0), age at implantation was 7.7 years (SD = 5.2, range: 2.0–25.0) and mean experience with device was 5.2 years (SD = 2.3, range: 0.3–11.0). Detailed demographic information is listed in Table 1. A control group of 21 NH listeners also participated in the experiment and completed all tests. All NH participants passed hearing screening at 20 dB HL from 250 to 8000 Hz in both ears. NH participants' mean age was 11.0 years (SD = 1.6, range: 8–14). Although the sample size was different between the two subject groups, a one-way Kruskal-Wallis analysis of variance (ANOVA) on ranked data showed no significant difference in age between groups (p = 0.161). Similarly a Fisher exact test showed no significant difference in the gender distribution between groups (p = 0.159).

CI participants were tested while wearing their clinically assigned speech processors and settings; once set, they were asked to not change these settings during the course of testing. As shown in Table 1, 11 CI subjects wore hearing aids (HAs) during their everyday listening experience. During testing, the HA was removed, and these subjects were tested using the CI only. The contralateral acoustic hearing ear was not plugged during testing.

Table 1. Demographic information of all CI participants.

Participant	Age (yrs)	Sex	Age at Implantation (yrs)	CI experience (yrs)	Pre/Post-lingually deafened	Hearing Aid Experience (yrs)	Duration of Deafness (yrs)
S1	15	F	4	11	Pre	0	15
S2	10	M	2	8	Pre	0	9
S3	6	F	2	4	Pre	0	5
S4	19	M	12	7	Pre	4	18
S5	11	M	3	8	Pre	0	10
S6	11	F	6	5	Pre	0	10
S7	8	F	4	4	Pre	0	7
S8	13	M	9	4	Pre	9	12
S9	9	F	4	5	Pre	2	9
S10	9	M	4	5	Pre	0	7
S11	7	F	5	2	Pre	3	6
S12	13	M	2	11	Pre	0	12
S13	9	M	4	5	Pre	0	6
S14	11	F	2	9	Pre	0	10
S15	13	M	2	11	Pre	0	12
S16	16	M	12	4	Pre	0	16
S17	11	M	2	9	Pre	0	10
S18	10	M	2	8	Pre	0	10
S19	10	M	4	6	Pre	0	9
S20	8	M	3	5	Pre	0	7
S21	8	F	3	5	Pre	2	7
S22	12	M	7	5	Post	1	8
S23	18	F	17	1	Post	7	2
S24	13	M	10	3	Post	0	4
S25	16	M	11	5	Post	8	13
S26	23	M	22	1	Post	21	21
S27	23	F	23	0.3	Post	11	11
S28	26	M	25	1	Post	0	24
S29	9	F	7	2	Post	0	4
S30	11	F	7	4	Post	0	8
S31	23	F	20	3	Post	8	17
S32	14	M	8	6	Post	0	9

Note: Yrs = years; F = female; M = male; CI = cochlear implant.

Test methods and materials

Assessment measures included a broad range of auditory and memory tasks. Working memory capacity was measured using forward digit span and backward digit span; working memory efficiency was measured using articulation rate. Speech perception was assessed with: (a) word-in-sentence recognition in quiet, (b) word-in-sentence recognition in noise, (c) Chinese disyllable recognition in quiet, (d) Chinese lexical tone recognition in quiet. Self-reported data were also collected regarding participants' performance in schoolwork. All testing was performed in a sound treated listening booth; participants were seated 1 m away from a single loudspeaker. All stimuli were presented at 65 dBA.

Auditory digit span. Forward and backward auditory digit span recall was measured using an adaptive (1-up/1-down) procedure. Stimuli included digits zero through nine produced by a single male talker. During testing, digits were randomly selected and presented in sequence in an auditory-only context (no visual cues). Participants responded by clicking on the response boxes (labeled "0" through "9") shown on a computer screen that in order of the sequence that they heard. The initial sequence contained three digits. Depending on the correctness of response, the number of digits presented was either increased or decreased (the sequence was adjusted by two digits for the first two reversals and by one digit size for the subsequent reversals). Each test run contained 25 trials. The digit span score represented the mean number of digits that could be correctly recalled averaged across all but the first two reversals. For the forward digit span test, participants were asked to recall the sequence of digits in the order presented. For the backward digit span test, participants were asked to recall the sequence of digits in reverse order from the original presentation.

Sentence recognition. Recognition of words in sentences in quiet and in noise was assessed using the Mandarin Speech Perception (MSP) materials, which consists of 10 lists of 10 sentences each, produced by a single female talker [32]. Each sentence contains seven monosyllabic words, resulting in a total of 70 monosyllabic words for each list. For testing in noise, steady noise was spectrally shaped to match the average spectrum across all sentences produced by the female talker. The signal-to-noise ratio (SNR) was fixed at +5 dB. During testing a sentence list was randomly selected, and a sentence from that list was randomly selected and presented to the participant, who repeated the sentence as accurately as possible. Subjects were instructed that each sentence contained seven words, and to guess at words they did not understand. If the participant gave no response or only a partial response, the tester repeated the sentence and tried to elicit a more complete repetition of all seven words in the sentence. Performance was scored in terms of the percentage of words in sentences correctly identified; two lists were tested for each participant, and scores were averaged across the two runs.

Articulation rate. Articulation rate was estimated from participant responses recorded during the assessment of word-in-sentence recognition in quiet. For each participant, the mean duration of the repetition of all seven syllables was used to calculate the articulation rate, similar to [10]. Participants were instructed that each sentence would contain seven syllables, and to guess at the syllables if they were unsure. Articulation rate measures were obtained for all sentence repetitions, whether or not they were repeated correctly.

Disyllable recognition. Mandarin disyllables, like spondees in English, consist of two stressed syllables, each of which contains a lexical tone. Disyllables are most widely used in daily life by Chinese Mandarin-speaking people. Disyllable recognition was assessed using the Mandarin Disyllable Recognition Test (DRT),

which consists of 10 lists of 35 disyllables each [33]. The disyllabic test lists were phonemically balanced in three dimensions: vowels, consonants and Chinese tones. During testing, a test list was randomly selected and stimuli were randomly selected from within the list (without replacement) and presented to the participant, who repeated the disyllable as accurately as possible. The tester calculated the percentage of syllables correctly identified in disyllabic words. All syllables in the DRT were scored, resulting in a total of 70 monosyllabic words for each list. No trial-by-trial feedback was provided during the test. Two of the 10 lists were randomly selected and used to test each participant.

Mandarin lexical tone recognition. Lexical tone recognition was measured for four tonal patterns: Tone 1 (flat fundamental frequency, or F0), Tone 2 (rising F0), Tone 3 (falling-rising F0), and Tone 4 (falling F0). Stimuli were taken from the Standard Chinese Database [34]. Sixteen Mandarin Chinese words (/ba/,/bo/,/bi/,/bu/ in Pinyin) were produced by two male and two female talkers, resulting in a total of 64 tokens. In each trial, a tone was randomly selected from the stimulus set and presented to the listener. Participants responded by clicking on one of four choices shown on a computer screen, labeled as "Tone 1", "Tone 2," "Tone 3", and "Tone 4". The mean percent correct was calculated across two runs for each participant. No training or trial-by-trial feedback was provided.

Self-reported school rank. Participants (or their parents) were asked to rate their performance in schoolwork. A five-point visual analog scale was used to obtain ratings, with 1 = 0–20% rank in class, 2 = 21–40% rank in class, 3 = 41–60% rank in class, 4 = 61–80% rank in class, and 5 = 81–100% rank in class.

Results

Figure 1 shows individual CI performance for forward (black bars) and backward digit span (red bars). Inter-subject variability was quite large, with performance ranging from 1.8 to 11 for forward digit span and from 2.1 to 9.7 for backward digit span.

Figure 2 shows the distribution of scores for forward digit span (left panels) and backward digit span (right panels) for CI (top panels) and NH participants (bottom panels). The mean CI score was 4.72 (SE = 0.33) for backward digit span and 6.10 (SE = 0.35) for forward digit span. The distribution of forward digit span scores was not significantly different from the normal distribution (p = 0.382). However, the distribution of backward digit span scores was significantly different from normal (p = 0.019). The mean NH score was 5.96 (SE = 0.30) for backward digit span and 7.39 (SE = 0.21) for forward digit span. The distribution of span scores was not significantly different from the normal distribution for both forward (p = 0.495) and backward digit span (p = 0.236). A split-plot repeated measures analysis of variance (RM ANOVA) with digit span (forward or backward) as the within-subject factor and group (CI or NH) as the between-subject factor was performed on the CI and NH digit span data. Results showed that forward digit span scores were significantly better than backward digit span scores [$F(1,51)$ = 72.81, p<0.001] and that NH performance was significantly better than CI performance [$F(1,51)$ = 8.14, p = 0.006]; there were no significant interactions [$F(1,51)$ = 0.027, p = 0.871].

Figure 3 shows speech performance for CI (left panel) and NH participants (right panel). The mean CI percent correct was 77.43 (SE = 4.11) for sentence recognition in quiet, 49.68 (SE = 5.38) for sentence recognition in noise, 82.94 (SE = 3.43) for disyllable recognition, and 80.96 (SE = 2.94) for lexical tone recognition. The mean NH percent correct was 100 (SE = 0.00) for sentence recognition in quiet, 99.83 (SE = 0.10) for sentence recognition in

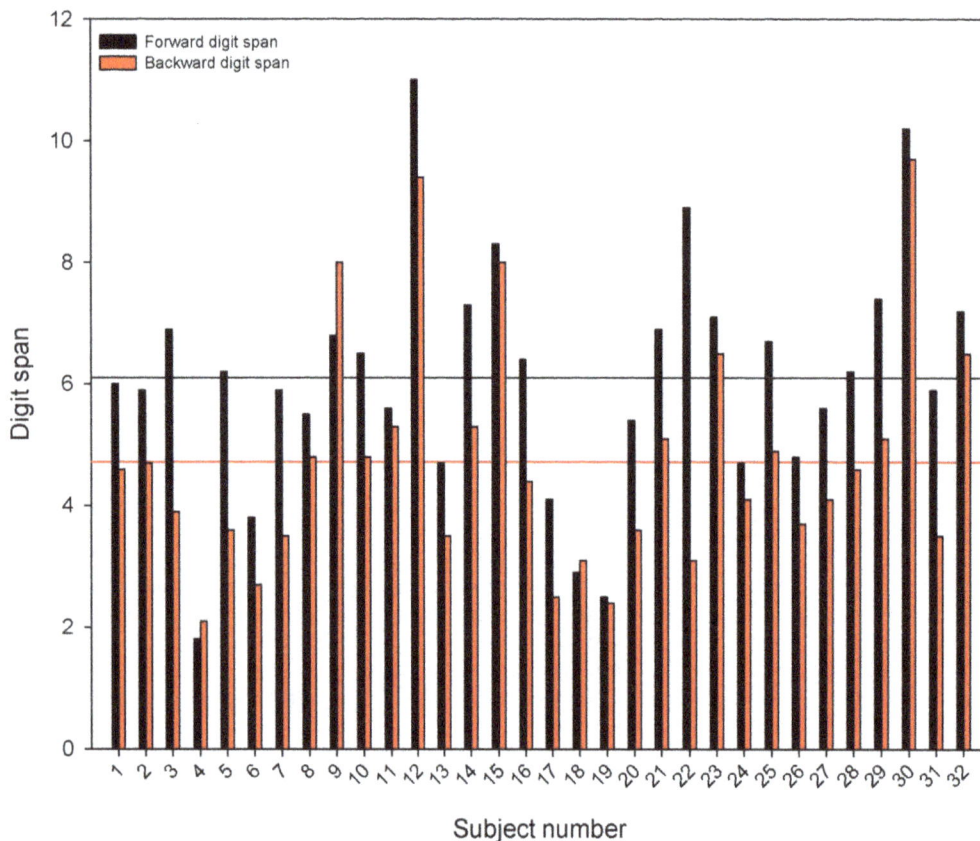

Figure 1. Forward and backward digit span scores for individual CI participants. The black bars show forward digit span data and the red bars show backward digit span data. The horizontal black line shows the mean forward digit span score and the horizontal red line shows the mean backward digit span score. CI = cochlear implant.

noise, 99.7 (SE = 0.12) for disyllable recognition, and 88.39 (SE = 3.60) for lexical tone recognition.

As shown in Table 1, 11 of the 32 CI subjects used a contralateral HA for everyday listening. The HA was removed during testing, but unfortunately the HA ear was not plugged; also no audiometric data was available for the acoustic hearing ear. A two-way ANOVA was performed on all the CI data, with everyday hearing status (CI-only or CI+HA) and speech test (sentence recognition in quiet, sentence recognition in noise, disyllable recognition, lexical tone recognition, forward digit span, backward digit span and articulation rate) as factors. Results showed a significant effect of test [$F_{(6,210)}$ = 179.188, p<0.001] but not for everyday hearing status [$F_{(1,210)}$ = 1.237, p = 0.267]; there were no significant interactions [$F_{(6,210)}$ = 1.407, p - 0.213]; Thus, while acoustic hearing without the HA may have been available to these subjects, there was no significant difference in performance between subjects who use only a CI in everyday listening and those who used a CI + HA.

A split-plot RM ANOVA with speech test (sentence recognition in quiet, sentence recognition in noise, disyllable recognition, and lexical tone recognition) as the within-subject factor and group (CI or NH) as the between-subject factor was performed on the CI and NH data. Results showed that significant effects for speech test [$F_{(1,153)}$ = 19.03, p<0.001] and subject group [$F_{(1,51)}$ = 1502.66, p<0.001]; there was a significant interactions [$F_{(3,153)}$ = 30.35, p<0.001]. Because there was a significant interaction, within-subject effects were tested independently for each group. For CI participants, a one-way RM ANOVA on ranked data showed a

significant effect of speech test (Chi-square = 45.56 with 3 degrees of freedom, p<0.001). Tukey pair-wise comparisons showed that performance for sentence recognition in quiet, disyllable recognition, and lexical tone recognition were all significantly better than for sentence recognition in noise (p<0.05). For NH participants, a one-way RM ANOVA on ranked data showed a significant effect of speech test (Chi-square = 49.40 with 3 degrees of freedom, p< 0.001). Tukey pair-wise comparisons showed that performance for sentence recognition in quiet, sentence recognition in noise, and disyllable recognition were all significantly better than for lexical tone recognition (p<0.05). One-way ANOVAs on ranked data showed that NH performance was significant better than CI performance for all speech tests (p<0.05 in all cases).

Table 2 shows simple bivariate correlations between demographic factors and speech measures. Age at testing, duration of deafness, and age at implantation were significantly correlated with sentence recognition in quiet and in noise, as well as with disyllable recognition. Duration of deafness was also significantly correlated with tone recognition. None of the demographic factors were significantly correlated with self-reported school rank.

Figure 4 shows forward (black circles) and backward (red circles) digit span as a function of articulation rate for CI (left panel) and NH participants (right panel). The mean CI articulation rate was 2526.1 ms (SE = 186.7), and the mean NH rate was 1951.2 ms (SE = 91.6). Because of the large variability in articulation rate values, especially for CI participants, articulation rate values were transformed to z-scores; the z-cores were used for subsequent analyses. Correlation analyses showed that CI participants'

CI participants

NH participants

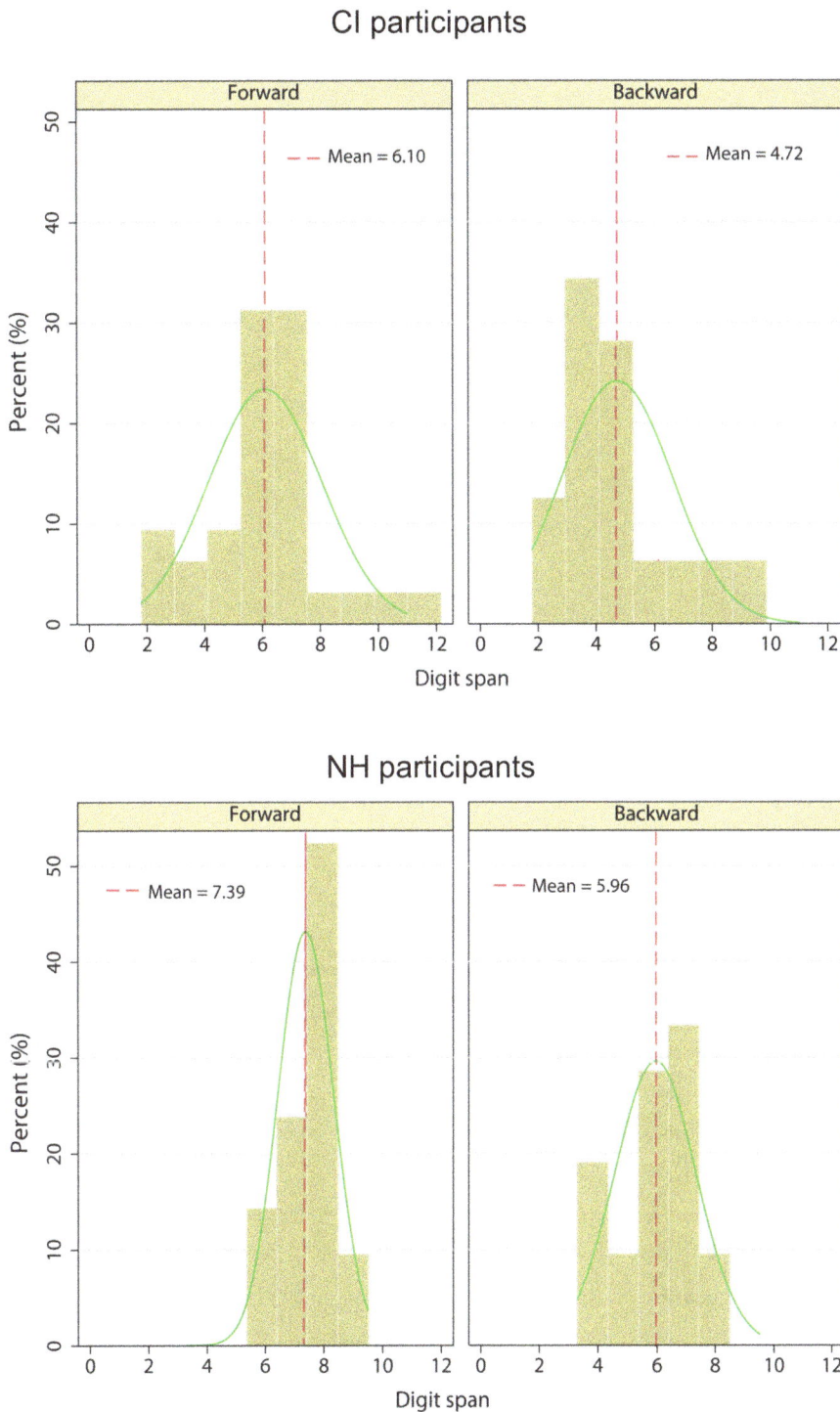

Figure 2. Distributions of forward and backward digit span scores for CI and NH participants. The left panels show forward digit span data and the right panels show backward digit span data. The top panels show CI data and the bottom panels show NH data. The vertical dashed lines show overall mean scores. The green lines show normal-density curve lines.

forward digit span was significantly correlated with articulation rate (r = −0.578, p = 0.001); the correlation between backward digit span and articulation rate failed to achieve significance (r = −0.348, p = 0.051). For NH participants, correlation analyses showed that articulation rate z-scores were significantly correlated

with both forward (r = −0.800, p<0.001) and backward digit span (r = −0.602, p = 0.004).

To better understand the relationship between working memory and speech performance, it is important to control for demographic variables likely to contribute to speech performance. As shown in Table 2, age at testing, duration of deafness, and age at

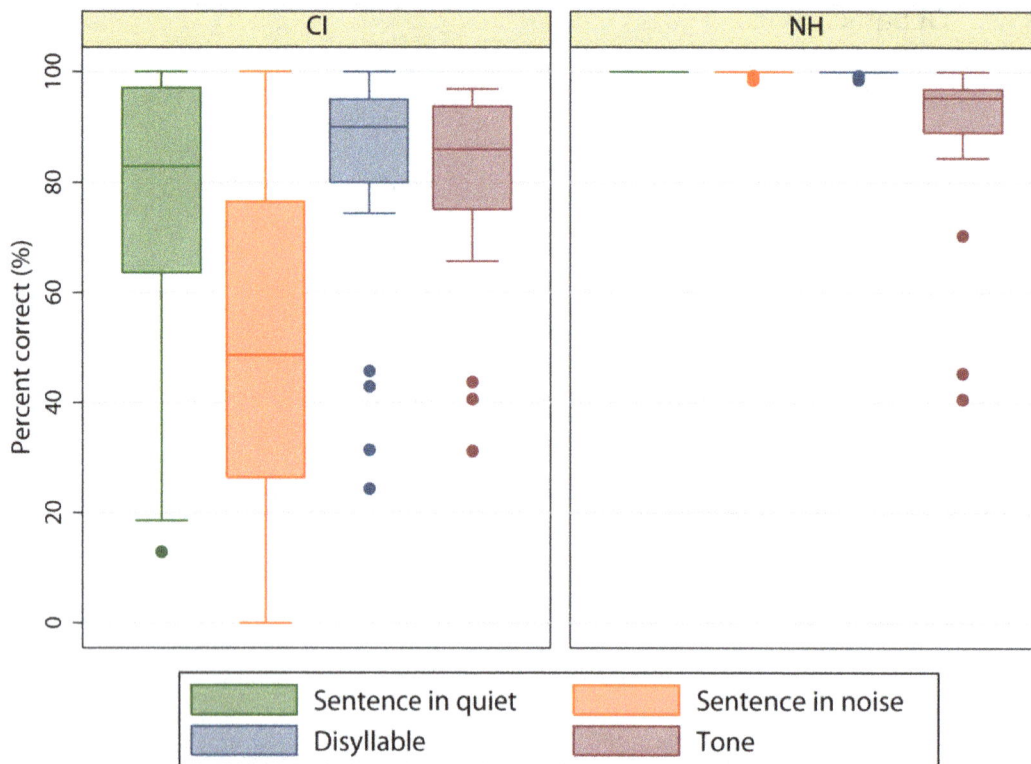

Figure 3. Boxplots of speech performance. The left panel shows CI data and the right panel shows NH data. Within each box, the horizontal line shows the mean, the error bars show the 10th and 90th percentiles, and the filled circles show outliers.

implantation were significantly correlated with most speech measures. Because these demographic factors may be inter-related, a factor analysis was performed to reduce the demo-graphic data. Factor extraction was performed using principal components analysis (PCA) for the following demographic factors: age at testing, age at implantation, duration of deafness, CI experience, and pre- or post-lingually deafened. Table 3 shows the correlations among five demographic variables. Figure 5 shows the factor loadings relating each demographic variable to each factor plotted in varimax rotated space. Because there were two components (factors), two PCA factor scores were used in the later correlation analyses between working memory and speech tests. Given a threshold of 0.7 for factor loadings, the data in Figure 5 suggest that CI experience, age at implantation, and pre- or post-lingual deafness were strongly represented by Component

1, and that age at testing and duration of deafness were strongly represented by Component 2.

Table 4 shows simple bivariate correlations and partial correlations between speech measures and working memory performance. The effects of demographic factors were partialled out using the PCA data in the partial correlations. For the simple bivariate correlation analyses, forward digit span and articulation rate were significantly correlated with sentence recognition in quiet, disyllable recognition, and tone recognition; backward digit span was correlated only with disyllable recognition. For the partial correlation analyses, most of the significant bivariate correlations persisted when statistically controlling for demograph-ic variables, except that articulation rate was no longer signifi-cantly correlated with sentence recognition in noise. Interestingly, after controlling for demographic variables, partial correlations

Table 2. Bivariate correlation between demographic variables and speech performance scores.

	SIQ	SIN	Disyllable	Tone	School rank
Age test	−0.56**	−0.63**	−0.65**	−0.39	−0.23
CI exp	0.31	0.41	0.44	0.19	0.10
Dur deaf	−0.55**	−0.51*	−0.57**	−0.47*	−0.40
Pre/post	−0.12	−0.26	−0.23	0.01	0.16
Age implant	−0.56**	−0.66**	−0.69**	−0.38	−0.22

r values are shown for each correlation. Age test = age at testing; CI exp = amount of experience with cochlear implant; Pre/Post = pre- or post-lingually deafened; Age implant = age at implantation; SIQ = sentence recognition in quiet; SIN = sentence recognition in noise.
*$p \leq 0.01$.
** $p \leq 0.001$.

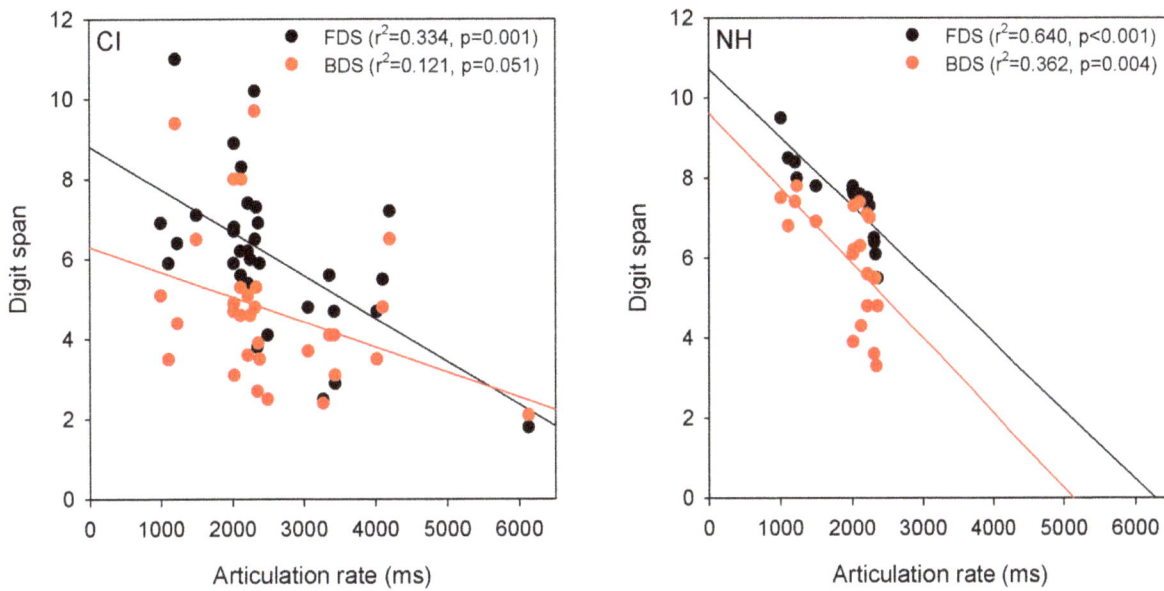

Figure 4. Forward and backward digit span as a function of articulation rate. The left panel shows CI data and the right panel shows NH data. The black circles show forward digit span data and the red circles show backward digit data. R squared values and *p* values are shown in the right of each panel. FDS = forward digit span; BDS = backward digit span.

showed that backward digit span was significantly correlated with sentence recognition in quiet (the simple bivariate correlation was not significant). For the simple bivariate correlations, forward digit span, backward digit span, and articulation rate were significantly correlated with self-reported school rank. After partialling out demographic variables, only forward and backward digit span remained significantly correlated with school rank.

Forward digit span was significantly correlated with backward digit span for both CI (r = 0.796; p<0.001) and NH participants (r = 0.647; p = 0.002). Table 5 shows correlations between working memory and speech performance while partialling out demographic factors using PCA data (as in Table 4) and partialling out either working memory capacity (forward and backward digit span) or efficiency (articulation rate). Because forward and backward digit span were significantly correlated, PCA data from factor analysis was used to reduce the working memory capacity data. When working memory capacity was partialled out, working memory efficiency was significantly correlated only with sentence recognition in quiet (r = −0.69; p<0.001). When working memory efficiency was partialled out, working memory capacity was significantly correlated only with disyllable recognition in quiet (r = 0.48; p = 0.006); working memory capacity was also significantly correlated with school rank (r = 0.61; p<0.001).

Discussion

Speech performance was significantly poorer for CI users than for NH listeners, for all speech measures. Mean CI subjects' Mandarin tone recognition, disyllable recognition and sentence recognition in quiet were all fairly good, better than 80% correct. However, sentence recognition in quiet was the most variable, with scores ranging from 12.9% to 100% correct. CI performance was poorest for sentence recognition in noise. Consistent with previous studies [9,10,22,35], forward and backward digit span scores were significantly poorer for CI than for NH participants, although there was some overlap in the distributions of digit span scores. Articulation rate was also significantly longer for CI than for NH participants. Taken together, these measures of auditory working memory suggest that CI users may experience poorer and less efficient auditory information processing than NH listeners [23]. These findings support our hypothesis that Mandarin-speaking CI participants may exhibit deficits in phonological information-processing capacity and efficiency compared with NH participants that would be reflected in the present digit span and articulation rate tasks.

CI users' sentence recognition in noise was not significantly correlated with working memory measures (see Table 4). In

Table 3. Correlation coefficents matrix from Principle Component Analysis (PCA).

	Age implant	Dur deaf	CI exp	Pre/Post
Age test	0.91	0.75	−0.33	0.59
Age implant		0.56	−0.69	0.71
Dur deaf			0.03	0.11
CI exp				−0.59

Age test = age at testing; Age implant = age at implantation; Dur deaf = duration of deafness, CI exp = amount of experience with cochlear implant; Pre/Post = pre- or post-lingually deafened;

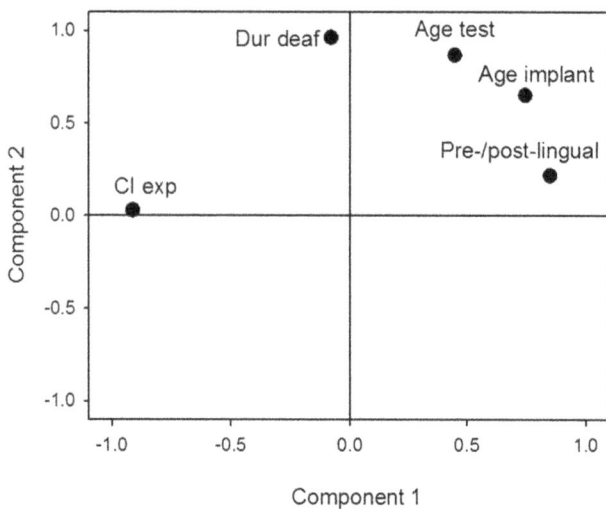

Figure 5. Factor loadings of demographic variables on two components. A varimax method was used to rotate the space. Age implant = age at implantation; Age test = age at testing; Dur deaf = duration of deafness; CI exp = CI experience; Pre-/post-lingual = pre- or post-lingually deafened.

contrast, articulation rate was significantly correlated with sentence recognition in quiet after controlling for demographic variables. The lack of correlation between sentence recognition in noise and working memory measures may have been due to masking of syllables in the sentences. As such, the items could not be reliably stored in the short-term working memory. Digit span recall and articulation rate were measured in quiet, where no such masking was present. The +5dB SNR proved very difficult for many of the present CI subjects, but has been used in previous CI studies. In Friesen et al. [36] study, sentence recognition in noise was tested at 0, +5, +10, and +15 dB SNR in adult CI users and NH listeners listening to acoustic CI simulations. With 8 channels, NH subjects scored ~60% correct while CI users scored only ~25% correct. Perhaps a better approach would have been to use an adaptive procedure to measure the speech reception threshold (SRT) - i.e., 50% correct words in sentences. Alternatively, a wider range of SNRs could have been tested.

Mean NH performance with disyllables and sentences in quiet or noise was nearly perfect, while mean performance with lexical

tones was nearly 11 points poorer. Compared with the contextual cues available for sentence and disyllable recognition, the monosyllable words used to test tone recognition contained fewer contextual cues. Also, intelligibility among the four lexical tones is not evenly distributed. Lee and Lee [37], testing NH Mandarin-speaking musicians, found that Tone 1 was most easily identified, followed by Tone 3, Tone 4, and Tone 2. Tones 2 and 3 were most easily confused, with some confusion between Tones 1 and 4. Confusion among the present tone stimuli may have similarly reduced performance relative to the context-heavy sentence and disyllable stimuli.

Forward and backward digit span scores were significantly correlated in both CI and NH participants, consistent with previous studies [9,10,22,38,39]. Because digit span data scales positively (better performance with more digits recalled) and articulation rate scales negatively (better performance with lower rate), correlations between digit span and articulation rate were negative, also consistent with previous CI studies [9,10,22,35,39]. In a study by Pisoni and colleagues [25], mean articulation rate for adolescent English-speaking CI users was 2002 ms. Interestingly, this was a follow-up study for articulation rate data collected in the same subjects 8 years earlier. At the initial measure, articulation rates were higher (mean = 3720 ms), suggesting that these CI users improved their working memory efficiency as they developed and gained experience with their device. In a recent study by Geers et al. [38], the mean articulation rate was 2024 ms for teenage CI users and 1777 ms for NH participants. In the present study, the articulation rate was slower for CI participants (mean = 2526 ms, SE = 186.7) than for NH participants (mean = 1951 ms, SE = 91.6). Some differences in methodology between this study and the Pisoni and Geers studies may explain the slower articulation rates found here. In the Pisoni studies, subjects were provided with some visual cues (e.g., lip-reading and/or the text of the sentence), which most likely improved understanding before repeating the sentence. In the present study, no visual cues or feedback was provided, which may have made speech understanding more difficult and the articulation rate slower. In the Geers study, the mean CI subject age was 16.7 years and the mean CI experience was 13.3 years. In the present study the mean CI subject age was 13.0 years and the mean CI experience 5.2 years, which may have also contributed to the slower articulation rate.

The correlation analyses shown in Table 4 showed significant correlations between many working memory and speech measures, with some exceptions (e.g., forward and backward digit span versus speech in noise; backward digit span versus tone

Table 4. Correlations between working memory and speech performance scores.

	Simple Bivariate Correlations			Partial Correlations		
	FDS	BDS	AR	FDS	BDS	AR
SIQ	0.70**	0.43	−0.79**	0.70**	0.54*	−0.77**
SIN	0.43	0.18	−0.50*	0.42	0.28	−0.41
Disyllable	0.71**	0.49*	−0.62**	0.80**	0.72**	−0.58**
Tone	0.65**	0.41	−0.54*	0.60**	0.43	−0.46*
SR	0.69**	0.63**	−0.46*	0.64**	0.64**	−0.40

r values are shown for each correlation. For the partial correlations, the reduced data from the PCA were used to statistically control for demographic variables. SIQ = sentence recognition in quiet; SIN = sentence recognition in noise; SR = self-reported school rank; FDS = forward digit span; BDS = backward digit span; AR = articulation rate.
*$p \leq 0.01$.
** $p \leq 0.001$.

Table 5. Partial correlations between working memory and speech performance scores.

	WM efficiency	WM capacity
	(partial out WM capacity)	(partial out WM efficiency)
SIQ	−0.69**	0.40
SIN	−0.30	0.10
Disyllable	−0.37	0.48*
Tone	−0.28	0.40
SR	−0.13	0.61**

Working memory efficiency was represented by articulation rate data. Working memory capacity was represented by combined forward and digit span data, using PCA data from factor analysis. The reduced data from the PCA were used to statistically control for demographic variables. Each column shows r values when one of the working memory measures was partialled out. WM = working memory; SIQ = sentence recognition in quiet; SIN = sentence recognition in noise; SR = self-reported school rank.
*$p \leq 0.01$.
** $p \leq 0.001$.

recognition). The subsequent analyses in Table 5 showed the relationship between working memory capacity, working memory efficiency, and speech performance. After controlling for demographic factors and partialling out working memory capacity (forward and backward digit span), working memory efficiency (articulation rate) was significantly correlated only with sentence recognition in quiet (Table 5). Working memory efficiency explained 48% of the variance in sentence recognition in quiet. Similarly, after partialling out working memory efficiency, working memory capacity was significantly correlated with disyllable recognition, also measured in quiet (Table 5). However, working memory capacity only explained 23% of the variance in disyllable recognition. Thus, the contribution of working memory capacity or efficiency seems to depend on the speech measure. For sentence recognition in quiet, the present findings are largely in agreement with Pisoni and colleagues [10], who argued that working memory efficiency explained a significant portion of the variability in CI speech performance. The results with disyllable recognition are more in agreement with Nittrouer et al [31], who argued that working memory capacity contributed to the variability in pediatric CI speech performance.

We hypothesized that the pattern of results might be different between Mandarin- and English-speaking populations, given the importance of F0 cues to tonal languages such as Mandarin Chinese. However, the main findings from the present study were consistent with previous studies in English-speaking participant populations. The correlation analyses in Table 4 showed significant correlations between tone recognition and forward digit span, as well as articulation rate. However, after partialling out either working memory capacity or efficiency, there was no significant correlation between tone recognition and working memory (Table 5). This finding is similar to that of Pisoni and Cleary [10], who found no significant correlation between monosyllabic word recognition and working memory capacity after partialling out working memory efficiency. Different from our hypothesis, the present data suggest that the relationship between speech performance and working memory may not be affected by perception of F0 cues important to tonal languages such as Mandarin Chinese.

In this study, self-reported school rank was used to estimate participants' learning abilities. After controlling for demographic variables, working memory capacity explained 37% of the variance in CI participants' self-reported school rank when working memory efficiency was partialled out, consistent with

findings by Alloway et al. [40]. However, school rank was not significant correlated with working memory efficiency when capacity was partialled out. Limitations to working memory can vary widely among NH children and is closely associated with children's learning ability [41,42], and deficits in working memory have been associated with learning difficulties [28,40,43–44]. When the acoustic input is degraded as in the CI case, it is unclear how the reduced working memory may interact with CI users' learning capabilities. The present data suggest that learning difficulties for young Mandarin-speaking CI users may be associated with limited working memory capacity instead of efficiency.

Conclusions

We compared auditory working memory measures with speech performance and in 32 Mandarin-speaking CI users and 21 NH participants. Major findings include:

1. Working memory performance was significantly poorer for CI than for NH participants, suggesting that Mandarin-speaking CI users experience limited working memory capacity (as measured with forward and backward digit span) and efficiency (as measured with articulation rate).

2. After controlling for demographic factors, CI users' forward digit span was significantly correlated with sentence recognition in quiet, disyllable recognition, tone recognition and school rank. Backward digit span was significantly correlated with sentence recognition in quiet, disyllable recognition, and school rank. Articulation rate was significantly correlated with sentence recognition in quiet, disyllable recognition, and tone recognition. Sentence recognition in noise was not significantly correlated with any working memory measure, possibly due the relatively low SNR used for testing.

3. After controlling for demographic factors and partialling out working memory capacity, working memory efficiency was significantly correlated only with sentence recognition in quiet. After partialling out working memory efficiency, working memory capacity was significantly correlated with disyllable recognition and school rank. This suggests that the contribution of working memory capacity and efficiency may depend on the speech measure.

4. The importance of F0 cues for tonal languages such as Mandarin Chinese did not appear to influence the relationship between working memory and speech understanding observed in previous studies with English-speaking listeners.

Acknowledgments

We are grateful to the subjects who participated in this research. Address for correspondence: Bing Chen, Department of Otology and Skull Base Surgery, Eye Ear Nose and Throat Hospital, Fudan University, 83 Fenyang Road, Shanghai 200031, China. E-mail: entdtao@gmail.com.

Author Contributions

Conceived and designed the experiments: QF BC DT. Performed the experiments: DT RD YJ. Analyzed the data: DT JG. Contributed reagents/materials/analysis tools: QF JG YJ. Wrote the paper: DT JG.

References

1. Niparko JK, Blankenhorn R (2003) Cochlear implants in young children. Ment Retard Dev Disabil Res Rev 9: 267–275.
2. Bodmer D, Shipp DB, Ostroff JM, Ng AH, Stewart S, et al. (2007) A comparison of postcochlear implantation speech scores in an adult population. Laryngoscope 117: 1408–1411.
3. Santarelli R, De Filippi R, Genovese E, Arslan E (2008) Cochlear implantation outcome in prelingually deafened young adults. A speech perception study. Audiol Neurootol 13: 257–265.
4. Bruce IA, Broomfield SJ, Melling CC, Green KM, Ramsden RT (2011) The outcome of cochlear implantation in adolescents. Cochlear Implants Int 12 Suppl 1: S82–83.
5. Lenarz M, Sonmez H, Joseph G, Buchner A, Lenarz T (2012) Cochlear implant performance in geriatric patients. Laryngoscope 122: 1361–1365.
6. Semenov YR, Martinez-Monedero R, Niparko JK (2012) Cochlear implants: clinical and societal outcomes. Otolaryngol Clin North Am 45: 959–981.
7. Berrettini S, Baggiani A, Bruschini L, Cassandro E, Cuda D, et al. (2011) Systematic review of the literature on the clinical effectiveness of the cochlear implant procedure in adult patients. Acta Otorhinolaryngol Ital 31: 299–310.
8. Forli F, Arslan E, Bellelli S, Burdo S, Mancini P, et al. (2011) Systematic review of the literature on the clinical effectiveness of the cochlear implant procedure in paediatric patients. Acta Otorhinolaryngol Ital 31: 281–298.
9. Pisoni DB, Geers AE (2000) Working memory in deaf children with cochlear implants: correlations between digit span and measures of spoken language processing. Ann Otol Rhinol Laryngol Suppl 185: 92–93.
10. Pisoni DB, Cleary M (2003) Measures of working memory span and verbal rehearsal speed in deaf children after cochlear implantation. Ear Hear 24: 106S–120S.
11. Pisoni DB (2000) Cognitive factors and cochlear implants: some thoughts on perception, learning, and memory in speech perception. Ear Hear 21: 70–78.
12. Baddeley A (1992) Working memory. Science 255: 556–559.
13. Baddeley A (2003) Working memory and language: an overview. J Commun Disord 36: 189–208.
14. Smyth MM, Scholey KA (1996) The relationship between articulation time and memory performance in verbal and visuospatial tasks. Br J Psychol 87 (Pt 2): 179–191.
15. Burkholder R, Pisoni D (2004) Digit span recall error analysis in pediatric cochlear implant users. Int Congr Ser 1273: 312–315.
16. Kronenberger WG, Pisoni DB, Harris MS, Hoen HM, Xu H, et al. (2012) Profiles of Verbal Working Memory Growth Predict Speech and Language Development in Children with Cochlear Implants. J Speech Lang Hear Res.
17. Kronenberger WG, Pisoni DB, Harris MS, Hoen HM, Xu H, et al. (2013) Profiles of verbal working memory growth predict speech and language development in children with cochlear implants. J Speech Lang Hear Res 56: 805–825.
18. Oba SI, Galvin JJ 3rd, Fu QJ (2013) Minimal effects of visual memory training on auditory performance of adult cochlear implant users. J Rehabil Res Dev 50: 99–110.
19. Alloway TP, Gathercole SE, Pickering SJ (2006) Verbal and visuospatial short-term and working memory in children: are they separable? Child Dev 77: 1698–1716.
20. Pickering SJ (2001) The development of visuo-spatial working memory. Memory 9: 423–432.
21. McGarr NS (1983) The intelligibility of deaf speech to experienced and inexperienced listeners. J Speech Hear Res 26: 451–458.
22. Pisoni DB, Kronenberger WG, Roman AS, Geers AE (2011) Measures of digit span and verbal rehearsal speed in deaf children after more than 10 years of cochlear implantation. Ear Hear 32: 60S–74S.
23. Cowan N, Wood NL, Wood PK, Keller TA, Nugent LD, et al. (1998) Two separate verbal processing rates contributing to short-term memory span. J Exp Psychol Gen 127: 141–160.
24. Gathercole SE, Hitch GJ, Service E, Martin AJ (1997) Phonological short-term memory and new word learning in children. Dev Psychol 33: 966–979.
25. Gupta P, MacWhinney B (1997) Vocabulary acquisition and verbal short-term memory: computational and neural bases. Brain Lang 59: 267–333.
26. Baddeley A, Gathercole S, Papagno C (1998) The phonological loop as a language learning device. Psychol Rev 105: 158–173.
27. Adams AM, Gathercole SE (2000) Limitations in working memory: implications for language development. Int J Lang Commun Disord 35: 95–116.
28. Gathercole SE, Pickering SJ, Ambridge B, Wearing H (2004) The structure of working memory from 4 to 15 years of age. Dev Psychol 40: 177–190.
29. Stiles DJ, McGregor KK, Bentler RA (2012) Vocabulary and working memory in children fit with hearing aids. J Speech Lang Hear Res 55: 154–167.
30. Watson DR, Titterington J, Henry A, Toner JG (2007) Auditory sensory memory and working memory processes in children with normal hearing and cochlear implants. Audiol Neurootol 12: 65–76.
31. Nittrouer S, Caldwell-Tarr A, Lowenstein JH (2013) Working memory in children with cochlear implants: problems are in storage, not processing. Int J Pediatr Otorhinolaryngol 77: 1886–1898.
32. Fu QJ, Zhu M, Wang X (2011) Development and validation of the Mandarin speech perception test. J Acoust Soc Am 129: EL267–273.
33. Zhu M, Wang X, Fu QJ (2011) Development and validation of the Mandarin disyllable recognition test. Acta Otolaryngol 132: 855–861.
34. Wang RH (1993) The standard Chinese database. University of Science of Technology of China, internal materials.
35. Geers AE, Pisoni DB, Brenner C (2013) Complex working memory span in cochlear implanted and normal hearing teenagers. Otol Neurotol 34: 396–401.
36. Friesen LM, Shannon RV, Baskent D, Wang X (2001) Speech recognition in noise as a function of the number of spectral channels: comparison of acoustic hearing and cochlear implants. J Acoust Soc Am 110: 1150–1163.
37. Lee CY, Lee YF (2010) Perception of musical pitch and lexical tones by Mandarin-speaking musicians. J Acoust Soc Am 127: 481–490.
38. Cleary M, Pisoni DB, Kirk KI (2000) Working Memory Spans as Predictors of Spoken Word Recognition and Receptive Vocabulary in Children with Cochlear Implants. Volta Rev 102: 259–280.
39. Harris MS, Kronenberger WG, Gao S, Hoen HM, Miyamoto RT, et al. (2013) Verbal short-term memory development and spoken language outcomes in deaf children with cochlear implants. Ear Hear 34: 179–192.
40. Alloway TP, Gathercole SE, Kirkwood H, Elliott J (2009) The cognitive and behavioral characteristics of children with low working memory. Child Dev 80: 606–621.
41. Caplan D, Waters G (2013) Memory mechanisms supporting syntactic comprehension. Psychon Bull Rev 20: 243–268.
42. Diller G (2010) The role of working memory in the language-learning process of children with cochlear implants. Cochlear Implants Int 11 Suppl 1: 286–290.
43. Andersson U (2008) Working memory as a predictor of written arithmetical skills in children: the importance of central executive functions. Br J Educ Psychol 78: 181–203.
44. Bull R, Scerif G (2001) Executive functioning as a predictor of children's mathematics ability: inhibition, switching, and working memory. Dev Neuropsychol 19: 273–293.

7

A Novel DFNA36 Mutation in *TMC1* Orthologous to the Beethoven (*Bth*) Mouse Associated with Autosomal Dominant Hearing Loss

Yali Zhao[1,2], Dayong Wang[1], Liang Zong[1], Feifan Zhao[1], Liping Guan[3], Peng Zhang[3], Wei Shi[1], Lan Lan[1], Hongyang Wang[1], Qian Li[1], Bing Han[1], Ling Yang[4], Xin Jin[3,5], Jian Wang[3], Jun Wang[3], Qiuju Wang[1]*

1 Chinese PLA Institute of Otolaryngology, Chinese PLA General Hospital, Beijing, China, 2 Beijing Institute of Otorhinolaryngology, Beijing Tongren Hospital, Capital Medical University, Beijing, China, 3 BGI-Shenzhen, Shenzhen, China, 4 BGI-Tianjin, Tianjin, China, 5 School of Bioscience and Biotechnology, South China University of Technology, Guangzhou, China

Abstract

Mutations in the transmembrane channel-like gene 1 (*TMC1*) can cause both DFNA36 and DFNB7/11 hearing loss. More than thirty DFNB7/11 mutations have been reported, but only three DFNA36 mutations were reported previously. In this study, we found a large Chinese family with 222 family members showing post-lingual, progressive sensorineural hearing loss which were consistent with DFNA36 hearing loss. Auditory brainstem response (ABR) test of the youngest patient showed a special result with nearly normal threshold but prolonged latency, decreased amplitude, and the abnormal waveform morphology. Exome sequencing of the proband found four candidate variants in known hearing loss genes. Sanger sequencing in all family members found a novel variant c.1253T>A (p.M418K) in *TMC1* at DFNA36 that co-segregated with the phenotype. This mutation in *TMC1* is orthologous to the mutation found in the hearing loss mouse model named *Bth* ten years ago. In another 51 Chinese autosomal dominant hearing loss families, we screened the segments containing the dominant mutations of *TMC1* and no functional variants were found. *TMC1* is expressed in the hair cells in inner ear. Given the already known roles of *TMC1* in the mechanotransduction in the cochlea and its expression in inner ear, our results may provide an interesting perspective into its function in inner ear.

Editor: Berta Alsina, Universitat Pompeu Fabra, Spain

Funding: This work was supported by the grants of the National Key Basic Research Program of China, No. 2014CB943001, the National Natural Science Foundation of China, Major Project, No. 81120108009. The funders had no role in study design, data collection and analysis, decision to publish, or preparation of the manuscript.

Competing Interests: The authors have declared that no competing interests exist.

* E-mail: wqcr@263.net

Introduction

Hearing loss is the most common sensory disorder affecting one in 1000 births [1] and the prevalence rises to 2.7 per 1000 by the age of four [2]. More than 60% of cases can be attributed to genetic causes and inherited across generations. Hereditary hearing loss is a highly heterogeneous disorder. So far, a total of 76 non-syndromic hearing loss genes have been identified, including 31 autosomal dominant, 47 autosomal recessive and four X-linked genes (http://hereditaryhearingloss.org). Among these genes, eight of them are inherited in both autosomal dominant and recessive patterns, such as *TMC1* (http://hereditaryhearingloss.org/).

TMC1 was identified as a causative gene for both autosomal dominant (DFNA36) and autosomal recessive (DFNB7/11) non-syndromic hearing loss by Kurima and colleagues in 2002[3]. Based on their results, Vreugde and colleagues screened the *Tmc1* gene and found the p.M412K mutation in a hearing loss mouse model named *Bth* which was arisen in a large-scale ENU mutagenesis program [4,5]. Since then, more than 30 autosomal recessive mutations in *TMC1* have been reported in DFNB7/11 families. *TMC1* is identified as a common gene associated with non-syndromic hearing loss with a frequency up to 6.6% in

Turkey [3,6–17]. In contrast, only two amino acid residues with three mutations have been reported to be associated with autosomal dominant hearing loss [3,14,18,19]. One is the amino acid-572 with two mutations at this site, p.D572N and p.D572H. These two mutations have been observed in three unrelated North American families with non-syndromic, post-lingual, progressive sensorineural hearing loss [3,18,19]. The other residue is the amino acid-417 with mutation p.G417R [14]. This mutation is adjacent to the *Bth* mouse mutation in the *Tmc1* gene, which may have similar function consequences. However, the mutation orthologous to p.M412K in murine *Tmc1* has yet to be found in human hearing loss family since it has been reported in 2002 [5]. Here, in a large Chinese family (1304) of six-generation with autosomal dominant hereditary hearing loss, we identified a novel mutation of p.M418K in *TMC1* through sequencing the whole exome of the proband, which is important and beneficial to discover the pathologic mechanism of DFNA36 hearing loss caused by *TMC1* mutation.

Methods

Ethics Statement

The study was approved by the Committee of Medical Ethics of Chinese People's Liberation Army (PLA) General Hospital. All the

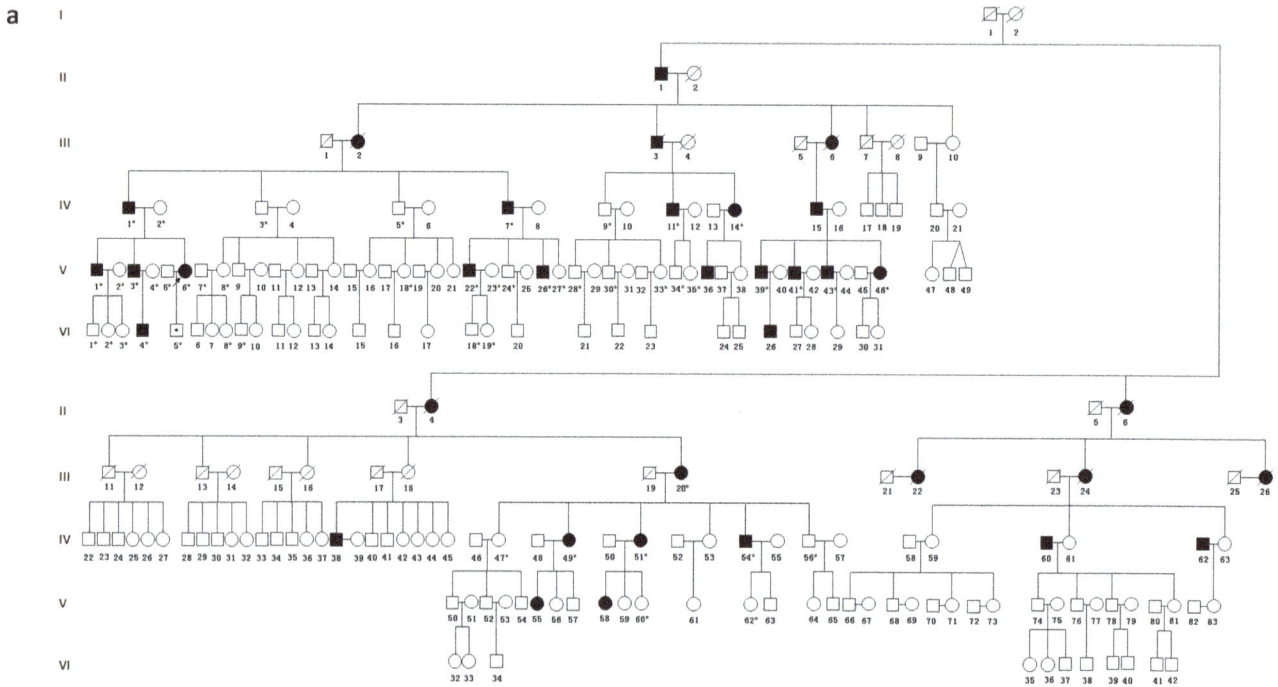

Figure 1. Pedigree of family 1304. Filled symbols for males (squares) and females (circles) represent affected individuals, and empty, unaffected ones. An arrow denotes the proband. A symbol with dot indicates the individual younger than the average age of onset, who is mutation carrier but does not present hearing loss (a mutation carrier). Symbols with asterisk are individuals who have had clinical and genetic tests.

samples were analyzed under the appropriate ethical approvals, and written informed consents were obtained from all subjects or caregivers. Next of kin, care takers or guardians consented on the behalf of minors/children participants whose capacity to consent was compromised.

Family Recruitment and Clinical Evaluations

Family 1304 were ascertained from the Department of Otolaryngology, Head and Neck Surgery, at the Institute of Otolaryngology of PLA, Chinese PLA General Hospital. Members of this family were interviewed by a team of experienced ear, nose and throat doctors, and physicians to identify either personal or

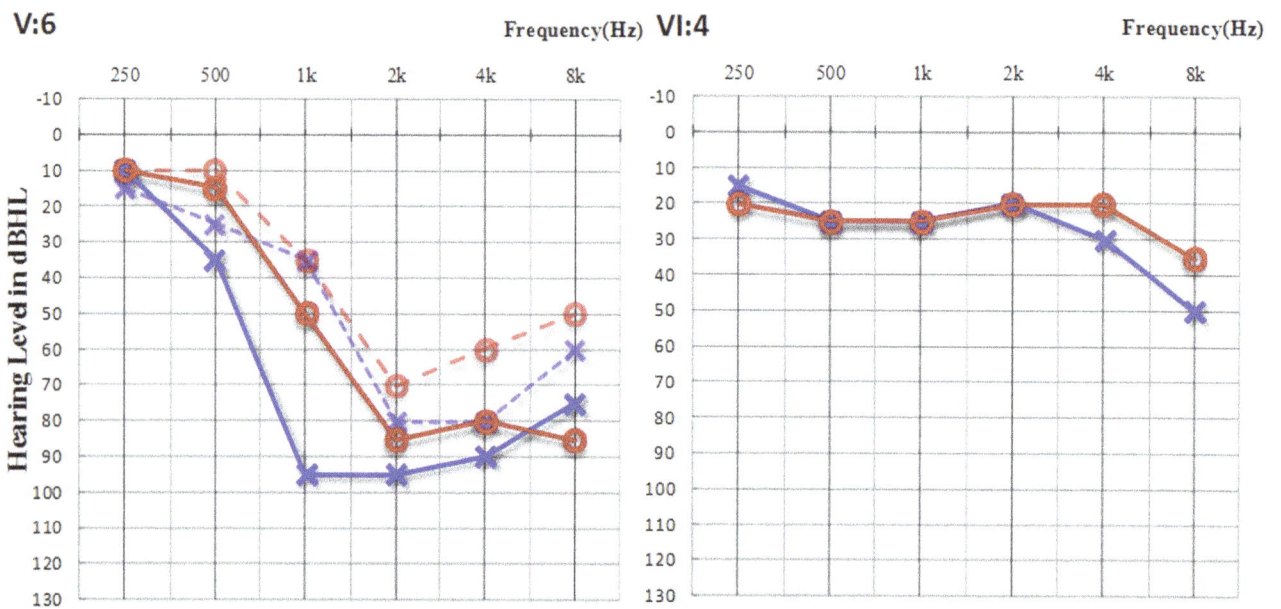

Figure 2. Audiograms of the proband (V:6) and the a five-year-old patient (VI:4). Symbols "o" and "x" denote air conduction pure-tone thresholds at different frequencies in the right and left ear. dB, decibels; Hz, Hertz. The dashed line represent the audiograms detected in 2005 when the proband (V:6) was 23 years old. Audiological examination with solid line was performed in 2012.

Table 1. Summary of the clinical data for all individuals with p.M418K in family 1304.

ID	Gender	Age of test (years)	Age of onset (years)	PTA	Severity of hearing loss	Tinnitus	Genotype
III:20	Female	70	NA	L:80.00	severe	L:durative	T/A
				R:83.75	severe	R:durative	
IV:1	Male	62	20	L:105.00	profound	L:durative	T/A
				R:107.50	profound	R:durative	
IV:7	Male	53	17	L:68.75	moderate	L:durative	T/A
				R:75.00	severe	R:durative	
IV:11	Male	44	24	L:83.75	severe	L:durative	T/A
				R:71.25	severe	R:no	
IV:14	Female	52	20	L:92.50	severe	L:no	T/A
				R:93.75	severe	R:no	
IV:49	Female	46	5	L:98.75	profound	L:durative	T/A
				R:101.25	profound	R:durative	
IV:51	Female	42	13	L:77.50	severe	L:durative	T/A
				R:81.25	severe	R:durative	
IV:54	Male	38	20	L:55.00	moderate	L:durative	T/A
				R:60.00	moderate	R:durative	
IV:60	Male	64	20	L:76.25	severe	L:durative	T/A
				R:77.50	severe	R:durative	
V:1	Male	37	18	L:80.60	severe	L:intermittence	T/A
				R:93.75	severe	R:intermittence	
V:3	Male	26	15	L:73.75	severe	L:durative	T/A
				R:71.25	severe	R:durative	
V:6	Female	23	13	L:55.00	moderate	L:durative	T/A
				R:43.75	moderate	R:durative	
V:22	Male	27	15	L:62.50	moderate	L:intermittence	T/A
				R:66.25	moderate	R:intermittence	
V:26	Male	20	15	L:62.50	moderate	L:intermittence	T/A
				R:66.25	moderate	R:intermittence	
V:39	Male	53	10	L:105.00	profound	L:durative	T/A
				R:105.00	profound	R:durative	
V:41	Male	45	28	L:73.75	severe	L:durative	T/A
				R:82.50	severe	R:durative	
V:43	Male	35	20	L:75.00	severe	L:durative	T/A
				R:71.25	severe	R:durative	
VI:4	Male	5	5	L:25.00	mild	L:no	T/A

Table 1. Cont.

ID	Gender	Age of test (years)	Age of onset (years)	PTA	Severity of hearing loss	Tinnitus	Genotype
VI:5	Male	2	NA	R:22.50	mild	R:no	T/A
				L:NA	NA	NA	
				R:NA	NA	NA	

PTA, Pure Tone Average. NA, Not Available. L, left ear; R, right ear; T/A in "Genotype" column indicates the genotype of the patient in the mutation of c.1253T>A (p.M418K).

family medical evidence of hearing loss, tinnitus, vestibular symptoms, use of aminoglycosides, and other clinical abnormalities. Audiometric evaluations included pure tone audiometry using Madsen Orbiter 922 audiometer (Denmark), auditory brainstem responses (ABR) and distortion product otoacoustic emissions (DPOAE) using SmartEP of Intelligent Hearing system (USA). The audiological data were evaluated based on the criteria established by European Working Group on Genetics of Hearing loss [20]. High resolution computed tomography (HRCT) was also performed on some subjects to verify whether the family members had other complications in addition to hearing disorders.

A total of 51 unrelated autosomal dominant hearing loss families were chosen as the other affected set for further analysis. In these families, mutations in common genes associated with hearing loss, such as *GJB2*, *SLC26A4* and mitochondrial DNA A1555G, were all excluded. As a comparison group, 100 unaffected individuals of matched geographical ancestry were recruited in this study.

DNA Sample and Exome capture

Peripheral blood samples were obtained and genomic DNA was extracted according to standard procedures. Qualified genomic DNA samples (6 ug) of the proband were sheared by sonication. Then the fragment of each shared genomic DNA sample was hybridized to the SureSelect Biotiny lated RNA Library (BAITS) for enrichment.

NGS, reads mapping and SNPs detection

The enriched libraries were loaded on the HiSeq 2000 platform to be sequenced. Raw image files were processed by Illumina Pipeline v1.6 for base-calling with default parameters and the sequences of each individual were generated as 90 bp paired-end reads. Then the sequenced raw data was aligned to the NCBI human reference genome (NCBI 36.3) using SOAPaligner [21]. After that, the duplicated reads were filtered out and the clean reads located in the target region were collected. The consensus of genotype and quality were estimated by SOAPsnp (version1.03) using the clean reads. The variations of low quality were filtered out according to the following criteria: (i) quality score < 20 (Q20); (ii) average copy number at the allele site > = 2; (iii) distance of two adjacent SNPs <5 bp; and (iv) sequencing depth <4 or >500.

Detection of insertions and deletions

Insertions and deletions (indels) in the exome regions were identified through the sequencing reads. We aligned the reads to the reference genome by Burrows-Wheeler Aligner (BWA0.5.8) [22], and passed the alignment results to the Genome Analysis Toolkit (GATK1.0.4705) to identify the breakpoints. Finally, we annotated the genotypes of insertions and deletions [23].

Sequencing analysis of candidate gene

Candidate variants located in previously reported hearing loss genes found in exome sequencing were screened in all available members from family 1304. Genotype of the variant c.1253T>A (p.M418K) in *TMC1* was found to be co-segregated with the hearing loss in family 1304. As the candidate gene, the variant in *TMC1* was screened in 100 unaffected individuals geographically matched. In addition, 51 unrelated autosomal dominant hearing loss families without *GJB2*, *SLC26A4* and mitochondrial DNA A1555G mutations were chosen as another affected set for further analysis. For this cohort, exon16, exon19 and their flank sequences containing all the four mutations associated with dominant

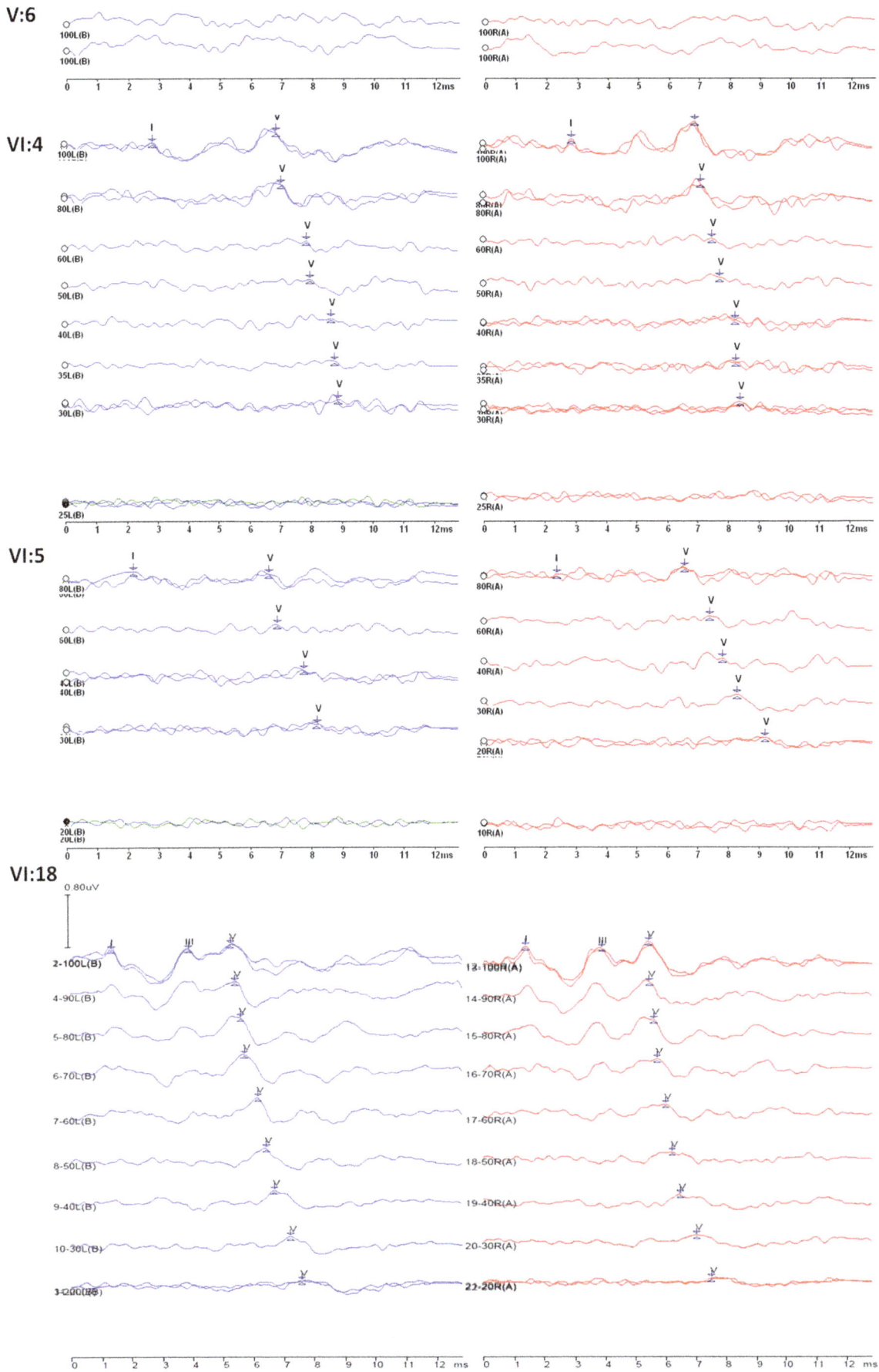

Figure 3. ABR results performed to the proband (V:6), a five-year-old patient (VI:4), a two-year-old carrier (VI:5) of p.M418K and a five-year-boy (VI:18) with normal hearing and wildtype genotype. ABR was performed using click stimulus.

hearing loss were sequenced applying Sanger sequencing. Primer pairs were designed using the online Primer 3.0 software and synthesized by Invitrogen (Table S1, Beijing, China) to amplify each exon and boundaries.

Results

Clinical description

Family 1304 was a six-generation pedigree with 222 members, 35 of whom suffered hearing loss (Figure 1). This family was originated from Hebei province in North China. In this study, 48

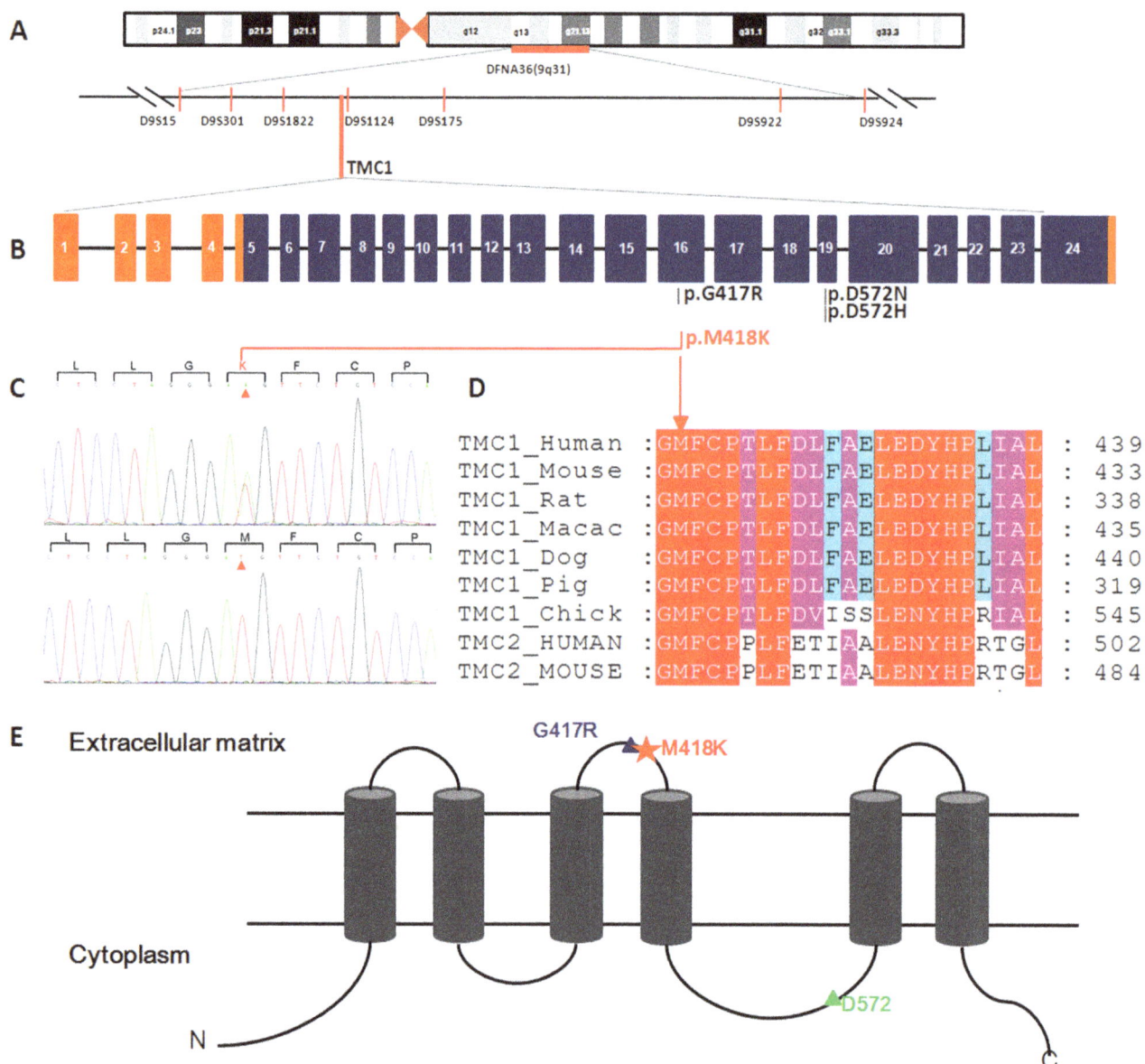

Figure 4. Gene identified in family 1304 with autosomal dominant progressive hearing loss. A: Schematic physical and genetic maps of DFNA36 locus on the 9q31chromosomal region. The *TMC1* gene is indicated. B: Schematic structure of *TMC1* gene. *TMC1* gene has 24 exons. Mutation of p.M418K and p.G417R locate in exon16, and mutation of p.D572N and p.D572H are in exon19. C: Sequencing chromatograms of *TMC1* showing the heterozygous substitution, c.1253A>T in affected individuals (upper panel) compared with that of normal control (lower panel). The mutated nucleotides are marked by triangles. The predicted amino acid changes and surrounding ones are indicated above the sequences. D: Multiple amino acid sequences alignment of *TMC1* and its paralog of *TMC2* using ClustalW software. The conservation analysis shows that p.M418K(arrow) mutation in *TMC1* located in a highly conserved position comparing with the corresponding sequences of human, mouse, rat, macaque, dog, pig, chick, human *TMC2* and mouse *Tmc2*. E: A schematic diagram of *TMC1* protein predicted by TMHMM2.0 containing six transmembrane domains, a cytoplasmic N and C termini. All reported DFNA36 mutations or residual are indicated. Mutation of p.M418K found in this study is located in the second extracellular loop between the third and the fourth transmembrane domain.

Table 2. Filter process for the variants found by whole exome sequencing.

Filter process	V:6
Functional_variations	7477
Against_dbSNP_132	1051
Against_dbSNP_1000 Genomes	723
Against_dbSNP_1000 Genomes _Hapmap 8	639
Against_dbSNP_1000 Genomes _Hapmap 8_YH	635
Variants in genes associated with hearing loss	4

The number of functional variants (non-synonymous/splice acceptor and donor site/insertions or deletions) is listed under various filters. Variants were filtered by presence in dbSNP, 1000 Genomes, HapMap 8 or YH.

members were under detailed physical examinations and audiometric evaluations (Figure 1), and 18 of them showed post-lingual, progressive, and symmetric sensorineural hearing loss with high frequency tinnitus (Figure 2, and Table 1). The onset age ranged from 5 to 28 years old. Hearing loss appeared to initially affect high frequencies with mild or moderate levels at the onset age and progressed to profound levels by the fifth or sixth decade. The low-frequency hearing deteriorated to profound levels and the audiometric graph changed to flat pattern eventually.

The proband (V:6) was a 23-year-old female suffering from hearing loss accompanied by tinnitus when she first visit the outpatient clinic in the year of 2005. She showed a severe hearing loss at 2 kHz and 4 kHz and a moderate hearing loss at 1 kHz and 8 kHz. Seven years later, the threshold increased about 15–30 dB HL at 1 kHz–8 kHz in the right ear, 10–15 dB HL at 2 kHz–8 kHz in the left ear (Figure 2). The threshold of the left ear at 1 kHz increased 60 dB HL within seven years. ABR could not be evoked in both ears (Figure 3). DPOAEs were absent at all frequencies. The youngest patient of this family (VI:4) was 5 years old. And behavior audiometry to him showed bilaterally mild hearing loss (Figure 2). The threshold of ABR was 30 dB nHL. The latencies of wave I, III and V were prolonged and the I-to-V interwave latencies were normal in both ears. The waveform morphology was abnormal and the amplitudes were lower compared to normal waveform morphology (Figure 3). DPOAEs were present from 2.5 kHz to 8 kHz and other frequencies were absent in the left ear, while in the right ear, it was evoked from 2 kHz to 8 kHz and other frequencies were not elicited. High resolution CT scan showed normal middle and inner ear structure, including normal vestibular aqueduct and internal auditory canal.

Exome sequencing

Whole exome of the proband was sequenced and an average of 4.7 billion bases of sequence were generated as paired-end, 90 bp reads, about 63.4% of the total bases were mapped to the targeted bases with a mean coverage of 53.7-fold. At this depth of coverage, 98.3% of the targeted regions were sufficiently covered to pass our thresholds for variant calling (Table S2, Figure S1 and Figure S2). A total of 38130 single nucleotide variants and 2220 indels were identified by exome sequencing (Table S3 and Table S4). Among these variants, we focused on non-synonymous (NS) variants, splice acceptor and donor site variants (SS), and short, frame-shift coding indels that were more likely to be pathogenic mutations than other variants. A total of 7477 variants following the above inclusion criteria were detected in the proband of family 1304 (Table 2). Hereditary hearing loss is a monogenic and always caused by rare variants, frequency of which may be rare or absent in the general population. Therefore, we compared all identified

NS/SS/Indel variants in the proband against dbSNP132, the 1000 Human Genome Project (201003 released), eight previously exome-sequenced HapMap samples (HapMap 8), and YH SNPs (Table 2), and removed the shared SNPs. After this filter process, the candidate list reduced to 635 NS/SS/Indel variants. Four of the 635 NS/SS/Indel variants, p.M418K (*TMC1*), p. R382C (*ESRRB*), p.S385P (*ESPN*) and p.D2E (*WFS1*) located in the known hearing loss genes, which may attribute to the phenotypes of the family. Then these four variants were sequenced in all available members of family 1304 by Sanger sequencing. It was found that the mutation of c.1253T>A (p.M418K, NM_138691) in *TMC1* gene completely co-segregated with the phenotype and all 18 patients were heterozygous on this site (Figure 4A, 4B, 4C). In addition to the clinically diagnosed patients, there was a two-year-old boy (VI:5) who carried this mutation without hearing loss (Figure 1). This mutation was not detected in any of the 100 geographical matched controls. The other three candidate variants did not co-segregate with the members of family. To access the likelihood that whether the variant p.M418K in *TMC1* gene is functional or not, we used SIFT software (vision 4.0.3) to predict the biophysical consequences of this substitution and found that this variant is likely to be deleterious. Alignments of the amino acid sequences of *TMC1* in human species, mouse, rat, macaque, dog, pig and chick as well as with human *TMC2* and mouse *Tmc2* showed that the mutation is located in a highly conserved position, which is homologous to the p.M412K mutation in the *Bth* mouse inherited in autosomal dominant pattern (Figure 4D).

To further analyze the contribution of *TMC1* for autosomal dominant hearing loss, we successfully screened the exon16 and exon19 in another 51 autosomal dominant hearing loss families. No functional variants were found to be associated with hearing loss in these families.

Discussion

In this study, we identified a novel mutation p.M418K in *TMC1* in a Chinese family of six generation using the strategy of exome sequencing to the proband. Screening of this mutation in family members showed that all patients were heterozygous and individuals with normal hearing were homozygous in the wild type, which indicated that p.M418K in *TMC1* was responsible for the hearing loss in this autosomal dominant family. *TMC1*, the transmembrane cochlear-expressed gene 1, was reported as the causative gene for both dominant and recessive hearing loss at the DFNA36 and DFNB7/11 [3]. Patients in this family (1304) showed post-lingual, bilateral, symmetric sensorineural hearing loss initially affected the mid and high frequency with mild level, followed by progression to severe or profound levels along with increasing ages, which was consistent with the phenotype of DFNA36 families reported previously [3,14,18,19]. Alignments of the amino acid sequences of transmembrane channel-like gene 1 in different species showed that mutation in family 1304 was an orthologous to the p.M412K mutation reported in the hearing loss mouse model named Beethoven [5]. All these results strongly supported that the mutation of p.M418K in *TMC1* was associated with the hearing loss of patients in family 1304.

Notably, for the first time, our study reported a dominant mutation of *TMC1* in a large family from Chinese. During the past ten years, three dominant mutations in *TMC1* (p.D572N, p.D572H and p.G417R) from four DFNA36 hearing loss families have been reported [5,14,18,19], i.e., the mutation of p.D572N and p.D572H were found in North American families [5,18,19]. The p.G417R mutation was found in an Iranian family [14].

TMC1 is predicted to encode a transmembrane protein containing at least six membrane spanning domains, a cytoplasmic N- and C-termini, and a large cytoplasmic loop named TMC domain [24,25]. The mutation found in this study, p.M418K, and the adjacent DFNA36 mutation of p.G417R, lie within a predicted second extracellular loop between the third and the fourth transmembrane domain (Figure 4E) [14,24], while the amino acid, D572, is located in the region of TMC domain (Figure 4E) [24]. These dominant mutations must act via a gain-of-function or dominant-negative mechanism. The cluster of these dominant mutations of *TMC1* indicates that this region should be important for the proper function of the protein.

It's noteworthy that, for the first time, we have found a family in human with the mutation orthologous to p.M412K in *Tmc1* of *Bth* mouse model since it was found in 2002 [5]. The *Bth* mouse showed progressive loss of the Preyer reflex from around P30 with appeared normal structure of middle ear and inner ear[5], which was similar with the phenotype of late-onset and progressive hearing loss in family 1304. In-situ hybridization on mouse cochlear showed that *Tmc1* is expressed in both outer and inner hair cells from early stage of development [3,5]. It may be required for cochlear hair-cell mechanotransduction as the integral components of the mechanotransduction complex [26]. Studies on the mutant mice that expressing the *Tmc1*[Bth] allele implicated that *Tmc1* was the component of the mechanotransduction channel in auditory hair cells of the inner ear [27]. And cells with the p.M412K point mutation in *Tmc1* reduced calcium permeability and single-channel currents [27]. Therefore, *TMC1* should act as a pore-forming subunit of the transduction channel and be involved in determining permeation properties [27].

To summarize, we found ABRs of the patients carrying the p.M418K mutation in *TMC1* showed a prolonged latency and abnormal waveform morphology for wave I to V, which was most likely a direct and causative link, although the mechanism was still obscure. The identification of the p.M418K in *TMC1* in family 1304 makes the *Bth* mouse an excellent animal model to study the mechanism for autosomal dominant hearing loss caused by *TMC1* mutation.

References

1. Morton NE (1991) Genetic epidemiology of hearing impairment. Ann N Y Acad Sci 630: 16–31.
2. Morton CC, Nance WE (2006) Newborn hearing screening—a silent revolution. N Engl J Med 354: 2151–2164.
3. Kurima K, Peters LM, Yang Y, Riazuddin S, Ahmed ZM, et al. (2002) Dominant and recessive deafness caused by mutations of a novel gene, TMC1, required for cochlear hair-cell function. Nat Genet 30: 277–284.
4. Hrabe de Angelis MH, Flaswinkel H, Fuchs H, Rathkolb B, Soewarto D, et al. (2000) Genome-wide, large-scale production of mutant mice by ENU mutagenesis. Nat Genet 25: 444–447.
5. Vreugde S, Erven A, Kros CJ, Marcotti W, Fuchs H, et al. (2002) Beethoven, a mouse model for dominant, progressive hearing loss DFNA36. Nat Genet 30: 257–258.
6. Kalay E, Karaguzel A, Caylan R, Heister A, Cremers FP, et al. (2005) Four novel TMC1 (DFNB7/DFNB11) mutations in Turkish patients with congenital autosomal recessive nonsyndromic hearing loss. Hum Mutat 26: 591.
7. Meyer CG, Gasmelseed NM, Mergani A, Magzoub MM, Muntau B, et al. (2005) Novel TMC1 structural and splice variants associated with congenital nonsyndromic deafness in a Sudanese pedigree. Hum Mutat 25: 100.

Supporting Information

Figure S1 The distribution of per-base sequencing depth in target regions for each sample. Y-axis indicated the percentage of total target region under a given sequencing depth.

Figure S2 Cumulative depth distribution in target regions for each sample. X-axis denotes sequencing depth, and y-axis indicated the fraction of bases that achieves at or above a given sequencing depth. From the figure above, we can see about 75.50% of target region bases obtains at least 20x fold coverage, that is to say, about 75.50% of target region was covered by more than 20 reads. And about 89.10% of target region achieved at least 10x.

Table S1 Primer sequences for p.M418 in exon16 and p.D572 in exon19.

Table S2 Summary of effective data for exome sequencing. * The region near target refers to flanking region within 200 bp of target regions. ** Total effective reads is the same meaning as the unique mapped reads which was stated in the pipeline above. Here the effective reads consist of two parts: i) the reads have only one best hit in the alignment. These reads comes from the unique region of genome ii) the reads have multiple best hits on the genome (the number of hits between 1 and 20), and they were randomly aligned onto the target regions. These reads mainly come from low complex genomic region, such as repetitive sequences, and account for about 4% of total effective reads. *** Target regions used here refer to genomic regions that the Exome array actually covered. The aggregate length of target is about 37.8 Mb.

Table S3 Summary of SNPs in Exome Sequencing for each Sample. * Consensus genotype with quality score of at least 20. ** Intronic SNPs within 4 bp of exon/intron boundary. *** 5' UTR refers to 200 bp upstream of initiation codon, 3'UTR is defined as 200 bp downstream of termination codon.

Table S4 Summary of Indels in Exome Sequencing for each Sample.

Author Contributions

Conceived and designed the experiments: QW YZ. Performed the experiments: YZ. Analyzed the data: LG PZ LY XJ. Contributed reagents/materials/analysis tools: DW LZ FZ WS LL HW QL BH. Wrote the paper: YZ. Critical reading and discussion of manuscript: Jian Wang Jun Wang QW.

8. Santos RL, Wajid M, Khan MN, McArthur N, Pham TL, et al. (2005) Novel sequence variants in the TMC1 gene in Pakistani families with autosomal recessive hearing impairment. Hum Mutat 26: 396.

9. Kitajiri SI, McNamara R, Makishima T, Husnain T, Zafar AU, et al. (2007) Identities, frequencies and origins of TMC1 mutations causing DFNB7/B11 deafness in Pakistan. Clin Genet 72: 546–550.

10. Hilgert N, Alasti F, Dieltjens N, Pawlik B, Wollnik B, et al. (2008) Mutation analysis of TMC1 identifies four new mutations and suggests an additional deafness gene at loci DFNA36 and DFNB7/11. Clin Genet 74: 223–232.

11. Sirmaci A, Duman D, Ozturkmen-Akay H, Erbek S, Incesulu A, et al. (2009) Mutations in TMC1 contribute significantly to nonsyndromic autosomal recessive sensorineural hearing loss: a report of five novel mutations. Int J Pediatr Otorhinolaryngol 73: 699–705.

12. Ben Said M, Hmani-Aifa M, Amar I, Baig SM, Mustapha M, et al. (2010) High frequency of the p.R34X mutation in the TMC1 gene associated with nonsyndromic hearing loss is due to founder effects. Genet Test Mol Biomarkers 14: 307–311.

13. Hildebrand MS, Kahrizi K, Bromhead CJ, Shearer AE, Webster JA, et al. (2010) Mutations in TMC1 are a common cause of DFNB7/11 hearing loss in the Iranian population. Ann Otol Rhinol Laryngol 119: 830–835.

14. Yang T, Kahrizi K, Bazazzadeghan N, Meyer N, Najmabadi H, et al. (2010) A novel mutation adjacent to the Bth mouse mutation in the TMC1 gene makes this mouse an excellent model of human deafness at the DFNA36 locus. Clin Genet 77: 395–398.

15. Brownstein Z, Friedman LM, Shahin H, Oron-Karni V, Kol N, et al. (2011) Targeted genomic capture and massively parallel sequencing to identify genes for hereditary hearing loss in middle eastern families. Genome Biol 12: R89.

16. de Heer AM, Collin RW, Huygen PL, Schraders M, Oostrik J, et al. (2011) Progressive sensorineural hearing loss and normal vestibular function in a Dutch DFNB7/11 family with a novel mutation in TMC1. Audiol Neurootol 16: 93–105.

17. Duman D, Sirmaci A, Cengiz FB, Ozdag H, Tekin M (2011) Screening of 38 genes identifies mutations in 62% of families with nonsyndromic deafness in Turkey. Genet Test Mol Biomarkers 15: 29–33.

18. Kitajiri S, Makishima T, Friedman TB, Griffith AJ (2007) A novel mutation at the DFNA36 hearing loss locus reveals a critical function and potential genotype-phenotype correlation for amino acid-572 of TMC1. Clin Genet 71: 148–152.

19. Hilgert N, Monahan K, Kurima K, Li C, Friedman RA, et al. (2009) Amino acid 572 in TMC1: hot spot or critical functional residue for dominant mutations causing hearing impairment. J Hum Genet 54: 188–190.

20. Mazzoli M, Van Camp G, Newton V, Giarbini N, Declau F, et al. (2003) Recommendations for the description of genetic and audiological data for families with nonsyndromic hereditary hearing impairment. Audiol Med 1: 148–150.

21. Li R, Li Y, Kristiansen K, Wang J (2008) SOAP: short oligonucleotide alignment program. Bioinformatics 24: 713–714.

22. Li H, Durbin R (2010) Fast and accurate long-read alignment with Burrows-Wheeler transform. Bioinformatics 26: 589–595.

23. McKenna A, Hanna M, Banks E, Sivachenko A, Cibulskis K, et al. (2010) The Genome Analysis Toolkit: a MapReduce framework for analyzing next-generation DNA sequencing data. Genome Res 20: 1297–1303.

24. Keresztes G, Mutai H, Heller S (2003) TMC and EVER genes belong to a larger novel family, the TMC gene family encoding transmembrane proteins. BMC Genomics 4: 24.

25. Kurima K, Yang Y, Sorber K, Griffith AJ (2003) Characterization of the transmembrane channel-like (TMC) gene family: functional clues from hearing loss and epidermodysplasia verruciformis. Genomics 82: 300–308.

26. Kawashima Y, Geleoc GS, Kurima K, Labay V, Lelli A, et al. (2011) Mechanotransduction in mouse inner ear hair cells requires transmembrane channel-like genes. J Clin Invest 121: 4796–4809.

27. Pan B, Geleoc GS, Asai Y, Horwitz GC, Kurima K, et al. (2013) TMC1 and TMC2 are components of the mechanotransduction channel in hair cells of the mammalian inner ear. Neuron 79: 504–515.

8

Need for Supplemental Oxygen at Discharge in Infants with Bronchopulmonary Dysplasia Is Not Associated with Worse Neurodevelopmental Outcomes at 3 Years Corrected Age

Abhay Lodha[1,2,3,4]*, Reg Sauvé[1,2,3,4], Vineet Bhandari[5], Selphee Tang[3], Heather Christianson[2,3], Anita Bhandari[6], Harish Amin[1,3], Nalini Singhal[1,3,4]

1 Department of Pediatrics, Foothills Medical Centre, Peter Lougheed Centre, Alberta Children's Hospital, Calgary, Canada, 2 Community Health Sciences, University of Calgary, Calgary, Canada, 3 Alberta Health Services, Calgary, Canada, 4 Alberta Children's Hospital Institute of Child & Maternal Health, Calgary, Canada, 5 Department of Pediatrics, Yale University School of Medicine, New Haven, Connecticut, United States of America, 6 Department of Pediatric Pulmonology, Connecticut Children's Medical Center, Hartford, Connecticut, United States of America

Abstract

Objectives: To determine if chronic oxygen dependency (discharge home on supplemental oxygen) in children with bronchopulmonary dysplasia (BPD; defined as requirement for supplemental O_2 at 36 weeks postmenstrual age) predicts neurodevelopmental disability rates and growth outcomes at 36 months corrected age (CA).

Study Design: Longitudinal cohort study.

Setting: Southern Alberta regional center located at high altitude.

Participants: Preterm infants weighing ≤1250 grams with no BPD, BPD, and BPD with chronic oxygen dependency.

Main outcome measures: Neurodevelopmental and growth outcomes.

Results: Of 1563 preterm infants admitted from 1995–2007, 1212 survived. Complete follow-up data were available for 1030 (85%) children. Children in BPD and BPD with chronic oxygen dependency groups had significantly lower birth weights, gestational ages, prolonged mechanical ventilation and oxygen supplementation and received more postnatal steroids, compared to those without BPD. Children with BPD and BPD with chronic oxygen dependency were more likely to be below the 5th centile in weight and height compared to those without BPD but there was little difference between the BPD and BPD with chronic oxygen dependency groups. After controlling for confounding variables, children who had BPD and BPD with chronic oxygen dependency had higher odds of neurodevelopmental disability compared to those without BPD [OR (odds ratio) 1.9 (95%CI 1.1 to 3.5) and OR 1.8 (1.1 to 2.9), respectively], with no significant difference between BPD and BPD with chronic oxygen dependency [OR 0.9 (95% CI 0.6 to 1.5)].

Conclusions: BPD and BPD with chronic oxygen dependency in children predicts abnormal neurodevelopmental outcomes at 36 months CA. However, the neurodevelopmental disability rates were not significantly higher in BPD with chronic oxygen dependency children compared to children with BPD only. Compared to those without BPD, growth is impaired in children with BPD and BPD with chronic oxygen dependency, but no difference between the latter two groups.

Editor: Pascal Lavoie, University of British Columbia, Canada

Funding: This work was supported by the University of Calgary and Department of Pediatrics. The funders had no role in study design, data collection and analysis, decision to publish, or preparation of the manuscript.

Competing Interests: The authors have declared that no competing interests exist.

* E-mail: aklodha@ucalgary.ca

Introduction

Bronchopulmonary dysplasia (BPD) is a common and serious problem in very preterm infants. It is characterized by early lung injury and can progress to severe BPD [1]. The incidence of BPD in preterm infants has varied from 4.6% to 72% depending on birth weight and gestational age category, definitions used [2], neonatal assisted ventilation strategies [3] and site of care [2,3]. Shannon et al. [4] defined BPD based on oxygen dependency at 36 weeks postmenstrual age (PMA) as opposed to Northway's definition [5] of BPD based on oxygen requirement at 28 days of life. This change in definition based on longer duration of oxygen requirement has had an impact on predicting preterm infants' long term neurodevelopmental outcomes. Frequent episodes of hypoxemia in BPD infants may affect growth, cardiac functions and long term neurodevelopmental outcomes [6]. Therefore, the purpose of home oxygen therapy is to prevent the effects of hypoxemia and to prevent pulmonary and bronchial vasoconstriction leading to alteration in the airway causing obstruction and impairment in growth of pulmonary and ocular vasculature and their effects on long term neurodevelopmental outcomes [3,7–9].

In a study by Majnemer et al., it was found that preterm infants with BPD who required home oxygen therapy were at a greater risk of poor neurodevelopmental outcomes at school age [10]. In a recent study, Trittmann et al. revealed that at 18 months corrected age, the need for supplemental oxygen at discharge was not associated with an increased risk of neurodevelopmental disability [11]. However, there are no reports of large longitudinal single center studies that examine the long term impact of chronic oxygen dependency in preterm infants with BPD, differentiating between infants with and without chronic oxygen dependency, on the risk for adverse neurodevelopmental outcomes at 36 months corrected age (CA).

We hypothesized that for preterm infants, the incidence of poor growth, neurodevelopmental disability, and abnormal language outcomes increases as the severity of BPD increases from no BPD, to BPD, and BPD with chronic oxygen dependency.

The primary objective of this study was to determine the relationship between BPD severity in preterm infants based on chronic oxygen dependency and neurodevelopmental disability rates. Secondary objectives examined the relationship between BPD severity with growth and language outcomes at 36 months CA.

Methods

Premature infants with birth weight ≤1250 grams born between January 1995 and December 2007 and admitted to the single largest tertiary Neonatal Intensive Care Unit (NICU) in Southern Alberta were included in the study. These infants were followed longitudinally from birth at a regional Perinatal Follow-up Program that serves the geographic catchment area of Southern Alberta, Canada. Infants with major congenital malformations or chromosomal disorders were excluded from this study. This study was approved by the institutional ethics review board of the University of Calgary, and signed consent was obtained from the parents of all study participants.

Standardized demographic, perinatal and neonatal data were collected from patients' charts by a by research coordinator and entered into a computerized database when the premature infants were discharged from the NICU. Occupations of fathers were ranked according to the Blishen socioeconomic index for occupations in Canada [12].

The specific guidelines for discharging an infant home from NICU are presented in Table 1. According to Alberta Health Provincial guidelines (page no. 34), a dated hard copy of pulse oximetry results 48 hours before discharge showing room air SpO2≤89% was required to discharge the baby home on oxygen. http://www.health. alberta.ca/documents/AADL-Manual-R-Respiratory.pdf.

At discharge the infants were categorized as having no BPD, BPD (O$_2$ dependency at 36 weeks PMA but not at the time of discharge home), and BPD with chronic oxygen dependency (O$_2$ supplementation at 36 weeks PMA and discharged home on O$_2$). We have had the same research coordinator in our Southern Alberta Perinatal follow-up program for the last 30 years and she has been consistently collecting the data from patients' charts and entering them into the database. Outcome definitions did not change during the study period in our perinatal follow-up clinic.

Perinatal and neonatal data were defined according to the Canadian Neonatal Network manual. (http://www.canadianneonatalnetwork. org/Portal/LinkClick.aspx?fileticket = I3jnvN9fGfE%3D&tabid = 69) Gestational age (GA) was defined as the best estimate based on obstetric history, obstetric examination and first prenatal ultrasound examination [13]. Bronchopulmonary dysplasia was defined as supplemental oxygen utilization at 36 weeks PMA [4]. Diagnosis of patent ductus arteriosus (PDA) was made clinically, with or without echocardiography [13]. Intraventricular hemorrhage (IVH) was diagnosed and classified based on the Canadian Pediatric Society's Cranial Ultrasound Statement [14]. Severe neurological injury defined as the presence of grade 3 or 4 intraventricular hemorrhage (IVH) or parenchymal echolucency [13]. Retinopathy of prematurity (ROP) grade 3 or 4 was defined according to the International Classification for ROP [13]. Necrotizing enterocolitis (NEC) was defined according to Bell's criteria (stage≥2) [13]. Small for gestational age (SGA) was defined as birth weight <10th percentile for the given GA [13]. Duration of mechanical ventilation was defined as the total number of days during which the infant was on mechanical ventilation during any part of the day. Total duration of oxygen use was defined as the total number of days during which the infant received supplemental oxygen. Length of stay was defined as the total number of days that an infant stayed in the NICU. These definitions remained constant throughout the study period.

All surviving preterm infants were routinely followed prospectively and underwent comprehensive developmental assessment by a multidisciplinary team (consisting of a neonatologist/developmental pediatrician, psychologist, occupational therapist, physiotherapist, dietician, speech therapist, social worker, nurse, ophthalmologist, audiologist) at 4, 8, and 18 and at 36 months CA, with referrals to treatment made as required. The cognitive assessments were performed by a trained psychologist using the Wechsler Preschool and Primary Scale of Intelligence, Third Edition (WPPSI-III) or the Stanford-Binet Intelligence Test, Fourth Edition (SB-IV). Formal speech and language assessments were completed by a speech and language pathologist using a battery of standardized test measures including the Preschool Language Scale (PLS 3 or 4) and the Clinical Evaluation of Language Fundamentals (CELF-P2). An audiologist examined each child using visual reinforcement audiometry, otoscopic evaluation and tympanometry at 4 months of CA. Members of the multidisciplinary team were not blinded to the details of the infant's neonatal hospital course.

For the primary outcome, neurodevelopmental disability at 36 months CA was classified using three categories: i) no disability, ii) mild disability, and iii) severe disability.

Classification of Disability

Disability was classified into two groups based on severity of disability: mild or severe. Mild disability was considered present if a child had one or more of the following conditions: mild, ambulant cerebral palsy, borderline cognitive scores of 1–2 standard deviations (SD) below the mean on standardized tests, visual or hearing disabilities, but were not blind or deaf. Severe disability was defined as one or more of: moderate-severe cerebral palsy, cognitive score >2 SD below the mean on standardized tests, blindness or deafness.

Detailed definitions of disability outcomes are described below.

Cerebral palsy. (CP) refers to a non-progressive disability of movement and posture and was diagnosed on the basis of abnormal muscle tone and reflexes on the physical and neurological examination. Severity of motor dysfunction in cerebral palsy was classified into two categories: mild or moderate-severe. Mild CP was defined as having abnormal tone

Table 1. Discharge criteria of infant from NICU.

Criteria
a. Corrected gestational age >34 weeks
b. Able to maintain body temperature (>36.4°C) in an open crib
c. Competent suckle feeding (breast or bottle) without cardiorespiratory compromise and gaining weight
d. Physiologically mature
e. Stable cardiorespiratory function
f. No apnea of prematurity
g. No active medical problems
h. Receipt of appropriate immunizations
i. Appropriate metabolic screening and car seat testing performed
j. In addition to the above criteria, family readiness

and reflexes with no limiting effects on daily activities and functions. Moderate-severe CP was defined as motor dysfunction requiring appliances or assistance with performance of daily activities and functions [15].

Cognitive delay. Delayed cognitive function was diagnosed if there was a cognitive score >2 SD below the mean on age appropriate standardized testing. Borderline cognitive function was diagnosed if there was a cognitive score 1–2 SD below the mean on age appropriate standardized testing.

Blindness. was considered present if the infant had bilateral blindness with corrected visual acuity of <20/200 in the better eye. Mild vision disability refers to those infants who had corrected visual acuity <20/60 but >20/200 in the better eye, significant refractive errors such as severe myopia or significant hypermetropia, or unilateral blindness.

Deafness. was defined as a bilateral sensorineural loss requiring amplification or cochlear implants. Mild hearing disability was defined as neurosensory hearing loss not requiring amplification or implants, or unilateral hearing loss requiring amplification.

Secondary Outcomes

Poor growth. Poor growth was considered present if weight, height, or head circumference was <5th centile at 36 months CA based on the Centers for Disease Control and Prevention (CDC 2000) growth curves [16].

Abnormal language. Overall abnormal communication was defined as receptive, expressive, or overall language scores >1 SD below the mean on standardized language tests, or if articulation was unintelligible. Abnormal receptive or expressive language was based on a score of >1 SD below the mean on the receptive or expressive component of standardized language tests respectively.

Statistical Analysis

The sample size estimation was based on the primary objective of this study: to examine the relationship between no BPD, BPD, and BPD with chronic oxygen dependency and neurodevelopmental disability. We used the method derived by Whitehead [17] for the estimation of sample size for ordinal data, where the cumulative odds ratio is the effect size. The cumulative odds ratio is calculated using the cumulative probability. In this case, the dependent variable consisted of three categories: no, mild, and severe disability. Thus, the two cumulative probabilities are the probability of any disability (mild or severe) and the probability of severe disability. The two cumulative odds are the probability of

any disability divided by the probability of no disability and the probability of severe disability divided by the probability of mild or no disability. In order to detect an ordinal odds ratio of at least 2.0 with alpha = 0.05 and 80% power, we estimated a sample size of at least 120 children in each of the three categories. Our total sample size was 1030 eligible infants, which allowed us to adjust for covariates.

The infant and maternal characteristics of the cohort were compared across the three groups using Pearson Chi-square or Fisher's exact test for categorical variables, and, since they were not normally-distributed with homogeneous variances, the Kruskal-Wallis test for continuous variables. To assess the three pairwise differences between groups (no BPD vs. BPD, no BPD vs. BPD with chronic oxygen dependency, and BPD vs. BPD with chronic oxygen dependency), confidence intervals for differences in proportion or Hodges-Lehmann median differences were calculated. To adjust for multiple comparisons, the Bonferroni correction was applied, and confidence intervals reported at the (1–0.05/3) level.

Given that our primary outcome was ordinal, a proportional odds model was used to determine the effect of the three levels of BPD status (independent variable) on neurodevelopmental disability (dependent variable). This approach considers the scale over the levels of disability and models the 'odds of greater disability' (the odds of mild or severe disability versus no disability, and the odds of severe disability versus mild or no disability). Candidate covariates were identified based on the association with BPD status from the univariate analyses. Covariates considered were: maternal race, caesarean section, maternal antihypertensive medications use, GA, birth weight (BW), sex, small for gestational age (SGA), duration of neonatal hospital stay, days on ventilation, days on oxygen, number of blood transfusions, postnatal steroids, diuretics, PDA, respiratory distress syndrome (RDS), sepsis, NEC, IVH, and ROP. In order to determine the most parsimonious model, we started with a model with all candidate variables included, and any non-statistically significant variables at the alpha = 0.05 level, aside from BPD status, were considered for elimination. The likelihood ratio test and Akaike's Information Criterion were used to assess whether a variable could be removed from the model without significantly affecting model fit. Once the final model was obtained, we included GA and BW separately, as these are clinically important covariates. The Score test was used to test the proportional odds assumption of the final model.

Secondary outcomes of poor growth and abnormal language were explored using the Chi-square test to compare the three

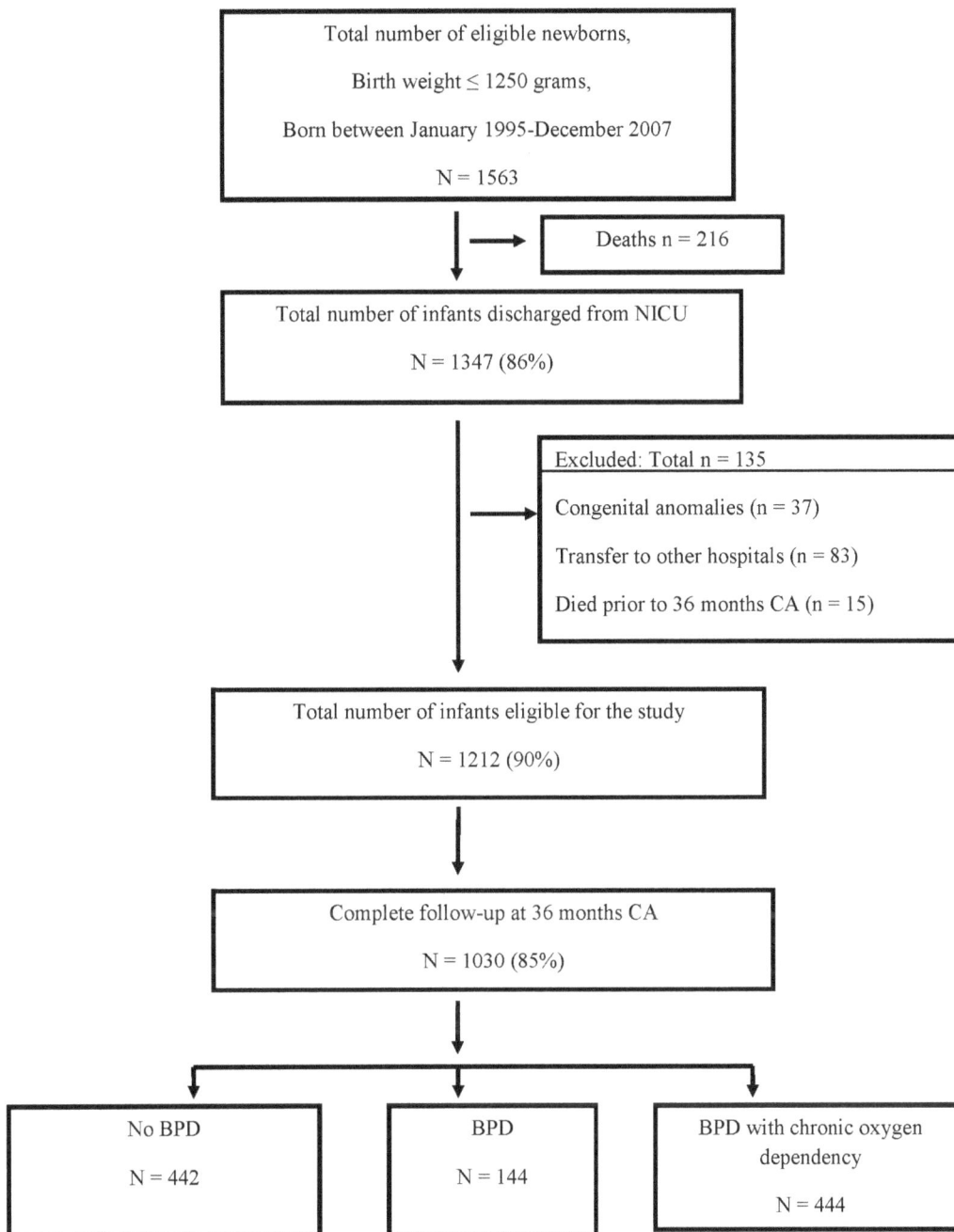

Figure 1. Flow diagram of the study cohort.

groups, along with the Bonferroni-corrected confidence intervals to assess pairwise differences between groups. Growth z-scores were compared across the three groups using ANOVA. All results were generated using SAS 9.3 (SAS Institute, Cary, NC, USA) and a significance level of 0.05 was used for all analyses.

Results

A total of 1563 infants weighing ≤1250 g were eligible at birth for study entry. A flow diagram of our study cohort is shown in **Figure 1**. After excluding infants who died prior to 36 months CA, congenital anomalies and unknown BPD status due to transfers to other hospitals, a total of 1212 children were eligible

for study entry. In this cohort, almost 90% of children were seen at least once over the three year follow-up period but at 36 months CA the follow-up rate was reduced to 85% (1030 children). These children were divided into three groups: 442 (43%) with no BPD, 144 (14%) with BPD, and 444 (43%) with BPD with chronic oxygen dependency.

Demographic characteristics and socio-economic status of the study population are shown in **Table 2**. Children lost to follow-up at 36 months CA of age (n = 182) and those followed up (n = 1030) were not significantly different in BW (median 983 vs. 950 g, p = 0.101) or GA (median 28 vs. 27 weeks, p = 0.096). Children lost to follow-up were more likely to have a shorter hospital stay (median 71 vs. 75 days, p = 0.019) and duration of mechanical

Table 2. Characteristics of the Follow-up Cohort and Their Mothers.

Characteristic	No BPD (n = 442)	BPD (n = 144)	BPD with chronic oxygen dependency (n = 444)	p-value†	Confidence Intervals for Pairwise Differences*		
					No BPD vs. BPD	No BPD vs. BPD with chronic oxygen dependency	BPD vs. BPD with chronic oxygen dependency
Infants							
Birth weight-grams, median (IQR)	1070 (930, 1180)	885 (750, 1060)	820 (690, 1000)	<0.001	(90 to 180)	(180 to 245)	(20 to 120)
Gestational age -wk, median (IQR)	29 (27, 30)	27 (26, 28)	26 (25, 28)	<0.001	(1 to 2)	(2 to 3)	(0 to 1)
Gestational age at discharge-wk, median (IQR)	37 (35, 38)	40 (38, 41)	39 (37, 41)	<0.001	(−4 to −2)	(−3 to −2)	(0 to 1)
Male sex, no. (%)	201 (45.5)	68 (47.2)	256 (57.7)	<0.001	(−0.13 to 0.10)	(−0.20 to −0.04)	(−0.22 to 0.01)
Singleton, no. (%)	311 (70.4)	90 (62.5)	317 (71.4)	0.121	(−0.03 to 0.19)	(−0.08 to 0.06)	(−0.20 to 0.02)
Inborn, no. (%)	396 (89.6)	124 (86.1)	391 (88.1)	0.496	(−0.04 to 0.11)	(−0.04 to 0.07)	(−0.10 to 0.06)
Small for gestational age (<10th %ile), no. (%)	95 (21.5)	18 (12.5)	70 (15.9)	0.019	(0.01 to 0.17)	(−0.01 to 0.12)	(−0.11 to 0.04)
Surfactant, no. (%)	168 (38.2)	95 (66.0)	333 (75.2)	<0.001	(−0.39 to −0.17)	(−0.44 to −0.30)	(−0.20 to 0.01)
Positive pressure ventilation, (CMV+HFO) no. (%)	250 (56.6)	133 (92.4)	424 (95.5)	<0.001	(−0.44 to −0.28)	(−0.45 to −0.33)	(−0.09 to 0.03)
NCPAP, no. (%)	170 (38.5)	107 (74.3)	368 (82.9)	<0.001	(−0.46 to −0.26)	(−0.51 to −0.37)	(−0.18 to 0.01)
Hospital stay-days, median (IQR)	56 (43, 71)	93 (76, 103)	92 (74, 109)	<0.001	(−39 to −30)	(−39 to −32)	(−7 to 4)
Total ventilation-days, median (IQR)	1 (0, 6)	21 (8, 39)	36 (18, 52)	<0.001	(−20 to −12)	(−34 to −27)	(−17 to −6)
Total suppl. oxygen-days, median (IQR)	6 (2, 37)	78 (62, 93)	209 (153, 277)	<0.001	(−68 to −56)	(−200 to −177)	(−144 to −112)
Total blood transfusions-times, median (IQR)	0 (0, 1)	3 (1, 4)	4 (2, 6)	<0.001	(−3 to −2)	(−4 to −3)	(−2 to 0)
Postnatal steroids, no. (%)	21 (4.8)	29 (20.3)	144 (32.5)	<0.001	(−0.24 to −0.07)	(−0.34 to −0.22)	(−0.22 to −0.03)
Diuretics, no. (%)	139 (31.6)	114 (79.7)	384 (86.5)	<0.001	(−0.58 to −0.38)	(−0.61 to −0.48)	(−0.16 to 0.02)
Patent ductus arteriosus, no. (%)	117 (26.5)	89 (61.8)	307 (69.3)	<0.001	(−0.46 to −0.24)	(−0.50 to −0.36)	(−0.19 to 0.04)
Respiratory distress syndrome, no. (%)	224 (50.7)	123 (85.4)	386 (87.1)	<0.001	(−0.44 to −0.26)	(−0.43 to −0.30)	(−0.10 to 0.06)
Confirmed sepsis, no. (%)	42 (9.7)	39 (27.3)	110 (25.0)	<0.001	(−0.27 to −0.08)	(−0.21 to −0.09)	(−0.08 to 0.12)
Necrotizing enterocolitis, no. (%)	40 (9.1)	24 (16.7)	54 (12.2)	0.037	(−0.16 to 0.01)	(−0.08 to 0.02)	(−0.04 to 0.13)
Intraventricular hemorrhage grade ≥ III, no. (%)	10 (2.3)	11 (7.7)	41 (9.2)	<0.001	(−0.11 to 0.002)	(−0.11 to −0.03)	(−0.08 to 0.05)
Periventricular leukomalacia, no. (%)	10 (2.3)	6 (4.2)	7 (1.6)	0.196	(−0.06 to 0.02)	(−0.02 to 0.03)	(−0.02 to 0.07)
Retinopathy of prematurity stage ≥III, no. (%)	14 (3.6)	28 (20.4)	119 (28.0)	<0.001	(−0.25 to −0.08)	(−0.30 to −0.19)	(−0.17 to 0.02)
Maternal							
Maternal education more than high school, no. (%)	252 (60.9)	79 (57.3)	253 (59.8)	0.753	(−0.08 to 0.15)	(−0.09 to 0.07)	(−0.14 to 0.09)
Single parent, no. (%)	29 (6.6)	7 (4.9)	29 (6.6)	0.735	(−0.03 to 0.07)	(−0.04 to 0.04)	(−0.07 to 0.03)
Blishen score, median (IQR)	41 (33, 56)	46 (33, 57)	44 (33, 57)	0.227	(−6 to 1)	(−4 to 1)	(−3 to 4)
Maternal race Caucasian, no. (%)	274 (70.8)	93 (79.5)	280 (77.6)	0.047	(−0.19 to 0.02)	(−0.14 to 0.01)	(−0.08 to 0.12)
Maternal antihypertensive, no. (%)	101 (23.2)	14 (10.3)	75 (17.3)	0.002	(0.05 to 0.21)	(−0.01 to 0.12)	(−0.15 to 0.01)
Smoking during pregnancy, no. (%)	121 (28.3)	39 (27.7)	102 (23.8)	0.302	(−0.10 to 0.11)	(−0.03 to 0.12)	(−0.06 to 0.14)
Antenatal corticosteroids, no. (%)	378 (86.7)	116 (82.9)	366 (83.8)	0.367	(−0.05 to 0.12)	(−0.03 to 0.09)	(−0.10 to 0.08)

Table 2. Cont.

Characteristic Infants	No BPD (n = 442)	BPD (n = 144)	BPD with chronic oxygen dependency (n = 444)	p-value†	Confidence Intervals for Pairwise Differences*		
					No BPD vs. BPD	No BPD vs. BPD with chronic oxygen dependency	BPD vs. BPD with chronic oxygen dependency
Maternal antibiotics, no. (%)	247 (57.2)	84 (60.4)	262 (60.5)	0.572	(−0.15 to 0.08)	(−0.11 to 0.05)	(−0.11 to 0.11)
Chorioamnionitis, no. (%)	94 (22.3)	37 (27.4)	93 (21.5)	0.354	(−0.15 to 0.05)	(−0.06 to 0.08)	(−0.04 to 0.16)
Caesarean section, no. (%)	303 (68.7)	94 (65.3)	246 (55.5)	<0.001	(−0.07 to 0.14)	(0.05 to 0.21)	(−0.01 to 0.21)

†Kruskal-Wallis test for continuous variables; Pearson χ^2 test for categorical variables.
*Bonferroni correction applied to adjust for the three pairwise comparisons, thus confidence intervals are reported at the (1−0.05/3) % level.
BPD: bronchopulmonary dysplasia; CMV: conventional mechanical ventilation; HFO: high frequency oscillatory ventilation; NCPAP: nasal continuous airways pressure.

ventilation (median 6 vs. 13 days, p = 0.031). Follow-up rates were similar among the three groups of children.

Maternal and neonatal characteristics are presented in **Table 2**. There were significant differences between preterm infants with no BPD, BPD, and BPD with chronic oxygen dependency for GA, BW, duration of ventilation, duration of supplemental oxygen, postnatal steroid use, diuretic use, and number of blood transfusions. Premature infants with BPD were discharged from NICU at a median of 39 weeks CA, whereas those without BPD were discharged at a median of 37 weeks (p<0.001).

Figure 2 shows that children with BPD and BPD with chronic oxygen dependency were more likely to have weights less than the 5th centile and height less than 5th centile compared to children with no BPD at 36 months CA (p = 0.018 and p = 0.047, respectively). However, the proportion with head circumferences below the 5th centile was not significantly different. Mean weight, height, and head circumference z-scores were not significantly different between groups (**Table 3**).

Neurodevelopmental outcomes in children with no BPD, BPD, and BPD with chronic oxygen dependency are summarized in **Table 4 and Figure 3**. BPD status was found to be significantly associated with disability (p<0.001). Six percent of those with no BPD had a severe disability, compared to 16% of children with BPD, and 18% of children with BPD with chronic oxygen dependency.

In the final model (**Table 5**), after adjusting for GA, maternal race, number of blood transfusions, postnatal steroids, NEC, and IVH grade 3 or 4, the proportional odds ratio (OR) for increasing disability for children with BPD with chronic oxygen dependency compared to no BPD was 1.8 (95% confidence intervals (CI): 1.1 to 2.9). The adjusted OR for increasing disability comparing children with BPD to no BPD was 1.9 (95% CI: 1.1 to 3.5). However, the adjusted OR for increasing disability comparing children with BPD with chronic oxygen dependency versus BPD was not significant at 0.9 (95% CI: 0.6 to 1.5). Replacing GA with BW in the final adjusted model gave us similar results (data not shown).

Overall abnormal communication was not significantly different between the BPD groups (59% in BPD with chronic oxygen dependency group, 59% in BPD group, and 51% in the no BPD group) (**Table 6**). The proportion of children with abnormal receptive and expressive language was not statistically significantly different between the 3 groups.

Discussion

This study found a large number of preterm infants with BPD who were discharged home on oxygen to facilitate early transition from hospital to home from the single largest level III NICU located at high altitude in Southern Alberta. Our percentage (43%) of BPD with chronic oxygen dependency infants is lower than those reported by other investigators (60–79%) [18], but higher than other reports (36%) [19]. This could be reflective of our study population, the fact that Calgary is 1,100 m (3,600 ft) above sea level and/or our clinical practice [18,20].

In our study, growth delay at 36 months CA was significantly more frequent in children with BPD and BPD with chronic oxygen dependency following discharge from NICU than those who had no BPD. Other investigators have also noted that impaired weight and height growth parameters occur in infants with BPD and BPD with chronic oxygen dependency [21],[22].

We found no difference in poor language outcomes between children with BPD and BPD with chronic oxygen dependency

Growth <5th centile

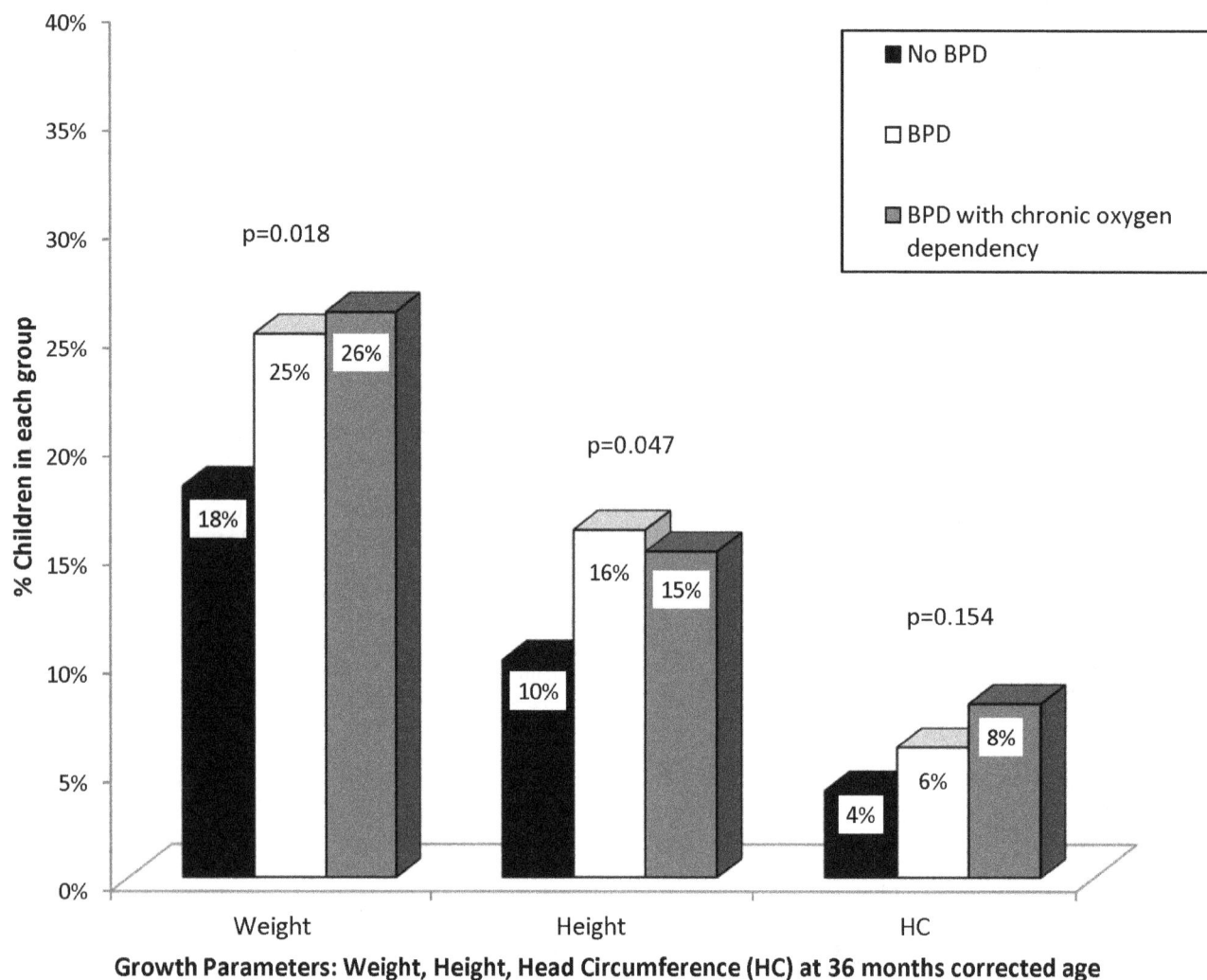

Growth Parameters: Weight, Height, Head Circumference (HC) at 36 months corrected age

Figure 2. Growth parameters (weight, height and head circumference) in the No BPD, BPD and BPD with chronic oxygen dependency groups at 36 months corrected age.

compared to children without BPD. These language findings are consistent with previous studies [23,24].

In this study, neurodevelopmental disability, particularly cognitive impairment, at 36 months CA was significantly more

frequent in children with BPD and BPD with chronic oxygen dependency following discharge from NICU than those who had no BPD. Even after adjusting for a variety of perinatal and neonatal factors, the significantly increased disability rate in

Table 3. Growth at 36 months corrected age.

Growth Parameter	No BPD (n = 409/442)	BPD (n = 139/144)	BPD with chronic oxygen dependency (n = 407/444)	p-value*
Weight z-score, mean (SD)	−0.64 (1.1)	−0.83 (1.6)	−0.81 (1.3)	0.082
Height z-score, mean (SD)	−0.30 (1.0)	−0.47 (1.1)	−0.46 (1.2)	0.078
Head circumference z-score, mean (SD)	−0.08 (1.0)	−0.07 (1.2)	−0.11 (1.1)	0.892

*ANOVA F-test. Welch's ANOVA F-test reported if variances were non-homogeneous according to Levene's test.
BPD: bronchopulmonary dysplasia.

Table 4. Disability Status at 36 Months Corrected Age (No., %).

Disability Type	Disability Severity	No BPD	BPD	BPD with chronic oxygen dependency	p-value[†]
		n = 442	n = 144	n = 444	
Cerebral Palsy	None	418 (94.6)	127 (88.2)	396 (89.2)	0.033
	Mild	10 (2.3)	6 (4.2)	17 (3.8)	
	Moderate-Severe	14 (3.2)	11 (7.6)	31 (7.0)	
Blindness	None	422 (96.1)	133 (93.0)	395 (89.6)	<0.001
	Visual Disability	15 (3.4)	10 (7.0)	34 (7.7)	
	Legally Blind	2 (0.5)	0 (0.0)	12 (2.7)	
Deafness	None	438 (99.8)	140 (97.9)	417 (94.6)	<0.001
	Hearing Disability	1 (0.2)	2 (1.4)	5 (1.1)	
	Deaf	0 (0.0)	1 (0.7)	19 (4.3)	
Cognitive Function	Normal	372 (84.9)	110 (76.9)	307 (69.9)	<0.001
	Borderline	44 (10.1)	19 (13.3)	78 (17.8)	
	Delay	22 (5.0)	14 (9.8)	54 (12.3)	
Any Disability	None	343 (79.4)	93 (65.5)	254 (58.3)	<0.001
	Mild	62 (14.4)	27 (19.0)	102 (23.4)	
	Severe	27 (6.3)	22 (15.5)	80 (18.4)	

[†]Pearson χ^2 test or Fisher's Exact test.
BPD: bronchopulmonary dysplasia;

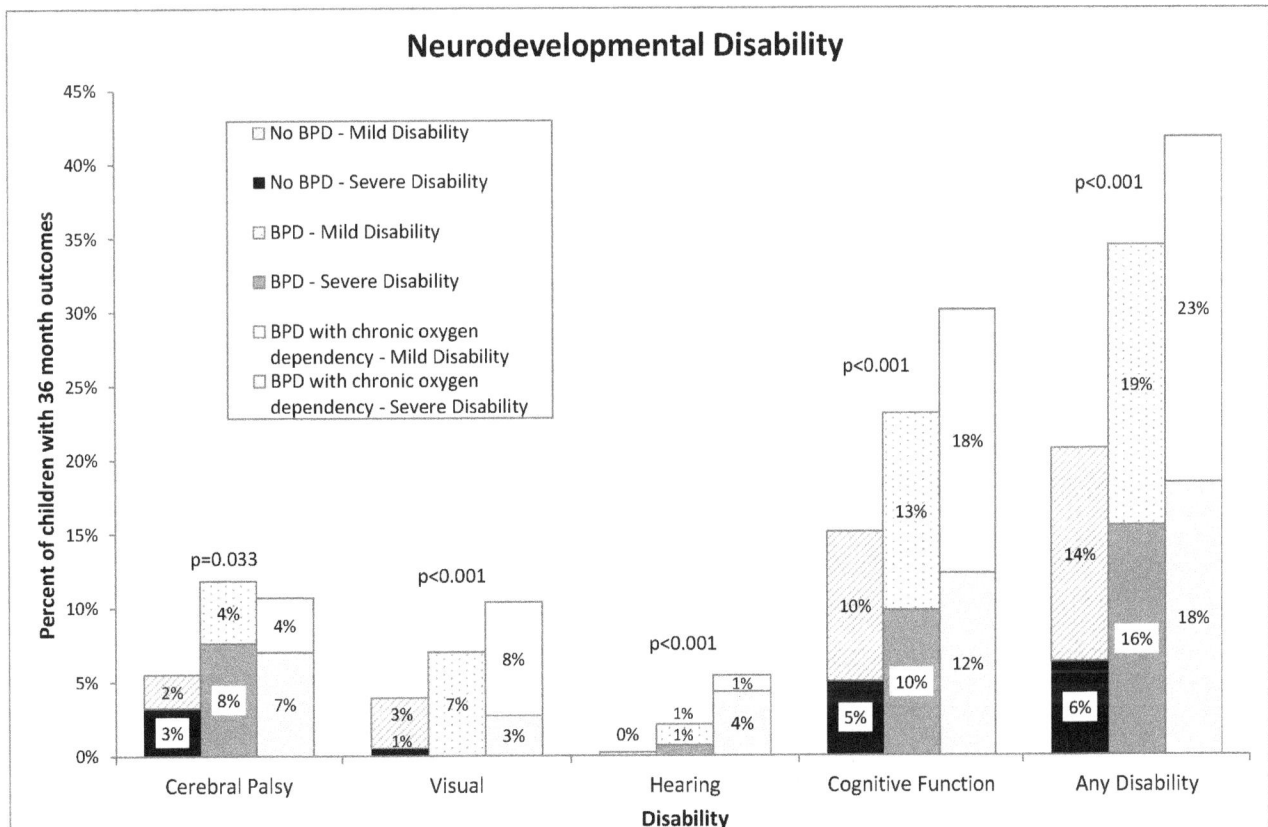

Figure 3. Disability Status at 36 Months Corrected Age.

Table 5. Proportional odds model of factors associated with neurodevelopmental disability.

Predictors	p-value	Odds ratio (OR) for increasing disability*
BPD with chronic oxygen dependency vs. No BPD[§]	0.013	1.8 (1.1 to 2.9)
BPD vs. No BPD[§]	0.022	1.9 (1.1 to 3.5)
BPD with chronic oxygen dependency vs. BPD[§]	0.755	0.9 (0.6 to 1.5)
Maternal Race (Non-Caucasian vs. Caucasian)	0.005	1.8 (1.2 to 2.6)
Blood transfusions (per unit increase in no. of times)	0.001	1.1 (1.1 to 1.2)
Postnatal steroids	0.029	1.6 (1.1 to 2.5)
NEC	0.017	1.9 (1.1 to 3.1)
IVH grade III or IV	<0.001	9.6 (5.0 to 18.8)
Gestational age (per 1 week increase)	0.535	1.0 (0.9 to 1.1)

*Estimated odds ratios from proportional odds model; odds of mild or severe disability versus no disability, and odds of severe disability versus milder or no disability; Score test for the proportional odds assumption: $p = 0.149$; Likelihood ratio test for overall model significance: $p < 0.001$.
[§]The model was first run with No BPD as the reference category. In order to obtain estimates for BPD with chronic oxygen dependency versus BPD, the model was run a second time, using BPD as the reference category.
BPD: bronchopulmonary dysplasia; NEC: necrotizing enterocolitis; IVH: intraventricular hemorrhage; SGA: small for gestational age; PDA: patent ductus arteriosus; RDS: respiratory distress syndrome; ROP: retinopathy of prematurity.

children with BPD and BPD with chronic oxygen dependency versus those with no BPD still remained. To our surprise, there was no difference in outcomes, going against the pre-conceived notion that supplemental oxygen is a surrogate marker for a more severe form of BPD and is potentially contributing to increased neurodevelopmental disability even after discharge home, compared to non-oxygen dependent BPD.

While caffeine [25] and non-invasive ventilation approaches [26] are being frequently utilized early in the NICU in an attempt to decrease BPD [27], the use of supplemental oxygen in these premature infants, while significantly contributing to the pathogenesis of BPD, is a fairly constant clinical practice as it is critical for their survival [28]. While attempts have been made to limit the dose and duration of exposure of supplemental oxygen to the immature lungs [29–32], given the decreased capacity of the preterm infants to combat oxidative stress, it is not surprising that supplemental oxygen that is required for prolonged periods in this population results in significant medical consequences. The duration of exposure to supplemental oxygen has been associated with delayed head growth [33], and need for supplemental oxygen at 36 weeks PMA has been associated with significant neurodevelopmental delays at 12–24 months CA [34–37]. In contrast, a recent study has noted that BPD accompanied by invasive mechanical ventilation at 36 weeks PMA strongly predicted the more common bilateral CP phenotypes (assessed at 2 years), but BPD without invasive mechanical ventilation (i.e. only requiring supplemental oxygen at 36 weeks PMA) was not associated with any form of CP [38]. Potential explanations for neurodevelopmental disability include: excessive production of reactive oxygen species [39], fluctuations in blood oxygen levels [40]; occurrence of pneumothorax; lung dysfunction and brain injury due to infection and associated therapies [41]. Long-term follow-up studies of infants with BPD, up to 8 years of age, have reported an association with the severity classification of BPD [42] and the duration of oxygen therapy in the NICU [8]. Our finding of an increased incidence of both mild and severe CP in children who had BPD and BPD with chronic oxygen dependency is similar to Anderson and Doyle's findings [43]. Our study supports the speculation that hypoxic brain damage and IVH ≥ grade III are more robust underlying mechanisms associated with adverse

neurodevelopmental outcomes in infants with BPD and chronic oxygen dependency [7,44].

Our data reaffirms BPD as an independent factor leading to increased neurodevelopmental disability in infants with BPD and BPD with chronic oxygen dependency, versus those with no BPD. The increased risk of neurodevelopmental disability in children with BPD/BPD with chronic oxygen dependency could be related to severe lung injury caused by prolonged hyperoxia and invasive ventilation-induced injury which possibly further exacerbates the risk of adverse neurodevelopmental outcomes secondary to severe brain injuries [10,44]. A multi-faceted and interdisciplinary approach [45] to prevent BPD early in the course in the NICU by favoring increased antenatal steroid use [25], use of caffeine [46], non-invasive ventilation techniques [47], and enhanced nutritional support to improve growth [48,49], offers a practical approach to also improve neurodevelopmental outcomes in such infants.

As an adjunct to clinical management of infants with BPD, home oxygen therapy at the time of discharge has been recommended in an attempt to prevent hypoxic pulmonary vasoconstriction and to allow for adequate growth [50,51]. In our study cohort, despite almost similar median hospital stay, infants with BPD with chronic oxygen dependency versus BPD required more blood transfusions and postnatal steroids. They also had a higher incidence of PDA, IVH (grade >3) and ROP (stage ≥ III). Yet, contrary to our hypothesis, these infants with BPD with chronic oxygen dependency did not have a higher incidence of neurodevelopmental disability at 3 years CA. While earlier studies had predicted worse neurodevelopmental outcomes of infants with BPD sent home on supplemental oxygen [52], recent reports are more in line with our results [53,54]. In one study, there was a difference in developmental scores at the 1 and 2 years follow up, but at 4 years CA, there were no differences in the BPD-room air and BPD-home oxygen groups, suggesting a catch-up between 2 and 4 years CA [53]. Taken together, these data suggest that the need for supplemental home oxygen therapy in infants with BPD does not predict increased neurodevelopmental disability over and above that of infants diagnosed with BPD at 36 weeks PMA. Importantly, even at 36 weeks PMA, it is the need for mechanical ventilation in addition to supplemental oxygen therapy that appears to be significantly associated with worse neurodevelop-

Table 6. Language outcomes at 36 months corrected age.

Language	No BPD	BPD	BPD with chronic oxygen dependency	p-value*	No BPD vs. BPD	No BPD vs. BPD with chronic oxygen dependency	BPD vs. BPD with chronic oxygen dependency
	(n = 385/442)	(n = 135/144)	(n = 398/444)				
Abnormal Overall Communication, no. (%)	195 (51.1)	80 (59.3)	234 (59.4)	0.053	(−0.20 to 0.04)	(−0.17 to 0.01)	(−0.12 to 0.12)
Abnormal Receptive Language, no. (%)	115 (32.9)	48 (39.3)	138 (39.3)	0.163	(−0.19 to 0.06)	(−0.15 to 0.02)	(−0.12 to 0.12)
Abnormal Expressive Language, no. (%)	144 (41.6)	55 (45.1)	158 (44.8)	0.654	(−0.16 to 0.09)	(−0.12 to 0.06)	(−0.12 to 0.13)

Confidence Intervals for Pairwise Differences§

*Pearson χ^2 test or Fisher's Exact test.
§Bonferroni correction applied to adjust for the three pairwise comparisons, thus confidence intervals are reported at the (1−0.05/3) % level.
BPD: bronchopulmonary dysplasia;

mental outcomes and CP. This has important implications in the prognostication of patients with BPD being sent home on oxygen therapy and has a bearing in alleviating parental anxiety in such circumstances [55].

This study has some limitations. The definitions of BPD proposed by NICHD Network [8] based on the concentrations of fraction of inspired oxygen (FiO_2) at various postnatal ages could not be applied retrospectively. Presently, the majority of Canadian centers affiliated with the Canadian Neonatal Net Work (CNN) are using this definition. It was felt that having a similar definition at the national level would be useful to compare the outcome data and for quality improvement purposes. Management practices, especially neonatal ventilation in the NICU, changed between 1995 and 2007; however, we still had a high number of infants with BPD being discharged home on oxygen. During the study period, there were changes in institutional practices especially in increased use of antenatal corticosteroids, the type of ventilation used specifically from intermittent mandatory ventilation to patient triggered/high frequency ventilation or nasal continuous positive air way pressure (NCPAP) use, early use of parentral nutrition, caffeine prior to extubation, early PDA ligation, restricted use of blood transfusions and postnatal steroids. Since 2001, however, there has been no change regarding our policies for discharging infants home on oxygen. Postnatal steroids prescriptions in the NICU require consultation of two neonatologists and verbal consent from parents for the infants with BPD and chronic oxygen dependency with a proper documentation of risk associated with postnatal steroids use in the patients' charts. No changes were made in the definitions of covariate morbidities and outcome measures over the period of study. We do not have information about marital status of mother and number of siblings. Blishen index reflects only the occupation of father which may not reflect actual socioeconomic status of the family. The assessors of the neurodevelopmental outcomes were not blinded to the status of BPD; hence, there is a potential risk of an assessment bias. During the study period, the Gross Motor Function Classification System was not used in our follow-up clinic to classify severity of cerebral palsy. Different cognitive tests were used over the study period and therefore, cognitive outcomes categories were used. Results of our study will be useful to the units those are located at higher altitudes [56]; therefore, generalizability is lacking especially to units located at sea level. The impact of our loss to follow-up is unknown, however, we believe it would not change the overall results as the population lost to follow-up was not significantly different in BW or GA, and a 15% loss of follow up is not an unusually high rate for such long term studies. The strength of our study is the follow-up period of 36 months. We know from past studies that 18 month outcomes are not as definitive and predictive of 3 year and 5 year outcomes. An additional strength of our study is that, to our knowledge, it is the largest single-centre, longitudinal cohort study followed prospectively that determined the impact of chronic oxygen dependency in premature infants with BPD on long-term neurodevelopmental outcomes.

Conclusions

Chronic oxygen dependency in infants with BPD is not associated with significantly increased rates of neurodevelopmental disability at 36 months CA, compared to infants with BPD not requiring supplemental oxygen at the time of discharge home from the NICU. However, compared to children with no BPD, children with BPD and BPD with chronic oxygen dependency have a higher incidence of growth failure and cognitive delay.

Acknowledgments

We acknowledge Dr. Alberto Nettel-Aguirre, PhD, PStat, Departments of Paediatrics and Community Health Sciences, University of Calgary, Dr. M. Sarah Rose, PhD, Biostatistician, Department of Community Health Sciences, University of Calgary, Dr. Marilyn Ballantyne PhD (Clinical Epidemiology) McMaster University, Hamilton, Ontario, Dr. Nidhi Lodha and Dr. Dianne Creighton, PhD (Psychology) University of Calgary for their help in the analysis of data and scientific review of this manuscript.

Author Contributions

Conceived and designed the experiments: AL RS HC ST VB NS. Performed the experiments: AL ST. Analyzed the data: AL ST VB NS. Contributed reagents/materials/analysis tools: AL ST HC VB. Wrote the paper: AL ST VB. Critically reviewed the manuscript: AL RS VB HA AB NS. Final approval of the version to be published: AL RS VB ST HC AB HA NS.

References

1. Ehrenkranz RA, Walsh MC, Vohr BR, Jobe AH, Wright LL, et al. (2005) Validation of the National Institutes of Health consensus definition of bronchopulmonary dysplasia. Pediatrics 116: 1353–1360.
2. Vohr BR, Wright LL, Dusick AM, Perritt R, Poole WK, et al. (2004) Center differences and outcomes of extremely low birth weight infants. Pediatrics 113: 781–789.
3. Van Marter LJ, Allred EN, Pagano M, Sanocka U, Parad R, et al. (2000) Do clinical markers of barotrauma and oxygen toxicity explain interhospital variation in rates of chronic lung disease? The Neonatology Committee for the Developmental Network. Pediatrics 105: 1194–1201.
4. Shennan AT, Dunn MS, Ohlsson A, Lennox K, Hoskins EM (1988) Abnormal pulmonary outcomes in premature infants: prediction from oxygen requirement in the neonatal period. Pediatrics 82: 527–532.
5. Northway WH Jr., Rosan RC, Porter DY (1967) Pulmonary disease following respirator therapy of hyaline-membrane disease. Bronchopulmonary dysplasia. N Engl J Med 276: 357–368.
6. Singer L, Martin RJ, Hawkins SW, Benson-Szekely LJ, Yamashita TS, et al. (1992) Oxygen desaturation complicates feeding in infants with bronchopulmonary dysplasia after discharge. Pediatrics 90: 380–384.
7. Chess PR, D'Angio CT, Pryhuber GS, Maniscalco WM (2006) Pathogenesis of bronchopulmonary dysplasia. Semin Perinatol 30: 171–178.
8. Short EJ, Klein NK, Lewis BA, Fulton S, Eisengart S, et al. (2003) Cognitive and academic consequences of bronchopulmonary dysplasia and very low birth weight: 8-year-old outcomes. Pediatrics 112: e359.
9. Fitzgerald DA, Massie RJ, Nixon GM, Jaffe A, Wilson A, et al. (2008) Infants with chronic neonatal lung disease: recommendations for the use of home oxygen therapy. Med J Aust 189: 578–582.
10. Majnemer A, Riley P, Shevell M, Birnbaum R, Greenstone H, et al. (2000) Severe bronchopulmonary dysplasia increases risk for later neurological and motor sequelae in preterm survivors. Dev Med Child Neurol 42: 53–60.
11. Trittmann JK, Nelin LD, Klebanoff MA (2013) Bronchopulmonary dysplasia and neurodevelopmental outcome in extremely preterm neonates. Eur J Pediatr 172: 1173–1180.
12. Blishen B, Carroll W, Moore C (1987) The 1981 socioeconomic index for occupations in Canada. Canad Rev Soc & Anth 24(4): 465–488.
13. Lodha A, Zhu Q, Lee SK, Shah PS (2011) Neonatal outcomes of preterm infants in breech presentation according to mode of birth in Canadian NICUs. Postgrad Med J 87: 175–179.
14. (2001) Routine screening cranial ultrasound examinations for the prediction of long term neurodevelopmental outcomes in preterm infants. Paediatr Child Health 6: 39–52.
15. Russman BS, Gage JR (1989) Cerebral palsy. Curr Probl Pediatr 19: 65–111.
16. Kuczmarski RJ, Ogden CL, Grummer-Strawn LM, Flegal KM, Guo SS, et al. (2000) CDC growth charts: United States. Adv Data: 1–27.
17. Whitehead J (1993) Sample size calculations for ordered categorical data. Stat Med 12: 2257–2271.
18. Lagatta J, Clark R, Spitzer A (2012) Clinical predictors and institutional variation in home oxygen use in preterm infants. J Pediatr 160: 232–238.
19. Hennessy EM, Bracewell MA, Wood N, Wolke D, Costeloe K, et al. (2008) Respiratory health in pre-school and school age children following extremely preterm birth. Arch Dis Child 93: 1037–1043.
20. Lee SK, Ye XY, Singhal N, De La Rue S, Lodha A, et al. (2012) Higher Altitude and Risk of Bronchopulmonary Dysplasia among Preterm Infants. Am J Perinatol.
21. Madden J, Kobaly K, Minich NM, Schluchter M, Wilson-Costello D, et al. (2010) Improved weight attainment of extremely low-gestational-age infants with bronchopulmonary dysplasia. J Perinatol 30: 103–111.
22. Wang LY, Luo HJ, Hsieh WS, Hsu CH, Hsu HC, et al. (2010) Severity of bronchopulmonary dysplasia and increased risk of feeding desaturation and growth delay in very low birth weight preterm infants. Pediatr Pulmonol 45: 165–173.
23. Lewis BA, Singer LT, Fulton S, Salvator A, Short EJ, et al. (2002) Speech and language outcomes of children with bronchopulmonary dysplasia. J Commun Disord 35: 393–406.
24. Singer LT, Siegel AC, Lewis B, Hawkins S, Yamashita T, et al. (2001) Preschool language outcomes of children with history of bronchopulmonary dysplasia and very low birth weight. J Dev Behav Pediatr 22: 19–26.
25. Bhandari A, Bhandari V (2009) Pitfalls, problems, and progress in bronchopulmonary dysplasia. Pediatrics 123: 1562–1573.
26. Bhandari V (2013) The potential of non-invasive ventilation to decrease BPD. Semin Perinatol 37: 108–114.
27. Botet F, Figueras-Aloy J, Miracle-Echegoyen X, Rodriguez-Miguelez JM, Salvia-Roiges MD, et al. (2012) Trends in survival among extremely-low-birth-weight infants (less than 1000 g) without significant bronchopulmonary dysplasia. BMC Pediatr 12: 63.
28. Bhandari V (2010) Hyperoxia-derived lung damage in preterm infants. Semin Fetal Neonatal Med 15: 223–229.
29. Carlo WA, Finer NN, Walsh MC, Rich W, Gantz MG, et al. (2010) Target ranges of oxygen saturation in extremely preterm infants. N Engl J Med 362: 1959–1969.
30. Stenson BJ, Tarnow-Mordi WO, Darlow BA, Simes J, Juszczak E, et al. (2013) Oxygen saturation and outcomes in preterm infants. N Engl J Med 368: 2094–2104.
31. Schmidt B, Whyte RK, Asztalos EV, Moddemann D, Poets C, et al. (2013) Effects of targeting higher vs lower arterial oxygen saturations on death or disability in extremely preterm infants: a randomized clinical trial. Jama 309: 2111–2120.
32. Bizzarro MJ, Li FY, Katz K, Shabanova V, Ehrenkranz RA, et al. (2013) Temporal quantification of oxygen saturation ranges: an effort to reduce hyperoxia in the neonatal intensive care unit. J Perinatol.
33. Nesterenko TH, Nolan B, Hammad TA, Aly H (2008) Exposure to oxygen and head growth in infants with bronchopulmonary dysplasia. Am J Perinatol 25: 251–254.
34. Karagianni P, Tsakalidis C, Kyriakidou M, Mitsiakos G, Chatziioanidis H, et al. (2011) Neuromotor outcomes in infants with bronchopulmonary dysplasia. Pediatr Neurol 44: 40–46.
35. Natarajan G, Pappas A, Shankaran S, Kendrick DE, Das A, et al. (2012) Outcomes of extremely low birth weight infants with bronchopulmonary dysplasia: impact of the physiologic definition. Early Hum Dev 88: 509–515.
36. Jeng SF, Hsu CH, Tsao PN, Chou HC, Lee WT, et al. (2008) Bronchopulmonary dysplasia predicts adverse developmental and clinical outcomes in very-low-birthweight infants. Dev Med Child Neurol 50: 51–57.
37. Schmidt B, Asztalos EV, Roberts RS, Robertson CM, Sauve RS, et al. (2003) Impact of bronchopulmonary dysplasia, brain injury, and severe retinopathy on the outcome of extremely low-birth-weight infants at 18 months: results from the trial of indomethacin prophylaxis in preterms. Jama 289: 1124–1129.
38. Van Marter LJ, Kuban KC, Allred E, Bose C, Dammann O, et al. (2011) Does bronchopulmonary dysplasia contribute to the occurrence of cerebral palsy among infants born before 28 weeks of gestation? Arch Dis Child Fetal Neonatal Ed 96: F20–29.
39. Sola A, Rogido MR, Deulofeut R (2007) Oxygen as a neonatal health hazard: call for detente in clinical practice. Acta Paediatr 96: 801–812.
40. Sedowofia K, Giles D, Wade J, Cunningham S, McColm JR, et al. (2008) Myelin expression is altered in the brains of neonatal rats reared in a fluctuating oxygen atmosphere. Neonatology 94: 113–122.
41. Laughon M, O'Shea MT, Allred EN, Bose C, Kuban K, et al. (2009) Chronic lung disease and developmental delay at 2 years of age in children born before 28 weeks' gestation. Pediatrics 124: 637–648.
42. Short EJ, Kirchner HL, Asaad GR, Fulton SE, Lewis BA, et al. (2007) Developmental sequelae in preterm infants having a diagnosis of bronchopulmonary dysplasia: analysis using a severity-based classification system. Arch Pediatr Adolesc Med 161: 1082–1087.
43. Anderson PJ, Doyle LW (2006) Neurodevelopmental outcome of bronchopulmonary dysplasia. Semin Perinatol 30: 227–232.
44. Luchi JM, Bennett FC, Jackson JC (1991) Predictors of neurodevelopmental outcome following bronchopulmonary dysplasia. Am J Dis Child 145: 813–817.
45. Shepherd EG, Knupp AM, Welty SE, Susey KM, Gardner WP, et al. (2012) An interdisciplinary bronchopulmonary dysplasia program is associated with improved neurodevelopmental outcomes and fewer rehospitalizations. J Perinatol 32: 33–38.
46. Schmidt B, Roberts RS, Davis P, Doyle LW, Barrington KJ, et al. (2007) Long-term effects of caffeine therapy for apnea of prematurity. N Engl J Med 357: 1893–1902.
47. Bhandari V, Finer NN, Ehrenkranz RA, Saha S, Das A, et al. (2009) Synchronized nasal intermittent positive-pressure ventilation and neonatal outcomes. Pediatrics 124: 517–526.
48. Ehrenkranz RA, Dusick AM, Vohr BR, Wright LL, Wrage LA, et al. (2006) Growth in the neonatal intensive care unit influences neurodevelopmental and

growth outcomes of extremely low birth weight infants. Pediatrics 117: 1253–1261.

49. Ehrenkranz RA, Das A, Wrage LA, Poindexter BB, Higgins RD, et al. (2011) Early nutrition mediates the influence of severity of illness on extremely LBW infants. Pediatr Res 69: 522–529.

50. Bancalari E, Wilson-Costello D, Iben SC (2005) Management of infants with bronchopulmonary dysplasia in North America. Early Hum Dev 81: 171–179.

51. Lagatta JM, Clark RH, Brousseau DC, Hoffmann RG, Spitzer AR (2013) Varying Patterns of Home Oxygen Use in Infants at 23–43 Weeks' Gestation Discharged from United States Neonatal Intensive Care Units. J Pediatr.

52. Sauve RS, McMillan DD, Mitchell I, Creighton D, Hindle NW, et al. (1989) Home oxygen therapy. Outcome of infants discharged from NICU on continuous treatment. Clin Pediatr (Phila) 28: 113–118.

53. Moon NM, Mohay HA, Gray PH (2007) Developmental patterns from 1 to 4 years of extremely preterm infants who required home oxygen therapy. Early Hum Dev 83: 209–216.

54. Trittmann JK, Nelin LD, Klebanoff MA (2013) Bronchopulmonary dysplasia and neurodevelopmental outcome in extremely preterm neonates. Eur J Pediatr.

55. Zanardo V, Freato F (2001) Home oxygen therapy in infants with bronchopulmonary dysplasia: assessment of parental anxiety. Early Hum Dev 65: 39–46.

56. Britton JR (2012) Altitude, oxygen and the definition of bronchopulmonary dysplasia. J Perinatol 32: 880–885.

9

Tinnitus and Other Auditory Problems – Occupational Noise Exposure below Risk Limits May Cause Inner Ear Dysfunction

Ann-Cathrine Lindblad[1]*, Ulf Rosenhall[2], Åke Olofsson[1], Björn Hagerman[1]

1 Department of Clinical Science, Intervention and Technology, Division of Ear, Nose and Throat Diseases, Unit of Technical and Experimental Audiology, Karolinska Institutet, Stockholm, Sweden, 2 Department of Clinical Science, Intervention and Technology, Division of Ear, Nose and Throat Diseases, Karolinska Institutet; and Department of Audiology and Neurotology, Karolinska University Hospital, Stockholm, Sweden

Abstract

The aim of the investigation was to study if dysfunctions associated to the cochlea or its regulatory system can be found, and possibly explain hearing problems in subjects with normal or near-normal audiograms. The design was a prospective study of subjects recruited from the general population. The included subjects were persons with auditory problems who had normal, or near-normal, pure tone hearing thresholds, who could be included in one of three subgroups: teachers, *Education*; people working with music, *Music*; and people with moderate or negligible noise exposure, *Other*. A fourth group included people with poorer pure tone hearing thresholds and a history of severe occupational noise, *Industry*. $N_{total} = 193$. The following hearing tests were used: − pure tone audiometry with Békésy technique, − transient evoked otoacoustic emissions and distortion product otoacoustic emissions, without and with contralateral noise; − psychoacoustical modulation transfer function, − forward masking, − speech recognition in noise, − tinnitus matching. A questionnaire about occupations, noise exposure, stress/anxiety, muscular problems, medication, and heredity, was addressed to the participants. Forward masking results were significantly worse for *Education* and *Industry* than for the other groups, possibly associated to the inner hair cell area. Forward masking results were significantly correlated to louder matched tinnitus. For many subjects speech recognition in noise, left ear, did not increase in a normal way when the listening level was increased. Subjects hypersensitive to loud sound had significantly better speech recognition in noise at the lower test level than subjects not hypersensitive. Self-reported stress/anxiety was similar for all groups. In conclusion, hearing dysfunctions were found in subjects with tinnitus and other auditory problems, combined with normal or near-normal pure tone thresholds. The teachers, mostly regarded as a group exposed to noise below risk levels, had dysfunctions almost identical to those of the more exposed *Industry* group.

Editor: Manuel S. Malmierca, University of Salamanca- Institute for Neuroscience of Castille and Leon and Medical School, Spain

Funding: This project was supported by AFA Insurance, T-50:05, www.afaforsakring.se; and by the Swedish Council for Working Life and Social Research (2003-0154), www.fasarbetsliv.se. The funders had no role in study design, data collection and analysis, decision to publish, or preparation of the manuscript.

Competing Interests: This project was partly supported by AFA Insurance. This does not alter the authors' adherence to PLOS ONE policies on sharing data and materials.

* E-mail: anncat.lindblad@ki.se

Introduction

Hearing problems are not just a matter of reduced ability to recognize speech and other sounds, but also of tinnitus, abnormal sensitivity to loud sound and sound distortion. Hearing loss, as measured by pure tone audiometry, is often accompanied by tinnitus. However, tinnitus occurs without concurrent self-reported hearing loss in about 1/3rd of all cases[1] (but bear in mind that self-reported hearing loss is poorly correlated to audiometric status). There are some reasons for this: 1) Tinnitus can be a non-auditory symptom, not involving the peripheral auditory system[2]; 2) Tinnitus can occur in conjuncture with a subclinical dysfunction of the cochlea[3,4], e.g. as a symptom at an early stage of noise-induced hearing loss (NIHL).

In a study of risk factors for tinnitus in a population 55 years and older Sindhusake et al[5] described a number of extrinsic and health factors that could be linked to tinnitus. The factor with the largest attributable risk was self-reported work-related noise exposure (almost 14%). The largest single factor was self-reported tolerable occupational noise exposure (9.3%). This means that a number of occupations with less noise burden than industrial exposure are at risk for noise-induced tinnitus. Teachers/preschool teachers are exposed to sudden slamming of for example lids, doors or toys, and preschool teachers may also suffer sudden screams near to the ear, although the mean noise levels are not excessive[6,7]. In occupations related to music the noise often varies around the sound level above which there is a risk of NIHL according to the international standardisation[8]. However, music sounds can be very loud, and alterations in the audiogram indicative of NIHL have been reported[9,10]. In other studies no relationship between music exposure and hearing loss, in terms of pure tone thresholds, has been found (for a review, see Zhao et al[11]). Tinnitus is common among rock/jazz musicians, also when the audiogram is similar to that of a reference group not exposed to excessive music[12].

These days when tinnitus is being paid so much attention, it may not be provocative to claim that hearing problems can be more than, or different from, having bad pure tone thresholds. Therefore there should be a demand for diagnostic test methods for identifying or excluding dysfunctions associated to the cochlea as the origin(s) of the hearing problems. Results from such tests could form the basis for individual treatment plans.

A test protocol, intended to be sufficiently sensitive to detect dysfunctions associated to minute cochlear lesions that cannot be diagnosed by routine clinical audiological tests, was developed. The protocol now consists of six auditory physiological tests, a Békésy audiogram, and a questionnaire.

In a first study, with fewer tests and test subjects (n = 46), who had tinnitus and normal or near-normal hearing-thresholds, we found that certain results could be associated with certain backgrounds[4]: 1) Persons exposed to impulse noise or other sudden loud sounds showed characteristic results. 2) Irregularities in the regulatory system may be a trustworthy sign of the cause of the tinnitus in persons well below middle-age, and with suspected hereditary tinnitus. 3) Subjects working with music had a variety of dysfunctions, but no features making them stand out from persons with other backgrounds. 4) Persons with suspected non-auditory tinnitus, on the other hand, showed very few dysfunctions.

The aim of the current study was to use the full test protocol to possibly identify dysfunctions associated with cochlear lesions in persons with up to moderate noise levels at work, with hearing problems, and without apparent deteriorations in the audiogram. If we found dysfunctions, would professions with different types of noise show their own characteristics?

The main finding of the current study was that teachers had characteristic results for two measurements not used in the first study. Those results were similar to results from industry workers tested for comparison, although the teachers had about 20 dB better pure tone thresholds. However, there were still no characteristic features to be found for musicians.

Materials and Methods

Ethics statement

The investigation was approved by the Regional ethical review board in Stockholm, no. 04-228/4. All test subjects gave their informed consents (written) to participate in the study.

Test subjects

Altogether 272 subjects of working age with tinnitus or other hearing problems, and not wearing a hearing aid, were tested in the study. About half of them were recruited by announcements in hearing clinics in Stockholm. The other half was recruited by an announcement at the home page of Karolinska University Hospital, and participants came from all over the country. The subjects were recruited and measured during a period of three years. There was no medical examination of the test subjects. The characterization of symptoms and exposure to e.g. noise was entirely based on the questionnaire. As it happened, very few professions were represented among these volunteers. Thus groups were formed to fit the assortment of volunteers regarding the amount and characteristics of noise exposure. It was not possible to match the participants regarding gender and age. Therefore the results should be interpreted with caution. However, some of the results have been compared with results for groups of persons of similar ages, but without hearing problems, or with internationally standardised pure tone thresholds. Reported here are results of subjects, who fulfilled the threshold criterion of having normal or near-normal hearing thresholds and who could be included in one

of three groups of professions. Results of a fourth group with industrial noise and worse hearing thresholds are also reported for comparison. This study may have found dysfunctions that are characteristic for these groups before the audiogram is affected, but it will not give us a general overview of the effects of noise on hearing for these groups of professions at later stages of deterioration of the audiogram. Neither can it tell how common the detected dysfunctions are.

The groups were: 1) teachers, with 1/3rd of them preschool teachers, forming the group *Education*; 2) people working professionally with music, the group *Music*; and 3) subjects with low or, in a few cases, moderate occupational noise exposure, mostly medical staff and students, the group *Other*. The group *Other* seemed the least homogenous regarding noise exposure. In these groups (1–3) pure tone thresholds on both ears had to be ≤25 dB hearing level (HL) at the frequencies 500, 1000, 1500 and 2000 Hz, and ≤ 40 dB HL at 4000 Hz. The average threshold at the frequencies 3000, 4000, and 6000 Hz on both ears had to be ≤35 dB HL. The threshold fence defining normality or near-normality was chosen to include the effect of normal aging for all the test subjects. At the higher frequencies it corresponds to the median thresholds of otologically normal 66 year old men with no history of undue noise exposure[13].

For comparison a fourth group was selected 4) constituted of persons with blue-collar occupations, having audiograms with high- (and sometimes mid-) frequency hearing impairments, indicative of noise-induced hearing loss, and also having tinnitus, the group *Industry*.

After omission of data from people not conforming to the threshold criterion or being unsuitable for the chosen groups of professions there was a total of 193 subjects, 102 men and 91 women, 18 to 66 years of age, to be analysed. The groups are presented in Table 1. The proportion of genders in the profession groups seems roughly the same as in working life in our country. Mean audiograms for the four test groups are shown in Figure 1.

Reference groups

"Normal" reference results for our methods and our equipment were used for comparison. These results were meant to be to be used in several projects. A *middle-aged reference group* consisted of fifty-seven 41–60 year old subjects, all without hearing problems and with hearing thresholds no worse than the median for 50-year-old men[13]. (In the 5-year age intervals there were 8 women and 8 men who were 41 to 45 years old, 7 women and 7 men who were 46 to 50, 7 women and 9 men who were 51 to 55, and 8 women and 4 men who were 56 to 60.) Another group consisted of twenty-seven young women, 18–24 years old, considering themselves normal and unexposed, and with normal hearing thresholds (< 20 dB HL 125–8000 Hz except for four individual thresholds exceeding 20 but not 23 dB HL). The mean pure tone thresholds for the group turned out to be 5 dB HL. A comparison to the ISO-standard above tells that 80% of unexposed women at those ages have better thresholds than our group of young women. Several of these young women often went to discos or pop concerts and had tinnitus. Thus they were not an ideal, "normal", "unexposed" group.

Equipment and measurements

A computer-controlled Tucker-Davis Technologies (System III) module system was used with Sennheiser HDA 200 headphones at the psychoacoustical tests, and with amplifiers plus probe systems ER-10C from Etymotic Research on both ears for the measurements of otoacoustic emissions. The HDA 200 headphones were

Table 1. Number, age, and gender of subjects in groups.

Profession	Group name	Number	Mean age (SD)	No. of men	No. of women
Teachers	*Education*	48	45.4 (10.6)	9	39
Musicians	*Music*	32	37.8 (11.5)	20	12
Other	*Other*	97	39.2 (13.5)	57	40
Noisy industry	*Industry*	16	54.4 (9.3)	16	0
TOTAL		193	45.0 (13.0)	102	91

calibrated according to ISO 389-8 and the ER-10C probe systems were calibrated in an ear simulator according to IEC 60711.

The software for all the methods, for the computer and the Tucker-Davis equipment, was written in our laboratory. The TDT system was programmed to produce and present stimuli, for example the OAE stimuli and the contralateral noise, as well as collect and store the responses. However, the speech test used stored sound files for the words and their respective noise stimuli. The adaptive procedure of the speech test was controlled by the computer. All tests were performed in a sound proof audiometric test room.

Basic otoscopy and tympanometry were performed. When necessary, cerumen was removed.

The hearing measurements took about three and a half hours including a coffee break. All the participating subjects performed all the tests. However, individual test subjects were allowed to exclude stimulus levels they considered too high.

Questionnaire. In the intermission between the measurements the subjects were given a questionnaire. Apart from questions about age and profession there were 22 questions with two to eight response alternatives, sometimes also with a possibility of an open response. The questions regarded hearing problems, tinnitus, sensitivity to loud sounds, noise exposure at work and in their leisure time, musical activities, impulse noise incidents, military service, medication (pain relieving and tinnitus medicine), eye and hair colour, smoking, neck problems, headache, stress, and relatives with hearing problems. The questions on tinnitus and

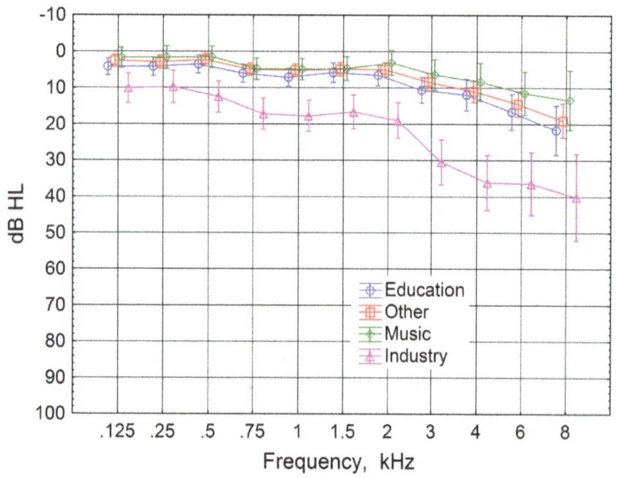

sensitivity to loud sounds had the response alternatives: never, only after a loud sound, at certain occasions, often, and constantly. The questions on headache and neck problems had only the response alternatives yes and no. The question "Do you feel stressed/anxious?" had the five response alternatives: never, seldom, sometimes, often and always. A translation of the questionnaire, including number of responses to each alternative, is presented in Appendix S1.

From the responses to the questions about profession, different types of noise exposure and exposure times, figures of noise exposure were estimated. The underlying principles for the judgements are found in Appendix S2. A summary is presented here: The range for 1) work noise exposure was 0 to 4, for 2) leisure time 0 to 3, and for 3) military service 0 to 2. Persons with only marginal noise exposure in compulsory military service, being well protected during a few initial shooting exercises, got the estimate 0, the same as persons not having been in military service. The total noise exposure was calculated as the sum of the three figures, which gave a scale from 0 to 9. However, the highest value for an individual in this study was 4. Within each profession group the figures were fairly equal. 4) Self-reported incidents with impulse noise were treated separately, range 0 to 3.

Békésy audiometry. Pure tone thresholds for left and right ears separately were measured at 125, 250, 500, 750, 1000, 1500, 2000, 3000, 4000, 6000, and 8000 Hz.

A pulsating tone is presented. The duration is 225 ms, including attack and release times, and with a 175 ms long interval between pulses. The level of the tone is increased by 2.8 dB/s until the subject detects the tone and starts pressing the button. The level of the tone decreases with the same speed until the button is released again, etc. Thus a zigzag pattern is formed around the threshold level. The turning-points are registered by the computer. The measurement is concluded after 10 turning points. The first two turning points are not used in the calculation. The threshold is calculated as the mean value of the medians of the remaining upper and lower turning points, and presented with the resolution of 1 dB. These parameters should give high accuracy with a standard deviation of repeated measures not exceeding 1.8 dB[14].

Otoacoustic emissions, TEOAEs. Transient evoked otoacoustic emissions, TEOAEs, were measured at two input levels without or with contralateral noise. Normally the contralateral noise will make the efferent system controlling the outer hair cells, OHCs, reduce, suppress, the response amplitude. We measure the response correlated to the stimulus signal, but also the uncorrelated response.

Clicks with the duration of 80 µs were repeated with a frequency of 50 Hz. The measurement was performed in a nonlinear mode to enhance those components in the response, which have a nonlinear dependence of the stimulus level, and to suppress the linear components. To accomplish this, the polarity of

Figure 1. Mean audiograms for the profession groups. Group names as shown in Table 1. Please note that the group *Industry* had no threshold restrictions. The vertical bars represent 95% confidence intervals. The data points are horizontally displaced for clarity.

every fourth click is reversed and the sound pressure level is increased by a factor of 3. After removal of the primary click by windowing technique, the acoustical responses from 1000 clicks are averaged. The stimulus level is specified as so called peak equivalent sound pressure level, peSPL. TEOAEs were measured at 70 and 85 dB peSPL with and without contralateral masking consisting of a 70 dB SPL broadband noise. The RMS-values for the correlated and uncorrelated responses, over the interval of measurement, are used as variables in the analyses and so are the RMS-values in three different frequency areas, Low (500–2500 Hz), Mid (2500–5000 Hz), and High (5000–8000 Hz).

Otoacoustic emissions, DPOAEs. When measuring distortion product otoacoustic emissions, DPOAEs, two stimulus tones are given, with frequencies near each other, $f_2/f_1 = 1.25$, and near the measurement frequency. The measurements were performed on both ears at an input level, L, of f_1 of 65 dB SPL, $L_{f1}/L_{f2} = 10$ dB, nominal frequency $\sqrt{f_1}*\sqrt{f_2}$. A weak response is measured at the frequency $2f_1-f_2$. Two measurements were done, the first one at the nominal frequency 1000 Hz and the second one at 2000 Hz. To avoid measuring in a notch of the DPOAE microstructure an automatic procedure measured at a few frequencies between 0.95 and 1.05 times the nominal frequency with an increment of 0.01 times the nominal frequency. The measurements were then performed at the frequency with the largest response. To estimate the background noise from equipment and ear, the level in narrow frequency areas below and above the response tone frequency was measured.

The measurements were made without and with contralateral noise. We made 20 3s long measurements of the response from the two tones without contralateral noise. We calculated the individual standard deviation of these responses to test the stability.

Measurements were also made with on-off noise (12 s on, and 12 s off, 5 times) on the contralateral ear in order to investigate the ability of the ear to regulate the sensitivity of the other ear. The response normally decreases somewhat when the contralateral noise is on. The difference between the medians of the five off-periods and the medians of the five on-periods shows the ability and endurance of the ear to suppress the response when the noise is on.

Psychoacoustical modulation transfer function, PMTF. The active nonlinear process in the cochlea is mediated by the OHCs and facilitates the perception of the complex sound patterns in speech. These patterns are characterized by rapid sound variations combined with slow modulations caused by speech syllables, words and intonation. A measurement termed the psychoacoustical modulation transfer function (PMTF) reflects the functioning of the inner ear when handling slow intensity variations like those of speech. PMTF measures the thresholds of brief tones placed at the peaks or in the valleys of a fully, sinusoidally intensity-modulated, octave-band noise at various sound pressure levels centred at the test tone frequency[15], thus involving simultaneous, forward and backward masking. The measurements were performed with Békésy-technique at various sound pressure levels of the noise. The test has been shown to measure more subtle qualities of hearing, and there is evidence that it reflects hair cell function[15].

PMTF measurements: The measurements were performed with the brief tone, 4 ms with raised cosine flanks, first with the octave-band filtered noise at 2000 Hz, and with a modulation frequency of 2.5 Hz; and then with the octave-band filtered noise at 4000 Hz, and with a modulation frequency of 10 Hz. The noise levels were 35 to 85 dB SPL in steps of 10 dB. Initially, the threshold for the brief tone was measured without noise to familiarize the subject with the brief tone. Both ears were

measured, with the left ear first. When the subject expressed tiredness or discomfort, only one ear, mostly the left ear, was measured.

Typical PMTF results: Figure 2 shows a few stylized, but characteristic PMTF curves. The normal PMTF curves are nonlinear, with a maximum in signal-to-noise-ratio, S/N, for the peak threshold, occurring at a noise level around 55 dB SPL (Figure 2A). (The term *peak threshold* is used for the threshold of the brief tone when the tone is placed at the peak of the noise. The term *valley threshold* is used when the tone is placed in the valley of the noise.) For the valley threshold there is a corresponding maximum at about 65 dB SPL (Figure 2A).

For a sensorineural hearing loss of cochlear origin, the nonlinearity is weaker. Both maxima have lower S/N and they occur at higher noise levels (Figure 2B). This type of pattern indicates *reduced nonlinearity*. However, in this study we focused on the effects described in the following paragraphs.

A second type of abnormal PMTF pattern is presented in (Figure 2D). The S/N maxima of the peak and valley threshold curves have markedly increased amplitudes and occur at the same, low noise level (35–45 dB SPL). The peak and valley curves are almost identical, which implicates that the affected ear can hardly take advantage of the silent interval around the brief tone in the valley. The term "hyper-PMTF" was coined for this pattern, which can appear after unprotected exposure to impulse noise or other sudden, loud noise with a rapid onset[4]. We speculate that there are lesions in the inner hair cell, IHC, region, since impulse noise by itself or embedded in continuous noise causes a larger proportion of damage to IHCs than continuous noise[16].

There are also intermediate varieties between normal and hyper-PMTF. A mildly abnormal variety is shown in Figure 2C. Like in the hyper-PMTF the S/N maxima of the peak and valley curves are positioned at the same noise level, but here they occur at a normal noise level (>45 dB SPL), and they are not as high as in the hyper-PMTF. The level dependence for peak and valley curves is the same. At every noise level used the S/N for the peak threshold is a roughly constant number of dB higher than the S/N for the valley threshold.

It is evident from the examples above that there are two main types of abnormal PMTF results: The positions of the maximum peak and valley thresholds can occur at higher (Figure 2B) or lower (Figure 2D) than normal noise levels (horizontal position in graph), and the corresponding S/N maxima are then either lower (Figure 2B) or higher (Figure 2D) than normal (vertical position in graph). Therefore, a practical way of analysis is to use a qualitative method to define certain typical patterns, for example the hyper-PMTF.

Depending on combinations of shapes and positioning of the peak and valley curves (relative each other and regarding the noise levels of the maxima) we divided the PMTF curves into classes depending on the likeness to hyper-PMTF. We called them P-type, and numbered them 0 to 3. A few P-types are exemplified in Figure 2. Curves denoted P-type = 3, called hyper-PMTF, indicate dysfunction, possibly from impulse noise or other sudden, loud noise with a rapid onset, Figure 2D. P-type = 0 means normal, or typical sensorineural loss that is still measurable at fairly low noise levels, Figure 2A and 2B. P-type = 1, seen in Figure 2C, and P-type = 2 fall in between: P-type = 1 looks more like P-type = 0; and P-type = 2 looks more like P-type = 3 by showing curves with maxima at low noise levels but not as high and/or regular as in the typical hyper-PMTF, i.e. "suspected hyper-PMTF". P-type = NM means not measurable, i.e. the peak and valley thresholds for the brief tone are entirely determined by the threshold for the brief

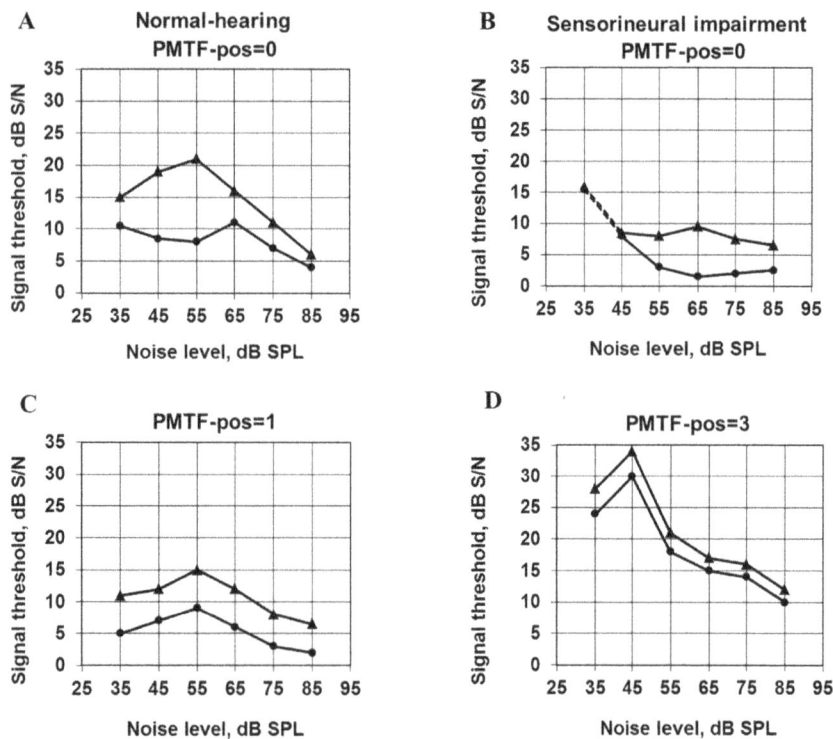

Figure 2. Characteristic PMTF-curves. The PMTF-curves are classified as four different P-types. 0 = normal PMTF-curves (2A) or typical sensorineural loss (2B) that is still measurable; 1 = mildly abnormal (2C), see text; 2 = suspected hyper-PMTF (not shown in the figure); 3 = hyper-PMTF (2D), indicates damage from impulse noise or other sudden, loud noise with a rapid onset; NM = not measurable (not shown in the figure). Triangles indicate peak thresholds. Round markers indicate valley thresholds.

tone without noise at the low noise levels where the characteristics of the hyper-PMTF are seen.

Forward masking. Experiments on mice, using auditory brainstem responses[17], have suggested that forward masking results indicate the status of the IHCs. After the offset of a noise burst the masking effect on a brief tone decreases rapidly in a good ear, but, according to that article, not in an ear with loss of IHCs. In our project a brief tone, 4 ms, at 2000 Hz (the same as used in the PMTF measurements), is presented 5 or 50 ms after the offset of an octave-band noise burst of 400 ms duration and a repetition interval of 800 ms at 65, 75 or 85 dB SPL, and the corresponding thresholds are measured with Békésy technique for one ear at a time, both ears. The difference between the thresholds for 5 and 50 ms interval between noise burst and tone at the same noise level is calculated. A small difference means that the masking effect from the noise burst has not decreased much after 50 ms, which has been attributed to less well-functioning IHCs[17,18]. Our middle-aged reference group showed a threshold difference of 27 ±9 dB. The median was also 27 dB, with lower quartile 22 dB, and a maximum of 49 dB. With results at the lower quartile the speech recognition in noise seemed to start to be degraded. For the group of young women the threshold difference was just 1 dB larger, 28 ±11dB, but the median was 30 dB, and the maximum threshold difference 51 dB.

Speech recognition threshold in modulated noise. The speech recognition threshold in modulated noise was measured on the self-reported worst ear. Hagermans 5-word sentences in noise were used with the original versions of the various words stored in the computer[19]. The noise was modulated to a degree of 100%, i.e. as much as possible without getting overflow[20], and had a long-term average spectrum identical to that of the speech read by a female voice. The modulating signal was a noise with most of its energy between 1 and 5 Hz, and a spectrum similar to the modulation spectrum of normal speech[19]. An adaptive method was used for the threshold measurement, with the change of the speech level after each sentence depending on number of correct words obtained. For a more detailed description see [20]. The threshold is defined as S/N for 40% correct words. The measurements were performed at noise levels 70 and 85 dB SPL. When 85 dB SPL was considered too loud, both ears were measured at 70 dB SPL. For the *middle-aged reference group* the S/N at threshold, over both ears, were −13.6 ±2.1 dB, at 70 dB SPL presentation level, and −15.5 ±2.2 dB, at 85 dB SPL. Corresponding values for the *group of young women*, for the left ear only, were −15.4 ±0.9 and −16.3 ±1.1 dB.

Tinnitus matching. The subjects were asked to compare pure tones from a modified version of the Békésy audiometry program to match the pitch of their tinnitus. The level was changed in steps of 1 dB, and the frequency in steps of 1 Hz. The participants were asked to: "Try to match the frequency of the tone in the earphone with the pitch of your tinnitus. After that, match the level of the tone to that of your tinnitus". The drawback with this method is that it is only applicable to tinnitus with a tonal character. The matching is less accurate for those perceiving their tinnitus as noise or other non-tonal sounds.

Statistical analyses. The program Statistica 9.1 was used for statistical analyses. For the hearing measurements, all of them resulting in continuous variables, analysis of variances was used, often with subsequent Tukey's post hoc tests. To find relations between continuous variables linear regression with age as covariate was used. However, in analyses where age was not significant, results from ANOVAS without age as covariate are presented. For the variables from the questionnaire, with rank order variables, where no information is given in the text, Kruskal-Wallis ANOVA by ranks was used, sometimes with subsequent multiple comparisons. Other statistical tests are mentioned in Results and Discussion.

Results and Discussion

Questionnaire

Hearing problems. Among the 193 subjects analysed, 69% had tinnitus and were also hypersensitive to loud sound, 22% had tinnitus only, 7% were only hypersensitive to loud sound and 2% had neither of these two symptoms, but felt they had difficulties hearing in noise. On a general question about hearing problems 25% answered that their hearing symptoms disturb them always: affect sleep, affect their whole life; 28% that their symptoms affect them in normal sound environments, but their tinnitus is masked by louder sounds; 25% that their symptoms affect them only in a quiet environment; 7% that they have symptoms but no problems (although the criterion for participating was having problems); 13% said they have problems, but did not specify to what extent. There was no statistical difference between the profession groups in this respect. Neither was there any difference between groups regarding hypersensitivity to loud sound.

Noise exposure. Very rough estimates of noise exposure based on the individual responses to the questionnaire indicated that the groups *Education* and *Other* were significantly different from the groups *Music* and *Industry* by being judged less noise exposed ($p < 0.05$). This was the result of a Kruskal-Wallis ANOVA by ranks with estimated noise exposure as the dependent variable and with profession group as the between subjects factor. The questions referred to regarded profession, number of years working, leisure activities, and military service.

Regarding self-reported incidents with impulse noise or sudden very loud noise, a corresponding analysis showed that the exposure estimate for the *Industry* group was significantly higher than for the three other groups ($p < 0.01$). Another group, which might have reported incidents for example with positive feedback in electronic systems, is the *Music* group. In our study, however, the musicians claimed that they were not using electronic amplification. This should have decreased the risk of unexpected sudden changes of the sound level. And the number of reported incidents did not differ significantly from those of the groups *Education* and *Other*.

The *Other* group included mainly hospital staff, and students. Only few of the participants had been exposed to occupational noise. In those cases, they handled medical devices.

Other data from the questionnaire. Regarding neck problems, *Education* had significantly higher values than *Industry* ($p < 0.0005$, Pearson Chi-square). The *Education* group had significantly more self-reported tension headaches than the groups *Other* and *Industry* ($p < 0.05$, Pearson Chi-square). The groups *Education* and *Music* had similar, slightly higher values for stress/anxiety than *Industry* and *Other*, but the differences were not significant. There were no significant differences between groups regarding pain relieving medication, eye and hair colour, smoking, and relatives with hearing problems. Tinnitus medicine was only used by ten subjects. Therefore it was not subjected to analyses. There was no difference in stress problems between the subgroups preschool teachers and other teachers.

Some relations between data from the questionnaire. Self-reported stress seemed to give tension headache and neck problems ($p < 0.05$, $p < 0.005$; binomial logit model). Headaches and neck problems influenced the use of medication ($p < 0.0001$, $p < 0.05$, Kruskal-Wallis ANOVA by

ranks). The amount of medication was not influenced by age (ordinal logit model), gender or stress.

Békésy audiometry

An ANOVA was performed with hearing threshold as the dependent variable, with profession group as a between subjects factor, and with ear and frequency as within subjects factors. The group *Industry*, the blue-collar group without threshold restrictions, chosen to have worse noise exposure than the other groups, was significantly different from all the other groups for left and right ears combined ($p < 0.00001$, Tukey's HSD), Figure 1. For the *Industry* group the right ear was on average 2.8 dB worse than the left ear for all frequencies, but the difference was not significant. This group had worse pure tone thresholds than those of unexposed men of the same age[13].

TEOAES

An ANOVA with the correlated TEOAE response as the dependent variable, with profession group as between subjects factor; and with ear, stimulus level, and frequency area as within subjects independent factors; showed no significant difference between the various professions or between left and right ear. For normal ears the response increases when the stimulus level is increased from 75 to 85 dB peSPL. There was such increases of 4.4 dB for each of the groups *Education*, *Other* and *Music*, and they were highly significant ($p < 0.00005$, Tukey's HSD). However, when compensated for age they were not, and the response of the *Industry* group at the higher level was just marginally higher, 1.4 dB, than at the lower level. For the uncorrelated response signal, on the other hand, the *Industry* group showed a 6 dB higher response than *Education*, *Other* and *Music* ($p < 0.005$ for all the three comparisons, Tukey's HSD). The TEOAE results of the *Industry* group may be explained by dysfunctional OHCs with reduced ipsilateral restraining regulation.

The contralateral suppression effect was very small, the means for the groups ranging from 0.22 dB to -0.26 dB without significant differences, although age was a significant factor.

DPOAES

An ANOVA with the DPOAE response level without contra-lateral noise as the dependent variable, with profession group as between subjects factor; with ear and frequency as within subjects factors, and age as covariate, showed that the mean response level was significantly higher at 1000 Hz than at 2000 Hz, 7.5 and 3.7 dB SPL respectively ($p < 0.00001$). There was a strongly significant age dependence ($p < 0.00001$). From the right ear *Industry* had a very weak mean response over frequencies, -1.9 dB SPL, which was significantly lower than the responses of the other groups ($p < 0.005$, Tukey's HSD).

To estimate the background noise from equipment and ear, the level in narrow frequency areas below and above the response tone frequency was measured. A statistical analysis corresponding to the one above was performed, now with this noise level as the dependent variable. In the left ear this noise level was about 3 dB higher than in the right ear ($p < 0.00001$). Furthermore, the group *Industry* had an almost 3 dB higher value of that noise in the left ear than the groups *Education*, *Other*, and *Music* ($p < 0.05$, Tukey's HSD).

A corresponding statistical analysis was also performed with the individual standard deviation of 20 consecutive measurements as the dependent variable. Also for this standard deviation the group *Industry* had a significantly higher value, 4.0 dB, than the groups *Education*, *Other*, and *Music* (2.0–2.1 dB), when averaged over ears and frequencies ($p < 0.00005$). Age had a significant influence, but compensation for age did not change any values. Thus, the group *Industry* differed from the other groups by low DPOAE responses on the right ear, a high noise level around the tone response on the left ear, and a large variation in the 20 measurements without contralateral noise. It looks like the DPOAE response from this group mostly consists of noise. Compare to TEOAE results.

There was no significant influence of any of the factors ear, frequency or profession group on the suppression effect using the contralateral on-off noise. The range of suppression for the groups was 0.4 to 0.6 dB.

OAEs in short. As the *Industry* group was chosen to have a noise induced hearing loss it was a natural finding that *both types of OAEs* for the *Industry* group were marginal, unstable and considerably noisy. There were deteriorations in the contralateral regulatory system for all groups, but considerably more so in the *Industry* group. A few individuals in the other three groups had abnormally high emissions at some frequencies suggesting impaired ipsilateral regulatory function.

As a whole our results regarding OAEs did not give much information, probably because most of our test subjects were middle-aged. One should keep in mind that there is a normal degradation of OAEs and regulatory efferent system with age, which may obscure for example noise induced degradation [21].

PMTF

The stimulus noise levels at which the maximum values of the threshold curves were found, were used as dependent variables in a multivariate ANOVA with profession group as between subjects factor; and with peak/valley curve and frequency as within subjects factors. Those noise levels did not differ significantly between the groups. This was true for both peak and valley curves and both ears.

The corresponding analyses, with the maximum value of the PMTF threshold curve on the left ear as dependent variable, showed that the maximum of the valley curve was significantly higher for the *Education* group than for *Other* and *Music* (p<0.05, Tukey's HSD). The same tendency was found on the right ear, but without statistical significance. An analysis for different types of teachers showed a tendency to higher maxima for preschool teachers than for other teachers. In this context it should be noted that a high maximum, especially on the valley curve, is one characteristic of a hyper-PMTF, Figure 2D. Although one cannot be certain that the results of the *Education* group are caused by sudden loud sounds, they definitely indicate a reduced ability to detect short sounds in silent intervals of a complicated signal, poor temporal processing.

Very few subjects with fully developed hyper-PMTFs (P-type = 3), suggesting exposure to impulse noise possibly associated to damage in the inner hair cell area [4,16,22], were found in this study. Although the *Industry* group had more self-reported impulse noise incidents (p<0.01) than the other groups, this did not result in significantly more hyper-PMTFs than in the other groups. One reason may be that some of the test subjects, especially in the *Industry* group, could not be measured at the low levels of the modulated noise at which the characteristics of the hyper-PMTF are seen. Measurements closer to the incidents, before the characteristics in our PMTF-measurements had been obscured by further deterioration of pure tone thresholds, would have clarified if there was a hyper-PMTF. Those actually classified with P-type = 3, hyper-PMTF showed fairly flat audiogram curves. See Figure 3. In the figure there is one curve showing the mean pure tone thresholds for the two subjects among the 193 who had P-type = 3 on the left ear. This curve shows thresholds around 10 dB HL. There is also an extra curve for these two subjects plus four

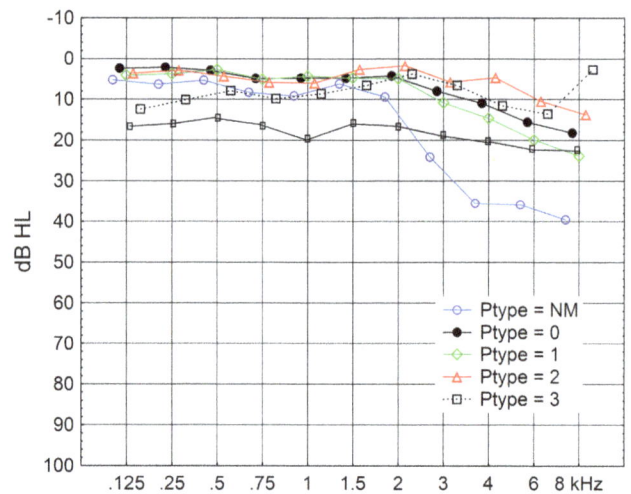

Figure 3. Mean audiograms for subjects with different types of PMTF-curves, 4000 Hz, left ear. See legend of Figure 2 about the PMTF classification. Numbers of subjects for P-types NM, 0, 1, 2, and 3 are 12, 40, 54, 13, and 2, respectively. An extra curve, black continuous line with smaller markers, black boxes, is added, which includes 4 more subjects with hyper-PMTF (P-type = 3), but outside the threshold criterion limiting to 193 subjects. Note that the two curves for hyper-PMTF are fairly flat. The data points are horizontally displaced for clarity.

more subjects with P-type = 3, left ear, from the total of 272 subjects measured. Most thresholds forming this curve are slightly better than 20 dB HL. Also the curve representing the 13 ears with P-type = 2, suspected hyper-PMTF, is fairly flat.

Audiograms with similar hearing thresholds for all frequencies have also been observed in conscripts sent to us for measurements after severe shooting incidents, unpublished data. It is not unusual that all thresholds have positions around 10 dB HL, i.e. totally normal. This may be a warning flag when a person with normal thresholds complains of hearing problems. In experiments on chinchilla, Wang[23] and El-Badry[24] have shown that as much as 70 – 85% of the IHCs could be damaged before threshold levels became abnormal. Another paper[25] shows that at sound levels well above threshold, other hearing functions, including forward masking, were strongly deteriorated before such a degree of degeneration.

Forward masking

An ANOVA was performed with the forward masking threshold difference (difference between the thresholds of the brief tone at 5 ms and at 50 ms after the noise burst) as the dependent variable, with profession group as a between subjects factor, and with ear and level as within subjects factors. The two older groups *Industry*, mean age 54, and *Education*, mean age 45, showed significantly worse forward masking mean results (over ears and levels), 19 and 21 dB threshold difference, than the about five years younger groups *Music* and *Other*, 32 and 30 dB, (p<0.005, Tukey's HSD). These results could be compared to the threshold difference, 27 ±9 dB (median 27 dB, lower quartile 22 dB) for our *middle-aged reference group* without hearing problems. Most notable is that the median of the teachers, the *Education* group, 23 dB, was almost as low as the lower quartile of the *middle-aged reference group*, 22 dB. The lower quartile of *Education* was 12 dB.

On the other hand one may note that the results of *Music* and *Other* are as good as the median result of the (much younger) *group of young women*, 30 dB. Walton[26] found that aging changed forward masking for the worse. This was also the general effect over all our test subjects. The change was 3 dB per decade (p< 0.00001 in all six linear regressions, i.e. two ears times three sound levels). However, in our study the significant differences between profession groups became even stronger when compensated for age (p<0.001, Tukey's HSD with age as covariate).

Figure 4 shows individual audiograms for six subjects with a threshold difference less than 5 dB for 5 and 50 ms delay between short tone and noise, on the left ear. Three of them came from the *Industry* group, two from *Education* and one from *Other*. Their PMTF results suggested either exposure to impulse noise or other sudden loud noise or they could not be measured at the levels of the modulated noise at which the characteristics of the hyper-PMTF are seen.

If an analogy with research animals is proposed, abnormal forward masking results may indicate IHC dysfunction or radial dendrite damage, independent of OHC status[18]. Later research on animals has found other damage in the IHC area [27–31], from earlier noise exposure not causing permanent threshold shifts, but with supra-threshold effects. If the speculation is true, that the ears of the research animals and humans work in a similar way, the results of this study suggest that some persons with professions considered less noise exposed may have considerable damage in the IHC area – and more such damage than in normal aging. However, this remains a speculation until more research has been carried out in humans.

Speech in noise

In the speech-in-noise test some subjects regarded 85 dB SPL listening level too loud and were measured at the lower level on both ears. Three subjects found even the lower listening level too loud and did not complete any speech test at all. The resulting number of measurements on the left ear was 125 at 70 dB SPL and 83 at 85 dB SPL, and on the right ear 108 and 72, respectively. ANOVAs were performed separately for the left and right ears with the S/N threshold as the dependent variable, with profession group as a between subjects factor, and with sound level as a within subjects factor.

Industry and *Education* were, on the left ear, significantly worse (p<0.05, Tukey's HSD) than *Music*, the only group that was normal at both levels. *Industry* was also significantly worse than *Other* (p<0.05, Tukey's HSD). However, when age was introduced as a covariate all the significant group differences disappeared. (The change in S/N at threshold per decade was 1 dB.)

More important was that, still on the left ear, *Industry* and *Education* were markedly worse than the *middle-aged reference group* (p<0.0001 for both groups at 85 dB SPL, t-tests), see Figure 5, like in the forward masking results. The group *Other* was normal at 70, but not at 85 dB SPL. Note that both the *middle-aged reference group* and the *group of young women* had considerably better results on the speech-in-noise test at the presentation level 85 dB SPL than at 70 dB SPL. Also the test groups in the current study had better results at the higher level, but the improvement was smaller due to larger deteriorations at the higher level than at the lower level.

On the right ear all group means except *Industry*'s were within normal limits compared to the mean over right and left ear of our *middle-aged reference group* without hearing problems. However, only two subjects in *Industry* were tested on the right ear.

Tinnitus matching

An ANOVA was performed with the matched tinnitus level as the dependent variable, with profession group as a between subjects factor and with ear as a within subjects factor. The group *Industry* had significantly louder tinnitus than *Music* and *Other* (p< 0.05, Tukey's HSD) according to the matching, but not significantly louder than *Education*. Figure 6 shows a histogram of the matched tinnitus levels for the left ear (n = 110). The results of the right ear were similar, as many subjects located their tinnitus in the centre of the head or in both ears. The subjects who did no matching to the test tone (n = 83) either had no pitch in their tinnitus or, for most of them; they had no tinnitus to match to at the test moment.

Relations between measurements

Relations between measurements were tested with linear regression. When forward masking was involved it was used as

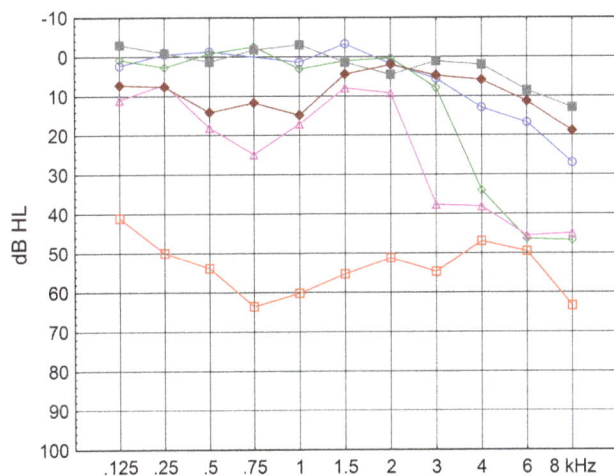

Figure 4. Individual audiograms for subjects with a forward masking threshold difference of less than 5 dB. Left ear, n=6. The three worst audiograms come from the group *Industry* without restrictions on pure tone thresholds.

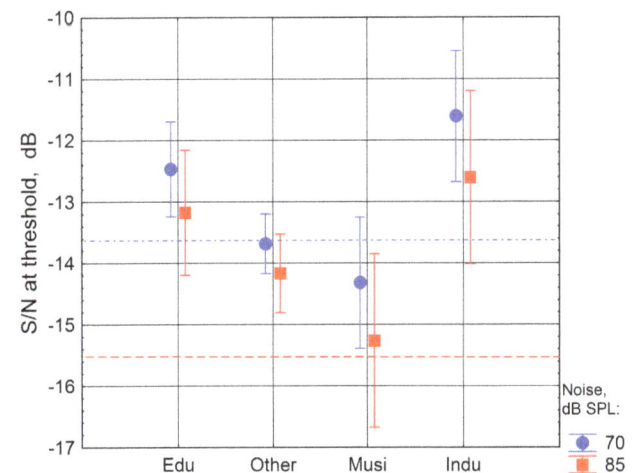

Figure 5. Mean of the speech recognition thresholds in noise. S/N at threshold for the profession groups, two noise levels 70 and 85 dB SPL, left ear. The vertical bars show 95% confidence intervals. Numbers of subjects in the different groups are from left to right 23, 58, 12, and 12. The horizontal lines show values for a *middle-aged reference group* without hearing problems for the noise levels 70 (dashed) and 85 (dotted) dB SPL. (The means and the numbers of measurements were obtained from the ANOVA, which explains the discrepancy from the number of measured ears.)

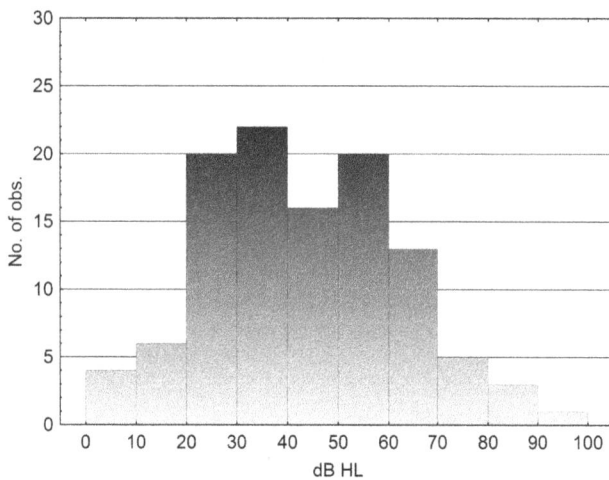

Figure 6. Histogram of matched tinnitus level, left ear, n = 110.
Right ear's histogram (n = 89) was similar. Median levels for left and right ears were 40 and 38 dB HL, respectively.

the independent variable. There were significant negative, and similar, correlations between *forward masking* results at each of the three test levels and *matched tinnitus level* for both ears (at best r = −0.36, p<0.001 at 65 dB SPL, right ear). This means that louder tinnitus was correlated to poor forward masking. The two groups with louder tinnitus, *Industry* and *Education*, had significantly worse forward masking results than *Music* and *Other*. That subjects with worse forward masking had louder matched tinnitus is in concordance with reports of increased gain at higher levels in the auditory system following loss of IHCs[32]. This is also in accordance to the assumption that there is an increased risk of tinnitus and abnormal sensitivity to loud sound in case of neural degeneration proximal to intact IHCs[27,28].

There was a significant correlation between the threshold difference in *forward masking* and the *speech recognition threshold in noise*. The groups with the poorest forward masking results (possibly also with the worst IHC status) had the worst speech recognition in noise. The correlation was strongest for both speech-in-noise levels on the right ear, and for the lower noise level on the left ear with correlations between −0.5 and −0.6 (p<0.00001) for relevant level combinations of speech-in-noise and forward masking results (with forward masking level equal to or lower than the noise level in the speech test). For the left ear at the higher speech-in-noise level the correlation was −0.3 to −0.4 (p<0.005).

Unlike the difference between the groups in the forward masking test, the differences between the groups in the speech-in-noise test were not significant when compensated for age. One may speculate that forward masking may be a basic measure of the status of receptor hair cells and a neural degeneration beyond, which has been shown to be a long-term after-effect of noise exposure[27,28,30], whereas speech recognition also has an added age-dependent component of cognition.

There were strongly significant correlations between *forward masking* results, only measured at 2000 Hz, and *PMTF*-results at the same frequency, indicating characteristics of the PMTF-curves concordant with hyper-PMTF (P-type = 3) or suspected hyper-PMTF (P-type = 2): Small forward masking threshold differences were accompanied by high maximum valley thresholds (r = −0.44, p<0.0001 for both ears and forward masking at 65 dB), and by positioning of the maximum valley thresholds at low noise level (r = 0.31, p<0.005 for both ears and forward masking at 65 dB

SPL). The bond between forward masking and PMTF regarding incidents with sudden loud sound was further strengthened by the fact that high maximum valley thresholds were accompanied by positioning of the maximum valley thresholds at low noise level (p<0.00001, r = −0.49 for the left ear, r = −0.54 for the right ear), both typical for the hyper-PMTF, Figure 2D. There were also significant correlations between the forward masking variables and the corresponding PMTF variables at 4 kHz on the left ear.

Relations between results of questionnaire and hearing tests

Forward masking proved to be the hearing test that showed the most revealing differences (or similarities) between persons with different professions. Therefore it was considered suitable to investigate if non-auditory factors could influence the forward masking results. Thus ANOVAs were performed with the forward masking threshold difference (difference between the thresholds of the brief tone at 5 ms and at 50 ms after the noise burst) as the dependent variable, and with ear and one non-auditory factor at a time as within subjects factors. The non-auditory factors were self-reported medication, headaches, neck problems, smoking or stress. The only non-auditory factor with a possible influence on forward masking was *medication* (p<0.05, p = 0.05, Kruskal-Wallis). The dose response indicates that this is not a spurious finding: The mean threshold difference for individuals taking more than 50 pain relieving tablets/year was 22 dB. For those taking 1–50 tablets/year the mean was 28 dB, and for those taking 0 tablets/year it was 29 dB. However, we have no explanation to this correlation between medication and forward masking. The fact that the *Education* group had forward masking results similar to the *Industry* group and not to the less noise exposed groups *Music* or *Other* could not be explained by this correlation, since there was no difference whatsoever in use of medication between any of the groups.

Hypersensitivity to loud sound as reported in the questionnaire (no or yes response) was related to *speech recognition in noise* at the lower test level, 70 dB SPL, right ear (p<0.005, simple ANOVA). Persons, who were hypersensitive to loud sound, had a better S/N, −14.1 dB, than persons who were not so sensitive, S/N = −12.4 dB. This effect may be caused by healthy OHCs combined with ipsilateral and contralateral regulatory systems with defective restraining capacity, resulting in higher levels in the cochlea [4,33,34]. OAE data showed such tendencies, but no significances. The hypothesis that persons hypersensitive to loud sound may have worse results on speech recognition in the 85 dB SPL noise than those not so sensitive could not really be tested, since there were too few persons tested at that level. Neither could any differences between the two categories in the amount of improvement with noise level be reliably analysed.

Complementary discussion

The hearing tests in this study show, that individuals with hearing problems in the profession group *Other*, consisting mainly of medical staff and students, have small deviations from results normal for their age, and that the group *Industry*, used for comparison, has substantial deviations in all tests. This might have been suspected from the self-estimated noise exposure including profession and other risk factors.

In our previous study musicians had some dysfunctions associated to damage to OHCs and the regulatory system, and a few of them showed the typical signs of incidents with sudden loud noise[4]. In the present study the group *Music* showed the same indications, but in addition the results were very normal for the two new measurements, forward masking and speech recognition in noise. The forward masking results were even as good as the results of the (much younger) *group of young women*. Thus the *Music*-group, except a few individuals exposed to incidents, had good results regarding measurements associated to IHC-function. Musicians are acknowledged to work at sound levels at which there is a risk of NIHL according to the international standard-isation[8], and our estimations of noise exposures suggested that the musicians should have more dysfunctional hearing than the teachers. However, the participating musicians seemed to have come from fairly controlled soundscapes without unexpected loud sounds from electronic systems. The changes in sound level in the music are expected by the musicians.

In contrast the *Education* group showed results similar to those of the *Industry* group, and worse than normal for middle-aged persons, regarding forward masking, and speech recognition in noise. The self-reported tinnitus level was about the same and worse than for the other two groups. There were also PMTF-results that may be associated to exposure to sudden loud sounds. According to animal research, one may speculate that there are lesions in the inner hair cell area as referred to in the result/discussion section. Although there is an uncertainty of the location of the possible lesions, this study has clearly shown that our *Education* group had poor temporal processing. Regarding the location of possible lesions in the hair cell areas and the regulatory system we have based the discussions on the literature. Unfortu-nately there is hitherto less literature regarding inner hair cells than outer hair cells, because of physiological difficulties to measure. Our findings seem to justify more studies in this area.

Our assumption was that the participants of the *Education* group had been exposed to lower noise levels than the *Industry* and *Music* groups. In the questionnaire, the estimates of self-assessed noise exposure supported that assumption. However, recent results from noise measurements in preschools show that preschool teachers are exposed to considerable noise levels[6]. In the seventeen preschools in that study the mean equivalent sound level over a working day was less than 80 dB(A), but the maximum was 85 dB(A), The mean rating of the noise was between "somewhat troublesome" and "very troublesome". About 80% of the 101 teachers judged unexpected sudden changes of the sound level to occur "several times per day" to "several times per hour". It is reasonable that noise levels and noise characteristics, e.g. the content of sudden, unexpected loud noises, depend on type of school, age of pupils, classroom acoustics and cultural factors. The teachers in our study had not used hearing protection, although it may be used by for example woodwork teachers.

It is possible that many of the teachers may have come from soundscapes like the one described above, with noise described as troublesome but still tolerable, with several unexpected sudden changes of the sound level every working day. Other reasons for the *Education* group having worse results than the *Music* group could not be found in the analyses of answers to the questionnaire. Self-reported neck problems, pain relieving medication, eye and hair colour, smoking, and relatives with hearing problems were about the same in the two groups. The self-reported amounts of stress and tension headaches were slightly higher for these two groups than for the other groups.

In the study of risk factors for tinnitus in a population 55 years and older a number of extrinsic and health factors that could be linked to tinnitus were described[35]. The largest single factor was reported occupational tolerable noise exposure (9.3%), which may correspond to what Sjödin reported for preschools[6]. The conclusion was that a number of occupations with less noise burden than industrial exposure are at risk for noise-induced tinnitus. Another study found poor temporal processing and

speech recognition in adverse listening conditions in individuals exposed to occupational noise more than 80 dB(A), but still with pure tone thresholds less than 25 dB HTL[36]. Those skills deteriorated with age, but were worse for exposed groups than for unexposed controls. Also that study seems to have relevance for the tested groups of teachers.

Our results show that persons exposed to moderate noise levels at work may run the risk of hearing dysfunction. Mean results of the 48 teachers in two measurements as well as of individual musicians and hospital staff with moderate noise exposure seem to prove that.

This study may have found dysfunctions that are characteristic for these groups before the audiogram is affected, but it will not give us a general overview of the effects of noise on hearing for these groups of professions at later stages of deterioration of the audiogram. Neither can it tell how common the dysfunctions are.

Conclusions

In this study, individuals having auditory problems and normal or near-normal hearing thresholds were divided into groups of subjects with similar noise exposure, and measured with advanced hearing tests. For each type of measurement there were individuals with abnormal results possibly indicating cochlear dysfunction.

For many of the subjects these dysfunctions caused less improvement than normal when the listening level in the speech in noise test was increased. Subjects sensitive to loud noise had significantly better speech recognition in noise at the lower test level than subjects not sensitive.

There were characteristic results:
Teachers had results suggesting substantial dysfunction in the auditory system reflected in far worse forward masking and speech recognition in noise than a group of middle-aged without hearing problems. These results, suggesting poor temporal processing, were about equally poor as those of a group exposed to industrial noise. The latter group was tested for comparison and had about 20 dB worse pure tone thresholds. The matched tinnitus level was correlated to the forward masking results and those two groups had the loudest matched tinnitus, possibly caused by dysfunction in the inner hair cell area.

Musicians showed some deficits normally associated to outer hair cells and had good results for their age at forward masking, and so did a group mainly consisting of hospital staff and students. The musicians had normal speech recognition in noise at both listening levels.

The study suggests that persons exposed to occupational noise below or around risk levels may risk hearing dysfunction. Several of the teachers in this study are examples of that, possibly because of combinations of unfavourable working environment and individual susceptibility. Medication or other self-reported non-auditory factors could not explain the poor results of the teachers.

Acknowledgments

We want to express our gratitude to Karin Erikson, and Eva B Svensson, who performed the measurements, and to our test subjects.

Author Contributions

Conceived and designed the experiments: ACL UR BH ÅO. Performed the experiments: ACL ÅO. Analyzed the data: ACL BH. Wrote the paper: ACL UR BH ÅO. Designed the software used for hearing tests: ÅO.

References

1. Axelsson A, Ringdahl A (1989) Tinnitus-a study of its prevalence and characteristics. Br J Audiol 23: 53–62.
2. Cacace AT (2003) Expanding the biological basis of tinnitus: crossmodal origins and the role of neuroplasticity. Hear Res 175: 112–132.
3. Attias J, Bresloff I, Furman V (1996) The influence of the efferent auditory system on otoacoustic emissions in noise induced tinnitus: clinical relevance. Acta Otolaryngol 116: 534–539.
4. Lindblad AC, Hagerman B, Rosenhall U (2011) Noise-induced tinnitus: a comparison between four clinical groups without apparent hearing loss. Noise Health 13: 423–431.
5. Sindhusake D, Golding M, Newall P, Rubin G, Jakobsen K, et al. (2003) Risk factors for tinnitus in a population of older adults: the blue mountains hearing study. Ear Hear 24: 501–507.
6. Sjödin F, Kjellberg A, Knutsson A, Landström U, Lindberg L (2012) Noise exposure and auditory effects on preschool personnel. Noise Health 14: 72–82.
7. McAllister AM, Granqvist S, Sjölander P, Sundberg J (2009) Child voice and noise: a pilot study of noise in day cares and the effects on 10 children's voice quality according to perceptual evaluation. J Voice 23: 587–593.
8. ISO1999 (1990) Acoustics – Determination of occupational noise exposure and estimation of noise-induced hearing impairment. Geneva: International Organization for Standardization.
9. Jansen EJ, Helleman HW, Dreschler WA, de Laat JA (2009) Noise induced hearing loss and other hearing complaints among musicians of symphony orchestras. Int Arch Occup Environ Health 82: 153–164.
10. Schmuziger N, Patscheke J, Probst R (2006) Hearing in nonprofessional pop/rock musicians. Ear Hear 27: 321–330.
11. Zhao F, Manchaiah VK, French D, Price SM (2010) Music exposure and hearing disorders: an overview. Int J Audiol 49: 54–64.
12. Kähäri K, Zachau G, Eklöf M, Sandsjö L, Möller C (2003) Assessment of hearing and hearing disorders in rock/jazz musicians. Int J Audiol 42: 279–288.
13. ISO7029 (2000) Acoustics - Statistical distribution of hearing thresholds as a function of age. Geneva: International Organization for Standardization.
14. Berninger E, Karlsson KK (1999) Clinical study of Widex Senso on first-time hearing aid users. Scand Audiol 28: 117–125.
15. Lindblad A-C, Hagerman B (1999) Hearing tests for selection of sonar operators. ACUSTICA - Acta acustica 85: 870–876.
16. Davis RI, Qiu W, Hamernik RP (2009) Role of the kurtosis statistic in evaluating complex noise exposures for the protection of hearing. Ear Hear 30: 628–634.
17. Duan ML, Canlon B (1996) Forward masking is dependent on inner hair cell activity. Audiol Neurootol 1: 320–327.
18. Duan ML, Canlon B (1996) Outer hair cell activity is not required for the generation of the forward masking curve. Audiol Neurootol 1: 309–319.
19. Hagerman B (1982) Sentences for testing speech intelligibility in noise. Scand Audiol 11: 79–87.
20. Hagerman B (2002) Speech recognition threshold in slightly and fully modulated noise for hearing-impaired subjects. Int J Audiol 41: 321–329.
21. Jacobson M, Kim S, Romney J, Zhu X, Frisina RD (2003) Contralateral suppression of distortion-product otoacoustic emissions declines with age: a comparison of findings in CBA mice with human listeners. Laryngoscope 113: 1707–1713.
22. Lindblad AC, Rosenhall U, Olofsson Å, Hagerman B (2011) The efficacy of N-acetylcysteine to protect the human cochlea from subclinical hearing loss caused by impulse noise: a controlled trial. Noise Health 13: 392–401.
23. Wang J, Powers NL, Hofstetter P, Trautwein P, Ding D, et al. (1997) Effects of selective inner hair cell loss on auditory nerve fiber threshold, tuning and spontaneous and driven discharge rate. Hear Res 107: 67–82.
24. El-Badry MM, McFadden SL (2007) Electrophysiological correlates of progressive sensorineural pathology in carboplatin-treated chinchillas. Brain Res 1134: 122–130.
25. McFadden SL, Kasper C, Ostrowski J, Ding D, Salvi RJ (1998) Effects of inner hair cell loss on inferior colliculus evoked potential thresholds, amplitudes and forward masking functions in chinchillas. Hear Res 120: 121–132.
26. Walton J, Orlando M, Burkard R (1999) Auditory brainstem response forward-masking recovery functions in older humans with normal hearing. Hear Res 127: 86–94.
27. Kujawa SG, Liberman MC (2009) Adding insult to injury: cochlear nerve degeneration after "temporary" noise-induced hearing loss. J Neurosci 29: 14077–14085.
28. Lin HW, Furman AC, Kujawa SG, Liberman MC (2011) Primary neural degeneration in the Guinea pig cochlea after reversible noise-induced threshold shift. J Assoc Res Otolaryngol 12: 605–616.
29. Wang Y, Ren C (2012) Effects of repeated "benign" noise exposures in young CBA mice: shedding light on age-related hearing loss. J Assoc Res Otolaryngol 13: 505–515.
30. Liu L, Wang H, Shi L, Almuklass A, He T, et al. (2012) Silent damage of noise on cochlear afferent innervation in guinea pigs and the impact on temporal processing. PLoS One 7: e49550.
31. Shi L, Liu L, He T, Guo X, Yu Z, et al. (2013) Ribbon synapse plasticity in the cochleae of Guinea pigs after noise-induced silent damage. PLoS One 8: e81566.
32. Qiu C, Salvi R, Ding D, Burkard R (2000) Inner hair cell loss leads to enhanced response amplitudes in auditory cortex of unanesthetized chinchillas: evidence for increased system gain. Hear Res 139: 153–171.
33. El-Badry MM, McFadden SL (2009) Evaluation of inner hair cell and nerve fiber loss as sufficient pathologies underlying auditory neuropathy. Hear Res 255: 84–90.
34. Sztuka A, Pospiech L, Gawron W, Dudek K (2010) DPOAE in estimation of the function of the cochlea in tinnitus patients with normal hearing. Auris Nasus Larynx 37: 55–60.
35. Sindhusake D, Mitchell P, Newall P, Golding M, Rochtchina E, et al. (2003) Prevalence and characteristics of tinnitus in older adults: the Blue Mountains Hearing Study. Int J Audiol 42: 289–294.
36. Kumar UA, Ameenudin S, Sangamanatha AV (2012) Temporal and speech processing skills in normal hearing individuals exposed to occupational noise. Noise Health 14: 100–105.

10

Pharmacological Inhibition of Cochlear Mitochondrial Respiratory Chain Induces Secondary Inflammation in the Lateral Wall: A Potential Therapeutic Target for Sensorineural Hearing Loss

Masato Fujioka[1,2], Yasuhide Okamoto[3,6], Seiichi Shinden[4,6], Hirotaka James Okano[2,5], Hideyuki Okano[2], Kaoru Ogawa[1], Tatsuo Matsunaga[6]*

1 Department of Otolaryngology, Head and Neck Surgery, Keio University, School of Medicine, Shinjuku, Tokyo, Japan, 2 Department of Physiology, School of Medicine, Keio University, School of Medicine, Shinjuku, Tokyo, Japan, 3 Department of Otorhinolaryngology, Inagi Municipal Hospital, Inagi, Tokyo, Japan, 4 Department of Otolaryngology, Saiseikai Utsunomiya Hospital, Utsunomiya, Tochigi, Japan, 5 Division of Regenerative Medicine, Jikei University School of Medicine, Tokyo, Japan, 6 The Laboratory of Auditory Disorders and Division of Hearing and Balance Research, National Institute of Sensory Organs, National Tokyo Medical Center, Meguro, Tokyo, Japan

Abstract

Cochlear lateral wall has recently been reported as a common site of inflammation, yet precise molecular mechanisms of the inflammatory responses remain elucidated. The present study examined the inflammatory responses in the lateral wall following acute mitochondrial dysfunction induced by a mitochondrial toxin, 3-nitropropionic acid (3-NP). Reverse-transcription (RT)-PCR revealed increases in the expression of the proinflammatory cytokines interleukin (IL)-1β and IL-6. Immunohistochemistry showed an increase in the number of activated cochlear macrophages in the lateral wall, which were in close proximity to IL-6-expressing cells. A genome-wide DNA microarray analysis of the lateral wall revealed that 35% and 60% of the genes showing >2-fold upregulation at 1 d and 3 d post-3-NP administration, respectively, were inflammatory genes, including CC- and CXC-type chemokine genes. High expression of CCL-1, 2, and 3 at 1 d, and of CCL-1, 2, 3, 4, and 5, CCR-2 and 5, and CX3CR1 at 3 d post-3-NP administration, coupled with no change in the level of CX3CL1 expression suggested that macrophages and monocytes may be involved in the inflammatory response to 3-NP-mediated injury. Quantitative (q)RT-PCR showed a transient induction of IL-1β and IL-6 expression within 24 h of 3-NP-mediated injury, followed by sustained expression of the chemoattractants, CCL-2, 4 and 5, up until 7 d after injury. The expression of CCL-2 and IL-6 was higher in animals showing permanent hearing impairment than in those showing temporary hearing impairment, suggesting that these inflammatory responses may be detrimental to hearing recovery. The present findings suggest that acute mitochondrial dysfunction induces secondary inflammatory responses in the lateral wall of the cochlear and that the IL-6/CCL-2 inflammatory pathway is involved in monocyte activation. Therefore, these secondary inflammatory responses may be a potential post-insult therapeutic target for treatments aimed at preventing the damage caused by acute mitochondrial dysfunction in the cochlear lateral wall.

Editor: Partha Mukhopadhyay, National Institutes of Health, United States of America

Funding: This work was supported by a Grant-in-Aid for Scientific Research (C) from MEXT/JSPS KAKENHI grant number 24592560 to M.F. by a Grant-in-Aid for Scientific Research (B) from MEXT/JSPS KAKENHI grant number 24390390 to K.O. and by a Health Labour Sciences Research Grant from the Ministry of Health Labour and Welfare to T.M. The funders had no role in study design, data collection and analysis, decision to publish, or preparation of the manuscript.

Competing Interests: The authors have declared that no competing interests exist.

* E-mail: matsunagatatsuo@kankakuki.go.jp

Introduction

Mitochondrial dysfunction in the cochlea is a well-known cause of sensorineural hearing loss. Mutations in mitochondrial DNA cause both syndromic and nonsyndromic deafness, and the inner ear is considered highly susceptible to mitochondrial dysfunction [5,11,19]. Recently, we established a novel rat model of acute mitochondrial dysfunction in the cochlea by applying 3-nitropropionic acid (3-NP) directly to the round window membrane [10]. 3-NP irreversibly inhibits the mitochondrial complex II enzyme, succinate dehydrogenase, by blocking the mitochondrial electron transport chain [1,3]. Using the aforementioned model, primary histological changes were detected in the lateral wall spiral ligament with a degeneration of its mitochondria, in which the endocochlear potential is produced [17]. Treatment with 300 mM 3-NP resulted in temporary hearing loss (temporary threshold shift (TTS) model), whereas treatment with 500 mM 3-NP resulted in profound and permanent hearing loss (permanent threshold shift (PTS) model) [10,17]. Because local ATP deprivation in the inner ear results from inhibition of inner ear mitochondrial function. this model replicates the etiology of inner ear energy failure caused by ATP deprivation due to inner ear ischemia. It has been reported that inner ear ischemia that results from occlusion of the anterior inferior cerebellar artery causes sensorineural hearing loss [14,24].

In addition, circulatory disturbances (most often vertebrobasilar ischemia) and inflammation (most often viral) are the most common etiologies in sudden deafness [8,16].

3-NP blocks cellular energy production by disrupting the mitochondrial electron transport chain. Therefore, we speculated that the primary pathophysiology in the rat model was apoptosis. Indeed, systemic application of a pan-caspase inhibitor (Z-VAD-FMK) prior to 3-NP treatment reduces the number of apoptotic cells in the lateral wall and significantly ameliorates hearing impairment [15]. However, this effect is observed only when the inhibitor is administered prior to the insult. The results suggest that apoptosis occurs at the early pathophysiological stage, and that a secondary event occurs at a later stage; this secondary event may be a potential therapeutic target after the onset of deafness.

Because the damaged spiral ligament is a common site of inflammation induced by various types of insult, including surgical stress, noise exposure, and immune-mediated treatments [6,9,18,21], the present study examined the inflammatory responses following acute mitochondrial dysfunction in the cochlea using both TTS and PTS models induced by treatment with 3-NP. IL-6 is a cytokine that is critical for the recruitment of inflammatory cells. The expression of IL-6 and other proinflammatory cytokines was detected in the lateral wall, along with prominent infiltration of the cochlear macrophages adjacent to the IL-6-expressing type III fibrocytes by cochlear macrophages. Genome-wide microarray analyses of the lateral wall revealed upregulation of numerous inflammatory genes related to the infiltration of monocytes and to the activation of macrophages. qRT-PCR showed a transient induction in the expression of IL-1β and IL-6 within 24 h of 3-NP administration, followed by sustained expression of the chemoattractants, CCL-2, 4 and 5, up until 7 d after 3-NP administration. The IL-6/CCL-2 signaling pathway was activated in both the PTS and TTS models, although the levels of activation were higher in the PTS model. The present findings show that inflammatory responses play an important role in the mitochondrial dysfunction observed in the cochlear lateral wall. Differences in the inflammatory responses between the PTS and TTS models suggest that the secondary inflammatory responses may be a potential therapeutic target, leading to a treatment for deafness caused by cochlear energy failure.

Results

1. Expression of proinflammatory cytokines in the 3-NP-injured cochlea

To detect inflammation in the 3-NP-injured cochlea, we measured the expression of TNF-α, IL-1α, IL-1β, IL-1RA, IL-6 and IL-12 p40 mRNA (all proinflammatory cytokines) using RT-PCR. We observed a temporal upregulation in IL-6 expression 1 d after 3-NP treatment; no such increase was noted in the controls. IL-1β was expressed in both 3-NP-injured and saline-treated cochlea; however, TNF-α was downregulated after treatment with 3-NP (Fig. 1). No expression of IL-1α, IL-1RA or IL-12 p40 mRNA was detected (data not shown). Whole cochlea were harvested from each animal for use in the assay.

2. Quantitative analysis of IL-6 expression in the cochlea

Time-dependent changes in IL-6 mRNA expression were quantified by qRT-PCR. In the TTS model (induced with 300 mM of 3-NP), significant expression of IL-6 was observed from Day 1 (P<0.01) and was maintained up until Day 3 (P<0.01). Expression of IL-6 was also observed in the saline-treated controls from 3 h post-surgery and it gradually decreased to undetectable levels by Day 3. Similar levels of IL-6 expression

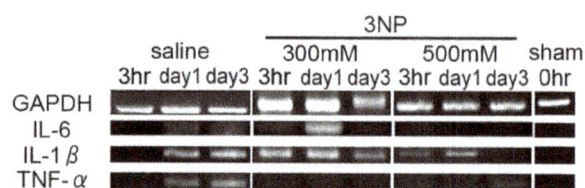

Figure 1. Expression of proinflammatory cytokines in 3-NP-injured cochlea. RT-PCR data for three major proinflammatory cytokines, IL-6, IL-1β, and TNF-α, and the house-keeping gene GAPDH. There was a significant difference in IL-6 expression in the 3-NP-treated cochleae compared with the saline-treated controls. Whole cochleae were harvested and used for the assay.

were observed in all three groups, saline control, TTS and PTS models, at 3 h post-surgery. In the PTS model (induced with 500 mM of 3-NP), IL-6 expression increased at 3 h post-3-NP administration but decreased to the saline-treated control level at Day 1; weak expression was sustained until Day 3 (Fig. 2). Note that the expression was not detected in the cochlea without any treatment or pre-treatment. Whole cochleae were used for the assays.

3. Emergence of cochlear macrophages in the damaged lateral wall, adjacent to the IL-6 expressing cells

We next performed immunohistochemical analyses to examine the expression of IL-6 (Fig. 3a and c) and the cochlear macrophage marker, Iba-1 (Fig. 3b and d), in the TTS model at Day 1 (when the induction of IL-6 was maximal). IL-6 was expressed by type III fibrocytes (Fig. 3a and c; blue arrows) and by the mesenchyme cells beneath the basement membrane (Fig. 3c, black arrows). Iba-1-expressing cochlear macrophages were observed in the same areas as type II fibrocytes, and were most frequently observed on the lateral side, adjacent to the IL-6-

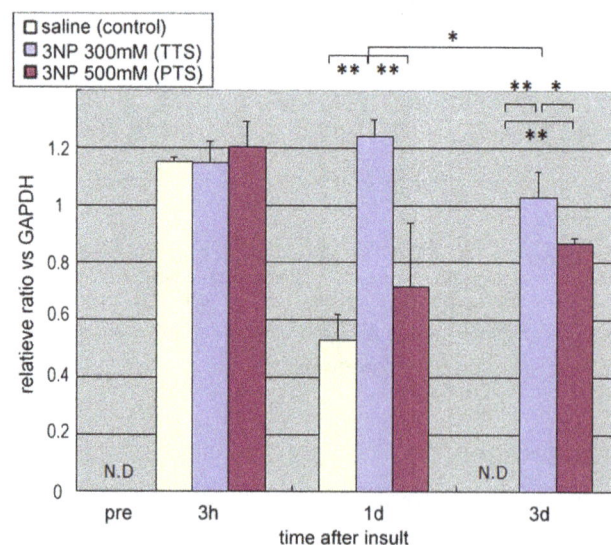

Figure 2. IL-6 expression in 3-NP-injured cochlea. Expression of IL-6 mRNA in whole cochlea. The temporal threshold shift (TTS) model (induced with 300 mM 3-NP) showed a significant induction of IL-6 mRNA from Day 1, which was sustained up until Day 3. The expression of IL-6 mRNA at Day 3 was also significantly higher in the permanent threshold shift (PTS) model (induced by 500 mM 3-NP) than in the saline-treated controls (*p<0.01, **p<0.05; N.D: not detected).

expressing type III cells (Fig. 3**b and d**; orange arrows); however, they were not observed in the same area as type III fibrocytes (blue arrows in Fig. 3**a and b**). Many Iba-1-expressing cells in the cochlea lateral wall had cellular processes, indicating that the macrophages had been activated. Iba-1-positive cells were also observed beneath the mesenchyme of the basilar membrane, but these cells did not have cellular processes (Fig. 3**d**, black arrows).

4. Genome-wide gene expression profiling of the lateral wall spiral ligament

Immunostaining revealed an inflammatory response to 3-NP in the cochlear lateral wall, particularly in the apical side of the basal turn. The molecular mechanism(s) underlying this inflammatory reaction remains to be elucidated. The spiral ligaments of the upper basal turns of the 3-NP-injured cochlea were harvested 1 d and 3 d post-administration of either 300 mM of 3-NP or saline, and subjected to genome-wide gene expression profiling (GEO accession number: 02708065). In the TTS model, 35% (26 of 74) and 60% (18 of 30) of the genes upregulated at Day 1 and Day 3 post-3-NP administration, respectively, were inflammatory genes, including CXC-type chemokines (Table 1) and CC-type chemokines (Table 2). Both types of chemokine induce chemotaxis by binding to their respective receptors, which are expressed on the surfaces of their target immune cells. We found high expression of CCL-1, 2 and 3 at Day 1, and high expression of CCL-1, 2, 3, 4, and 5, CCR-2 and 5, and CX3CR1 at Day 3 post-3-NP administration; however, there was no change in the expression of CX3CL1 (Tables 1 and 2). CCR-2 is an essential receptor for chemotaxis and is abundantly expressed on the surface of monocytes. CCL-2, a chemokine ligand for CCR-2, was upregulated in the 3-NP-injured lateral wall (Table 2). IL-1β and IL-6 were also detected. A>2-fold increase in gene expression compared with that in the saline-treated control was used as the cut-off threshold.

5. Acute IL-6 induction and sustained chemokine expression in the damaged cochlea lateral wall

Next, time-dependent changes in the expression of proinflammatory genes, chemokines, and chemoattractants in the lateral wall were examined by qRT-PCR. IL-6 was significantly upregulated in both the TTS and PTS models, before being rapidly downregulated to normal levels (Fig. 4**a**: p<0.01). The peak level of IL-6 expression was significantly higher in the PTS model than in the TTS model (Fig. 4**a**; p<0.01). Chemokines and chemoattractants, including the CCL and/or the CXCL families, play an essential role in recruiting inflammatory cells to the peripheral tissues. Many of these are induced by proinflammatory cytokines such as IL-6 (and were also detected in the genome-wide assay; Tables 1 and 2). Thus, we next examined the expression of several CCL-type chemokines, including CCL-2 (MCP-1), CCL-5 (RANTES) and CCL-4 (MIP-1β). All of these chemokines were expressed in the lateral wall of the cochlea from 6 h to 7 d after 3-NP administration, and their expression was sustained for longer than that of IL-6, which was upregulated at the early stages and then quickly downregulated in a time-dependent manner (Fig. 4**a–d**). The levels of CCL-2 in the PTS and TTS models were significantly different, being greater in the PTS model than in the TTS model (Fig. 4**b**; p<0.01). We also found the expression of TNF-α but was not as much induced as IL-6 (Fig. 4**e**).

Discussion

The pathology in the model of acute mitochondrial dysfunction described in the present study begins with the degeneration of the lateral wall of the cochlear. Fibrocytes maintain the homeostatic circulation of ions and the endocochlear potential of the lateral wall, whereas mitochondria integrate the apoptotic pathways and the production of reactive oxygen species, which cause cell damage [7]. Both apoptosis and the formation of reactive oxygen species are involved in the pathophysiological mechanisms underlying ischemia-, ototoxin-, and noise-induced cochlear damage [12,22,23]. Thus, mitochondrial dysfunction is likely to

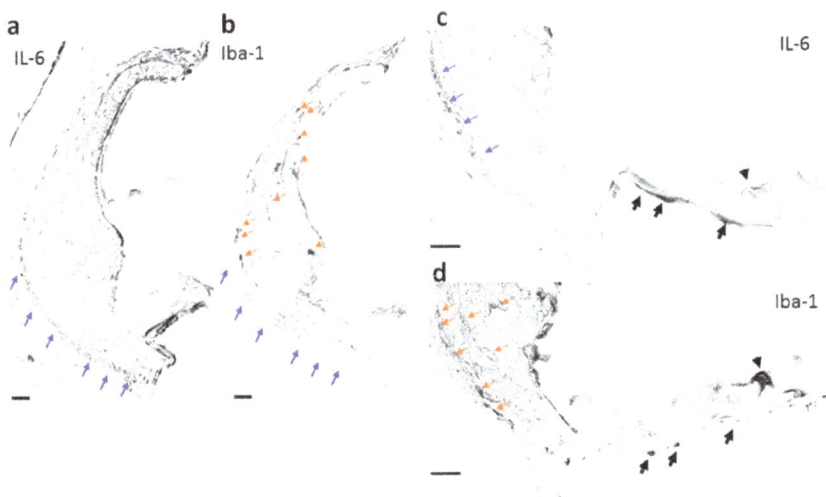

Figure 3. IL-6-expressing cells in 3-NP-injured cochlea were accompanied by macrophages. Cells expressing IL-6 (**a** and **c**) or Iba-1 (**b** and **d**) in the temporal threshold shift (TTS) model were examined by immunohistochemistry at Day 1 by using neighboring sections. IL-6 was expressed in type III fibrocytes (**a** and **c**; blue arrows) and in the mesenchyme cells beneath the basement membrane (**c**; black arrows). Cochlear macrophages expressing Iba-1 were identified adjacent to cells expressing IL-6, including in the lateral portion of the type II fibrocyte region that contacts type III cells (**b** and **d**; orange arrows), and were seen infiltrating the cells beneath the mesenchyme of the basilar membrane (**d**; black arrows). Iba-1-expressing cells were not observed in the type III area in which IL-6 was expressed (blue arrows in Fig. 3**a** and **b**).

Table 1. Upregulated CXC-type chemokine genes in the lateral wall of 3-NP-injured cochlea.

Receptor and its cell types	Chemokine Ligands	Day1	Day3
CXCR2 (not detected)	CXCL1	7	2.9
neutrophils	CXCL2	3.5	2.2
monocytes	CXCL3	NC	NC
	CXCL5	NC	NC
CXCR3 (not detected)	CXCL9	8.2	4.1
various cell types	CXCL10	6.5	NC
	CXCL11	6.3	NC
CXCR4	CXCL12	2	NC
widely expressed			
CX3CR1	CX3CL1	NC	NC
macrophages			

The values displayed refer to the -fold changes compared with the saline-treated controls.
Genes showing >2-fold changes are listed.
NC: no change compared with control.

play a critical role in hearing loss. One critical feature of the model used in this study is that infusion of a lower concentration of 3-NP leads to TTS, despite the fact that the drug irreversibly blocks mitochondrial complex II. This suggests that there may be cellular and/or intra-cellular sources that may help the recovery of injured fibrocytes. A comparison between the TTS and PTS models may be a useful strategy in the search for potential therapies.

The inner ear had been believed as an "immune-privileged organ" and it is true that sensorineural hearing loss models show no evidence of neutrophil infiltration in the absence of complete destruction of the cochlear structure. However, recent studies of several different cochlear damage models show the presence of other types of inflammatory cell in the injured cochlear lateral wall. Hirose and colleagues reported the infiltration of mononuclear cells into cochleae subjected to noise-induced damaged, as demonstrated by immunostaining for the leukocyte common antigen, CD45 [9]. Based on the observation of phagocytic macrophages, they claimed that the infiltrating marrow-derived cells may have "cleared" the dead cells that resulted from noise [9]. Schulte and colleagues showed that marrow-derived cells or hematopoietic stem cells could migrate and differentiate into cochlear lateral wall cells, including sodium/potassium/chloride co-transporter (NKCC)- or Na/K-ATPase-positive fibrocytes, in

normal adult rodents [13]. Okano and colleagues showed that cells migrating from the bone marrow constitutively resided in the cochlea and could be identified by staining for macrophage markers such as Iba-1 [18]. They also used an elegant chimeric assay to show that the Iba-1-positive cells were continuously resupplied from the bone marrow [18]. Although all three of these groups showed the migration of circulating hematopoietic cells or marrow-derived cells into the cochlea, the mechanisms underlying this phenomenon were not examined. The present study showed that the expression of inflammatory genes, including those for chemokines and chemoattractants, was induced in the damaged lateral wall of the cochlea in comparison with the saline- treated control. These genes were expressed in the areas in which infiltrating cells are most frequently observed [9,13,18]. Therefore, we speculate that the intrinsic program that controls gene expression in the lateral wall cells provides a mechanism for the infiltration of inflammatory cells.

Based on our microarray analyses, it is also true that the infiltration of neutrophils is lacking, as neutrophil-specific markers, such as CXCR2, could not be detected, while their ligands, CXCL1 and 2, were induced in the damaged lateral wall (Table 1). By contrast, many other chemokines, and the receptors for other types of immune cells, were detected. The monocyte receptors

Table 2. Upregulated CC-type chemokine genes in the lateral wall of 3-NP-injured cochlea.

Receptor and its cell types	Chemokine ligands	Day 1	Day 3
CCR2	CCL2	6.6	3.5
monocytes	CCL7	NC	NC
dendritic cells	CCL8	NC	NC
	CCL13	NC	NC
CCR5	CCL3	3..8	2.1
monocytes	CCL4	NC	2.3
T lymphcyte	CCL5	NC	2.6

The values displayed refer to the -fold changes compared with the saline-treated controls.
Genes showing >2-fold changes are listed.
NC: no change compared with control.

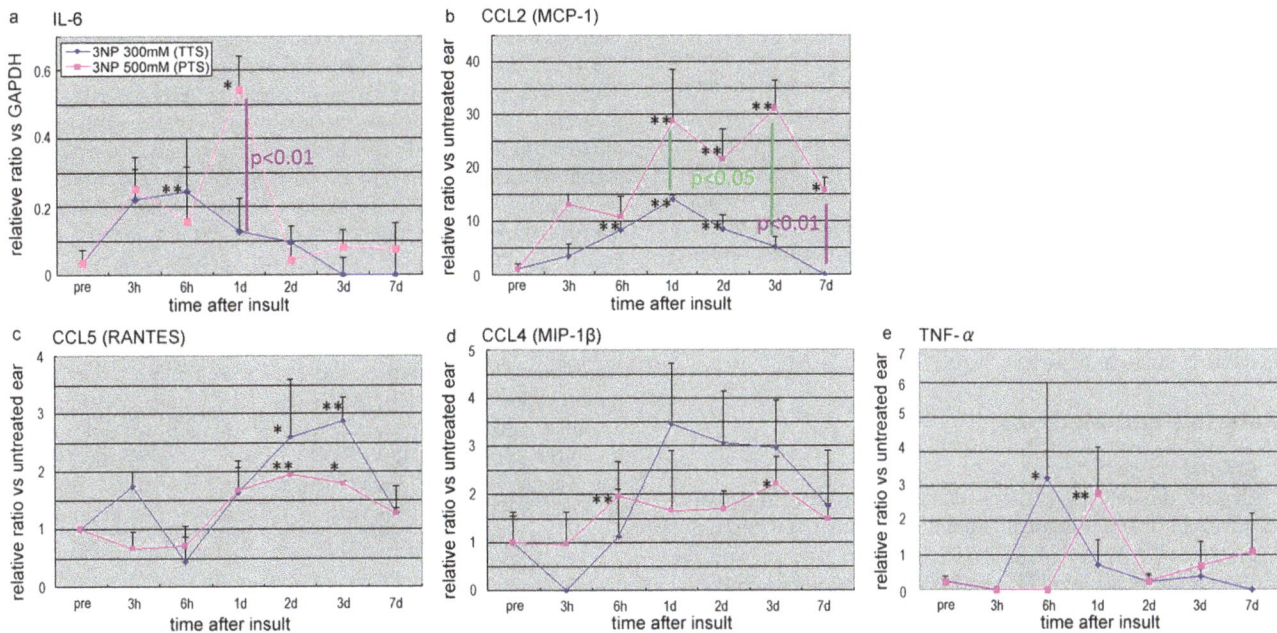

Figure 4. Time-dependent expression of IL-6 and chemokines in the 3-NP-injured cochlea lateral wall. Quantitative RT-PCR to examine the expression of IL-6 and chemokines, including CCL2 (MCP-1), CCL5 (RANTES) and CCL4 (MIP-1β), in the injured cochlear lateral wall. The expression of IL-6 was induced 3 h after 3-NP administration. IL-6 expression was higher in the PTS model (blue lines) than in the temporal threshold shift model (pink lines) at Day 1 (**a**; p<0.01; purple), suggesting that IL-6 was a detrimental factor. IL-6 expression was high in the PTS model at Day 1 post-injury but was quickly downregulated. Chemokines were induced in the 3-NP-injured lateral wall from 6 h to 7 d post 3-NP administration. Chemokine expression was induced more slowly than that of proinflammatory cytokines, but it was sustained (**a–d**). The level of CCL2 expression in the PTS and TTS models was significantly different, being greater in the PTS model than in the TTS model (**b**; p<0.05 (green) and p<0.01 (purple)), suggesting that CCL2 was also a detrimental factor. * indicates p<0.05, ** indicates p<0.01.

CCR-2 and 5 were highly expressed, and their ligands (CCL-2 and CCL-3, 4, and 5, respectively) were upregulated after 3-NP administration. mRNA for the cochlear macrophage receptor CX3CR1 was also detected, which is consistent with the immunostaining data showing the presence of Iba-1 positive cells; however, its ligand, CX3CL1, was not induced at Day 1 or 3 post-3-NP administration. These results suggest that macrophages were not recruited from the peripheral blood via CS3CL1/CX3CR1-dependent chemotaxis, but were derived from their precursors or from monocytes, which were recruited by the CCR/CCL pathway and activated by cytokines produced by cells within the cochlear lateral wall.

The present study showed that IL-6 was expressed by type III fibrocytes, and that immune cells were most frequently observed in-between type III and type II fibrocytes. Interestingly, a similar pattern of distribution was seen in noise-induced damaged cochlea, in which IL-6 was expressed by type IV fibrocytes and immune cells were most frequently observed in between type III and type IV fibrocytes [6]. The findings in the two different models examined in the present study suggest that the induction of IL-6 in the lateral wall at the early stages of damage determines the inflammatory responses that occur in the lateral wall. We also found that CCL-2 (MCP-1) was induced upon IL-6 production. IL-6 is a strong inducer of chemokines or chemoattractants, such as CCL-2, which recruits inflammatory cells from the peripheral blood to the local injured area via its receptor, CCR-2. CCL-2 was the only CCR-2 ligand identified in the assay. Finally, both IL-6 and CCL-2 were expressed at higher levels in the permanent hearing loss model than in the temporary hearing loss model. These results lead us to believe that the IL-6/CCL-2 pathway contributes to the inflammatory response initiated by 3-NP-

induced damage to the cochlear lateral wall, and that the pathway is essential for the inflammatory reactions observed in this model. Therefore, manipulating this pathway would be a feasible approach to controlling cochlear inflammation. Further studies of this pathway should incorporate genetically-modified rodents to investigate these genes using 'loss of function' and 'gain of function' approaches.

It is widely accepted that excessive inflammation is harmful, and that blocking of the associated inflammatory responses is a potential therapeutic strategy. In the present model, the expression of IL-6 and CCL-2 in the lateral wall was significantly higher in the PTS model than in the TTS model, suggesting that excessive production of inflammatory cytokines and chemokines was detrimental to organ function. It is also widely known that an appropriate inflammatory response is essential for tissue recovery. Our previous studies showed that type II and IV fibrocytes in the spiral ligament divide after injury, and exogenous mesenchymal stem cell transplantation studies show that these cells promote fibrocyte proliferation both *in vivo* and *in vitro* [20]. CCL-type chemokines, such as CCL-2, are potent agents that recruit these cells [2,4]. Thus, in this context, appropriate activation of the local IL-6/CCL-2 pathway may contribute to the recovery of the lateral wall of the cochlea. The results presented herein indicate that treatment with anti-inflammatory agents would be a feasible strategy for treating acute energy failure in the cochlea; however, considerable thought and pre-clinical investigation is required to identify suitable regimens, along with appropriate timings and doses.

Conclusion

In conclusion, the present study shows that secondary inflammation occurs in the lateral wall of the cochlea after 3-NP-induced acute energy failure. Macrophage activation and the induction of inflammatory genes were detected following mitochondrial dysfunction. The expression of IL-6 and CCL-2 was higher in the permanent hearing damage model than in the temporary hearing damage model, suggesting that the inflammatory response is a potential therapeutic target for the treatment of deafness resulting from energy failure in the lateral cochlear wall. Further studies that focus on the inflammatory response in this organ will help us to understand the pathophysiology of the lateral wall damage involved in acute hearing loss.

Materials and Methods

1. Animal models

All experimental procedures described in this study were approved by the Institutional Animal Care and Use Committee of the National Tokyo Medical Center, in accordance with the Guide for the Care and Use of Laboratory Animals (National Institute of Health, Bethesda, MD). Female Sprague-Dawley rats weighing between 180 g and 210 g (8–10 weeks old) were used for the experiments. The surgical protocols have been described previously [10,17]. Briefly, after general anesthesia with pentobarbital (30–40 mg/kg, i.p.) and the local administration of lidocaine (1%), an incision was made posterior to the left pinna near the external meatus. The left otic bulla was opened and the round window niche was infused with 3-NP (500 mM or 300 mM; Sigma, St. Louis, MO, USA) dissolved in saline (pH adjusted to 7.4 with NaOH). Infusion with saline alone was used as a control. Following treatment, and before the wound was closed, a small piece of gelatin was placed onto the niche to keep the solution in place and to allow for head movement after the animals awoke. The right cochlea was surgically destroyed to avoid cross-hearing during the recording of auditory brain-stem responses. To confirm deafness, auditory brain-stem responses were recorded before and 3 h after 3-NP or saline administration, or at the end of the observation period (1, 7, and 14 d; Table S1).

2. RT-PCR, quantitative RT-PCR and DNA array analyses

Either the whole cochlea or the second turn of the lateral wall (excluding the stria vascularis) was harvested and reverse transcription was performed with an oligo-dT primer and a SuperScript II RT-PCR kit (Invitrogen) according to the manufacturer's protocol. The obtained cDNAs were used for RT-PCR (for whole cochlear samples taken 3 h, 1 d, and 3 d after the administration of 300 mM and 500 mM of 3-NP; n = 4 per group or samples without any treatment; n = 6) or qRT-PCR (for lateral wall samples taken before administration and 3 h, 6 h, 1 d, 2 d, 3 d, and 7 d after administration of 300 mM and 500 mM 3-NP; n = 3 per group). RT-PCR was performed over 37 cycles with primers supplied in the message Screen Rat Inflammatory Cytokine Set 2 Multiplex PCR Kits (BioSource International Inc., Camarillo, CA). The thermal cycling conditions for the Taq polymerase (Takara Biotechnology Co., Ltd., Otsu, Japan) were as stated in the manufacturer's protocol. Quantitative real-time RT-PCR reactions were carried out in a Mx3000p (Stratagene, La Jolla, CA) using FAM-conjugated TaqMan primers against IL-1β, IL-6, CCL-2, CCL-4, CCL-5 and SOCS-3, and a VIC-conjugated glyceraldehyde-3-phosphate dehydrogenase (GAPDH) probe as an internal control (Applied Biosystems, Foster City, CA).

As a reference, the fluorescent dye, ROX, was used to calibrate inter-sample variability. The relative expression levels of each cytokine were statistically compared across both groups (PTS and TTS) using a one-way analysis of variance (ANOVA). Repeated measures ANOVA was used to analyze differences in the results obtained pre- and at 3 h, 6 h, 1 d, 2 d, 3 d, and 7 d post-3-NP administration (within-subject variability) and the differences between the PTS and TTS groups (between subject variability). All procedures incorporated controls that did not undergo RT or lacked the PCR template. DNA array analyses were performed using samples obtained 1 d and 3 d after 3-NP or saline administration (n = 4) and the GeneChip Rat Expression Set 230 (AFFYMETRIX). All experiments were conducted using a GeneChip Fluidics Station 400 (AFFYMETRIX), a GeneChip hybridization Oven 640 (AFFYMETRIX), and a Gene array Scanner (Agilent). Raw data and its information was uploaded to the NIH database, GEO (GEO accession number: 02708065). The data were analyzed with Signet Viewer (Biomatrix). For each gene, the ratio of the signal in the TTS sample to that in the saline-treated control was calculated and the data were analyzed.

3. Histology

Histological analysis was performed 1 day after the administration of 300 mM 3-NP (n = 3). For tissue fixation, rats were deeply anesthetized with pentobarbital (as described above) and transcardially perfused with 4% paraformaldehyde. Paraffin sections were prepared as previously described [20]. Immunohistochemistry for Iba-1 and IL-6 was performed as previously described [6]. All slides were washed with PBS, incubated in 1.5% hydrogen peroxide for 15 min, rinsed three times in PBS, incubated with 10% normal goat serum for 1 h at room temperature, and then incubated overnight with the appropriate primary antibodies at 48°C. The primary antibodies used were a rabbit anti-IL-6 polyclonal antibody (diluted 1:150; Sigma) and a rabbit anti-Iba-1 polyclonal antibody (diluted 1:500; Wako Pure Chemicals). The slides were then incubated with biotinylated secondary antibodies (1:1000) at 37°C for 30 min, washed three times in PBS, and then incubated in VECTASTAIN Elite ABC reagent (Elite ABC kit, Vector Laboratories, Burlingame, CA) for 30 min at room temperature. After gentle washing in PBS (three times), staining was visualized by incubating the samples with diaminobenzidine solution (Wako Pure Chemical Industries). After a final wash with PBS, the samples were dehydrated and mounted under coverslips.

Acknowledgments

We are grateful to Dr. Yoshiaki Fujinami for assistance with the experiments.

Author Contributions

Conceived and designed the experiments: MF TM. Performed the experiments: MF YO SS. Analyzed the data: MF TM. Contributed reagents/materials/analysis tools: YO SS HJO HO KO TM. Wrote the paper: MF TM.

References

1. Alston TA, Mela L, Bright HJ (1977) 3-Nitropropionate, the toxic substance of Indigofera, is a suicide inactivator of succinate dehydrogenase. Proceedings of the National Academy of Sciences of the United States of America 74: 3767–71.

2. Belema-Bedada F, Uchida S, Martire A, Kostin S, Braun T (2008) Efficient homing of multipotent adult mesenchymal stem cells depends on FROUNT-mediated clustering of CCR2. Cell Stem Cell 5;2:566–75.

3. Coles CJ, Edmondson DE, Singer TP (1979) Inactivation of succinate dehydrogenase by 3-nitropropionate. The Journal of biological chemistry 254: 5161–7.

4. Dwyer RM, Potter-Beirne SM, Harrington KA, Lowery AJ, Hennessy E, et al. (2007) Monocyte chemotactic protein-1 secreted by primary breast tumors stimulates migration of mesenchymal stem cells. Clin Cancer Res 1;13:5020–7

5. Fischel-Ghodsian N (2003) Mitochondrial diseases. The New England journal of medicine 349: 1293–4; author reply 1293-4.

6. Fujioka M, Kanzaki S, Okano HJ, Ogawa K, Okano H et al. (2006) Proinflammatory cytokines expression in noise-induced damaged cochlea. Journal of neuroscience research 83: 575–83.

7. Green DR, Reed JC (1998) Mitochondria and apoptosis. Science 281: 1309–12.

8. Haberkamp TJ, Tanyeri HM (1999) Management of idiopathic sudden sensorineural hearing loss. Am J Otol 20:587–592; discussion 593-585.

9. Hirose K, Discolo CM, Keasler JR, Ransohoff R (2005) Mononuclear phagocytes migrate into the murine cochlea after acoustic trauma. The Journal of comparative neurology 489: 180–94.

10. Hoya N, Okamoto Y, Kamiya K, Fujii M, Matsunaga T (2004) A novel animal model of acute cochlear mitochondrial dysfunction. Neuroreport 15: 1597–600.

11. Hsu CH, Kwon H, Perng CL, Bai RK, Dai P, et al. (2005) Hearing loss in mitochondrial disorders. Annals of the New York Academy of Sciences 1042: 36–47.

12. Huang T, Cheng AG, Stupak H, Liu W, Kim A, et al. (2000) Oxidative stress-induced apoptosis of cochlear sensory cells: otoprotective strategies. International journal of developmental neuroscience : the official journal of the International Society for Developmental Neuroscience 18: 259–70.

13. Lang H, Ebihara Y, Schmiedt RA, Minamiguchi H, Zhou D, et al. (2006) Contribution of bone marrow hematopoietic stem cells to adult mouse inner ear: mesenchymal cells and fibrocytes. The Journal of comparative neurology 496: 187–201.

14. Lee H, Ahn BH, Baloh RW (2004) Sudden deafness with vertigo as a sole manifestation of anterior inferior cerebellar artery infarction. J Neurol Sci 222:105–107.

15. Mizutari K, Matsunaga T, Kamiya K, Fujinami Y, Ogawa K, et al. (2008) Caspase inhibitor facilitates recovery of hearing by protecting the cochlear lateral wall from acute cochlear mitochondrial dysfunction. Journal of neuroscience research 86: 215–22.

16. Mort DJ, Bronstein AM (2006) Sudden deafness. Curr Opin Neurol 19:1–3.

17. Okamoto Y, Hoya N, Kamiya K, Ogawa K, Matsunaga T, et al. (2005) Permanent threshold shift caused by acute cochlear mitochondrial dysfunction is primarily mediated by degeneration of the lateral wall of the cochlea. Audiology & neuro-otology 10: 220–33.

18. Okano T, Nakagawa T, Kita T, Kada S, Yoshimoto M, et al. (2008) Bone marrow-derived cells expressing Iba1 are constitutively present as resident tissue macrophages in the mouse cochlea. Journal of neuroscience research 86: 1758–67.

19. Pickles JO, et al. (2004) Mutation in mitochondrial DNA as a cause of presbyacusis. Audiology & neuro-otology 9: 23–33.

20. Sun GW, Fujii M, Matsunaga T (2012) Functional interaction between mesenchymal stem cells and spiral ligament fibrocytes : J Neurosci Res 90:1713–22

21. Wang Y, Hirose K, Liberman MC (2002) Dynamics of noise-induced cellular injury and repair in the mouse cochlea. Journal of the Association for Research in Otolaryngology : JARO 3: 248–68.

22. Yamane H, Nakai Y, Takayama M, Iguchi H, Nakagawa T, et al. (1995) Appearance of free radicals in the guinea pig inner ear after noise-induced acoustic trauma. European archives of oto-rhino-laryngology : official journal of the European Federation of Oto-Rhino-Laryngological Societies 252: 504–8.

23. Yamane H, Nakai Y, Takayama M, Konishi K, Iguchi H, et al. (1995) The emergence of free radicals after acoustic trauma and strial blood flow. Acta oto-laryngologica. Supplementum 519: 87–92.

24. Yamasoba T, Kikuchi S, Higo R (2001) Deafness associated with vertebrobasilar insufficiency. J Neurol Sci 187:69–75.

11

Risky Music Listening, Permanent Tinnitus and Depression, Anxiety, Thoughts about Suicide and Adverse General Health

Ineke Vogel[1,2]*, **Petra M. van de Looij-Jansen**[2], **Cathelijne L. Mieloo**[2], **Alex Burdorf**[1], **Frouwkje de Waart**[2]

1 Dept of Public Health, Erasmus MC University Medical Center, Rotterdam, the Netherlands, **2** Dept of Youth Policy, Municipal Public Health Service for Rotterdam Area, Rotterdam, the Netherlands

Abstract

Objective: To estimate the extent to which exposure to music through earphones or headphones with MP3 players or at discotheques and pop/rock concerts exceeded current occupational safety standards for noise exposure, to examine the extent to which temporary and permanent hearing-related symptoms were reported, and to examine whether the experience of permanent symptoms was associated with adverse perceived general and mental health, symptoms of depression, and thoughts about suicide.

Methods: A total of 943 students in Dutch inner-city senior-secondary vocational schools completed questionnaires about their sociodemographics, music listening behaviors and health. Multiple logistic regression analyses were used to examine associations.

Results: About 60% exceeded safety standards for occupational noise exposure; about one third as a result of listening to MP3 players. About 10% of the participants experienced permanent hearing-related symptoms. Temporary hearing symptoms that occurred after using an MP3 player or going to a discotheque or pop/rock concert were associated with exposure to high-volume music. However, compared to participants not experiencing permanent hearing-related symptoms, those experiencing permanent symptoms were less often exposed to high volume music. Furthermore, they reported at least two times more often symptoms of depression, thoughts about suicide and adverse self-assessed general and mental health.

Conclusions: Risky music-listening behaviors continue up to at least the age of 25 years. Permanent hearing-related symptoms are associated with people's health and wellbeing. Participants experiencing such symptoms appeared to have changed their behavior to be less risky. In order to induce behavior change *before* permanent and irreversible hearing-related symptoms occur, preventive measurements concerning hearing health are needed.

Editor: Joel Snyder, UNLV, United States of America

Funding: The authors have no support or funding to report.

Competing Interests: The authors have declared that no competing interests exist.

* E-mail: i.vogel@erasmusmc.nl

Introduction

According to the World Health Organization, adult onset hearing loss (HL) is the second leading cause of 'years lived with disability' (YLD) after depression at global level, accounting for 4.6% of total global YLDs [1]. Exposure to excessive noise is a major cause of hearing disorder worldwide; 16% of the disabling HL in adults is attributed to occupational noise [2].

Outside the workplace millions of adolescents and young adults are potentially at risk of permanent hearing symptoms through listening to their favorite music. The risks of excessive music-listening are most likely to result in hearing-related symptoms such as tinnitus – a perceived sound in the ears with no external source of sound being present [3–5]. Prevalence of permanent tinnitus increases with age; previous research indicates that only 1% of those under 45 years experience permanent tinnitus, while about 12% of those aged 60–69 years develop it [6]. However, it has

been reported that increasing numbers of adolescents and young adults now experience permanent symptoms indicative of poor hearing due largely to listening to music at high volumes [2,7,8].

It has been estimated that about 20% of Dutch adolescents aged 12–16 years are potentially at risk of developing hearing-related symptoms after 5 years because of listening to potentially hazardous music levels. Between 30.0% and 61.2% of them reported temporary hearing-related symptoms such as tinnitus after exposure to music from MP3 players and at discotheques [9]. If such exposure continues after the age of 16 years, temporary hearing-related symptoms will become more severe and even permanent.

Symptoms of poor hearing may lead to difficulties in future life. Because HL may influence communication and behavioral skills, it can adversely affect education and quality of life. Also, it is a growing social problem as more and more young people are

Table 1. Socio-demographic characteristics of study population (N = 943).

	Frequency in study population (unless otherwise specified)	
Mean age (years)	18 (sd 2; range 16–25)	
Gender		
Female	593	(62.9%)
Ethnicity		
Non-Dutch	625	(66.3%)
Home situation		
Living with parent(s)	745	(79.0%)

Characteristics adjusted from Vogel et al [17].

limited in their choice of or even rejected from jobs because of preventable HL. Furthermore, it may lead to reduced psychological and social function, such as increased feelings of isolation, depression, loneliness, anger, fear, frustration, stress and disappointment [2,8,10].

Among 12–16 year olds, mainly adolescents attending pre-vocational education report relatively high levels of music exposure [11,12]. Therefore, to investigate the prevalence of permanent hearing-related symptoms and its potential negative consequences among young people, we conducted a study among 16–25 year old students from lower educational levels. This group of students is assumed to be most and long enough exposed to potentially hazardous music levels, and thus the group most likely to experience permanent hearing-related symptoms such as tinnitus, muffled sounds, distortion or hyperacusis. We (1) estimated the extent to which these students' exposure to music through earphones or headphones with MP3 players or at discotheques and pop/rock concerts exceeded current occupational safety standards for noise exposure, (2) examined the extent to which these students reported temporary and permanent hearing-related symptoms, and (3) examined whether the experience of permanent symptoms was associated with adverse perceived general and mental health, symptoms of depression, and thoughts about suicide.

Methods

Ethics Statement

According to the Dutch Act on public health, the Municipal Executive has to acquire, based on epidemiological analysis, insight into the health situation of the population and has to take care of systematic monitoring and highlighting of developments in the health status of young people [13]. All data were gathered through questionnaires by the local Municipal Public Health Service within this government-approved research of youth healthcare. Administration of the questionnaires at schools was carried out by specially trained researchers and public health promoters of the Municipal Public Health Service and/or a teacher. Students received written and verbal information about the study and were free to refuse to participation. The research was conducted in accordance with the requirements of the Dutch act on protection of personal data. Only anonymous data were used and the questionnaires were completed on a voluntary basis by students. Informed consent from parents is not required for people aged 16 and over [14]. Observational research with data does not fall within the ambit of the Dutch Act on research involving human subjects and does not require the approval of an

ethics review board [15]. This study conformed to the principles embodied in the Declaration of Helsinki [16].

Study Population and Procedure

A total of 1228 students (aged about 16–25 years) of 2 Dutch inner-city senior-secondary vocational schools were invited to complete questionnaires (Table S1) about their sociodemographics, music listening behaviors and health under supervision at school. All students that were present at the time of assessment completed the questionnaire. However, 272 students did not complete the questionnaire because of illness (27), visiting a doctor or nurse or stay away without leave (46), or because they were absent for unknown reasons (199); resulting in a total of 956 questionnaires, for a response of 77.9%. We excluded 13 more questionnaires because of an age outside the range of 16–25 years; thus, 943 questionnaires were used in the analyses. Participants' ages ranged from 16 to 25 years (mean = 18; SD = 2). Sixty three percent were female, 66.3% were of non-Dutch ethnicity and 79.0% were living with their parent(s). Table 1 gives an overview of the socio-demographic characteristics of the study population. This table is adjusted from a previous study [17].

Measures

Table S1 lists the survey items.

Sociodemographic characteristics. Sociodemographic characteristics included sex, age, ethnicity (Dutch; non-Dutch) and home situation (living with parent(s); not living with parent(s)). Ethnicity was determined on the basis of mother's and father's country/countries of birth according to definitions of Statistics Netherlands [18].

Risky music listening. Estimation of risky music listening behaviors – MP3 player listening and discotheque and pop/rock concert attendance – previously has been described in detail [9,17]. Average weekly exposure times to MP3 players and stereos were estimated by multiplying days per week and hours per day. Average exposure time per month during discotheque visits was estimated by multiplying the number of discotheque visits per month by average time spent per visit. Average exposure time per year during pop/rock concerts was estimated by multiplying numbers of visits per year by 2.5 hours.

Since we did not measure music volume levels, to be able to estimate the exposure to potentially hazardous music levels, we had to estimate the music-volume levels per music source. Portnuff and Fligor have evaluated the output levels of several most popular players [19]. We used their grand average output levels across all evaluated players, which are similar to estimations made by a Dutch evaluation of the output levels of MP3 players and earphones [20], to convert volume-control levels of MP3 players and stereos into decibel levels. For discotheques the average decibel level was assumed to be 100 dBA, for pop/rock concerts 105 dBA [21].

Within current European occupational safety standards [22], music volume levels equal to or exceeding the equivalent of 80 decibels (dB/dBA) for 40 hours per week are assumed to be potentially damaging. However, in the report of the Scientific Committee on Emerging and Newly Identified Health Risks it is assumed that listening for 1 hour a day to a sound level of over 89 dBA is potentially damaging [2]. By applying the principle that a doubling in level (+3 dB) can be offset by halving the permissible exposure duration [23,24], it can be calculated that listening 7 hours per week to a music level of 89 dB is equal to listening for 56 hours per week, or 8 hours per day, to a music level of 80 dBA. Therefore, we choose to use a loosened 56-hours criterion instead of the more stringent safety standard of 40 hours; i.e. 16 hours are added for the weekend days, because music listening is not restricted to working days.

To be able to estimate a weekly music dose (D) on the basis of reported exposure times and levels, we first calculated permissible exposure limits (PELs) for the estimated dBA levels of each participant per music source (MP3-player use and discotheque and pop/rock concert attendance) using the equation: $PEL_{(week)} = 56/2^{(L-80)/3}$; L stands for the estimated dBA level [24]. Secondly, each adolescent's actual exposure time per music source was divided by the PEL to compute his or her estimated weekly music dose per music source [24]. Thirdly, the estimated doses per music source were summed to calculate an estimated total weekly music dose for all music sources combined [24]. A dose that was missing for a certain source was assumed to be zero.

To evaluate potential risk behavior, we first dichotomized responses on the basis of the loosened safety standard into students who were estimated to not be exposed to potentially hazardous music levels (D<1; exposed to equivalent levels of <80 dBA during 8 hours per day) and those who were estimated to be exposed to potentially hazardous music levels (D≥1; exposed to equivalent levels of ≥80 dBA during 8 hours per day) [24]. As an additional quantification of the severity of the potential risk, we applied three categories that estimated whether students were exposed (by source and by all sources combined) to a potential hazardous level for 8 hrs per day equivalent to: 80–85 dBA (low risk); 85–90 dBA (moderate risk); ≥90 dBA (high risk).

Health indicators. Hearing symptoms included symptoms such as tinnitus, muffled sounds, distortion, hyperacusis or (temporary) hearing loss. Temporary hearing-related symptoms were categorized as 'I experienced hearing-related symptoms at least once in the past month after listening to an MP3 player' (yes; no) and 'I experienced hearing-related symptoms at least once in the past year after visiting discotheques and/or pop/rock concerts' (yes; no). Permanent hearing-related symptoms were categorized as 'I am constantly experiencing hearing symptoms' (yes; no).

'General health' was categorized as: 'My health in general is good or very good' (yes/no). 'Mental health' was measured with the five-item Mental Health Inventory (MHI-5) [25]. The MHI-5 measures general mental health and can be used to screen for depressive symptoms and feelings of anxiety [26]. Each item asks the respondent about a particular feeling during the past month. The duration is reported on a six-point scale ranging from 'all of the time' to 'none of the time'. Therefore, the score for each individual ranges between 5 and 30. This score is transformed into a variable ranging from 0–100 using a standard linear transformation, where a score of 100 represents optimal health. We used a cut-off score of <60 to define moderate-to-poor mental health.

This cut-off is widely used and provides the best sensitivity and specificity [25,27].

'Symptoms of depression' were measured with the Center for Epidemiologic Studies Depression Scale (CES-D) [28]. The CES-D was designed to measure current level of depressive symptomatology. It consists of 20 items that ask the respondent to indicate the frequency with which he/she experienced a symptom during the past week. One symptom, for example, is: 'During the past week I did not feel like eating; my appetite was poor'. The frequency is reported on a 4-point response scale ranging from 0 (rarely/none of the time; less than 1 day) to 3 (most/all of the time; 5 to 7 days). Therefore, the summative score ranges between 0 and 60. Scores of ≥16 are regarded as clinically significant levels of depressive symptoms in the general population [28]. 'Thoughts about suicide' were categorized as: 'I often or very often seriously thought to end my life during the past 12 months' (yes/no).

Statistical Analysis

Cross-sectional statistical analyses were performed using the SPSS program (version 19; SPSS Inc, Chicago, IL). Frequency tables were used to explore music listening, risky music listening and health of the total study population (N = 943), and females (n = 593) and males (n = 350); frequency differences were examined through chi-square statistics. Multivariate odds ratios (ORs) and their 95% confidence intervals (CIs) were calculated with multiple logistic regression analyses to explore the association between the estimated exposure to high-volume levels and both reported temporary and permanent hearing-related symptoms. Frequency tables and multiple logistic regression analyses were used to explore the associations between permanent hearing-related symptoms and the other health indicators (adverse perceived general and mental health, symptoms of depression, and thoughts about suicide). Any p values of <0.05 were considered to be statistically significant.

Results

Risky Music Listening

We estimated that 19.2% of participants were exposed to high-risk sound levels; they exceeded a sound level equivalent to 90 dBA for 56 hours per week for all sources of music combined; with regard to MP3 players alone, that figure was 15.4%, and for discotheques and pop/rock concerts 3.1% (Table 2).

Health Indicators

After listening to music on MP3 players 14.5% experienced temporary hearing-related symptoms; after visiting discotheques and/or pop/rock concerts 44.2%. Almost 10% of participants reported constant hearing-related symptoms; about one third of them consulted a physician for their hearing problems. Regarding the other four health indicators, (adverse perceived general health, adverse mental health, depressive symptoms and thoughts about suicide) frequencies for experiencing adverse outcomes ranged between 17.8% (thoughts about suicide) and 34.5% (mental unhealthy). For all indicators, in comparison with males, females reported more often adverse outcomes (Table 3).

Risky Music Listening and Hearing-related Symptoms

Temporary hearing-related symptoms – such as tinnitus, muffled sounds, distortion, hyperacusis or hearing loss – that occurred after using an MP3 player or going to a discotheque or pop/rock concert were associated with exposure to high-volume music (Table 4). Students that reported listening at high-risk levels experienced almost two times more often temporary hearing-

Table 2. Music exposure of study population[a] (N = 943).

	Total	Males	Females	p[b]
	N = 943	n = 350	n = 593	
Music exposure				
Listened to music on MP3 players (in past month)	88.0	83.6	90.7	***
Frequency of use				
7 d/wk (in past month)	35.4	34.6	35.9	
>3 h/d	15.4	17.9	14.0	
Used volume setting of more than three fourths	44.6	40.3	47.0	*
Visited discotheques (last year)	61.2	64.6	59.2	
Visited pop/rock concerts (last year)	39.8	43.2	37.9	
Risky music exposure[c]				
Risky exposure from combined sources (≥80 dBA)	61.5	64.0	59.9	
Low risk (80–85 dBA)	25.8	25.6	25.6	
Moderate risk (85–90 dBA)	16.5	18.7	15.3	
High risk (≥90 dBA)	19.2	19.6	18.9	
Risky exposure from MP3 players (≥80 dBA)	30.4	28.8	31.4	
Low risk (80–85 dBA)	11.6	13.8	10.3	
Moderate risk (85–90 dBA)	3.5	2.3	4.2	
High risk (≥90 dBA)	15.4	12.7	16.9	
Risky exposure from discotheques and pop/rock concerts (≥80 dBA)	48.1	54.8	44.2	***
Low risk (80–85 dBA)	30.1	30.0	30.0	
Moderate risk (85–90 dBA)	15.0	19.6	12.3	
High risk (≥90 dBA)	3.1	5.2	1.9	

[a]Values reported are percentages.
[b]Females compared to males.
*P<0.05.
***P<0.001.
[c]Average exposure equivalent to sound levels of 80 dBA during ≥56 hours per week.

related symptoms than students listening at sounds levels that were not risky. For discotheques and pop/rock concerts this was more than 15 times more often.

Compared to students experiencing such symptoms, students not experiencing permanent hearing-related symptoms listened more than 2.5 times more often to sound levels equivalent to ≥ 90 dBA for 56 hours per week (high-risk sound levels) (Table 4).

Table 3. Health indicators of study population[a] (N = 943).

Health indicators	Total	Males	Females	p[b]
	N = 943	n = 350	n = 593	
Temporary hearing-related symptoms[c]				
At least once in the prior month after listening to music on an MP3 player	14.5	14.1	14.7	
In the past year after going to a discotheque or pop/rock concert	44.2	46.7	43.0	
Permanent hearing-related symptoms[c]	9.2	8.1	9.9	
Consulted a physician for hearing	2.9	2.0	3.4	
Adverse perceived general health	30.9	22.2	36.1	***
Adverse mental health	34.5	25.9	39.5	***
Depressive symptoms	32.7	23.3	38.3	***
Thoughts about suicide (past year)	17.8	12.4	21.1	***

[a]Values reported are percentages.
[b]Females compared to males *P<0.05, ***P<0.001
[c]Hearing-related symptoms included symptoms such as tinnitus, muffled sounds, distortion, hyperacusis or (temporary) hearing loss.

Table 4. Prevalence (%) of self-reported hearing-related symptoms and the association with estimated exposure to potentially hazardous music levels.

	Temporary hearing-related symptoms (N = 856)[a]				Permanent hearing-related symptoms (N = 943)	
	MP3 players		Discotheques and pop/rock concerts			
	Frequency of hearing symptoms such as tinnitus 'at least once in the past month'		Frequency of hearing symptoms such as tinnitus 'at least once in the past year'			
	%	OR[b] (95% CI)	%	OR[b] (95% CI)	%	OR[b] (95% CI)
Total study population	16.0[a]		48.7[a]		9.2	
Music exposure						
Not at risk – reference (<80 dBA[c])	14.7	1.00	24.6	1.00	10.7	1.00
Low risk (80–85 dBA[c])	17.0	1.25 (0.69–2.25)	73.2	8.84 (6.18–12.63)***	9.9	0.86 (0.49–1.49)
Moderate risk (85–90 dBA[c])	9.7	0.62 (0.18–2.09)	74.2	8.69 (5.49–13.76)***	10.3	0.93 (0.50–1.75)
High risk (≥90 dBA[c])	22.3	1.70 (1.07–2.70)*	82.1	15.30 (5.62–41.65)***	4.4	0.39 (0.18–0.86)*

OR = Odds Ratio; CI = Confidence Interval; dBA = decibels.
[a]Participants with reported permanent hearing symptoms excluded (N = 87).
[b]Adjusted for age and gender.
[c]Equivalent sound level in dBA for 56 hrs per week.
*P<0.05.
***P<0.001.

Permanent Hearing-related Symptoms and other Health Indicators

All other health indicators – adverse perceived general health, adverse mental health, depressive symptoms and thoughts about suicide – were significantly related to permanent hearing-related symptoms (corrected for sociodemographics). Compared to participants not experiencing permanent hearing-related symptoms, those experiencing such symptoms reported at least two times more often symptoms of depression, thoughts about suicide and adverse self-assessed general and mental health (Table 5).

Discussion

An alarming percentage of almost 10% of this relatively young age group reported permanent hearing-related symptoms. Furthermore, experiencing such symptoms was related to adverse self-assessed general and mental health, and to having symptoms of depression and thoughts about suicide.

Our study is one of the first to provide a preliminary insight into the association between exposure of 15–25-year-old inner-city youth attending lower education to potentially hazardous music and temporary and permanent hearing symptoms, and into the association between permanent hearing-related symptoms and adverse health consequences. The results show that risky music-listening behaviors continue up to at least the age of 25 years among students attending lower educational levels. We estimated that by listening to high-volume music during leisure time, about 20% listened on average to sound levels that may cause permanent hearing-related symptoms such as tinnitus or even permanent hearing loss that is noticeable to individual people themselves after 5 years of such exposure [29].

As found previously [9,30], this study showed that participants exposed to potentially hazardous sound levels experienced

Table 5. Prevalence (%) of self-reported other adverse health indicators and the association with experiencing permanent hearing-related symptoms (N = 943).

| | Permanent hearing-related symptoms | |
	%	OR[a] (95% CI)
Total study population	9.2	
Health indicators		
Adverse perceived general health	47.1	2.03 (1.26–3.25)**
Adverse mental health	55.2	2.68 (1.66–4.33)***
Depressive symptoms	56.3	2.58 (1.60–4.16)***
Thoughts about suicide (past year)	31.0	1.99 (1.19–3.34)**

OR = odds ratio; CI = confidence interval.
[a]Adjusted for age, sex, ethnicity and home situation.
**P<0.01.
***P<0.001.

temporary hearing-related symptoms more often than those not exposed to such sound levels. Most people tend to underestimate the threat of music-induced hearing loss, probably because of the gradual development of hearing loss and because most people with mild high-frequency hearing loss are unaware of their impairment [31]. Repeated experiences of temporary hearing-related symptoms might be an indication that an individual's hearing is susceptible to noise-related damage and should be taken as warning signs for people to reduce their exposure to very high noise levels [31,32]. However, previous research has shown that young people attending lower educational levels who had experienced tinnitus did not consider this as a warning that their hearing was susceptible to damage from loud music and did not intend to change their behavior voluntarily [11,12,33].

Remarkably, most of the alarming percentage of almost 10% of this relatively young age group that reported permanent and thus irreversible hearing-related symptoms appeared to have changed their behavior: the more often permanent hearing-related symptoms were reported, the lower the reported average sound levels. Probably these people adjusted their behavior in order to prevent the symptoms from worsening and protect their hearing from further deterioration. Furthermore, experiencing permanent symptoms was related to adverse self-assessed general and mental health, and to having symptoms of depression and thoughts about suicide. These results show that permanent hearing-related symptoms occur considerably among certain groups of youth and are associated with young people's health and wellbeing comparable to what has been found among adults [6].

There is previous evidence that hearing problems are associated with depression and other serious mental health problems. An Australian study found that compared with population norms, hearing disability at all levels was associated with poorer mental health [34]. A meta-analysis reported that hearing impairment (HI) is among the most common chronic conditions associated with depression [35]. A systematic review of the literature demonstrated that HI children and adolescents were more prone to outcomes with lower quality of life and more mental health problems than normally hearing (NH) children and adolescents. For example, III individuals have more difficulties with making friends and are more socially isolated. It also consistently demonstrated that HI children en adolescents were more prone to developing depression, aggression, oppositional defiant disorder, conduct disorder, and psychopathy than their normally hearing peers [36]. A recent study [37] found - after accounting for health conditions and other factors - a strong association between HI and depression among US adults of all ages. The prevalence of depression increased as HI became worse, except among participants who, by self-report, were deaf and least likely to report depression [37].

On the other hand, previous studies have reported a reduction in depressive symptoms of people using hearing aids [38–40]. The finding that treated hearing loss improves mental health might be an indication that at least a part of mental health problems could be avoided by preventing hearing impairment. In combination with our results, this implies that hearing symptoms in youth need to be addressed and appropriately managed [41] and, preferably, be prevented to avoid such adverse consequences. In order to induce behavior change *before* permanent and irreversible hearing-related symptoms occur, we recommend that health authorities, those involved in presenting music venues, schools, parents, and young people should be informed about the potential risks of high-volume music via public health campaigns and the mass media, and should be alerted to the need for preventive hearing healthcare by health professionals such as practitioners of pediatrics, family medicine, audiology and youth health care. Real examples of peer-group people who had lost hearing through listening to loud music should be provided [33]. Previous research identified the following opportunities for protective measures concerning potentially hazardous music in music venues [21]: music venues could inform their visitors for the potential risk for hearing loss and inform and warn visitors about the potential dangers of exposure to high-volume music by clearly stating this on their advertisements, at the venue entrance, and on the tickets for admission. Furthermore, they could make available 'ear rest rooms' (areas with low-volume music), as well as hearing protection devices.

This study has several limitations. One was the use of a convenience sample of students attending senior-secondary vocational education. However, most of the characteristics of the study group reflected those of this subgroup of Dutch inner-city adolescents and emerging adults. The group of non-Dutch ethnicity (66.3%) consists of the following ethnicities: Surinam (15,3%) Antillean (9,0%) Moroccan (12%) Turkish (15,0%) other (15%). These percentages reflect those of the population of the Rotterdam inner-city senior-secondary vocational schools. Although the proportion of females attending inner-city senior-secondary vocational education is somewhat greater than the proportion of males, the proportion of females was relatively greater in our sample [18]. Also, we have no information about the music-listening behaviors of nonparticipants in the study. With regard to selective nonresponse, our nonparticipation was 22.1%; this may have affected the results. The data used in our study were cross-sectional and self-reported, which implies that no causal relationships can be inferred [42].

We did not report on the relation between drug use and both auditory symptoms and the other adverse health indicators. Drug use might increase the risk of noise induced hearing loss and/or other adverse health indicators [43,44]. However, after checking, we found no significant association between permanent hearing symptoms and both cannabis use and hard drug use in the past four weeks. We reanalyzed the data by additionally correcting the multiple logistic regression analyses of Table 5 for cannabis and hard drug use in the past four weeks. This resulted in only marginally lower odds ratios (results not shown).

We may have underestimated the exposure levels for several reasons. First, because we did not take into account other potentially hazardous sounds to which the participants in our study may have been exposed, which increase the risk of hearing loss. In a previous study we found that adolescents were also exposed to other potentially hazardous sounds, such as music through loudspeakers (88.0%) and through their own activities as musicians (21.5%), as well as the noise to which they were exposed when riding mopeds or scooters (27.1%) or when using firecrackers (60.8%) [9]. Future studies should also take account of such exposures. Furthermore, we did not ask participants whether they used earbud-style earphones or supra-aural earphones. The output level should be corrected by adding 5.5 decibels when using earbud-style earphones [2,45] and previously has been found that 93.2% of adolescents used earbud-style earphones [46]. Finally, in the absence of safety standards for leisure-time sound exposure, we relied on loosened occupational safety standards. However, there is no scientific evidence that social noise produces different NIHL levels compared to occupational noise [2,47].

In conclusion, as hearing problems tend to isolate people from friends, family and others because of a decreased ability to communicate, the impact of HI may be profound as it can impose a heavy social and economic burden on individuals, families, communities, and countries [37]. Our results show the need for structural action by both attention for future research regarding the consequences of music-listening behaviors for hearing, as well as for the development and implementation of strategies for prevention and intervention. This would also contribute to the development of safety standards for leisure-time noise exposure. If these findings are confirmed, such standards are essential to avoid the possibility that entire generations could be suffering severe hearing problems due to excessive high-volume music exposure in their childhood, adolescence and emerging adulthood.

Author Contributions

Conceived and designed the experiments: PMVDLJ CLM FDW. Performed the experiments: CLM. Analyzed the data: IV AB. Wrote the paper: IV. Revising article for important intellectual content: PMVDLJ CLM AB FDW.

References

1. World Health Organization (WHO) (2001) The world health report 2001. Mental health: new understanding, new hope. Geneva: World Health Organization.
2. Scientific Committee on Emerging and Newly Identified Health Risks (SCENIHR) (2008) Potential health risks of exposure to noise from personal music players and mobile phones including a music playing function. Available: http://ec.europa.eu/health/ph_risk/committees/04_scenihr/docs/scenihr_o_018.pdf. Accessed Oct 17 2008.
3. World Health Organization (1997) Prevention of noise-induced hearing loss. Report of an informal consultation heald at the World Helath Organization, Geneva on 28–30 October 1997. Available: http://www.who.int/pbd/deafness/en/noise.pdf. Accessed 31 May 2011.
4. Vernon JA (1987) Pathophysiology of tinnitus: a special case - hyperacusis and a proposed treatment. Am J Otol 8: 201–202.
5. Bläsing L, Goebel G, Flötzinger U, Berthold A, Kröner-Herwig B (2010) Hypersensitivity to sound in tinnitus patients: an analysis of a construct based on questionnaire and audiological data. Int J Audiol 49: 518–526.
6. Holmes S, Padgham ND (2009) Review paper: more than ringing in the ears: a review of tinnitus and its psychosocial impact. J Clin Nurs 18: 2927–2937.
7. Fausti SA, Wilmington DJ, Helt PV, Helt WJ, Konrad-Martin D (2005) Hearing health and care: the need for improved hearing loss prevention and hearing conservation practices. J Rehabil Res Dev 42: 45–62.
8. Niskar AS, Kieszak SM, Holmes AE, Esteban E, Rubin C, et al. (2001) Estimated prevalence of noise-induced hearing threshold shifts among children 6 to 19 years of age: the Third National Health and Nutrition Examination Survey, 1988–1994, United States. Pediatrics 108: 40–43.
9. Vogel I, Verschuure H, van der Ploeg CPB, Brug J, Raat H (2010) Estimating adolescent risk for hearing loss based on data from a large school-based survey. Am J Public Health 100: 1095–1100.
10. Serra MR, Biassoni EC, Richter U, Minoldo G, Franco G, et al. (2005) Recreational noise exposure and its effects on the hearing of adolescents. Part I: An interdisciplinary long-term study. Int J Audiol 44: 65–73.
11. Vogel I, Brug J, Van der Ploeg CP, Raat H (2010) Discotheques and the risk of hearing loss among youth: risky listening behavior and its psychosocial correlates. Health Educ Res 25: 737–747.
12. Vogel I, Brug J, Van der Ploeg CPB, Raat H (2011) Adolescents risky MP3-player listening and its psychosocial correlates. Health Educ Res 26: 254–264.
13. (2008) Wet publieke gezondheid [Dutch act on public health]. Bwb-id: BWBR00024705. http://wettenoverheidnl/BWBR0024705/geldigheidsdatum_26-05-2013.
14. (2000) Wet bescherming persoonsgegevens [Dutch act on protection of personal data]. Bwb-id: BWBR0011468. http://wettenoverheidnl/BWBR0011468/geldigheidsdatum_09-06-2013.
15. (1998) Wet medisch-wetenschappelijk onderzoek met mensen [Dutch act on research involving human subjects]. Bwb-id:BWBR0009408. http://wettenoverheidnl/BWBR0009408/geldigheidsdatum_26-05-2013.
16. World Medical Association (2008) Declaration of Helsinki. Ethical principles for medical research involving human subjects. Available: http://www.wma.net/en/30publications/10policies/b3/17c.pdf. Accessed 9 November 2011.
17. Vogel I, Van de Looij-Jansen PM, Mieloo CL, De Waart F, Burdorf A (2012) Risky music-listening behaviors and associated health-risk behaviors. Pediatrics 129: 1097–1103.
18. Statistics Netherlands (2007) Statline. Heerlen: Statistics Netherlands.
19. Portnuff CDF, Fligor BJ (2006) Sound output levels of the iPod and other MP3 players: is there potential risk to hearing? Available: http://www.hearingconservation.org/docs/virtualPressRoom/portnuff.htm. Accessed February 2 2007.
20. Dreschler WA, Körössy L, Kornegoor M, Griffioen B, Van Hooff R, et al. (2007) Luister je veilig? Technisch onderzoek naar geluidsniveaus MP3-spelers en bijbehorende oortelefoons. Rapport NHS 2007-1. Available: http://www.hoorstichting.nl/plaatjes/user/File/MP3%20rapport%20Luister%20je%20veilig%20pdf.pdf. Accessed 20 November 2007.
21. Vogel I, van der Ploeg CPB, Brug J, Raat H (2009) Music venues and hearing loss: Opportunities for and barriers to improving environmental conditions. Int J Audiol 48: 531–536.
22. European Parliament and Council (2003) Directive 2003/10/EC of the European Parliament and of the Council. Official J Europ Union 15.2.2003.
23. International Organization for Standardization (ISO) (1990) Acoustics - determination of occupational noise exposure and estimation of noise-induced hearing impairment. ISO 1999: 1990. Geneva: ISO.
24. American Academy of Audiology (2003) Position statement: preventing noise-induced occupational hearing loss. Available: http://www.audiology.org/resources/documentlibrary/Documents/niohlprevention.pdf. Accessed 31 December 2007.
25. Berwick DM, Murphy JM, Goldman PA, Ware JE Jr, Barsky AJ, et al. (1991) Performance of a five-item mental health screening test. Med Care 29: 169–176.
26. Rumpf HJ, Meyer C, Hapke U, John U (2001) Screening for mental health: validity of the MHI-5 using DSM-IV Axis I psychiatric disorders as gold standard. Psychiatry Res 105: 243–253.
27. Kelly MJ, Dunstan FD, Lloyd K, Fone DL (2008) Evaluating cutpoints for the MHI-5 and MCS using the GHQ-12: a comparison of five different methods. BMC Psychiatry 8: 10.
28. Radloff LS (1977) The CES-D scale: a self-report depression scale for research in the general population. Appl Psych Meas 1: 385–401.
29. Ward WD (1986) Auditory effects of noise. In: Berger EH, Ward WD, Morrill JC, Royster LH, editors. Noise & hearing conservation manual. Fairfax, Virginia: American Industrial Hygiene Association. 197–216.
30. Chung JH, Des Roches CM, Meunier J, Eavey RD (2005) Evaluation of noise-induced hearing loss in young people using a web-based survey technique. Pediatrics 115: 861–867.
31. Brookhouser PE (1994) Prevention of noise-induced hearing loss. Prev Med 23: 665–669.
32. Meyer-Bisch C (1996) Epidemiological evaluation of hearing damage related to strongly amplified music (personal cassette players, discotheques, rock concerts): high-definition audiometric survey on 1364 subjects. Audiol 35: 121–142.
33. Vogel I, Brug J, Hosli EJ, van der Ploeg CPB, Raat H (2008) MP3 players and hearing loss: adolescents' perceptions of loud music and hearing conservation. J Pediatr 152: 400–404.
34. Hogan A, O'Loughlin K, Miller P, Kendig H (2009) The health impact of a hearing disability on older people in Australia. J Aging Health 21: 1098–1111.
35. Huang CQ, Dong BR, Lu ZC, Yue JR, Liu QX (2010) Chronic diseases and risk for depression in old age: a meta-analysis of published literature. Ageing Res Rev 9: 131–141.
36. Theunissen SC, Rieffe C, Netten AP, Briaire JJ, Soede W, et al. (2014) Psychopathology and its risk and protective factors in hearing-impaired children and adolescents: a systematic review. JAMA Pediatr 168: 170–177.
37. Li CM, Zhang X, Hoffman HJ, Cotch MF, Themann CL, et al. (2014) Hearing impairment associated with depression in US adults, National Health and Nutrition Examination Survey 2005–2010. JAMA Otolaryngol Head Neck Surg doi:10.1001/jamaoto.2014.42. [Epub ahead of print]: E1–E10.
38. Boorsma M, Joling K, Dussel M, Ribbe M, Frijters D, et al. (2012) The incidence of depression and its risk factors in Dutch nursing homes and residential care homes. Am J Geriatr Psychiatry 20: 932–942.
39. Gopinath B, Wang JJ, Schneider J, Burlutsky G, Snowdon J, et al. (2009) Depressive symptoms in older adults with hearing impairments: the Blue Mountains Study. J Am Geriatr Soc 57: 1306–1308.
40. Seniors Research Group (1999) The consequences of untreated hearing loss in older persons. Washington, DC: National Council on the Aging.
41. Shetye A, Kennedy V (2010) Tinnitus in children: an uncommon symptom? Arch Dis Child 95: 645–648.
42. Rothman KJ, Greenland S (1998) Modern epidemiology. Philadelphia: Lippincott-Raven Publishers.
43. Rawool V, Dluhy C (2011) Auditory sensitivity in opiate addicts with and without a history of noise exposure. Noise Health 13: 356–363.
44. Rasic D, Weerasinghe S, Asbridge M, Langille DB (2013) Longitudinal associations of cannabis and illicit drug use with depression, suicidal ideation and suicidal attempts among Nova Scotia high school students. Drug Alcohol Depend 129: 49–53.
45. Portnuff CDF, Fligor BJ (2006) Sound output levels of the iPod and other MP3 players: is there potential risk to hearing? Available: http://www.hearingconservation.org/docs/virtualPressRoom/portnuff.htm. Accessed 2 February 2007.

12

Novel Compound Heterozygous Mutations in *MYO7A* Associated with Usher Syndrome 1

Xue Gao[1,2,4¶], **Guo-Jian Wang**[1,2¶], **Yong-Yi Yuan**[1], **Feng Xin**[1], **Ming-Yu Han**[1,2], **Jing-Qiao Lu**[3], **Hui Zhao**[1,2], **Fei Yu**[1], **Jin-Cao Xu**[4], **Mei-Guang Zhang**[4], **Jiang Dong**[5], **Xi Lin**[3*], **Pu Dai**[1,2*]

1 Department of Otolaryngology, Head and Neck Surgery, PLA General Hospital, Beijing, P. R. China, **2** Department of Otolaryngology, Hainan Branch of PLA General Hospital, Sanya, P. R. China, **3** Department of Otolaryngology, Emory University School of Medicine, Atlanta, Georgia, United States of America, **4** Department of Otolaryngology, the Second Artillery General Hospital, Beijing, P. R. China, **5** Xi'an Research Institute of Hi_tech, Hongqing, Xi'an, Shaanxi, P. R. China

Abstract

Usher syndrome is an autosomal recessive disease characterized by sensorineural hearing loss, age-dependent retinitis pigmentosa (RP), and occasionally vestibular dysfunction. The most severe form is Usher syndrome type 1 (USH1). Mutations in the *MYO7A* gene are responsible for USH1 and account for 29–55% of USH1 cases. Here, we characterized a Chinese family (no. 7162) with USH1. Combining the targeted capture of 131 known deafness genes, next-generation sequencing, and bioinformatic analysis, we identified two deleterious compound heterozygous mutations in the *MYO7A* gene: a reported missense mutation c.73G>A (p.G25R) and a novel nonsense mutation c.462C>A (p.C154X). The two compound variants are absent in 219 ethnicity-matched controls, co-segregates with the USH clinical phenotypes, including hearing loss, vestibular dysfunction, and age-dependent penetrance of progressive RP, in family 7162. Therefore, we concluded that the USH1 in this family was caused by compound heterozygous mutations in *MYO7A*.

Editor: Tiansen Li, National Eye Institute, United States of America

Funding: This work was supported by grants from the Project of the National Natural Science Foundation of China (Grant Nos. 30801285, 81230020, 81200751, 81070792, 81000415, 81360159), grants from China Postdoctoral Science Foundation (No. 2012M521878, No. 2013T60947), a grant from State 863 High Technology R&D Key Project of China (2011AA02A112, 2012AA020101), a grant from Minister of Science and Technology of China (2012BAI09B02), a grant from the National Basic Research Program of China (973 Program) (2014CB541706), a grant from Beijing technology new star project (2010B081) and a grant from Minister of Health of China (201202005). Work performed in the Lin lab was supported by a grant from NIH (R33 DC010476). We sincerely thank all the family members for their participation and cooperation in this study. The funders had no role in study design, data collection and analysis, decision to publish, or preparation of the manuscript.

Competing Interests: All authors have declared that no competing interests exist.

* Email: daipu301@vip.sina.com (PD); xlin2@emory.edu (XL)

¶ XG and GJW are co-first authors on this work.

Introduction

Usher syndrome is a clinically and genetically heterogeneous recessive disease with a worldwide prevalence of 1 in 16,000–50,000 [1]. Based on the severity and progression of hearing loss, age at onset of retinitis pigmentosa (RP), and presence or absence of vestibular impairment, the majority of Usher syndrome cases can be classified into three clinical subtypes. The most severe is Usher syndrome type 1 (USH1), which is characterized by severe-to-profound congenital hearing loss, absence of vestibular function in most cases, and prepubertal-onset retinal degeneration, with impaired night vision and gradual restriction of the visual fields diagnosed as RP. In most populations, USH1 accounts for approximately one-third of Usher syndrome patients. Usher syndrome type II (USH2) has moderate-to-severe sensorineural hearing loss that is stable in most cases, normal vestibular function, and RP, whereas patients with type III (USH3) have moderate sensorineural hearing loss with progression to acquired deafness, progressive vestibular dysfunction, and RP. Cohen et al has reported that among the deaf population, the proportion of patients with USH may be as high as 10%, making Usher

syndrome an important diagnosis in clinical practices [2]. Molecular genetic testing can confirm or exclude Usher syndrome at an early age, even before the onset of visual problems [3].

Seven loci have been mapped for USH1 (*USH1B-USH1H*). Five causative genes have been identified: *USH1B*, encoding myosin VIIa; *USH1C*, encoding harmonin (USH1C); *USH1D*, encoding cadherin 23 (CDH23); *USH1F*, encoding protocadherin 15 (PCDH15); and *USH1G*, encoding SANS. Mutations in these genes affect the pressure-sensitive stereocilia of the inner ear (Hereditary Hearing Loss Homepage, http://hereditaryhearingloss.org/) and do not occur at the same frequencies across ethnicities. Of all pathogenic mutations, 29~55% are in the *MYO7A* gene [4,5,6,7,8, 9,10,11].

Collectively, the five USH1 genes comprise 183 coding exons (http://www.genome.ucsc.edu/). A comprehensive molecular diagnosis of Usher syndrome has been hampered both by the genetic heterogeneity of the disease and the large number of exons of known Usher syndrome genes. Next-generation sequencing (NGS) is a revolutionary technology that allows the simultaneous screening of mutations in a large number of genes. It is cost effective compared to classical strategies of linkage analysis and

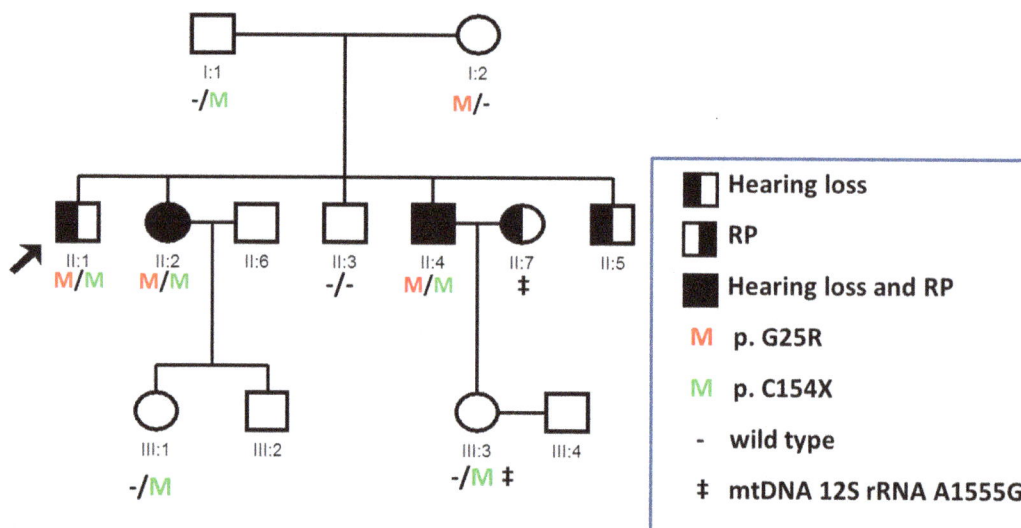

Figure 1. Pedigree of Chinese Family 7162 with Recessive USH1 and segregation of the mutations in *MYO7A*. The proband is indicated by an arrow. Subject I:1, I:2, II:1, II:2, II:3 and II:4 were tested by NGS. gDNA from II:5 is not available.

direct sequencing when the number or size of genes is large [12]. Therefore, targeted deafness gene capture combined with NGS provides opportunities to identify causative mutations and new Usher syndrome genes using a limited number of patient samples [13,14,15,16,17,18].

The *MYO7A* gene has 49 exons, spans approximately 87 kb of genomic sequence on chromosome 11q13.5, and encodes the actin-based motor protein myosin VIIa. The protein consists of 2215 amino acids and contains an N-terminal motor domain, a neck region containing several IQ motifs, a short predicted coiled coil domain, a MyTH4 domain, a FERM domain, an SH3 domain, and a second C-terminal MyTH4-FERM tandem domain [19]. In humans, myosin VIIa is expressed in a variety of cells, including the inner ear hair cells, retinal pigment epithelium, and photoreceptor cells of the retina [20]. Different roles have been postulated for myosin VIIa in the inner ear, such as participation in mechano-transduction in hair cells and differentiation and organization of hair cell stereocilia [21]. In the human retina, myosin VIIa functions actively in the migration of retinal pigment epithelium, photoreceptor cells, and opsin transport [22,23]. Mutations in this gene have been reported to cause Usher syndrome type 1B (USH1B) and non-syndromic deafness (DFNB2, DFNA11) [24,25,26].

In this study, we performed large-scale mutation screening of 131 known deafness-related genes, including 5 USH1 genes, in a Chinese family (no. 7162) diagnosed with USH1 and identified two compound heterozygous disease-segregating mutations in the *MYO7A* gene: a known missense mutation c.73G>A (p.G25R) and a novel nonsense mutation c.462C>A (p.C154X).

Materials and Methods

Clinical data

Family 7162 is a Chinese family clinically diagnosed with autosomal recessive USH1. To identify candidate mutations, DNA samples were obtained from eight members of family 7162 and 219 ethnicity-matched controls. Written informed consent was obtained from each subject or their guardians. The study protocol, including the consent procedure, was performed with the approval of the Ethics Committee of Chinese PLA General Hospital. A

medical history was obtained using a questionnaire regarding the following aspects: age at onset, evolution, symmetry of the hearing impairment, presence of tinnitus, medication, noise exposure, possible head or brain injury, use of aminoglycoside antibiotics, and other relevant clinical manifestations. A physical examination, otoscopy, and pure tone audiometric examination (at frequencies from 250 to 8000 Hz) were performed to identify the phenotype. Immittance testing was used to evaluate the middle-ear pressure, ear canal volume, and tympanic membrane mobility. Unaffected phenotype status was defined by a threshold lower than the age- and gender-matched 50th percentile values for all frequencies measured. The physical examinations of all members revealed no signs of systemic illness or dysmorphic features. Computed tomography (CT) of the temporal bone was performed in the index patient. A diagnosis of profound sensorineural hearing impairment was made according to the ICD-10 criteria based on the audiometric examination.

Vestibular functions were evaluated using the tandem gait and Romberg tests. The ocular examination included the best-corrected visual acuity, slit lamp examination, and detailed stereoscopic fundoscopy. The electroretinogram (ERG) was measured according to the standards of the International Society for Clinical Electrophysiology of Vision [27] beginning after

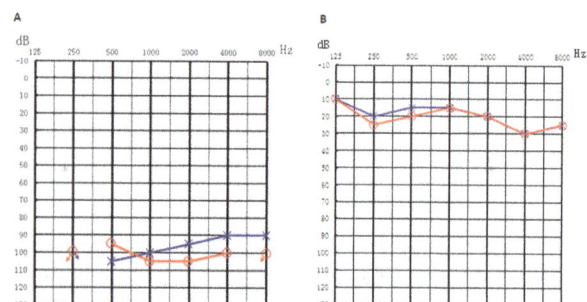

Figure 2. Audiogram showed bilateral profound sensorineural hearing loss of affected subjects II:4 and normal hearing of subject II:3 (red, right ear; blue, left ear).

30 min of dark adaption using 10-µs xenon flashes in a Ganzfeld bowl. The pupils were dilated fully using 10% phenylephrine HCl and 1% tropicamide, and Burian-Allen bipolar corneal electrodes were applied after topical anesthesia with 5% proparacaine HCl.

Deafness gene capture and Illumina library preparation

Genomic DNA (gDNA) was extracted from peripheral blood using a blood DNA extraction kit, according to the manufacturer's protocol (Tiangen, Beijing, China). Three prevalent deafness-associated genes, *GJB2*, *SLC26A4*, and mtDNA*12SrRNA,* were first screened for mutations in all participating family members. Then, we sequenced all of the coding exons plus ~100 bp of the flanking intronic sequences for 131 deafness genes and ~5 kilobases of *GJB2* regulatory sequences (Table S1) in three affected members (II:1, II:2, II:4) and three unaffected members (II:3, I:1, I:2) of family 7162.

gDNA quality was evaluated using the optical density ratio (260/280 ratio) and gel electrophoresis imaging. High-molecular-weight gDNA (~3 µg) was fragmented ultrasonically using an E210 DNA-shearing instrument (Covaris; Woburn, MA, USA) to an average size of 300 base pairs (bps). The Covaris protocol was set at 3-min total duration, duty cycle 10%, intensity 5, and 200 cycles per burst.

Fragmented gDNA libraries for Illumina GAII sequencing were prepared with the NEBNext™ DNA Sample Prep Master Mix set (E6040, New England BioLabs; Ipswich, MA). End repair of DNA fragments, the addition of a 3′ adenine (A), adaptor ligation, and reaction cleanup were performed following the manufacturer's protocol. The libraries were cleaned and size-selected using the AMPure DNA Purification kit (Beckman Agencourt; Danvers, MA, USA). The ligated product (20 ng) was amplified for 14 PCR cycles with the Illumina PCR primers InPE1.0, InPE2.0, and indexing primers, following the manufacturer's instructions.

For targeted enrichment of deafness genes, the Illumina library DNA was purified with a QIAquickMinElute column and eluted into 50 µL of hybridization buffer (HB, Roche NimbleGen; Madison, WI, USA). The barcoded Illumina gDNA libraries (0.5 µg) were incubated in with probes to enrich for the targets in solution. More details of capture probe validation and preparation

can be found in our previous study [28]. Nonspecific DNA fragments were removed after six washing steps in a washing buffer (Roche NimbleGen, Madison, WI). The DNA bound to the probes was eluted by incubating it with NaOH (425 mL, 125 mM) for 10 min. The eluted solution was transferred to a 1.5-mL Eppendorf tube containing 500 µL of neutralization buffer (QIAGEN PBI buffer). The neutralized DNA was desalted and concentrated on a QIAquick MinElute column and eluted into 30 µL in EB buffer. To increase the yield, we typically amplified 5 µL of eluted solution for 12 PCR cycles using the Illumina PCR primers InpE1.0 and 2.0. The enrichment of the targeted deafness gene sequences was assessed using quantitative PCR (qPCR) by comparing the growth curves of captured and non-captured samples [29]. Barcoded libraries of captured samples were pooled and paired-end Illumina sequencing was performed using the Illumina HiSeq system (Illumina; San Diego, CA, USA). Details of the bioinformatics analysis methods have been published [29]. Sequence read data of the affected subjects in family 7162 has been deposited into Sequence Read Archive (http://www.ncbi. nlm.nih.gov/sra webcite; accession number SRR1296682).

Mutational analysis of MYO7A

The segregation of the *MYO7A* c.73G>A and c.462C>A mutations was tested in eight family members (I:1, I:2, II:1, II:2, II:3, II:4, III:1 and III:3), including the five whose gDNAs have been subjected to 131 deafness-associated gene NGS analysis, using PCR (primer sequences available on request) followed by bidirectional Sanger sequencing of the amplified fragments (ABI 3100; Applied Biosystems). Nucleotide alterations were identified by sequence alignment with the *MYO7A* GenBank sequence using the GeneTools software. In addition, sequences from 219 ethnicity-matched negative samples were examined.

Multiple sequence alignment was performed using ClustalW2 with the default settings and the sequences *NP_000251.3* (Homo sapiens), *XP_001087868.2* (Macacamulatta), *XP_003313297.2* (Pan troglodytes), *XP_002693553.2* (Bostaurus), *XP_542292.3* (Canis lupus), *NP_001243010.1* (Musmusculus), *NP_703203.1* (Rattusnorvegicus), *XP_417277.3* (Gallusgallus), and *NP_694515.1* (Daniorerio).

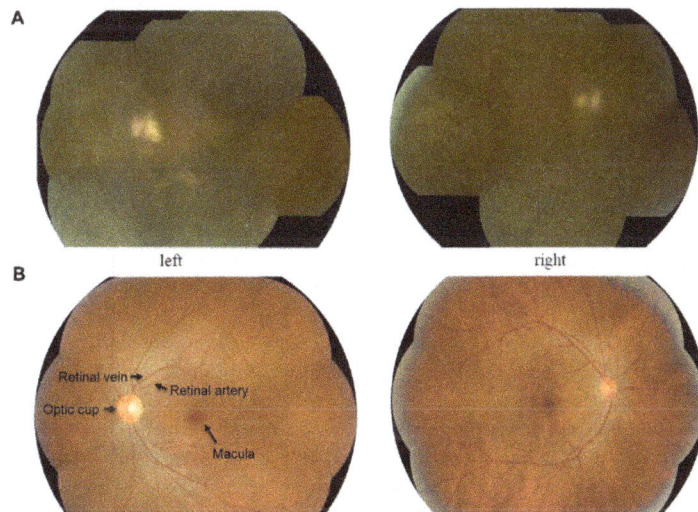

Figure 3. Composite image of the fundus photographs of individuals from family 7162. A: The appearance of the fundus in one patient (II:4) with RP at 54 year old shows typical retinal degeneration with obvious waxy pallor of the optic discs, attenuation of the retinal vessels, irregular pigment clumps in the retina. B: Fundus photographs of patient II:1 without RP at 62 years old shows bright optic disc where blood vessels converge.

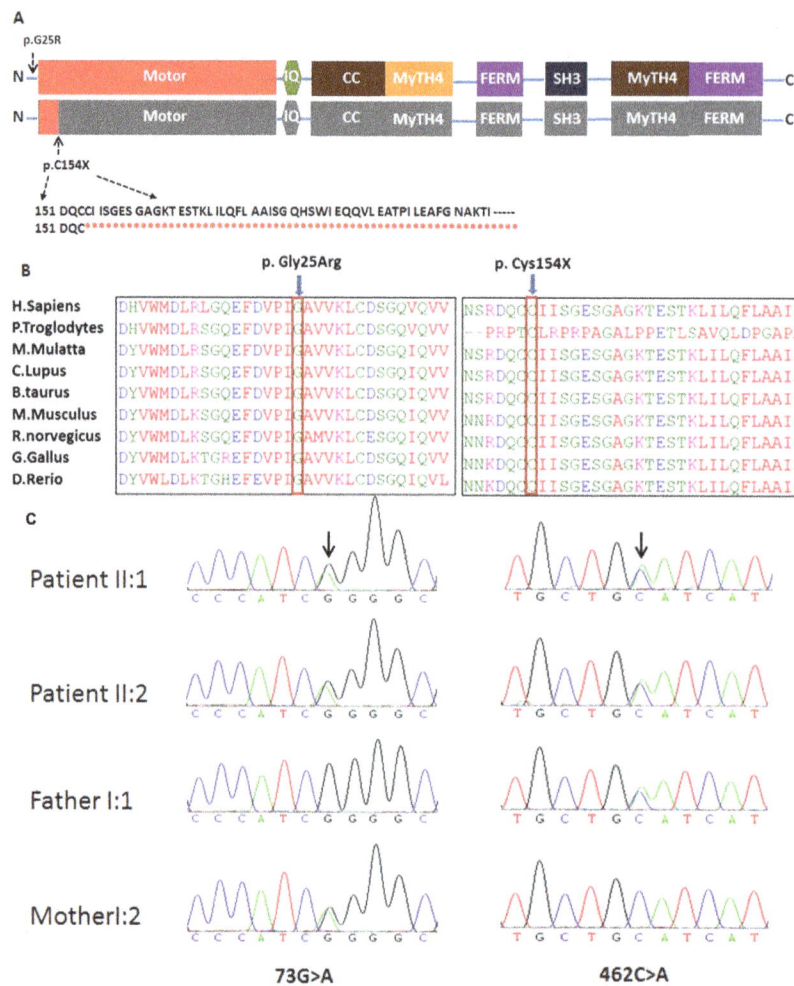

Figure 4. Domain structure, conservation analysis and mutational analysis of *MYO7A* in family 7162. A: Domain structure of myosin VIIa showing the nonsense mutation introduces a premature stop codon which is predicted to truncate the protein within the N-terminal motor domain. B: Protein alignment showing conservation of residues myosin VIIaG25 and C154 across nine species. Two mutations both occurred at evolutionarily conserved amino acids (in red box). C: DNA sequencing profile showing the c.73G>A and c.462C>A mutations in *MYO7A*. Both variants co-segregated with the clinical phenotype and c.462C>A were absent in 219 ethnicity-matched controls.

Model building and structural-based analysis

Three-dimensional (3D) modeling of the human wild-type and p.G25R mutation was carried out using SWISS-MODEL, an automated homology modeling program (http://swissmodel. expasy.org/workspace/). This study used the automatic modeling approach to model the complete human myosin VIIa protein, including its 2215 amino acids (NP_000251.3) with or without the mutations. Data obtained from the homology models were visualized using Swiss-PdbViewer 4.1.

Results

Family and clinical evaluations

We analyzed a Chinese USH1 family (no. 7162, Figure 1), which includes four affected siblings: II:1 (male, 62 years old), II:2 (female, 60 years old), II:4 (male, 54 years old) and II:5 (male, 52 years old), one unaffected siblings II:3 (male, 57 years old), two unaffected parents (I:1, 83 years old and I:2, 80 years old), and two unaffected daughters (III:1, 30 years old and III:3, 27 years old). For each subject, the diagnosis was established from the medical history and a detailed evaluation of vision, vestibular function, and

hearing. Hearing loss is congenital and stable. Audiograms of the affected siblings showed that the hearing loss was bilateral and profound (Figure 2). Immittance testing demonstrated normal and bone conduction values equal to the air conduction measurements, suggesting sensorineural hearing impairment. High-resolution CT of the temporal bone and the brain in the affected subject II:4 was normal, excluding inner-ear gross malformations. The physical examinations of all participating members revealed no signs of systemic illness or dysmorphic features. Affected individuals did not have obvious delayed gross motor development. This phenotype is consistent with that reported for USH1. For the affected subject II:5, gDNA and examinations were unavailable. The penetrance of hearing loss and RP was 100% and 50%, respectively (Figure 1).

For affected subject II:4, tandem walking was abnormal and the Romberg test was positive. Difficulty with night vision was observed at a very young age, and constriction of the visual field was apparent in the second decade of life, which likely occurred earlier. The ophthalmoscopic examination demonstrated obvious waxy pallor of the optic discs, attenuation of the retinal vessels, and

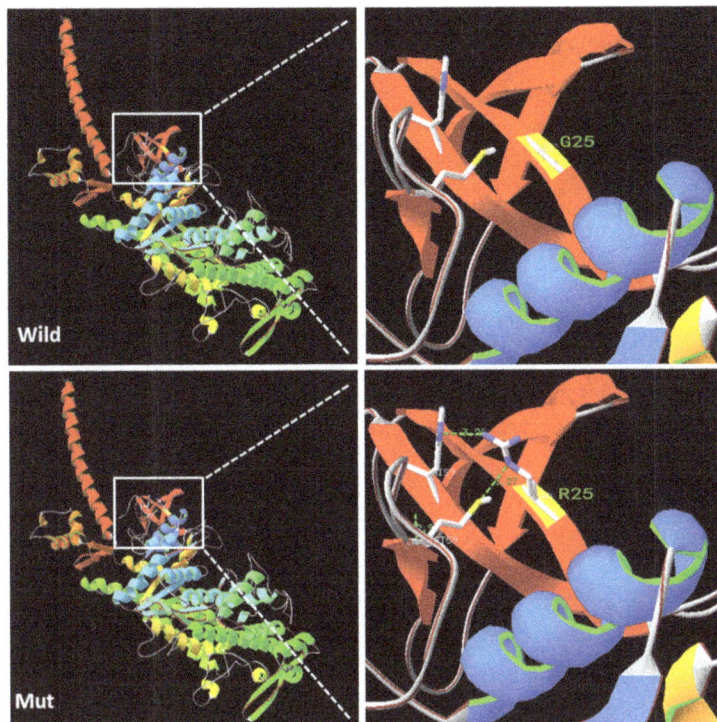

Figure 5. Structure of wild-type and mutant myosin VIIa. A: G25 in the wild-type protein has no side chain to interact with the His9 and Met59. B: The distance (dotted lines) between the long side chain of R25 and the residues H9 and M59 in the mutant protein were less than 3.5Å, which is shorter enough to form new hydrogen bonds (Created by SWISS-MODEL and shown with PY-MOL).

bone spicule-type pigment deposits (Figure 3). The ERG wave amplitudes of patient II:4 were undetectable from the baseline.

Targeted deafness gene capture and massively paralleled sequencing

One subject, II:7, is married to one of the sibling, II:4, and was identified to carry a homogeneous mtDNA*12S rRNA*A1555G mutation (Figure 1). This mutation was passed to daughter III:3. Subject II:7 had a history of aminoglycoside administration and is hearing impaired. All subjects were screened first for mutations of *GJB2* and *SLC26A4*, which have a predominant presence in genetic hearing loss. Both genes were excluded. We subsequently sequenced all of the coding exons plus ~100 bp of the flanking intronic sequence of 131 deafness genes in three affected (II:1, II:2, II:4) and two unaffected members of family 7162 (I:1, II:3). Four variants leading to amino acid change were detected in the *MYO7A*:c.73G>A (G25R), c.462C>A (C154X), c.47T>C (L16S), and c.4996A>T (S1666C). Of these, two variants c.47T>C (L16S) and c.4996A>T (S1666C) were found in the homozygous state in unaffected members as well as in the affected members, suggesting that these two variants are non-pathogenic. In contrast, the *MYO7A* compound heterozygous variants c.73G>A (p.G25R) and c.462C>A (p.C154X) co-segregated in all affected family members tested.

Mutation analysis

Using Sanger sequencing, eight participating members (three affected, five unaffected) in family 7162 were genotyped to identify the mutations. Compound heterozygous c.73G>A (p.G25R) and c.462C>A (p.C154X) variants of *MYO7A* were found in three affected family members (II:1, II:2, and II:4) (Figure 1 and 4C); these were considered pathogenic. In addition, *MYO7A* c.462C>

A (p.C154X) was found in three normal hearing family members, including the father and two grand-daughters (I:1, III:1, and III:3), while *MYO7A* c.73G>A (p.G25R) was found only in the mother (I:2) (Figure 1). The novel c.462C>A mutation in *MYO7A* was absent from 219 unrelated Chinese controls. Both amino acids are highly conserved across species (Figure 4B). The mutation of 73G>A causes a glycine to arginine change, and the 462C>A creates a premature stop codon at the position of amino acid 154 of the large myosin VIIa protein of 2215 amino acids.

SIFT and Polyphen2 were used as a filter to predict how the identified amino acid substitutions would affect protein function considering sequence homology and the physical properties of amino acids. Both *MYO7A* c.73G>A (p.G25R) and c.462C>A (p.C154X) were predicted to be damaging (according to GenBank accession number NM_000260.3) [9,30].

Mutation c.462C>A is a novel mutation (http://www.umd.be/MYO7A/) located within exon 4 that results in the nonsense mutation C154X. The premature stop codon apparently activates the nonsense-mediated mRNA decay response, leading to a decrease in *MYO7A* mRNA expression (Figure 4A). It is predicted that the two compound heterozygous mutations in the same subject caused complete dysfunction of myosin VIIa, leading to the observed phenotype in all three affected family members [9].

Structure modeling of p. G25R

A molecular model of myosin VIIa was constructed based on the crystal structure of myosin V motor (PDB ID: iw7jA). The constructed model covered the target sequence of myosin VIIa (residues 3–769). The sequence identity between the target and template was 39.51%, higher than the average 25%. Using Swiss-PdbViewer 4.1, the mutation was predicted to perturb an amino acid side chain due to the substitution of glycine by arginine and two extra hydrogen bonds. This region of the protein is predicted to be highly hydrophobic, as previously shown in a hydrophobicity plot (Figure 5).

These data, together with the clinical presentation of the four affected siblings and the consistent Mandelian inheritance of the variants in the affected and unaffected members, indicate that the *MYO7A* compound mutations c.73G>A (p.G25R) and c.462C>A (p.C154X) are the cause of USH1 in this family.

Discussion

Hundreds of different mutations of USH1 are listed in the Universal Mutation Database (UMD) USHbases, a comprehensive set of databases that records pathogenic mutations and unclassified variants in five genes causing USH1 [31]. However, due to the genetic heterogeneity of the disease and the large number of exons of the nine known Usher syndrome genes, the genetic causes for a large proportion of Usher syndrome remain unknown. Targeted deafness gene capture combined with NGS is suited to identify the causative mutations of Usher syndrome and hereditary hearing loss owing to the following advantages: 1) comprehensive coverage of large numbers of genes and large genes associated with the disease; 2) significant cost saving; 3) higher sequencing accuracy because of deeper achievable coverage; 4) a significantly shorter turnaround time and 5) more convincing dataset by excluding other deafness genes.

By sequencing the 366 coding exons and flanking regions of the nine known Usher syndrome genes, Bonnet *et al.* recently found mutations in 91% of the patients tested, improving the molecular diagnosis of Usher syndrome greatly [11]. We speculate that targeted deafness gene capture and NGS provides opportunities to identify causative mutations and new Usher syndrome genes efficiently.

In family 7162, four patients have deafness and vestibular dysfunction and two of them have RP, all symptoms compatible with USH1. Targeted NGS revealed two compound *MYO7A* mutations, c.73G>A and c.462C>A, segregating with disease in this family. The *MYO7A* compound mutations c.73G>A (p.G25R) and c.462C>A (p.C154X) were identified as pathogenic mutations in family 7162 with USH1. Mutation c.73G>A(p.G25R) was reported previously in a Caucasian population and is considered a recessive pathogenic mutation [9]. It located within exon 2 and changes the conserved uncharged hydrophilic Glycine to positively charged hydrophilic arginine at the highly conserved codon 25 in the N-terminal hydrophobic region, upstream from the motor head of myosin VIIa. In addition, the amino acid glycine does not have a side chain and is often found close to or at the surface in loop regions, conferring high flexibility

to these regions. Glycine residues are often highly conserved in protein families since they are essential for preserving a particular protein three-dimensional fold. With the p.G25R mutation, a small uncharged residue without a side chain is replaced by a big, hydrophilic, positively charged amino acid. *In silico* analysis indicated a pathogenic effect of this mutation, given that the region where it is located is highly conserved and structure modeling of G25R results in gaining two extra hydrogen bonds (Figure 5). Therefore, the mutation will lead to extra ionic interactions and other possible interactions of the arginine residue in the mutated-type *MYO7A*, such as creating additional hydrogen bonds, loss of structural flexibility conferred by Glycine, or alternation in protein localization.

The stop codon in exon 4 (c.462C>A [C154X]) identified in this study is close to the reported mutation c.448C>T (R150X) [9]. The mutation would lead to a truncated protein lacking 2061 amino acid residues that contain almost all of the important functional domains (Figure 4A). Therefore, the mutant myosin VIIa protein resulted from either mutation might lose the ability to link the proteins in the cell membrane to the proteins in the cytoskeleton, be misfolded, nonfunctional, or be much reduced.

In summary, we report the clinical and genetic characteristics of a non-consanguineous Chinese family (no. 7162) with autosomal recessive USH1. We identified two *MYO7A* compound heterozygous mutations, c.73G>A and c.462C>A, as disease-causing mutations through multiple deafness gene capture, NGS, and bioinformatic analysis. In the future, we will gather more samples from Chinese USH1 patients and determine the molecular background of USH1 in China to provide the patients and their families with precise, early molecular diagnoses, accurate genetic counseling, and optimal rehabilitation.

The English in this document has been checked by at least two professional editors, both native speakers of English. For a certificate, please see: http://www.textcheck.com/certificate/I3NwIG.

Author Contributions

Conceived and designed the experiments: XG PD XL. Performed the experiments: XG GJW YYY FX. Analyzed the data: MYH HZ FY JD JQL. Contributed reagents/materials/analysis tools: JCX MGZ. Wrote the paper: XG PD XL.

References

1. Rizel L, Safieh C, Shalev SA, Mezer E, Jabaly-Habib H, et al. (2011) Novel mutations of MYO7A and USH1G in Israeli Arab families with Usher syndrome type 1. Mol Vis 17: 3548–3555.
2. Cohen M, Bitner-Glindzicz M, Luxon L (2007) The changing face of Usher syndrome: clinical implications. Int J Audiol 46: 82–93.
3. Kimberling WJ, Hildebrand MS, Shearer AE, Jensen ML, Halder JA, et al. (2010) Frequency of Usher syndrome in two pediatric populations: Implications for genetic screening of deaf and hard of hearing children. Genet Med 12: 512–516.
4. Bharadwaj AK, Kasztejna JP, Huq S, Berson EL, Dryja TP (2000) Evaluation of the myosin VIIA gene and visual function in patients with Usher syndrome type I. Exp Eye Res 71: 173–181.
5. Jaijo T, Aller E, Oltra S, Beneyto M, Najera C, et al. (2006) Mutation profile of the MYO7A gene in Spanish patients with Usher syndrome type I. Hum Mutat 27: 290–291.
6. Ouyang XM, Yan D, Du LL, Hejtmancik JF, Jacobson SG, et al. (2005) Characterization of Usher syndrome type I gene mutations in an Usher syndrome patient population. Hum Genet 116: 292–299.

7. Roux AF, Faugere V, Le Guedard S, Pallares-Ruiz N, Vielle A, et al. (2006) Survey of the frequency of USH1 gene mutations in a cohort of Usher patients shows the importance of cadherin 23 and protocadherin 15 genes and establishes a detection rate of above 90%. J Med Genet 43: 763–768.
8. Nakanishi H, Ohtsubo M, Iwasaki S, Hotta Y, Takizawa Y, et al. (2010) Mutation analysis of the MYO7A and CDH23 genes in Japanese patients with Usher syndrome type 1. J Hum Genet 55: 796–800.
9. Levy G, Levi-Acobas F, Blanchard S, Gerber S, Larget-Piet D, et al. (1997) Myosin VIIA gene: heterogeneity of the mutations responsible for Usher syndrome type IB. Hum Mol Genet 6: 111–116.
10. Jaijo T, Aller E, Beneyto M, Najera C, Graziano C, et al. (2007) MYO7A mutation screening in Usher syndrome type I patients from diverse origins. J Med Genet 44: e71.
11. Bonnet C, Grati M, Marlin S, Levilliers J, Hardelin JP, et al. (2011) Complete exon sequencing of all known Usher syndrome genes greatly improves molecular diagnosis. Orphanet J Rare Dis 6: 21.
12. Metzker ML (2010) Sequencing technologies - the next generation. Nat Rev Genet 11: 31–46.

13. Kalay E, Yigit G, Aslan Y, Brown KE, Pohl E, et al. (2011) CEP152 is a genome maintenance protein disrupted in Seckel syndrome. Nat Genet 43: 23–26.
14. Krawitz PM, Schweiger MR, Rodelsperger C, Marcelis C, Kolsch U, et al. (2010) Identity-by-descent filtering of exome sequence data identifies PIGV mutations in hyperphosphatasia mental retardation syndrome. Nat Genet 42: 827–829.
15. Kuhlenbaumer G, Hullmann J, Appenzeller S (2011) Novel genomic techniques open new avenues in the analysis of monogenic disorders. Hum Mutat 32: 144–151.
16. Musunuru K, Pirruccello JP, Do R, Peloso GM, Guiducci C, et al. (2010) Exome sequencing, ANGPTL3 mutations, and familial combined hypolipidemia. N Engl J Med 363: 2220–2227.
17. Puente XS, Pinyol M, Quesada V, Conde L, Ordonez GR, et al. (2011) Whole-genome sequencing identifies recurrent mutations in chronic lymphocytic leukaemia. Nature 475: 101–105.
18. Simpson CL, Justice CM, Krishnan M, Wojciechowski R, Sung H, et al. (2011) Old lessons learned anew: family-based methods for detecting genes responsible for quantitative and qualitative traits in the Genetic Analysis Workshop 17 mini-exome sequence data. BMC Proc 5 Suppl 9: S83.
19. Chen ZY, Hasson T, Kelley PM, Schwender BJ, Schwartz MF, et al. (1996) Molecular cloning and domain structure of human myosin-VIIa, the gene product defective in Usher syndrome 1B. Genomics 36: 440–448.
20. Hasson T, Heintzelman MB, Santos-Sacchi J, Corey DP, Mooseker MS (1995) Expression in cochlea and retina of myosin VIIa, the gene product defective in Usher syndrome type 1B. Proc Natl Acad Sci U S A 92: 9815–9819.
21. Adato A, Michel V, Kikkawa Y, Reiners J, Alagramam KN, et al. (2005) Interactions in the network of Usher syndrome type 1 proteins. Hum Mol Genet 14: 347–356.
22. Udovichenko IP, Gibbs D, Williams DS (2002) Actin-based motor properties of native myosin VIIa. J Cell Sci 115: 445–450.
23. El-Amraoui A, Petit C (2005) Usher I syndrome: unravelling the mechanisms that underlie the cohesion of the growing hair bundle in inner ear sensory cells. J Cell Sci 118: 4593–4603.
24. Liu XZ, Walsh J, Mburu P, Kendrick-Jones J, Cope MJ, et al. (1997) Mutations in the myosin VIIA gene cause non-syndromic recessive deafness. Nat Genet 16: 188–190.
25. Liu XZ, Walsh J, Tamagawa Y, Kitamura K, Nishizawa M, et al. (1997) Autosomal dominant non-syndromic deafness caused by a mutation in the myosin VIIA gene. Nat Genet 17: 268–269.
26. Weil D, Blanchard S, Kaplan J, Guilford P, Gibson F, et al. (1995) Defective myosin VIIA gene responsible for Usher syndrome type 1B. Nature 374: 60–61.
27. Marmor MF, Holder GE, Seeliger MW, Yamamoto S (2004) Standard for clinical electroretinography (2004 update). Doc Ophthalmol 108: 107–114.
28. Tang W, Qian D, Ahmad S, Mattox D, Todd NW, et al. (2012) A low-cost exon capture method suitable for large-scale screening of genetic deafness by the massively-parallel sequencing approach. Genet Test Mol Biomarkers 16: 536–542.
29. Tang WS, Qian D, Ahmad S, Mattox D, Todd NW, et al. (2011) A low-cost exon capture method suitable for large-scale screening of genetic deafness by the massively-parallel sequencing approach. Genetic Testing & Mol Biomarker in press.
30. Le Quesne Stabej P, Saihan Z, Rangesh N, Steele-Stallard HB, Ambrose J, et al. (2012) Comprehensive sequence analysis of nine Usher syndrome genes in the UK National Collaborative Usher Study. J Med Genet 49: 27–36.
31. Baux D, Faugere V, Larrieu L, Le Guedard-Mereuze S, Hamroun D, et al. (2008) UMD-USHbases: a comprehensive set of databases to record and analyse pathogenic mutations and unclassified variants in seven Usher syndrome causing genes. Hum Mutat 29: E76–87.

13

Functional Abstraction as a Method to Discover Knowledge in Gene Ontologies

Alfred Ultsch[1], Jörn Lötsch[2,3]*

1 DataBionics Research Group, University of Marburg, Marburg, Germany, 2 Institute of Clinical Pharmacology, Goethe - University, Frankfurt am Main, Germany, 3 Fraunhofer Institute for Molecular Biology and Applied Ecology IME, Project Group Translational Medicine and Pharmacology TMP, Frankfurt am Main, Germany

Abstract

Computational analyses of functions of gene sets obtained in microarray analyses or by topical database searches are increasingly important in biology. To understand their functions, the sets are usually mapped to Gene Ontology knowledge bases by means of over-representation analysis (ORA). Its result represents the specific knowledge of the functionality of the gene set. However, the specific ontology typically consists of many terms and relationships, hindering the understanding of the 'main story'. We developed a methodology to identify a comprehensibly small number of GO terms as "headlines" of the specific ontology allowing to understand all central aspects of the roles of the involved genes. The Functional Abstraction method finds a set of headlines that is specific enough to cover all details of a specific ontology and is abstract enough for human comprehension. This method exceeds the classical approaches at ORA abstraction and by focusing on information rather than decorrelation of GO terms, it directly targets human comprehension. Functional abstraction provides, with a maximum of certainty, information value, coverage and conciseness, a representation of the biological functions in a gene set plays a role. This is the necessary means to interpret complex Gene Ontology results thus strengthening the role of functional genomics in biomarker and drug discovery.

Editor: Christian Schönbach, Nazarbayev University, Kazakhstan

Funding: This work was supported by the "Landesoffensive zur Entwicklung wissenschaftlich-ökonomischer Exzellenz": "LOEWE-Schwerpunkt: Anwendungsorientierte Arzneimittelforschung" (JL). The funders had no role in method design, data selection and analysis, decision to publish, or preparation of the manuscript.

Competing Interests: The authors have declared that no competing interests exist.

* E-mail: j.loetsch@em.uni-frankfurt.de

Introduction

The computational analysis of complex biological pathways has become an increasingly important part of biology. To reveal interaction networks of complex traits and diseases from sets of genes obtained from microarray analyses, proteomic research or thematic literature searches, the knowledge captured in cell biological ontologies is exploited. The gold-standard in this field is the Gene Ontology (GO; http://www.geneontology.org/) [1] where the major biological processes, cellular components or molecular functions of the genes respectively gene products are described by a controlled vocabulary (GO terms) [2]. A characterization of a gene set is obtained by statistical means identifying GO terms that are overrepresented in the gene list, i.e., annotated to the gene list more often than expected by chance [3,4].

However, the intended comprehension of main processes and interaction networks characterizing a gene set is often impeded by the complexity of the results of such an over-representation analysis (ORA) (Figure 1). A complete representation of the knowledge about the gene set's function as result of an ORA is contained in a specific ontology, which is a directed acyclic graph (DAG, knowledge representation graph). Such a specific ontology often contains hundreds of significant terms and therefore fails to provide a comprehensible selection of relevant information on the functionality of the given gene set. Therefore, an abstraction method is needed. Classical approaches, i.e., choosing most significant or most specialized terms, provided only narrowed

views on the functions represented in a gene set. Other approaches were focused on the decorrelation of GO terms [5].

The proposed methodology of functional abstraction aims at identifying a small number of GO terms (headlines) that confer the "big picture" of the biological functions of the genes in a set of genes. Its main goal was providing an informative representation that covers the different aspects of biological functions of a gene set at a human-understandable level [6].

Methods

Selection of Gene Sets

To demonstrate this knowledge discovery method on a real-life example, a set of genes which are known to be associated with a specific research topic is selected. Such a topical set of genes causally associated with hearing impairment [7] was retrieved mainly (n = 104 genes) from the "Hereditary Hearing Loss Homepage" at http://hereditaryhearingloss.org on September 20, 2013. The causal genotype phenotype associations in that data base correspond to the recommendations of the GENDEAF study group at http://hereditaryhearingloss.org/main.aspx?c = . HHH&n = 86638. Additional genes (n = 6) were obtained from [8] and from the Deafness Gene Mutation Database at http://hearing.harvard.edu/db/genelist.htm, and further genes (n = 9) were added from a recently actualized review [9]. The complete set of $n = 119$ genes (Table 1) is referred to as the Hereditary Hearing Impairment (HHI) gene set intended as a didactical example with therefore few genes in comparison to previous

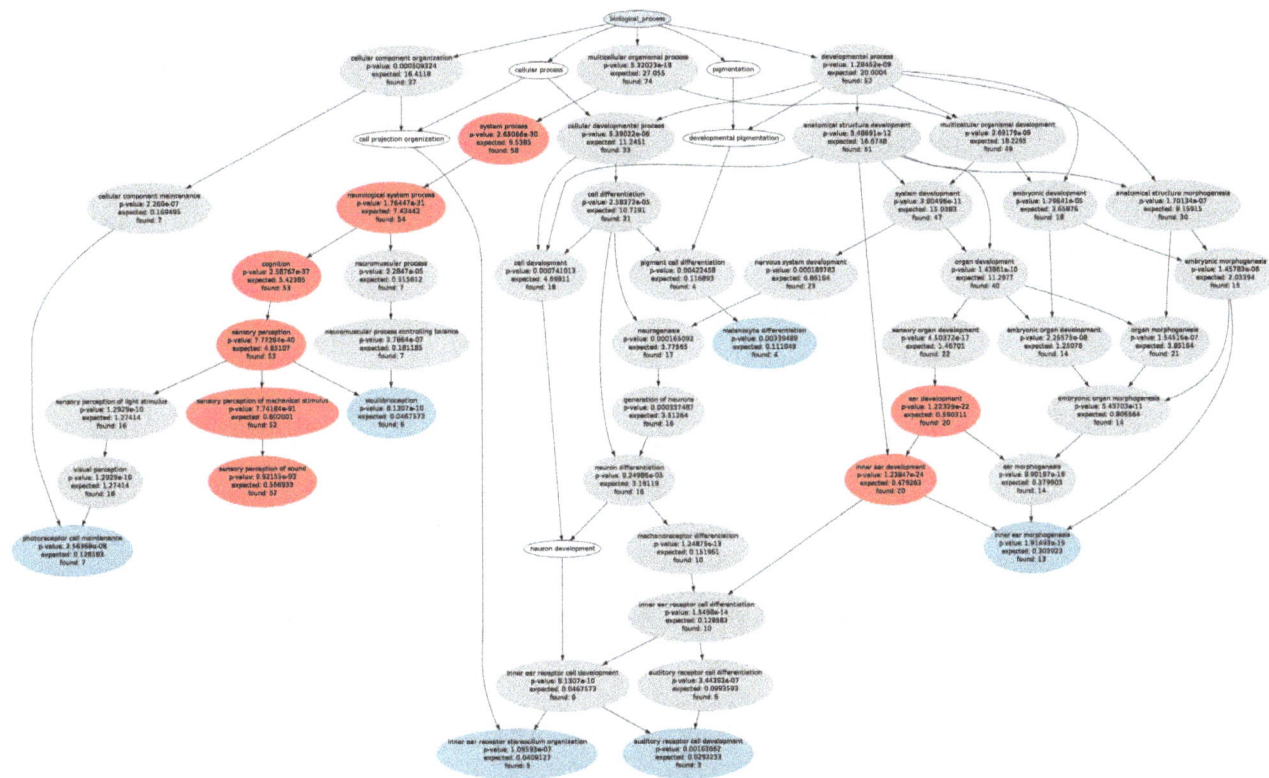

Figure 1. ORA results and functional areas obtained with the CLASSIC abstraction methods. Graphical representation of the specific ontology showing the polyhierarchy of functional annotations (GO terms) assigned to HHI gene set (G = 119, Table 1) and forming a directed acyclic graph (DAG). The figure was generated with the GeneTrail web-based analysis tool [12]. Significant GO terms were identified using ORA, which resulted in 71 terms at a significance level of p = 1.0 · 10^{-2} and Bonferroni α correction (grey ellipses in which the observed number of member genes, the expected number of genes by chance and the p-value of the significance of the deviation from the expectations (Fisher's exact test) are annotated). The CLASSIC p-value approach to the interpretation of ORA results is the selection of headline terms along descending statistical significance. When setting the p-value threshold at p = 10^{-20}, eight headlines resulted (red ellipses). The CLASSIC detail approach is the selection of the leaves of each ontology, which with the present ORA parameters resulted in seven details (blue ellipses plus "sensory perception of sound, the latter colored red since also selected by the p-value method).

methodologically similar analyses (e.g., 410 genes in a topical set of pain genes [10], 231 genes in the microarray derived expression pattern of the olfactory bulb [11]).

Gene Over-representation Analysis (ORA)

Subcategories of biological functions in which the genes of the example set are involved were identified by means of ORA [3] using the web-based GeneTrail [12] tool at http://genetrail.bioinf.uni-sb.de/. This compared the GO terms annotated to the expressed genes with the occurrence of terms among the set of all human genes. The significance of a GO term associated with the present list of genes was determined by means of a hypergeometric test that annotates the resulting GO terms with p-values. Subsequently, a correction for multiple testing was applied and only terms with a p-value lower than preset threshold t_p were considered as significant. For the HHI gene set, the threshold t_p, was set at 0.01 (similarly as elsewhere used [5]) and corrected for multiple testing according to Bonferroni, which resulted in a *significant term set* (for definitions, see Table 2).

ORA provided a representation of what is known (knowledge representation) about the roles of the genes in an organism. The significant term set may derive specific ontologies starting from either of the three possible root terms, i.e., "biological process", "cellular component" or "molecular function" [1]. In each specific ontology the terms are arranged in a polyhierarchy starting at the

root, with the broadest definition, and specializing toward the leaves, with the narrowest definition (details). For the present analysis, "biological process" was chosen (Figure 1). This consists of one or more ordered assemblies of molecular functions involving chemical or physical transformations, such as cell growth and maintenance or signal transduction [1].

The resulting specific ontology contained 48 significant terms, with the most detailed descriptions of the role of HHI gene set specified in seven leaves (Figure 1). A path from the root term to a particular detail, narrowing the definitions of the terms from universal to specific, is called "taxonomy" (Figure 1). For example the path "biological process", "multicellular organismal process", "system process", "neurological system process", "cognition", "sensory perception", "equilibrioception" is the taxonomy for the detail "equilibrioception".

Abstraction of ORA Results

With typical sets of several hundred genes the resulting specific ontologies typically also contain 100 and more significant terms [10,11]. Even for the present small HHI gene set of 119 genes and using restrictive multiple testing correction, the specific ontology contained approximately 50 significant terms. Identifying a manageable amount of terms as "**headlines**" of the "main story" will in the following be referred to as an **abstraction** of the specific ontology.

Table 1. The hereditary hearing impairment (HHI) example data set, consisting of G = 119 genes (for names and functional explanations, see http://www.genenames.org/or Table S1, HearingGenes119.xlsx) taken mainly from the Hereditary Hearing Loss Homepage at http://hereditaryhearingloss.org [7] on September 20, 2013 (104 genes) and completed from the Deafness Gene Mutation Database at http://hearing.harvard.edu/db/genelist.htm, and two publications, i.e., [8] and [9] with its last revision dating from January 3, 2013 (http://www.ncbi.nlm.nih.gov/books/NBK1434/).

ACTG1	CLRN1	DFNB31	FAM189A2	HARS2	LRTOMT	MYO15A	PCDH15	SLC17A8	TMC1
AGAP2	COCH	DFNB59	FOXI1	HGF	MARVELD2	MYO1A	PDZD7	SLC26A4	TMIE
ATP2B2	COL11A1	DIABLO	GIPC3	HSD17B4	MIR96	MYO1C	POU3F4	SLC26A5	TMPRSS3
BSND	COL11A2	DIAPH1	GJA1	ILDR1	MITF	MYO1F	POU4F3	SMPX	TMPRSS5
CABP2	COL2A1	DIAPH3	GJB1	KCNE1	MSRB3	MYO3A	PRPS1	SNAI2	TPRN
CCDC50	COL4A3	DSPP	GJB2	KCNJ10	MT-RNR1	MYO6	PTGS1	SOX10	TRIOBP
CDH23	COL4A4	EDN3	GJB3	KCNQ1	MT-TE	MYO7A	PTPRQ	SOX2	TRMU
CEACAM16	COL4A5	EDNRB	GJB6	KCNQ4	MT-TK	NDP	RDX	STRC	USH1C
CHD7	COL9A1	ESPN	GPR98	KIAA1199	MT-TL1	NF2	SEMA3E	TCOF1	USH1G
CIB2	COL9A2	ESRRB	GPSM2	LARS2	MT-TS1	OTOA	SERPINB6	TECTA	USH2A
CLDN14	CRYM	EYA1	GRHL2	LHFPL5	MYH14	OTOF	SIX1	TIMM8A	WFS1
CLPP	DFNA5	EYA4	GRXCR1	LOXHD1	MYH9	PAX3	SIX5	TJP2	

As quality criteria for understandable and informative subsets (abstractions) of significant GO terms (headlines) of a specific ontology, four dimensions were predefined, i.e., certainty, coverage, information value and conciseness.

Firstly, **certainty** requires that terms should be relevant for the gene set. For a term T_i in the significant term set, the certainty measure was defined as $Cert(T_i) = p(there\ is\ a\ Term\ with\ smaller\ P\text{-}Value) = (\#(T_k\ with\ p\text{-}value < pval(T_i)))/n_T$, where n_T denotes the number of significant GO terms annotated to the given set of genes. This reflects how safe it is to assume that the term T_i describes the gene set, with numerical values in the interval [0,1]. The certainty of the whole abstraction is the average certainty of all headlines in this abstraction.

Secondly, **coverage** requires the headlines to incorporate all the details of a specific ontology in the abstraction. A term T, which is not the root, covers a term T_d, if there is a path (in the direction from root to leaf) in the specific ontology from T to T_d. The coverage of an abstraction can be measured as the percentage of covered details in the ontology.

Thirdly, the **information** value requires that the identified headlines should be as informative as possible. To capture this dimension, the (partial) Shannon information of a term T_i in the significant term set was calculated. For each T_i, its gene frequency (probability) can be calculated: $p_i = n_{G(Ti)}/n_G$, where $n_{G(Ti)}$ denotes the number of genes of a set annotated to a term T_i and n_G denotes the total number of genes in the set. In information theory the (Shannon-) information or entropy of a probability distribution

Table 2. Definitions and notations used in the present functional abstraction process.

Gene set: a number of genes for which the genetic functionality is sought, often the result of other experiments such as microarray or proteomic analysis or database research for a certain topic such as "pain".

Overrepresentation analysis (ORA): calculation of a significant term set for a gene set. For all terms T_i of the GO p-values pval(T_i) are calculated with regard to the gene annotations of T_i and the gene set by using Fisher's exact test statistic [3]. To obtain a significant term set usually a predefined threshold t_p is used and only terms T_i with (pval(T_i)<t_p) are regarded, and corrections to control for multiple testing errors (e.g. Bonferroni, False Discovery Rate [19]) are applied.

Significant term set: the result of an ORA. The set of GO terms consisting of those terms that are annotated to the given gene set significantly more often than expected by chance. The significant terms set forms a specific ontology.

Specific Ontology: a subset of the GO, the polyhierarchy formed by the significant terms set within the thematic ontologies biological process, molecular function or cellular component.

Root term/top level term: the most general GO term of the thematic ontology from which all specific ontologies originate.

Details: the leaves of an ontology, describing the most specific pieces of knowledge.

Taxonomy: a path from the root term to a particular detail, narrowing the definitions of the terms from universal to specific details.

Remarkableness of a term: a non-negative number proportional to certainty and information value of a term.

Headline: the term with the largest remarkableness of taxonomy.

Subsumption: substitution of a set of headlines H = {T_1,..T_k} by a single term T. T must cover H i.e. all paths from the root term to any term in H must pass through T.

Detailization: substitution of a headline T by a set of terms H = {T_1,..T_k} which are covered by T.

Functional Areas: a set of terms FA = {T_1,…,T_n} covering all details of a specific ontology. FA optimizes certainty (P-values) and is most informative in an information theoretical sense. The size of the set is optimized such that human understanding is enhanced.

$P = \{p_1, ..., p_n\}$ is measured as [13,14]. The terms in the summation, i.e. $Info(T_i)$, measure the particular information *(information value)* that is contributed to the total entropy by the annotations of the particular term. Using the factor $c = e$ and the natural logarithm, i.e. $Info(T_i) = -e \cdot p_i \cdot ln(p_i)$, scales the values of $Info(T_i)$ to the interval $[0,1]$. The graph of this function is arc shaped (Figure 2) reflecting that maximum information value is provided neither by the root term of the specific ontology, e.g., "biological process" which is relevant for all genes and due to its low information cannot be selected, nor by the details which describe the role of only a small number of genes, such as "potassium transport" may be too detailed when "sodium transport" is also important and therefore "ion transport" should be preferred.

Fourthly, the dimension of **conciseness** aims at a number of headlines facilitating that humans can grasp the specific ontology, as few as possible, however not too few to avoid very abstract but general headlines covering all details. A suitable approach to this requirement is the Miller number [15] of seven headlines. If there are less than 7 - 5 headlines some terms should be replaced by more detailed terms. If there are more than 7–9 headlines some terms should be merged. Ideally a number of 5–9 terms enhances human comprehension [16].

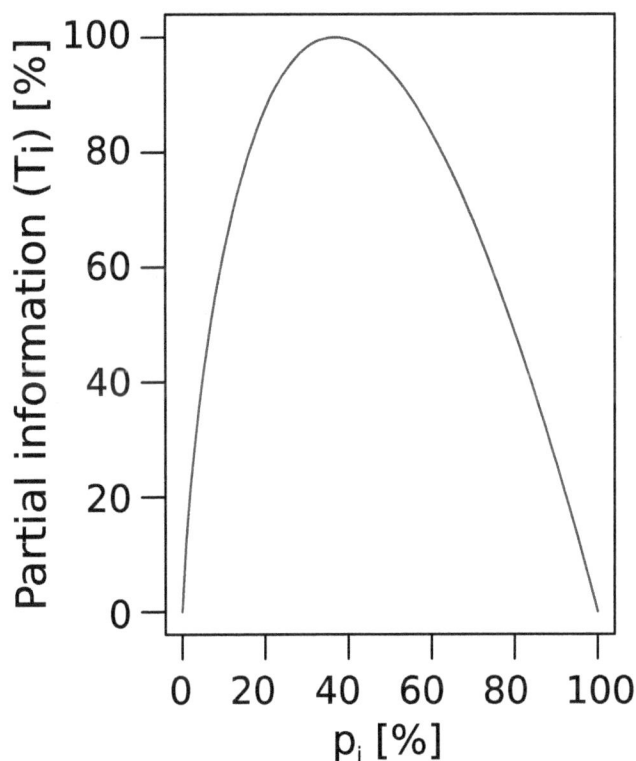

Figure 2. Graph of the Information value function $Info(T_i) = -e \cdot p_i \cdot ln(p_i)$, $p_i = n_{G(Ti)}/n_G$ **where** $n_{G(Ti)}$ **denotes the number of genes of a set annotated to a term** T_i **and** n_G **denotes the total number of genes in the set.** Derived from Shannon information [14], $Info(T_i)$ measures the contribution of the annotations of T_i to the total (Shannon) information of an specific ontology. Specifically, In bioinformatics, $IC(T_i) = -log(p_i)$ measures the information content (IC) of a GO term, [21], if p_i is the number of all genes annotated to T_i relative to all annotations in the GO. So $Info(T_i)$ can be interpreted as weighted Information Content of a specific ontology. $Info(T_i) = 0$ if term T_i does not possess any annotations ($p_i = 0$) and for the root of the ontology. $Info(T_i)$ has its maximum $Info(T_i) = 1$ at a gene probability of 37%.

Classical approaches at ORA abstraction. The current state-of-the-art approaches to a concise interpretation of ORA results mainly consist of (i) selections of the most significant terms as headlines (CLASSIC p-value), (ii) detail method taking the leaves of the ontology (CLASSIC detail), or (iii) ad hoc selection. Considering the shortcomings of current approaches, it becomes evident that a new method providing a comprehensive coverage of the functions of a gene set is needed.

The selection of the terms with the smallest p-values as headlines is a classical approach for the selection of a meaningful subset of headline terms (CLASSIC p-value). For example, a p-value limit of less than 10^{-20} selects the eight headline terms marked in red in Figure 1. One essential requirement of headline selection is complete coverage of details. In a specific ontology this means that the taxonomies of all details are covered. At least one of the headlines (other than the root) should be on the path from the detail to the root. Using the CLASSIC p-value method, however, there are several details which are not covered by these headlines.

However, this covered the ontology only poorly since more than half of the details lacked a headline (Figure 1). A possible workaround would be taking all the details as headlines (CLASSIC detail). However, this included several uninformative headlines such as "photoreceptor cell maintenance" and "melanocyte differentiation". This failed to provide an adequate overview about biologic functions concerned with hearing loss. Moreover, the results of these procedures critically depend on the parameters of the particular ORA. Therefore a different set of headlines would result from choosing other ORA significance levels. Sometimes the specific ontology is just eyeballed and a set of headline terms is ad hoc selected as particularly interesting. An example of such an approach can be found in [8]. There, for a gene set of 51 non-syndromic hereditary hearing loss genes, which is a subset of the present HHI, five headlines were identified in a specific ontology consisting of 42 terms (green circles in figure 4 of [8]). Four of these headlines are the details of the specific ontology, one is an arbitrarily chosen inner node.

Functional abstraction. To better meet the requirements at an abstraction than classical approaches and to obtain an understandable and informative set of GO terms from ORA, the following heuristic of functional abstraction (FA) was developed:

For each term T_i in the set of terms, its remarkableness, $Rem(T_i)$, was calculated as the product of **certainty** and **information value**, i.e., $Rem(T_i) = Cert(T_i) \cdot Info(T_i)$. **Coverage** was addressed by assuring that the taxonomies of all details of a specific ontology, i.e., all the different paths from the leaves (details) to the root, are being considered. Specifically, the most remarkable term in each taxonomy was headline candidate. From all candidate terms, C, redundancies were eliminated, i.e., if all parents of a term T in C were also members of C, then T was deleted as already represented in C, thereby addressing conciseness of the **abstraction**. The remaining headlines, H, of this FA are called "functional areas".

While these functional areas are a suitable comprehensive representation of the taxonomies of a specific ontology, a more global abstraction can be obtained by two methods: detailization or subsumption. Let T be a term in a specific ontology which covers the terms $T_1, .. T_k$. A set of headlines H containing T is detailed if T is replaced by the headlines $T_1, .. T_k$ in H. Alternatively, a set of headlines H containing $T_1, .. T_k$ is abstracted if $T_1, .. T_k$ are replaced by T in H. Detailization enlarges, subsumption reduces the number of headlines. Note that the root is never a headline, since it is excluded from the definition of coverage. To enhance human comprehensibility a number of 5–9 headlines correspond to the human capacity of information processing [15]. Thus, if the number of headlines in H is smaller than the Miller optimum, detailization is applied for the headline T with the largest remarkability, whereas subsumption will be applied if the number of headlines in H exceeds the Miller optimum.

Results

For the HHI sample gene set (n = 119) an ORA with p-value threshold of $t_p = 1.0 \cdot 10^{-2}$ and Bonferroni α correction resulted in the specific ontology of 71 significant terms (see Table S1) including seven details shown in figures 1 and 2. Functional abstraction identified a set H of $k = 8$ terms (Table 3, red in Figure 3) as headlines of the biological processes in which the 119 genes of hereditary hearing loss are involved. Subsequently, three headlines were eliminated since they were explained (covered) by other members of H. The final set of functional areas emerging from functional abstraction (FA) contained five terms (green circles in Figure 3). This improved the overall values of the four predefined major abstraction requirements substantially, i.e., certainty, coverage, information value and conciseness (Table 4), as compared to the currently most often used approaches to ORA interpretation (CLASSIC detail, CLASSIC p-value).

Discussion

A typical ORA results in an all-embracing, encyclopedical representation of the knowledge about biological processes, molecular functions or cellular components related with a given gene set. Human comprehension of this complex knowledge requires abstraction to a manageable number of headline terms as acknowledged previously [8]. The method of functional abstraction (FA) exceeds previous attempts of ad-hoc selections of suitable terms and uses quantifiable key requirements of an abstraction of a polyhierarchy, i.e., certainty, coverage, information value and conciseness. The method provided the comparatively highest overall values in these dimensions and identified headlines that reflect the definition of the trait exemplified by hereditary deafness [9].

The present FA method uses the term with the largest numerical value of remarkableness of each taxonomy as a candidate for a headline. The optimization of remarkableness encompasses both, the certainty that a GO term represents the taxonomy and its information value, because it is the product of both numerical values rescaled to the unit interval. By the selection of suitable terms for all taxonomies, FA also delivers the complete coverage of a selected ontology. By taking the Miller optimum into account, an abstraction of a set of headlines is obtained which explicitly aims at maximizing human understanding of the "big picture" of a specific ontology.

The process of abstraction may enable emergence [17] in the sense that novel, formerly unseen properties on a macroscopic level become visible on top of the only locally defined pieces of knowledge. Emergence in understanding might be obtained by integrating taxonomies into a more comprehensive view on the specific ontology as a whole, i.e., by the interactions of the locally defined headlines for the detail knowledge representations with the global structure of the specific ontology [17]. The procedures of detailization or subsumption provide a basis to obtain emergence in particular when in larger data sets the initial number of functional areas selected on the basis of remarkability and coverage differs from the Miller optimum [15].

In applications with larger sets of genes than in HHI this could be already observed and used for the discovery of new bits of knowledge: by a combined proteomic and transcriptomic analysis of a set of n = 231 genes were identified for the human olfactory bulb [11]. A suitable ORA identified for this gene set a set of 94 significant GO terms. By the functional abstraction method presented here the existence of neurogenesis in the adult human olfactory bulb emerged as a major finding [11]. An ORA on genes related to pain [18] resulted for the n = 410 genes causally involved in pain initially in 234 significant terms. Functional abstraction identified only 12 relevant functional areas that comprehensively describe the biology of pain from a genetics [18].

With its regard to several intuitively important dimensions of an abstraction of ORA results (certainty, coverage, information value and conciseness), FA exceeds the currently most often applied method of selecting the terms with the most significant p-values (CLASSIC), which, in contrast to FA, only aims at certainty. Such a limited focus may result in low values for coverage and information. This applied also to the present HHI example gene set. Similarly, another classical method consisting of selecting the leaves of the ontology (CLASSIC details) as an abstraction provides complete coverage. However, this method disregards information value and certainty. Moreover, the obtained headlines directly depend on the ORA parameters. In the extreme, those consist of just the root term if the chosen p-value threshold is very low, or in a great number of headlines in the opposite case. A typical example of the current state-of-the-art in the abstraction of specific ontologies is the selection of headlines for a set of 70 genes of which 55 are included in the present HHI set (Figure 4 in [8]). The specific ontology contains 49 terms and 3 details. These details and two other terms are marked as remarkable. That method of abstraction was ad hoc and involved a major subjective component.

As a consequence of this comprehensive and comprehension focused approach, FA improved the classical methods of ORA interpretation in two main ways. Firstly, it provided the number k of the functional areas covered by a given gene set as a result. By contrast, in the classical methods k depends on the selection of the p-value threshold. Secondly, FA avoided the selection of a set of terms mainly along the most important taxonomy. The reason why the CLASSIC method often results in a set covering only a single or a few but usually not all taxonomies originates from the semantics of the gene ontology. If a gene G is annotated to a certain term T, then by the rules of the GO all parents of T are automatically also annotated with gene G (http://www.geneontology.org/GO.annotation.conventions.shtml). Therefore, a large part of the genes annotated to term T will be also annotated to the parents (i.e. broader terms) P of T, resulting in correlated lists in T and P. If T is significant, the significance of P is consequently highly likely. This issue has previously been approached by a decorrelation method [5]. In their "TopGO" approach to ORA, these authors propose two different methods, ELIM and WEIGHT [5], for the recalculation of p-values based on different heuristics to eliminate correlations. Results these methods applied to the present HHI gene set are shown in the supporting information (Figures S1 and S2, respectively). The methods produced comparatively lower values in the quality dimensions of abstraction (Table 4). Moreover, GO terms emerged as significant which were not part of the original ORA results.

Conclusions

The method of functional abstraction (FA) aims at human comprehension of voluminous gene set specific ontologies. The idea was to select terms that provide a comprehensive, yet

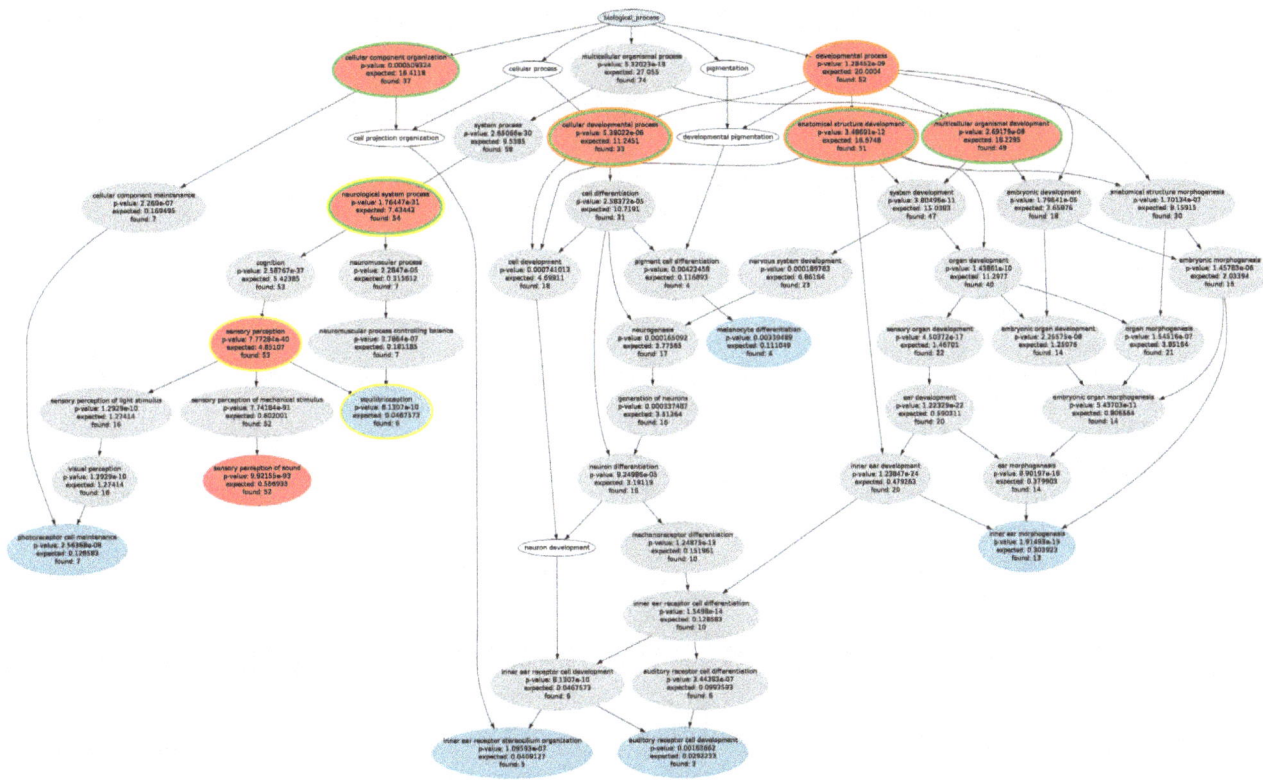

Figure 3. Functional abstraction of ORA results. Graphical representation of the specific ontology showing the polyhierarchy of functional annotations (GO terms) assigned to HHI gene set (G = 119, Table 1). ORA resulted in 71 terms at a significance level of p = 1.0 · 10^{-2} and Bonferroni α correction (grey ellipses). The functional abstraction approach to ORA results uses as a main measure the degree of remarkableness, calculated as the product (AND) of certainty, i.e., how safely one can assume that a GO term described the given set of genes, and information, calculated as Shannon information. Among most remarkable terms (n = 8, red ellipses), immediate redundancy is eliminated by deleting all terms that are already presented by others. This resulted in functional areas (red ellipses with green margins) conferring a comprehensive set of headline terms characterizing the biological functions of the HHI gene set. Although the present data set was of limited complexity, greater data sets may result in the initial identification of more than the desired up to nine functional areas. In this case, the method of subsumption can be applied to reduce this number. In the present case, this would, for example, join "cellular developmental process" and "anatomical structure development" to the next upper remarkable GO term "developmental process" (orange margins). In the opposite case, if the number of functional areas is low and an increase may be desirable, detailization may be applied. In this case, the terms downstream the hierarchy with the next highest remarkability are chose. For example, "neurological system process" would be split into "sensory perception and "equilibrioception" (yellow margins), which along the hierarchy have the next highest value of remarkability following the initial term. Note that the intermediate terms have lower remarkability and are therefore not chosen (Table S1).

complete coverage of the biological functions of a given gene set. The objective was achieved by (i) introducing a measure of remarkableness of a term addressing both, the certainty that a term indeed describes the functions of the gene set and the information content that avoids too general or too narrow descriptions, (ii) by selecting headlines from the most remarkable terms in order to obtain complete coverage of all parts of the polyhierarchical structure of the biological functions of the gen set,

Table 3. The headlines produced by functional abstraction resulted in these five headline terms or functional areas (green circled red ellipses in Figure 2).

Go Term ID	GO category	Info [%]	Certainty [%]	Remarkableness	Nr. Genes (and %)
GO:0050877	neurological system process	97	95	92	55 (46)
GO:0048856	anatomical structure development	98	77	75	54 (45)
GO:0007275	multicellular organismal development	98	65	64	52 (44)
GO:0048869	cellular developmental process	98	45	44	35 (29)
GO:0016043	cellular component organization	100	20	20	40 (34)

Significant GO terms are a result of over-representation analysis (ORA) of the n = 119 genes (Table 1) of the Hereditary Hearing Impairment (HHI) gene set. The precise definition of the GO terms can be obtained using AmiGO search tool for GO at http://amigo.geneontology.org/[20]. For a full list of significant terms and associated p-values, see Table S1. Remarkableness of a term is the product of the certainty that the term is not by chance associated with the GO biological process and the information of the particular subset of genes associated with the term. Genes is the number of genes annotated to the headline.

Table 4. Comparison of different abstraction methods, numerically quantified for the four required performance dimensions.

Method	Mean Certainty	Coverage	Information Value	Conciseness (ideal 5–9)
CLASSIC p-values ($<10^{-12}$)	94%	57%	94%	8
CLASSIC details	13%	100%	50%	7
Functional abstraction (FA)	**61%**	**100%**	**98%**	**5**

ORA conditions of classic approaches as in Figure 1. For results of FA, see Figure 3.

(iii) and by adjusting the number of headlines close to the Miller optimum of 5–9 to enhance human comprehension [15]. The result was an improvement of the current state-of-the art approaches to ORA interpretation in several ways. This included the identification of the number of informative headlines and the concise coverage of the original ORA. In this respect, FA exceeded the classical approaches at ORA abstraction (CLASSIC detail, CLASSIC p-value). By focusing on information rather than decorrelation of GO terms, it targeted towards human comprehension more than ELIM and WEIGHT [5] which aim at term decorrelation. On large gene sets typically obtained from topical searches or microarray analyses FA describes complex and unmanageable knowledge representations in a comprehensive manner [10,11]. This may lead to a stimulation of the research of new aspects strengthening functional genomics in biomarker and drug discovery.

Supporting Information

Figure S1   ORA results and functional areas obtained with the ELIM TopGO method [5]. Graphical representation of the specific ontology showing the polyhierarchy of functional annotations (GO terms) assigned to HHI gene set (G = 119) and forming a directed acyclic graph (DAG). The figure was generated with the GeneTrail web-based analysis tool [12]. Significant GO terms were identified using ORA, which resulted in 71 terms at a significance level of p = 1.0 · 10-2 and Bonferroni α correction (grey ellipses in which the observed number of member genes, the expected number of genes by chance and the p-value of the significance of the deviation from the expectations (Fisher's exact test) are annotated). The TopGO approach [5] to GO abstraction exploits the correlation of terms. The selection of the k terms of the smallest values is done from the recalculated p-values. The ELIM method investigates the nodes in the GO graph bottom-up and iteratively removes genes from significant nodes [5], recalculating the ORA with the remaining set of genes. This may result in the selection of terms that were not significant in the original ORA (given at the right bottom of the figure, in red to emphasize the formal equivalence with the functional areas in Figures 1 and 3 of the main report).

Figure S2   ORA results and functional areas obtained with the WEIGHT TopGO method [5]. Graphical represen-

tation of the specific ontology showing the polyhierarchy of functional annotations (GO terms) assigned to HHI gene set (G = 119) and forming a directed acyclic graph (DAG). The figure was generated with the GeneTrail web-based analysis tool [12]. Significant GO terms were identified using ORA, which resulted in 71 terms at a significance level of p = 1.0 · 10-2 and Bonferroni α correction (grey ellipses in which the observed number of member genes, the expected number of genes by chance and the p-value of the significance of the deviation from the expectations (Fisher's exact test) are annotated). The TopGO approach [5] to GO abstraction exploits the correlation of terms. The selection of the k terms of the smallest values is done from the recalculated p-values. In the WEIGHT method, significance scores of connected nodes (a parent and its child) are compared to detect locally most significant terms, which is achieved by down-weighting genes in less significant neighbors [5]. This may result in the selection of terms that were not significant in the original ORA (given at the right bottom of the figure, in red to emphasize the formal equivalence with the functional areas in Figures 1 and 3 of the main report).

Table S1   Significant GO terms are a result of over-representation analysis (ORA) of the n = 119 genes of the Hereditary Hearing Impairment (HHI) gene set. The precise definition of the GO terms can be obtained using AmiGO search tool for GO at http://amigo.geneontology.org/ [20]. Remarkableness of a term is the product of the certainty that the term is not by chance associated with the GO biological process and the information of the particular subset of genes associated with the term. Genes is the number of genes annotated to the headline.

Acknowledgments

We thank Dr. A. Doehring for her help in choosing the genetic sample data set.

Author Contributions

Conceived and designed the experiments: JL AU. Analyzed the data: AU. Wrote the paper: JL AU.

References

1. Ashburner M, Ball CA, Blake JA, Botstein D, Butler H, et al. (2000) Gene ontology: tool for the unification of biology. The Gene Ontology Consortium. Nat Genet 25: 25–29.
2. Camon E, Magrane M, Barrell D, Lee V, Dimmer E, et al. (2004) The Gene Ontology Annotation (GOA) Database: sharing knowledge in Uniprot with Gene Ontology. Nucleic Acids Res 32: D262–266.
3. Backes C, Keller A, Kuentzer J, Kneissl B, Comtesse N, et al. (2007) GeneTrail-advanced gene set enrichment analysis. Nucleic Acids Res 35: W186–192.
4. Khatri P, Draghici S (2005) Ontological analysis of gene expression data: current tools, limitations, and open problems. Bioinformatics 21: 3587–3595.
5. Alexa A, Rahnenfuhrer J, Lengauer T (2006) Improved scoring of functional groups from gene expression data by decorrelating GO graph structure. Bioinformatics 22: 1600–1607.
6. Gaines P (1996) Transforming Rules and Trees into Comprehensible Knowledge Structures. In: Fayyad UM, editor. Advances in knowledge discovery and data mining. Menlo Park, Calif. [u.a.]: AAAI Press [u.a.]. pp. XIV, 611 S.

7. Van Camp G, Smith RJH Hereditary Hearing Loss Homepage. Available: http://hereditaryhearingloss.org. Accessed 2014 Feb 3.

8. Accetturo M, Creanza TM, Santoro C, Tria G, Giordano A, et al. (2010) Finding new genes for non-syndromic hearing loss through an in silico prioritization study. PLoS One 5.

9. Smith RJH, Shearer AE, Hildebrand MS, Van Camp G (1993) Deafness and Hereditary Hearing Loss Overview. In: Pagon RA, Adam MP, Bird TD, Dolan CR, Fong CT et al., editors. GeneReviews. Seattle (WA).

10. Lötsch J, Doehring A, Mogil JS, Arndt T, Geisslinger G, et al. (2013) Functional genomics of pain in analgesic drug development and therapy. Pharmacol Ther.

11. Lötsch J, Schaeffeler E, Mittelbronn M, Winter S, Gudziol V, et al. (2013) Functional genomics suggest neurogenesis in the adult human olfactory bulb. Brain Struct Funct.

12. Keller A, Backes C, Al-Awadhi M, Gerasch A, Kuntzer J, et al. (2008) GeneTrailExpress: a web-based pipeline for the statistical evaluation of microarray experiments. BMC Bioinformatics 9: 552.

13. Cover TM, Thomas JA (1991) Elements of information theory New York: Wiley & Sons.

14. Shannon CE (1951) A mathematical theory of communication. Bell Syst Techn J 30: 50–64.

15. Miller GA (1956) The magical number seven plus or minus two: some limits on our capacity for processing information. Psychol Rev 63: 81–97.

16. Saaty TL, Ozdemir MS (2003) Why the magic number seven plus or minus two Mathematical and Computer Modelling 38: 233–244.

17. Ultsch A. Emergence in Self-Organizing Feature Maps. In: Ritter H, Haschke R, editors; 2007; Bielefeld, Germany. Neuroinformatics Group.

18. Lötsch J, Doehring A, Mogil JS, Arndt T, Geisslinger G, et al. (2013) Functional genomics of pain in analgesic drug development and therapy. Pharmacol Ther 139: 60–70.

19. Benjamini Y, Hochberg Y (1995) Controlling the false discovery rate - a practical and powerful approach to multiple testing. J R Stat Soc B 57.

20. Carbon S, Ireland A, Mungall CJ, Shu S, Marshall B, et al. (2009) AmiGO: online access to ontology and annotation data. Bioinformatics 25: 288–289.

21. Mazandu GK, Mulder NJ (2013) Information content-based gene ontology semantic similarity approaches: toward a unified framework theory. Biomed Res Int 2013: 292063.

14

Single- and Multi-Channel Modulation Detection in Cochlear Implant Users

John J. Galvin III[1,2,3,4]*, **Sandy Oba**[1,2], **Qian-Jie Fu**[1,2], **Deniz Başkent**[3,4]

1 Division of Communication and Auditory Neuroscience, House Research Institute, Los Angeles, California, United States of America, 2 Department of Head and Neck Surgery, David Geffen School of Medicine, University of California Los Angeles, Los Angeles, California, United States of America, 3 Department of Otorhinolaryngology, Head and Neck Surgery, University Medical Center Groningen, University of Groningen, Groningen, The Netherlands, 4 Research School of Behavioral and Cognitive Neurosciences, Graduate School of Medical Sciences, University of Groningen, Groningen, The Netherlands

Abstract

Single-channel modulation detection thresholds (MDTs) have been shown to predict cochlear implant (CI) users' speech performance. However, little is known about multi-channel modulation sensitivity. Two factors likely contribute to multichannel modulation sensitivity: multichannel loudness summation and the across-site variance in single-channel MDTs. In this study, single- and multi-channel MDTs were measured in 9 CI users at relatively low and high presentation levels and modulation frequencies. Single-channel MDTs were measured at widely spaced electrode locations, and these same channels were used for the multichannel stimuli. Multichannel MDTs were measured twice, with and without adjustment for multichannel loudness summation (i.e., at the same loudness as for the single-channel MDTs or louder). Results showed that the effect of presentation level and modulation frequency were similar for single- and multi-channel MDTs. Multichannel MDTs were significantly poorer than single-channel MDTs when the current levels of the multichannel stimuli were reduced to match the loudness of the single-channel stimuli. This suggests that, at equal loudness, single-channel measures may over-estimate CI users' multichannel modulation sensitivity. At equal loudness, there was no significant correlation between the amount of multichannel loudness summation and the deficit in multichannel MDTs, relative to the average single-channel MDT. With no loudness compensation, multichannel MDTs were significantly better than the best single-channel MDT. The across-site variance in single-channel MDTs varied substantially across subjects. However, the across-site variance was not correlated with the multichannel advantage over the best single channel. This suggests that CI listeners combined envelope information across channels instead of attending to the best channel.

Editor: Manuel S. Malmierca, University of Salamanca- Institute for Neuroscience of Castille and Leon and Medical School, Spain

Funding: Mr. Galvin, Ms. Oba, and Dr. Fu were supported by National Institutes of Health grant R01-DC004993. Dr. Baskent was supported by VIDI grant 016.096.397 from the Netherlands Organization for Scientific Research (NWO) and the Netherlands Organization for Health Research and Development (ZonMw), and a Rosalind Franklin Fellowship from University of Groningen, University Medical Center Groningen. The funders had no role in study design, data collection and analysis, decision to publish, or preparation of the manuscript.

Competing Interests: The authors have declared that no competing interests exist.

* E-mail: Jgalvin@ucla.edu

Introduction

Temporal amplitude modulation (AM) detection is one of the few psychophysical measures that have been shown to predict speech perception by users of cochlear implants (CIs) [1–2] or auditory brainstem implants [3]. Various stimulation parameters have been shown to affect modulation detection thresholds (MDTs) measured on a single electrode, including current level, modulation frequency, and stimulation rate [2], [4–14]. In these single-channel modulation detection studies, MDTs generally improve as the current level is increased and as the modulation frequency is reduced. However, given that nearly all CIs are multichannel, it is crucial to characterize multichannel MDTs and their relation to the single-channel MDTs.

One factor that may affect multichannel temporal processing is loudness summation. Clinical CI speech processors are generally fitted with regard to loudness (i.e., between barely audible and the most comfortable levels), and adjustments are often necessary to accommodate multichannel loudness summation. As such, current levels on individual channels may be lower when presented in a multichannel context compared to those when measured in isolation. Because MDTs are level-dependent [4], [6], [8–10], [15], modulation sensitivity on individual channels may be poorer after adjusting for multichannel loudness summation. Another factor that may affect multichannel temporal processing is across-site variability in single-channel modulation sensitivity. Garadat et al. [16] showed significant variability in single-channel MDTs across stimulation sites within and across CI subjects. It is unclear how single-channel across-site variability may contribute to multichannel modulation sensitivity. These two factors – loudness summation and across-site variability – may combine in some way such that CI users may attend to the channels with the best modulation sensitivity, but at lower current levels after adjusting for summation. Alternatively, CI users may combine temporal information from all channels when detecting modulation with multiple channels.

While single-channel temporal processing has been extensively studied, there are relatively few studies regarding multichannel temporal processing. Geurts and Wouters [17] measured single- and multi-channel AM frequency detection in CI users. They found that AM frequency detection was improved with multi-channel stimulation, relative to single-channel performance. However, no adjustment was made for multichannel loudness summation. Chatterjee and colleagues [15], [18] measured modulation detection interference (MDI) by fluctuating maskers in CI subjects. They found significant MDI, even when the maskers were spatially remote from the target, suggesting that CI users combined temporal information across distant neural populations (i.e., more central processing of temporal envelope information). Although their results supported the notion that central processes mediate envelope interactions, they did not find evidence for modulation tuning of the sort observed in normal-hearing (NH) listeners [19–20]. Kreft et al. [21] measured AM frequency discrimination in NH and CI listeners in the presence of steady-state and modulated maskers that were spatially proximate or remote to the target; the maskers were presented with or without a temporal offset relative to the target. Similar to the MDI findings by Chatterjee and colleagues, Kreft et al. [21] found significant interference by modulated maskers, but with some effect of masker location; temporal offset between the masker and target did not significantly reduce interference. The Chatterjee and Kreft studies present some evidence that central mechanisms result in combinations of and interactions between envelopes on remote spatial channels.

In this study, single- and multi-channel MDTs were measured in 9 CI subjects. MDTs were measured at relatively low and high presentation levels, and at low and high modulation frequencies. Single-channel MDTs were measured at 4 maximally spaced stimulation sites to target spatially remote neural populations, which would presumably result in greater across-site variability than with 4 closely spaced electrodes. Multichannel MDTs were measured using the same electrodes used to measure single-channel MDTs. To explore the effects of loudness summation on multichannel modulation sensitivity, multichannel MDTs were measured with and without adjustment for multichannel loudness summation.

Methods

Participants

Nine adult, post-lingually deafened CI users participated in this experiment. All were users of Cochlear Corp. devices and all had more than 2 years of experience with their implant device. Relevant subject details are shown in Table 1. All subjects previously participated in a related study [22].

Ethics Statement

All subjects provided written informed consent prior to participating in the study, in accordance with the guidelines of the St. Vincent Medical Center Institutional Review Board (Los Angeles, CA), which specifically approved this study. All subjects were financially compensated for their participation.

Single-channel Modulation Detection Thresholds (MDTs)

Stimuli

All stimuli were 300-ms biphasic pulse trains. The pulse phase duration was 100 µs; the inter-phase gap was 20 µs. Four test electrodes were selected and assigned to channel locations that spanned the electrode array from the base (A) to the basal-middle (B) to the middle-apical (C) to the apex (D). Table 1 lists the test electrode, channel assignment and stimulation mode for each subject. The stimulation rate was 500 pulses per second (pps). The

Table 1. CI subject demographic information.

Subject	Gender	Age at testing (yrs) (yrs)	CI exp (yrs)	Dur deafness (yrs)	Device	Stim mode	Experimental electrodes			
							A	B	C	D
S1	F	77	10	12	N-24	MP1+2	8	12	17	22
S2	F	67	7	20	N-24	MP1+2	2	8	14	20
S3	M	81	15	1	N-22	BP+1	2	8	14	20
S4	F	78	23	14	Freedom	MP1+2	3	9	15	21
S5	M	70	21	4	N-22	BP+1	2	8	14	20
S6	F	58	17	20	N-22	BP+1	5	10	15	20
S7	F	28	5	5	Freedom	MP1+2	2	8	14	20
S8	F	66	7	24	Freedom	MP1+2	2	8	14	20
S9	M	74	3	2	Freedom	MP1+2	2	8	14	20

The experimental electrode used as the reference for loudness-balancing in shown in column C. CI exp = experience with cochlear implant device; Dur deafness = duration of diagnosed severe-to-profound deafness prior to cochlear implantation; Stim mode = stimulation mode; MP1+2 = intracochlear monopolar stimulation with two extracochlear grounds; BP+1 = intracochlear bipolar stimulation with active and return electrode separated by one electrode.

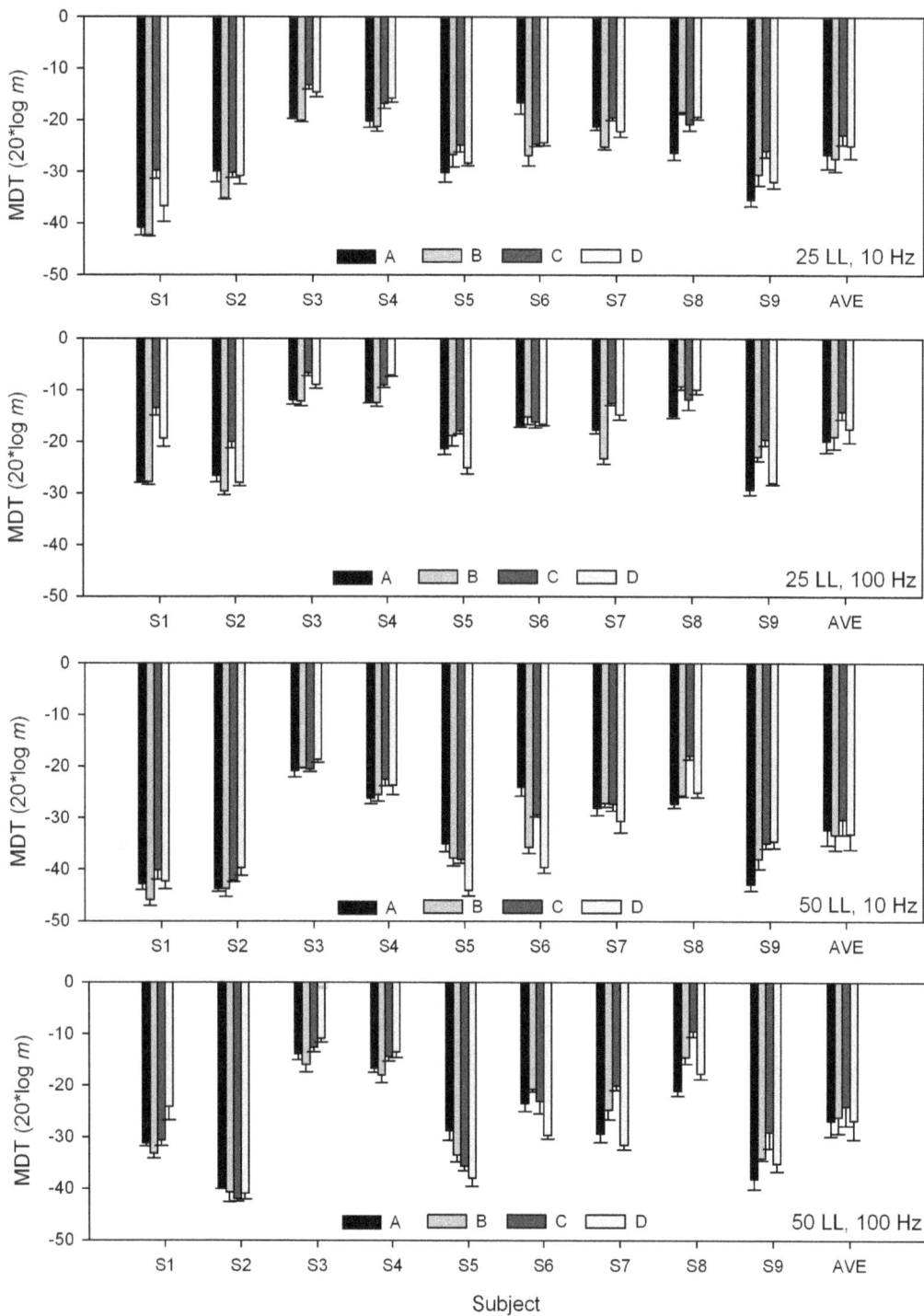

Figure 1. Single-channel MDTs for individual CI subjects. From top to bottom, the panels show 10-Hz MDTs at 25 LL, 100-Hz MDTs at 25 LL, 10-Hz MDTs at 50 LL, 100-Hz MDTs at 50 LL, respectively. The shaded bars show MDTs for the A, B, C, and D channels, respectively; the electrode-channel assignments are shown for each subject in Table 1. The error bars show the standard error.

presentation level was referenced to 25% or 50% of the dynamic range (DR) of a 500 pps stimulus. The modulation frequency was 10 Hz or 100 Hz.

Sinusoidal AM was applied as a percentage of the carrier pulse train amplitude according to [f(t)] [1+$m$sin(2πf$_m$t)], where f(t) is a steady-state pulse train, m is the modulation index, and f$_m$ is the modulation frequency. All stimuli were presented via research

interface [23], bypassing CI subjects' clinical speech processors and settings.

Dynamic Range Estimation

DRs were estimated for all single-channel stimuli, presented without modulation (non-AM). Absolute detection thresholds were estimated according to the "counting" method commonly used for

Table 2. Results of three-way ANOVAs performed on individual subjects' single-channel MDT data.

Subject	Stimulation level				Modulation frequency				Stimulation site			
	dF, res	F	p	Post-hoc p<0.05	dF, res	F	p	Post-hoc p<0.05	dF, res	F	p	Post-hoc p<0.05
S1	1, 3	65	0.004	50 LL>25 LL	1, 3	304	<0.001	10 Hz>100 Hz	3,3	25	0.012	A,B>C
S2	1, 3	134	<0.001	50 LL>25 LL	1, 3	10	0.052		3,3	2	0.29	
S3	1, 3	26	0.015	50 LL>25 LL	1, 3	113	0.002	10 Hz>100 Hz	3,3	10	0.044	
S4	1, 3	278	<0.001	50 L>25 LL	1, 3	634	<0.001	10 Hz>100 Hz	3,3	41	0.006	A,B>C, D
S5	1, 3	213	<0.001	50 LL>25 LL	1, 3	47	0.006	10 Hz>100 Hz	3,3	8	0.058	
S6	1, 3	220	<0.001	50 L>25 LL	1, 3	166	<0.001	10 Hz>100 Hz	3,3	27	0.011	A>D
S7	1, 3	54	0.005	50 LL>25 LL	1, 3	10	0.049	10 Hz>100 Hz	3,3	5	0.103	
S8	1, 3	22	0.019	50 LL>25 LL	1, 3	143	0.001	10 Hz>100 Hz	3,3	17	0.021	A>C
S9	1, 3	256	<0.001	50 LL>25 LL	1, 3	94	0.002	10 Hz>100 Hz	3,3	58	0.004	A>B, A,D>C

dF = degrees of freedom; res = residual error; F = F-ratio.

clinical fitting. Maximum acceptable loudness (MAL) levels, defined as the "loudest sound that could be tolerated for a short time," were estimated by slowly increasing the current level until reaching MAL. Threshold and MAL levels were averaged across a minimum of two runs, and the DR was calculated as the difference in current (in microamps) between MAL and threshold.

Loudness Balancing

The four test electrodes were loudness-balanced to a common reference using an adaptive two-alternative, forced-choice (2AFC), double-staircase procedure [24–25]. Stimuli were loudness-balanced without modulation. For each subject, the reference was the C channel (see Table 1) presented at 25% or 50% of its DR. The current amplitude of the probe was adjusted according to subject response (2-down/1-up or 1-down/2-up, depending on the track). The initial step size was 1.2 dB and the final step size was 0.4 dB. For each run, the final 8 of 12 reversals in current amplitude were averaged, and the mean of 2–6 runs was considered to be the loudness-balanced level. The low and high presentation levels were referenced to 25% DR or 50% DR of the reference electrode, and are referred to as the 25 loudness level (LL) and 50 LL, respectively. Thus, test electrodes A, B, C, and D were equally loud at the 25 LL and at the 50 LL presentation levels.

To protect against potential loudness cues in AM detection [14,26], an adaptive AM loudness compensation procedure was used during the adaptive MDT task, as in Galvin et al. [22]. The AM loudness compensation functions were the same as in Galvin et al. [22], as the subjects, reference stimuli, and loudness-balance conditions were the same. Briefly, non-AM stimuli were loudness-balanced to AM stimuli using an adaptive, 2AFC double-staircase procedure [24–25]. The reference was the AM stimulus (AM depths = 5%, 10%, 20%, or 30%) presented to electrode C at either 25% or 50% DR. The probe was the non-AM stimulus, also presented to electrode C. The current amplitude of the probe was adjusted according to subject response (2-down/1-up or 1-down/2-up, depending on the track). For each run, the final 8 of 12 reversals in current amplitude were averaged, and the mean of 2–6 runs was considered to be the current level needed to loudness-balance the non-AM stimulus to the AM stimulus. For each loudness balance condition, an exponential function was fit across the non-AM loudness-balanced levels at each modulation depth. The mean exponent across the exponential fits was used to customize an AM loudness compensation function for each subject. For more details, please refer to Galvin et al. [22].

Modulation Detection

MDTs were measured using an adaptive, 3AFC procedure. The modulation depth was adjusted according to subject response (3-down/1-up), converging on the threshold that corresponded to 79.4% correct [27]. One interval (randomly assigned) contained the AM stimulus and the other two intervals contained non-AM stimuli. Subjects were asked to indicate which interval was different. For each run, the final 8 of 12 reversals in AM depth were averaged to obtain the MDT; 3–6 test runs were conducted for each experimental condition.

MDTs were measured while controlling for potential AM loudness cues, as in Galvin et al. [22]. For each subject, the amount of level compensation y (in dB) was dynamically adjusted throughout the test run according to: $y = 20 \log_{10}\left(\dfrac{1+m}{1+am}\right)$,

where m is the modulation index of the modulated stimulus and α is the exponent (ranging from 0 to 1) of the exponential function fit to each subject's AM vs. non-AM loudness-balance data. After applying this level compensation to the non-AM stimuli, the

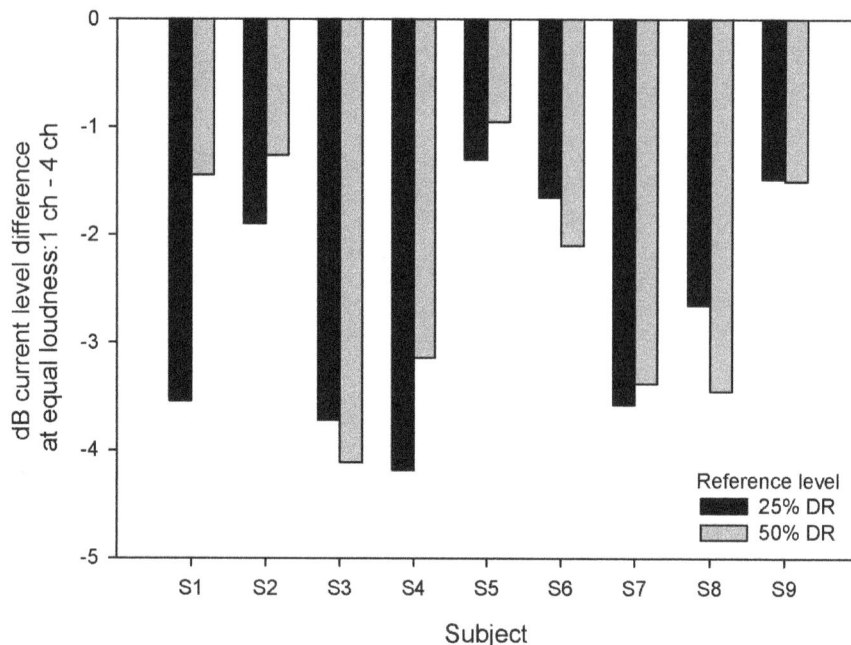

Figure 2. Loudness balancing between single- and multi-channel stimuli. The y-axis shows the current level adjustment needed to maintain equal loudness between 4-channel stimuli and the reference (single-channel, 500 pps, electrode C). The black bars show data referenced to 25% DR and the gray bars show data referenced to 50% DR. The error bars show the standard error.

current level of all stimuli in each trial was independently roved by a random value between −0.75 and +0.75 dB (±4 clinical units) as in Fraser and McKay [14].

Multichannel MDTs

Stimuli

All stimuli were 300-ms biphasic pulse trains. The pulse phase duration was 100 µs; the inter-phase gap was 20 µs. The stimulation rate was 500 pps/electrode (ppse), resulting in a cumulative stimulation rate of 2000 pps. The modulation frequency was 10 Hz or 100 Hz. The component electrodes for the 4-channel stimuli were the same as used for single-channel modulation detection. The loudness-balanced current levels for each component electrodes were used for the 4-channel stimulus. The four channels were interleaved in time with an inter-pulse interval of 500 µs. Because of multichannel loudness summation, the 4-channel stimulus was louder than the single-channel stimuli [28–29]. To see the effects of loudness summation on modulation sensitivity, multichannel MDTs were also measured after loudness-balancing the 4-channel stimulus to the same single-channel references used for the single-channel loudness balancing. Thus, 4-channel MDTs were measured with and without adjustment for loudness summation.

Coherent sinusoidal AM was applied to all four electrodes as a percentage of the carrier pulse train amplitude according to $[f(t)][1+m\sin(2\pi f_m t)]$, where $f(t)$ is a steady-state pulse train, m is the modulation index, and f_m is the modulation frequency. All stimuli were presented via research interface [23].

Loudness Balancing

The loudness-balanced current levels for the component electrodes were used as the initial stimulation levels for the 4-channel stimulus. The four-channel stimulus was loudness-balanced to the same single-channel reference stimuli used for

single-channel loudness balancing (channel C, 500 pps, 25% or 50% DR) using the same adaptive procedure as for the single-channel loudness balancing. The current amplitude of the 4-channel probe was globally adjusted (in dB) according to subject response, thereby adjusting the amplitude for each electrode by the same ratio. Thus, the 4-channel stimulus was equally loud to the single-channel stimuli at the 25 LL and at the 50 LL presentation levels.

Modulation Detection

Multichannel MDTs were measured using the same adaptive, 3AFC procedure as used for single-channel modulation detection. The modulation depth applied to all 4 electrodes was adjusted according to subject response. Potential AM loudness cues were controlled using the same AM loudness compensation and level roving methods used for single-channel modulation detection. Additionally, the reference current levels within the 4-channel stimulus were independently jittered by ±0.75 dB to reduce any loudness differences across the component electrodes.

Results

Figure 1 shows individual and mean single-channel MDTs for the different listening conditions. Overall MDTs were highly variable across subjects, with subjects exhibiting relatively good (S1, S2, S5, S9) or poor modulation sensitivity (S3, S4, S8). Across modulation frequencies, mean MDTs were 7.57 dB better (lower) at the higher presentation level than at the lower level. Across presentation levels, mean MDTs were 7.05 dB better (lower) with the 10 Hz modulation frequency than with the 100 Hz modulation frequency. MDTs were variable across channel locations. Mean MDTs (across subjects) differed by as much as 5.74 dB across channels. For individual subjects, MDTs differed across channels by as little as 1.77 dB (S6, 25 LL, 100 Hz) to as much as 15.55 dB (S6, 50 LL, 10 Hz). A three-way repeated-measures

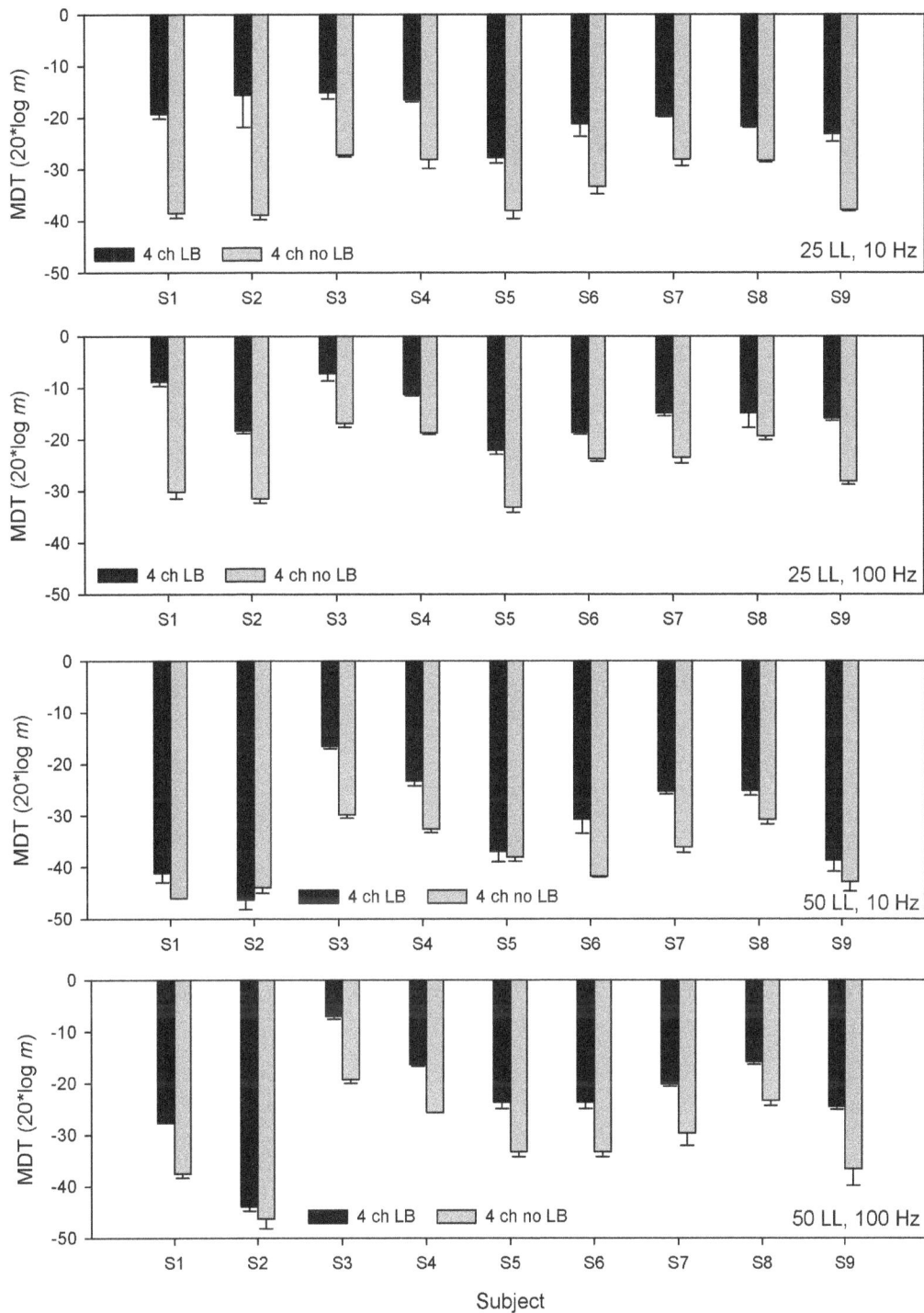

Figure 3. Multichannel MDTs for individual CI subjects. From top to bottom, the panels show 10-Hz MDTs at 25 LL, 100-Hz MDTs at 25 LL, 10-Hz MDTs at 50 LL, 100-Hz MDTs at 50 LL, respectively. The black bars show the MDTs for the 4-channel loudness-balanced stimuli (i.e., equally loud as the single-channel stimuli in Fig. 1) and the gray bars show MDTs for the 4-channel stimuli without loudness-balancing (i.e., louder than the single-channel stimuli in Fig. 1 and the 4-channel loudness-balanced stimuli). The error bars show the standard error.

analysis of variance (RM ANOVA) was performed on the data, with presentation level (25 LL, 50 LL), modulation frequency (10 Hz, 100 Hz), and stimulation site (A, B, C, or D) as factors. Results showed significant effects of presentation level [F(1,8) = 46.488, p<0.001], modulation frequency [F(1,8) = 39.665, p<0.001], and stimulation site [F(3,24) = 4.545,

p = 0.012]. There was a significant interaction only between presentation level and modulation frequency [F(1,8) = 7.043, p = 0.029], most likely due to ceiling effects with the higher presentation level, especially for the 10 Hz modulation frequency. At very small modulation depths, the amplitude resolution may limit modulation sensitivity as the current level difference between

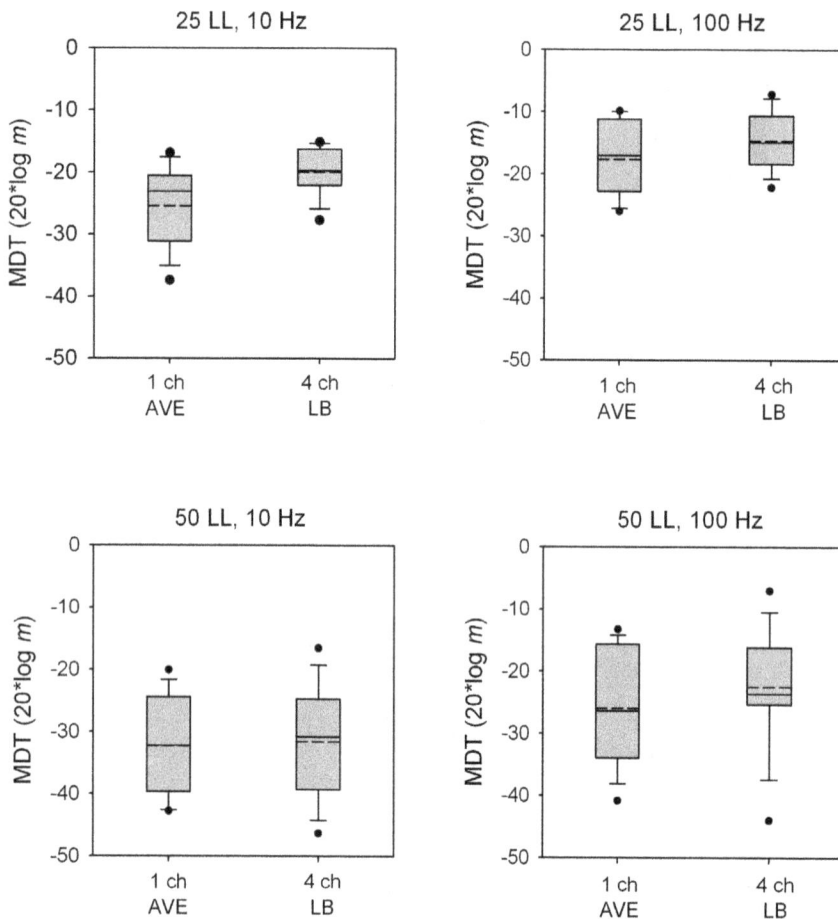

Figure 4. MDTs for equally loud single- and multi-channel stimuli. Box plots are shown for MDTs averaged across the best single channel or with the 4-channel loudness-balanced stimuli; note that all stimuli were equally loud. From left to right, the panels show data for the 25 LL/10 Hz, 25 LL/100 Hz, 50 LL/10 Hz, 50 LL/100 Hz conditions. In each box, the solid line shows the median, the dashed line shows the mean, the error bars show the 10th and 90th percentiles, and the black circles show outliers.

the peak and valley of the modulation may be the same as or even less than each current level unit, which is approximately 0.2 dB.

Although the 3-way RM ANOVA showed a significant main effect of channel, there were individual differences in terms of the across-site variability in MDTs, with different best and worst channels for individual subjects. Additional 3-way ANOVAs were performed on individual subject data, with presentation level, modulation frequency and stimulation site as factors; the results are shown in Table 2. Significant effects were observed for presentation level in all 9 subjects, modulation frequency in 8 of 9 subjects, and stimulation site in 6 of 9 subjects. Post-hoc analyses showed that the best and worst stimulation sites differed among subjects.

Figure 2 shows the current level adjustment to the 4-channel stimulus needed to maintain equal loudness to the 500 pps, single-channel reference (electrode C at 25% and 50% DR). For the 4-channel stimuli, the current level adjustments were highly variable, ranging from 0.95 dB (subject S5 at the 50% DR reference) to 4.95 dB (subject S4 at the 25% DR reference). A one-way RM ANOVA showed no significant effect for reference level [F(1,8) = 2.398, p = 0.160], suggesting that loudness summation was similar at the relatively low and high presentation levels.

Figure 3 shows individual subjects' multichannel MDTs for the different listening conditions. The black bars show MDTs for the 4-channel loudness-balanced stimuli, which were as loud as the

single-channel stimuli shown in Figure 1. The gray bars show MDTs for the 4-channel stimuli without loudness-balancing, which were louder than the single-channel stimuli shown in Figure 1 and the 4-channel loudness-balanced stimuli. As with the single-channel MDTs, multichannel MDTs were generally better with the higher presentation level (50 LL) and the lower modulation frequency (10 Hz). In every case, 4-channel MDTs were poorer when current levels were reduced to match the loudness of the single-channel stimuli. A three-way RM ANOVA was performed on the data, with presentation level (25 LL, 50 LL), modulation frequency (10 Hz, 100 Hz), and loudness summation (4-channel with or without loudness-balancing) as factors. Results showed significant effects of presentation level [F(1,8) = 18.13, p = 0.003], modulation frequency [F(1,8) = 54.967, p<0.001], and loudness summation [F(1,8) = 97.287, p<0.001].

Figure 4 shows boxplots for MDTs averaged across single channels or with the 4-channel loudness-balanced stimuli. Note that all stimuli were equally loud. Across all conditions, the average single-channel MDT was 3.13 dB better (lower) than with the 4-channel loudness-balanced stimuli; mean differences ranged from 0.70 dB for the 50 LL/10 Hz condition to 5.44 dB for the 25 LL/10 Hz condition. A Wilcoxon signed rank test showed that the average single-channel MDT was significantly better than that with the 4-channel loudness-balanced stimuli (p = 0.003). Similarly, a ranked sign test showed that MDTs with the best single

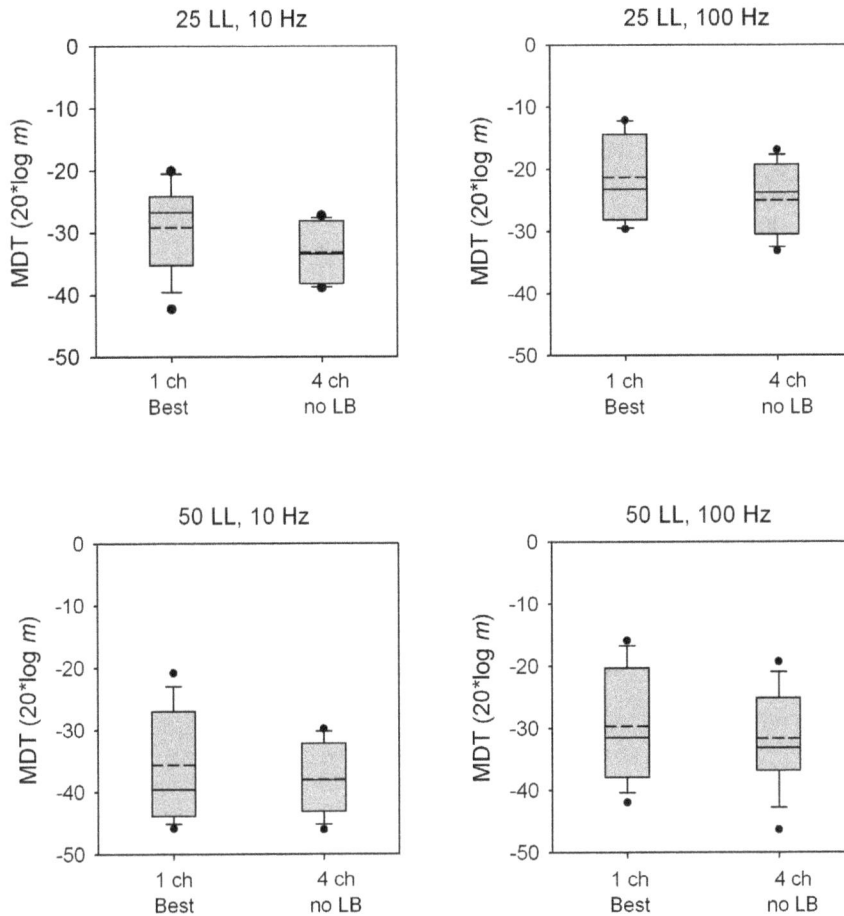

Figure 5. MDTs for single- and multi-channel stimuli without loudness summation compensation. Box plots are shown for MDTs with the best single-channel or with the 4-channel stimuli without loudness-balancing; note that the 4-channel stimuli without loudness-balancing were louder than the single-channel stimuli. From left to right, the panels show data for the 25 LL/10 Hz, 25 LL/100 Hz, 50 LL/10 Hz, 50 LL/100 Hz conditions. In each box, the solid line shows the median, the dashed line shows the mean, the error bars show the 10th and 90th percentiles, and the black circles show outliers.

channel were significantly better than those with the 4-channel loudness-balanced stimuli (p<0.001). Finally, a ranked sign test showed that the difference between MDTs with the worst single channel and with the 4-channel loudness-balanced stimuli failed to achieve significance (p = 0.052).

Figure 5 shows boxplots for MDTs with the best single channel or with the 4-channel stimuli with no loudness compensation. Thus, the 4-channel stimuli were louder than the single-channel stimuli. Across all conditions, the mean MDT was 3.01 dB better with the 4-channel stimuli than with the best single channel; mean differences ranged from 1.97 dB for the 50 LL/100 Hz condition to 3.97 dB for the 25 LL/10 Hz condition. A paired t-test across all conditions showed that MDTs were significantly better with the 4-channel stimuli than with the best single channel (p = 0.001).

As shown in Figure 1, across-site variability in MDTs differed greatly across subjects. It is possible that subjects with greater across-site variability may attend more to the single channel with the best modulation sensitivity when listening to the 4-channel stimuli. Similarly, subjects with less across-site variability may better integrate information across all channels in the 4-channel stimuli. The mean across-site variance in single-channel MDTs was calculated for individual subjects across the presentation level and modulation frequency test conditions, as in Garadat et al. [16]. Across all subjects, the mean variance was 10.08 dB^2, and

ranged from 3.91 dB^2 (subject S4) to 19.07 dB^2 (subject S1). Individual subjects' mean across-site variance was compared to the multichannel advantage (with no loudness compensation) in modulation detection over the best single channel without loudness-balancing (i.e., 4-channel MDT − best single-channel MDT). Linear regression analysis showed no significant relationship between the degree of multichannel advantage and across-site variance (r^2 = 0.181, p = 0.253).

As shown in Figure 3, performance with 4-channel stimuli was much poorer when the current levels were reduced to match the loudness of single-channel stimuli. Figure 2 shows great inter-subject variability in terms of multichannel loudness summation. It is possible that the degree of multichannel loudness summation may be related to the deficit in multichannel modulation sensitivity after compensating for loudness summation. The mean loudness summation across both presentation levels was calculated for individual subjects, and was compared to the difference in MDTs between 4-channel stimuli with and without loudness-balancing. Linear regression analysis showed no significant correlation between the degree of multichannel loudness summation and the difference in MDTs between the 4-channel stimuli with or without loudness compensation (r^2 = 0.014, p = 0.79).

Discussion

The present data suggest that, at equal loudness, MDTs were poorer with 4 channels than with a single channel, most likely due to the lower current levels in the 4-channel stimuli needed to maintain equal loudness to the single-channel stimuli. With no compensation for loudness multichannel summation, MDTs were significantly better with 4-channel stimuli than with the best single channel, suggesting some multichannel advantage. Below, we discuss the results in greater detail.

Effects of Presentation Level and Modulation Frequency

With single- or multi-channel stimulation, MDTs generally improved as the presentation level was increased and/or the modulation frequency was decreased, consistent with many previous studies [4], [6], [9–10], [12], [14–15], [22]. Across the single- and 4-channel conditions in Experiments 1 and 2, mean MDTs were 7.67 dB better with the 50 LL than with the 25 LL presentation level, and 7.07 dB better with the 10 Hz than with the 100 Hz modulation frequency.

Effect of Loudness Summation on Multichannel MDTs

At equal loudness, 4-channel MDTs were significantly poorer than the average single-channel MDT (Fig. 4); 4-channel MDTs were also significantly poorer after compensating for multichannel loudness summation (Fig. 3). In both cases, the deficits were presumably due to lower current levels on each channel needed to compensate for multichannel loudness summation. MDTs are very level dependent, especially at lower presentation levels [6], [8–10], [15]. The present data suggest that at equal loudness, single-channel estimates of modulation sensitivity may greatly over-estimate the functional sensitivity when multiple channels are stimulated. In clinical speech processors, current levels must often be reduced to accommodate multichannel loudness summation. The present data suggests that such current level adjustments may worsen multichannel modulation sensitivity.

Loudness summation was not significantly correlated with the difference in MDTs between 4-channel stimuli with or without loudness compensation. This may reflect individual subject variability in modulation sensitivity, especially at presentation low levels. Such variability has been reported in many studies [6], [8–10], [13–14]. Thus, some subjects may have been more susceptible than others to the level differences between the 4-channel stimuli with and without loudness compensation.

Note that in the present study, we were unable to measure single-channel MDTs at the component channel stimulation levels used in the 4-channel loudness-balanced stimuli. After the current adjustment to accommodate multichannel loudness summation, the component channel current levels were often too low (i.e., below detection thresholds) to measure single-channel MDTs.

Multichannel loudness summation may also explain some of the advantage of multichannel stimulation observed by Geurts and Wouters [17] in AM frequency discrimination. Similar to their findings, the present data showed that multichannel stimulation without loudness compensation offered a small but significant advantage over the best single channel. In Guerts and Wouters [17] there was no level adjustment to equate loudness between the single- and multi-channel stimuli. If such a level adjustment had been applied to the multichannel stimuli, AM frequency discrimination may have better with single than with multiple channels, as in the present study with modulation detection. Future studies may wish to examine how component channels contribute to AM frequency discrimination in a multichannel context in which loudness summation does not play a role.

Contribution of Single Channels to Multichannel MDTs

Across-site variability was not significantly correlated with the multichannel advantage over the best single channel, suggesting that CI subjects combined information across channels, instead of relying on the channels with best temporal processing, even when there was great variability in modulation sensitivity across stimulation sites. This finding is in agreement with recent multichannel MDI studies in CI users [18,21] that suggest that multichannel envelope processing is more centrally than peripherally mediated.

Implications for Cochlear Implant Signal Processing

The present data suggest that accommodating multichannel loudness summation, as is necessary when fitting clinical speech processors, may reduce CI users' functional modulation sensitivity. When high stimulation rates are used on each channel, the functional temporal processing may be further compromised, as the current levels must be reduced to accommodate summation due to high per-channel rates and multichannel stimulation. Selecting a reduced set of optimal channels (ideally, those with the best temporal processing) to use within a clinical speech processor may reduce loudness summation, allowing for higher current levels to be used on each channel. Such optimal selection of channels has been studied by Garadat et al. [16], who found better speech understanding in noise when only the channels with better temporal processing were included in the speech processor. In that study, subjects were allowed to adjust the speech processor volume for the experimental maps, which may have compensated for the reduced loudness associated with the reduced-electrode maps, possibly resulting in higher stimulation levels on each channel. Bilateral signal processing may also allow for fewer numbers of electrodes within each side, thereby reducing loudness summation, increasing current levels, and thereby improving temporal processing. The reduced numbers of channels on each ear may be combined, as the spectral holes on one side are filled in by the other. Such optimized "zipper processors" have been explored by Zhou and Pfingst [30], who found better speech performance in some subjects, presumably due to the increased functional spectral resolution. Using fewer channels within each speech processor may have also reduced loudness summation, resulting in higher current levels and better temporal processing.

Loudness summation and spatio-temporal channel interactions should be carefully considered to improve the spectral resolution and temporal processing for future CI signal processing strategies. It is possible that by selecting a fewer number of optimal electrodes (in terms of temporal processing and key spectral cues) within each stimulation frame would reduce the instantaneous loudness summation, allowing for higher current levels that might produce better temporal processing. Using relatively low stimulation rates (e.g., 250–500 Hz/channel) might help reduce channel interaction between adjacent electrodes. Zigzag stimulation patterns which maximize the space between electrodes in sequential stimulation (e.g., electrode 1, then 9, then 5, then 13, then 3, then 11, etc.) might also help to channel interaction.

Conclusions

Single- and multi-channel modulation detection was measured in CI users. Significant findings include:

1. Effects of presentation level and modulation frequency were similar for both single- and multi-channel MDTs; performance improved as the presentation level was increased or the modulation frequency was decreased.

2. At equal loudness, single-channel MDTs may greatly over-estimate multichannel modulation sensitivity, due to the lower current levels needed to accommodate loudness summation in the latter.

3. When there was no level compensation for loudness summation, multichannel MDTs were significantly better than MDTs with the best single channel.

4. There was great inter-subject variability in terms of multi-channel loudness summation. However, the degree of loudness summation was not significantly correlated with the deficit in modulation sensitivity when current levels were reduced to accommodate multichannel loudness summation.

5. There was also great inter-subject variability in the across-site variance observed for single-channel MDTs. However, across-site variability was not significantly correlated with the

multichannel advantage over the best single-channel. This suggests that CI listeners combined information across multiple channels rather that attend primarily to the channels with the best modulation sensitivity.

Acknowledgments

We thank all implant subjects for their participation, Joseph Crew for help with data collection, as well as Monita Chatterjee, David Landsberger, Bob Shannon, Justin Aronoff, and Robert Carlyon for helpful comments.

Author Contributions

Conceived and designed the experiments: JJG QF. Performed the experiments: JJG SO. Analyzed the data: JJG SO QF DB. Contributed reagents/materials/analysis tools: QF. Wrote the paper: JJG SO QF DB.

References

1. Cazals Y, Pelizzone M, Saudan O, Boex C (1994) Low-pass filtering in amplitude modulation detection associated with vowel and consonant identification in subjects with cochlear implants. J Acoust Soc Am 96: 2048–2054.

2. Fu QJ (2002) Temporal processing and speech recognition in cochlear implant users Neuroreport 13: 1635–1640.

3. Colletti V, Shannon RV (2005) Open set speech perception with auditory brainstem implant. Laryngoscope 115: 1974–1978.

4. Shannon RV (1992) Temporal modulation transfer functions in patients with cochlear implants. J Acoust Soc Am 91: 2156–2164.

5. Busby PA, Tong Y, Clark GM (1993) The perception of temporal modulations by cochlear implant patients. J Acoust Soc Am 94: 124–131.

6. Donaldson GS, Viemeister NF (2000) Intensity discrimination and detection of amplitude modulation in electric hearing. J Acoust Soc Am 108: 760–763.

7. Chatterjee M, Robert ME (2001) Noise enhances modulation sensitivity in cochlear implant listeners: stochastic resonance in a prosthetic sensory system? J Assoc Res Otolaryngol 2: 159–171.

8. Galvin JJ 3rd, Fu QJ (2005) Effects of stimulation rate mode and level on modulation detection by cochlear implant users. J Assoc Res Otolaryng 6: 269–279.

9. Galvin JJ 3rd, Fu QJ (2009) Influence of stimulation rate and loudness growth on modulation detection and intensity discrimination in cochlear implant users. Hear Res 250: 46–54.

10. Pfingst BE, Xu L, Thompson CS (2007) Effects of carrier pulse rate and stimulation site on modulation detection by subjects with cochlear implants. J Acoust Soc Am 121: 2236–2246.

11. Arora K, Vandali A, Dowell R, Dawson P (2011) Effects of stimulation rate on modulation detection and speech recognition by cochlear implant users. Int J Audiol 50: 123–132.

12. Chatterjee M, Oberzut C (2011) Detection and rate discrimination of amplitude modulation in electrical hearing. J Acoust Soc Am 130: 1567–1580.

13. Green T, Faulkner A, Rosen S (2012) Variations in carrier pulse rate and the perception of amplitude modulation in cochlear implant users Ear Hear 33: 221–230.

14. Fraser M, McKay CM (2012) Temporal modulation transfer functions in cochlear implantees using a method that limits overall loudness cues. Hear Res 283: 59–69.

15. Chatterjee M, Oba SI (2005) Noise improves modulation detection by cochlear implant listeners at moderate carrier levels. J Acoust Soc Am 118: 993–1002.

16. Garadat SN, Zwolan TA, Pfingst BE (2012) Across-site patterns of modulation detection: Relation to speech recognition. J. Acoust. Soc. Am 131: 4030–4041.

17. Geurts L, Wouters J (2001) Coding of the fundamental frequency in continuous interleaved sampling processors for cochlear implants. J Acoust Soc Am 109: 713–726.

18. Chatterjee M (2003) Modulation masking in cochlear implant listeners: envelope versus tonotopic components. J Acoust Soc Am 113: 2042–2053.

19. Dau T, Kollmeier B, Kohlrausch A (1997a) Modeling auditory processing of amplitude modulation. I. Detection and masking with narrow-band carriers. J Acoust Soc Am 102: 2892–2905.

20. Dau T, Kollmeier B, Kohlrausch A (1997b) Modeling auditory processing of amplitude modulation. II. Spectral and temporal integration. J Acoust Soc Am 102: 2906–2919.

21. Kreft HA, Nelson DA, Oxenham AJ (2013) Modulation frequency discrimination with modulated and unmodulated interference in normal hearing and in cochlear-implant users. J Assoc Res Otolaryngol 14: 591–601.

22. Galvin JJ 3rd, Fu QJ, Oba SI (2013) A method to dynamically control unwanted loudness cues when measuring amplitude modulation detection in cochlear implant users. J Neurosci Methods DOI information: 10.1016/j.jneumeth.2013.10.016.

23. Wygonski J, Robert ME (2002) HEI Nucleus Research Interface HEINRI Specification Internal materials.

24. Jesteadt W (1980) An adaptive procedure for subjective judgments. Percept Psychophys 28: 85–88.

25. Zeng FG, Turner CW (1991) Binaural loudness matches in unilaterally impaired listeners Quarterly. J Exp Psych 43: 565–583.

26. McKay CM, Henshall KR (2010) Amplitude modulation and loudness in cochlear implantees. J Assoc Res Otolaryng 11: 101–111.

27. Levitt H (1971) Transformed up-down methods in psychoacoustics. J Acoust Soc Am 49 Supp 2: 467.

28. McKay CM, Remine MD, McDermott HJ (2001) Loudness summation for pulsatile electrical stimulation of the cochlea: effects of rate, electrode separation, level, and mode of stimulation. J Acoust Soc Am 110: 1514–1524.

29. McKay CM, Henshall KR, Farrell RJ, McDermott HJ (2003) A practical method of predicting the loudness of complex electrical stimuli. J Acoust Soc Am 113: 2054–2063.

30. Zhou N, Pfingst BE (2012) Psychophysically based site selection coupled with dichotic stimulation improves speech recognition in noise with bilateral cochlear implants. J Acoust Soc Am 132: 994–1008.

15

Self-Esteem in Hearing-Impaired Children: The Influence of Communication, Education, and Audiological Characteristics

Stephanie C. P. M. Theunissen[1]*, Carolien Rieffe[2,3], Anouk P. Netten[1], Jeroen J. Briaire[1], Wim Soede[1], Maartje Kouwenberg[2], Johan H. M. Frijns[1,4]

1 Department of Otorhinolaryngology and Head & Neck Surgery, Leiden University Medical Center, Leiden, The Netherlands, 2 Department of Developmental Psychology, Leiden University, Leiden, The Netherlands, 3 Dutch Foundation for the Deaf and Hard of Hearing Child, Amsterdam, The Netherlands, 4 Leiden Institute for Brain and Cognition, Leiden, The Netherlands

Abstract

Objective: Sufficient self-esteem is extremely important for psychosocial functioning. It is hypothesized that hearing-impaired (HI) children have lower levels of self-esteem, because, among other things, they frequently experience lower language and communication skills. Therefore, the aim of this study was to compare HI children's self-esteem across different domains with those of normal hearing (NH) children and to investigate the influence of communication, type of education, and audiological characteristics.

Methods: This large (N = 252) retrospective, multicenter study consisted of two age- and gender-matched groups: 123 HI children and 129 NH controls (mean age = 11.8 years). Self-reports were used to measure self-esteem across four domains: perceived social acceptance by peers, perceived parental attention, perceived physical appearance, and global self-esteem.

Results: HI children experienced lower levels of self-esteem regarding peers and parents than NH controls. Particularly HI children who attended special education for the deaf were at risk, even after correcting for their language development and intelligence. Yet, levels of global self-esteem and self-esteem involving physical appearance in HI children equalled those of NH controls. Furthermore, younger age at implantation and longer duration of having cochlear implants (CIs) were related to higher levels of self-esteem.

Conclusion: HI children experience lower levels of self-esteem in the social domains. Yet, due to the heterogeneity of the HI population, there is high variability in levels of self-esteem.

Discussion: Clinicians must always be aware of the risk and protective factors related to self-esteem in order to help individual patients reach their full potential.

Editor: Brett Thombs, McGill University, Canada

Funding: This research was supported by the Innovational Research Incentives Scheme (a VIDI grant) by The Netherlands Organisation for Scientific Research (NWO), no. 452-07-004 to Carolien Rieffe. The funders had no role in study design, data collection and analysis, decision to publish, or preparation of the manuscript.

Competing Interests: The authors have declared that no competing interests exist.

* E-mail: s.c.p.m.theunissen@lumc.nl

Introduction

Self-esteem refers to one's general evaluation or appraisal of the self, including feelings of self-worth [1]. Besides an evaluation of the self, self-esteem also denotes how one values oneself. This basic appreciation of the self has effects on multiple dimensions in our lives, such as our friendships, our successes, and our academic career. Moreover, individuals with higher levels of self-esteem are better able to cope with stressful life events [1], whereas lower levels of self-esteem are associated with more loneliness, peer rejection, aggression, delinquency, and psychopathology [2–6]. Hence, it is of the utmost importance to have a sufficient level of self-esteem.

One would assume that hearing-impaired (HI) individuals encounter more difficulties regarding their self-esteem because they often face multiple challenges, such as speech and language delays, communication problems, and less or no access to the sound-dominated world [7]. These problems could potentially harm HI children's level of self-esteem, resulting in for example less stable friendships and more bullying [8]. Well-developed language and communication skills have been linked to higher levels of self-esteem [9]. Nowadays, deaf children who can have no or minimal benefit from conventional hearing aids receive cochlear implants (CIs), which considerably change and often improved outcomes for them in the aforementioned domains [10,11]. Recently, CI recipients have been found to have levels of self-esteem that equal those of NH children [12,13], which emphasizes the importance of adequate language development for self-esteem.

Studies that looked at levels of self-esteem in a more heterogeneous group of HI children showed inconsistent results. When compared to normal hearing (NH) peers, some researchers reported lower self-esteem in children with mild to profound hearing losses [14–16], while others demonstrated that levels of self-esteem were similar to those of NH counterparts [12,13,17–19]. In the literature, no consensus has been reached for the effect of type of education on HI children's self-esteem: some researchers showed higher self-esteem in HI children attending mainstream education than the ones attending special education, whereas others found no difference [19–21]. Possibly, HI children evaluate their abilities differently in different school contexts. Whilst HI children attending special schools evaluate themselves within a compatible peer group, HI children in a mainstream setting will compare themselves with their hearing peers. [21]. Conversely, it could also be argued that HI children attending mainstream schools actually feel a higher self-worth, because they are able to fit in with hearing peers, which can be perceived as a major achievement.

Self-esteem is often conceptualized as being multidimensional, consisting of several specific domains that are related to various facets of life (e.g. perceived parental attention, social acceptance by peers and physical appearance), as well as a more general view of oneself, often called 'global self-esteem' [3,22]. Levels of self-esteem can vary considerably across these different domains, particularly during adolescence, as this is a transition phase marked by crucial emotional and behavioral changes [3,23]. Parents become less influential, while close friends' and classmates' judgments become increasingly important [24]. Attention to and perception of one's physical appearance also increase. A child may be at risk of low self-esteem in one specific domain but not in another [21]. Although it has been postulated that self-esteem interventions do not directly improve outcomes, being aware of these distinctions can support the caregiver when helping or counseling the child [2].

Besides the contrasting findings of past research regarding differences in HI and NH children's levels of global self-esteem, there is a paucity of data concerning the more specific domains of self-esteem in HI children compared to NH children. Only a few studies have reported on specific domains of self-esteem in HI children when compared to NH controls. These found that the HI children had more difficulties regarding peer acceptance and family relations although they felt equally confident about their physical appearance [15,19,25]. To the best of our knowledge, no other studies have been performed to date in which these specific domains were studied and compared in both HI and NH children.

Hence, our goal here was not only to investigate the level of global self-esteem in a large and diverse sample of HI and NH children and adolescents, but also to examine three more specific domains of self-esteem: perceived social acceptance by peers, perceived parental attention and perceived physical appearance. Secondly, we wanted to study whether language development and communication skills, type of education, and audiological characteristics would influence the level of self-esteem. Based on (the majority of) the existing literature, we expected that adequate communication skills would result in higher self-esteem [9,12,13] and that children attending special education would have lower self-esteem than children in mainstream education [19–21]. Concerning audiological factors, no recent studies were available on which to base our predictions. Therefore, we have performed several explorative analyses to see whether relations between these factors and the different domains of self-esteem exist.

Materials and Methods

Participants

A total of 252 children (Mean age $= 11.8$ years, $SD = 1.7$) participated in this study of which 123 were HI children and 129 were NH controls. All children had a nonverbal IQ of at least 80, and no other known learning problems. Children were not included if they experienced comorbidities such as visual impairment or Autism Spectrum Disorders. The HI children were included if they experienced a loss of at least 40 decibels in the best ear, which was detected prelingually (<3 years) or perilingually (3–5 years). Table 1 shows the characteristics of all included children. For the CI recipients specifically, the mean age at implantation was 3.8 years ($SD = 2.7$; range $= 0.9$–10.8 years). The mean duration of CI use was 8.3 years ($SD = 2.6$; range 0.8–13.0 years). Most CI users ($n = 40$; 76%) had one CI, and 13 (24%) children were bilaterally implanted.

Procedure

The NH controls were recruited from primary and secondary mainstream schools across the Netherlands to reach a geographically and socio-economically diverse sample. To collect a sample that represented the complete spectrum of HI children, we recruited from 14 (both primary and secondary) mainstream schools and special schools for the HI (schools that supported development of auditory and oral skills, with or without the use of signs), 2 hospitals, 5 Speech and Hearing centers or residential schools, and via newsletters in the Netherlands and the Dutch-speaking part of Belgium.

The questionnaire was administered on a laptop. Questions appeared one by one on the screen. Instructions for all tests were provided in the child's preferred mode of communication to ensure that the child understood. The HI children could choose between two versions of the questionnaire: the first version which comprised written items exclusively, and the second version in which each item was presented in written text and sign language simultaneously by means of a video clip in the upper right-hand corner of the screen. Translation from spoken language into sign language was performed by a qualified interpreter and back translation of all signed items showed good convergence with the original items.

Parents or caregivers were requested to complete a questionnaire assessing demographic variables such as net income and level of education. In the HI group, several audiological variables were derived from the child's medical and audiological notes after informed consent was given. SES was calculated as the mean of parental education, job, and net income. Unfortunately, due to privacy reasons, almost half of the parents did not fill out the question concerning net income, so these were not taken into account.

Ethics statement and privacy regulation

Approval for the study was obtained by the Medical Ethics Committee of the Leiden University Medical Center under number P10.137, and carried out in accordance with the standards set out by the Declaration of Helsinki. All parents or caregivers gave written consent for their child's participation prior to data collection. Next to parents and caregivers, all children aged 12 or older gave written consent as well. Before the assessment started, all children were assured that their responses would be processed anonymously.

Table 1. Characteristics of all participants.

	Total sample (N = 252)		HI sample (n = 123)	
	Controls	HI	CI	Hearing aid
Number of children – n	129	123	53	70
Age mean in years (SD)	11.6 (1.3)	12.0 (1.8)	11.9 (2.1)	12.0 (1.7)
Gender - n (%)				
Male	58 (45%)	60 (49%)	24 (45%)	36 (51%)
Female	71 (55%)	63 (51%)	29 (55%)	34 (49%)
Socioeconomic status mean (SD)[a]	12.1 (2.4)	11.5 (2.3)	11.7 (2.3)	11.3 (2.4)
Nonverbal IQ				
IQ norm score Picture arrangement (SD)	10.6 (3.4)	10.2 (3.5)	9.9 (3.5)	10.4 (3.5)
IQ norm score Block design (SD)	10.6 (3.0)	10.4 (3.1)	10.3 (2.8)	10.5 (3.4)
Spoken language skills[b]				
Sentence comprehension (SD)	7.1 (2.3)	6.6 (3.1)	6.6 (3.1)	6.7 (3.1)
Story comprehension (SD)	7.0 (2.5)	6.3 (2.8)	5.6 (3.0)	6.8 (2.6)
Sign language skills[c]				
Sentence comprehension (SD)	-	2.3 (0.9)	2.1 (1.0)	2.3 (1.0)
Story comprehension (SD)	-	2.6 (0.7)	2.8 (0.8)	2.5 (0.7)
Children's Communication Checklist[d]				
General Communication Composite (SD)	73.9 (18.2)	91.3 (18.2)[1]	91.9 (18.4)	90.8 (18.2)
Pragmatic Composite (SD)	36.2 (9.1)	46.6 (8.7)[1]	47.3 (9.1)	46.1 (8.5)
Audiological variables				
Degree of hearing loss - n (%)[e]				
Moderate (40–60 dB)	-	29 (24%)	0 (0%)	29 (41%)[1]
Severe (61–90 dB)	-	25 (20%)	1 (2%)	24 (34%)[1]
Profound (>90 dB)	-	61 (50%)	50 (94%)	11 (16%)[1]
Unknown	-	8 (6%)	2 (4%)	6 (9%)
Preferred mode of communication - n (%)				
Oral language only	-	88 (71%)	36 (68%)	52 (74%)
Sign-supported language	-	33 (27%)	17 (32%)	16 (23%)
Sign language only	-	2 (2%)	0 (0%)	2 (3%)
Type of education – n (%)				
Regular education	-	74 (60%)	32 (60%)	42 (60%)
Special education	-	49 (40%)	21 (40%)	28 (40%)
Mean age at onset in years (SD)	-	1.6 (1.3)	1.2 (0.9)	1.9 (1.5)[2]
Age at onset of hearing loss - n (%)				
Prelingual (<3 yrs)	-	104 (85%)	49 (93%)	55 (79%)[3]
Perilingual (3–5 yrs)	-	12 (10%)	2 (4%)	10 (14%)[3]
Unknown	-	7 (6%)	2 (4%)	5 (7%)
Mean age at 1st hearing aid in years (SD)	-	2.1 (1.4)	1.5 (0.9)	2.6 (1.5)[1]

[a]Socioeconomic status score was measured by parental education, job, and net income. (Unfortunately, due to privacy reasons, almost half of the parents did not fill out the question concerning the net income, so these were not taken into account.)
[b]Spoken language skills were derived from the Clinical Evaluation of Language Fundamentals; see Materials section for more information.
[c]Sign language skills were derived from the Assessment Instrument for Sign Language of the Netherlands; see Materials section for more information.
[d]Higher scores indicate more (social) language problems. More than 70% of the parents responded.
[e]Degree of hearing loss was calculated by averaging unaided hearing thresholds at 500, 1,000, and 2,000 Hertz.
[1]$p < .001$;
[2]$p < .01$;
[3]$p < .05$.

Self-esteem questionnaire

To assess self-esteem, the self-report *Children's Self-Confidence and Acceptance Scale* [26,27] was used, which had only been used in NH children previously. The scale showed a strong convergent validity

with the CBSK, which is the well-established Dutch version of Harter's self-esteem scale (*The Self-Perception Profile for Children* [28,29]). Harter's scale was used because we wanted to address the different specific domains of self-esteem instead of the more general global self-esteem measured by the Rosenberg self-esteem scale [30]. The items of the questionnaire were formulated by a team of child psychologists, targeting key aspects of self-esteem. Sentences were formulated short and simple, so HI children with language comprehension problems would be able to understand these items and respond to them coherently. The reason for choosing a self-report instead of parent or teacher reports is that self-reports give the most accurate scores when measuring self-esteem [31,32].

The questionnaire represents three relevant domain-specific categories, and one overall category, that could be answered on a 3-point Likert scale:

1. The *perceived social acceptance by peers* ('peers', 5 items) domain examines the perception of the child of how well he or she is accepted by peers or feels popular (Example item: "Children ask to play with me").

2. The *perceived parental attention* ('parents', 7 items) domain assesses the self-perceived degree to which parents or caregivers are interested in and give support to the child's thoughts and needs ("My father or mother are happy with me").

3. The *perceived physical appearance* ('physical appearance', 5 items) domain reflects the child's idea of how good-looking or attractive he or she is ("Other children think my appearance is nice").

4. The *global self-esteem* ('global', 5 items) measures the child's perceptions of general statements concerning the self ("I am happy with myself"). These five items address comparable issues to those used in Rosenberg's self-esteem scale [30].

Children were asked to rate the items on a 3-point Likert-type scale (1 = *not true*, 2 = *sometimes true*, 3 = *often true*). The internal consistency was good for both the HI and the NH group (Table 2).

Language development and communication skills

Language development and communication skills were measured because of their known positive influence on self-esteem [9]. Two types of language development were assessed: *sentence comprehension* and *story comprehension*. HI children using spoken language and NH controls received two corresponding subtests of the Dutch version of the *Clinical Evaluation of Language Fundamentals - Fourth Edition* (CELF) [33,34]. HI children who use sign or sign-supported language received specific subtests of the *Assessment Instrument for Sign Language of the Netherlands* [35]. All original language scores were transformed to norm scores and these were corrected for chronological age. The sentence comprehension task was not administered to 10 HI and 16 controls and the story

comprehension task was not administered to 5 HI and 16 NH controls.

The *Children's Communication Checklist version 2* was used to evaluate communication skills indicated by the parents or caregivers [36]. This questionnaire, consisting of 70 items, has been predominantly designed to assess social and pragmatic language of children aged 4 to 16, although it also assesses other qualitative aspects of language. The checklist contains eight scales: speech production, syntax, semantics, coherence, inappropriate initiation, stereotyped conversation, use of context, and non-verbal communication. Two composite scores are conventionally obtained from these scales: the general communication composite (GCC) and the pragmatic composite (PC). Each item can be scored from 0 (*never or less than once a week*) to 3 (*several times a day or always*). Higher scores indicate more (social) language problems. To the parents of the HI children using sign or sign-supported language, the speech production and syntax scales were not administered.

Intelligence

An index of the nonverbal intelligence was obtained with two tests from the *Wechsler Intelligence Scale for Children - Third Edition*: block design by copying geometric designs with cubes, and picture arrangement by sequencing pictures to make logical stories [37,38]. All raw scores were converted into age-equivalent norm scores based on Dutch standards (10 = average). A random sampling ($n = 23$) across HI children who were previously assessed with a complete intelligence test (either the Snijders-Oomen nonverbal intelligence test [39] or the WISC) showed a high correlation between the scores of our tests and the IQ score, $r = .79$, $p < .001$. The tasks were not administered to 8 HI and 17 NH children, due to time constraints.

Statistical analyses

First, in order to compare the levels of the specific domains of self-esteem between HI and NH children, Multivariate Analysis of Variance (MANOVA) and Multivariate Analysis of Covariance (MANCOVA) were used. In the MANCOVAs, several covariates were incorporated one by one, including intelligence, socio-economic status (SES) and language and communication skills. For the second and third research questions (i.e., influence of communication skills and type of education on the different domains of self-esteem, respectively) MANCOVAs were performed, and confounding variables were included one by one in case of group differences. Several continuous audiological factors (e.g., duration of CI use, age at implantation) and their association with the different domains of self-esteem were addressed by Pearson's correlations. Nominal variables (uni- or bilateral CI, pre-

Table 2. Psychometric properties of the four domains of self-esteem.

	Range	Number of items	Inter-item correlation	Cronbach's Alpha	
				HI	NH controls
Domains of self-esteem					
Perceived social acceptance by peers	1–3	5	.75	.74	.75
Perceived parental attention	1–3	7	.34	.76	.75
Perceived physical appearance	1–3	5	.46	.83	.78
Global self-esteem	1–3	5	.25	.66	.60

or perilingual onset of HI) were compared by means of MANOVAs. When a score or variable was not available, the participant was excluded from the analysis concerned. It was checked whether there were group differences on age, gender, SES, and type of hearing device between those who completed and those who did not complete all the questionnaires and this was not the case. The program *Statistical Packages for the Social Sciences* (version 20.0) was used.

Results

Self-esteem in HI versus NH children

Regarding global self-esteem, the scores of NH and HI children did not significantly differ ($\Delta = -.007$, $p = .881$). To compare the groups with respect to their specific domains of self-esteem, a MANOVA was carried out with group (NH or HI) as the between-subjects variable and the levels of self-esteem in each of the specific domains as the within-subjects variable. This analysis revealed a main effect for self-esteem $F_{HF}(1.62, 403.73) = 56.78$, $p<.001$ $\eta_p^2 = .19$, and for group $F(1, 250) = 11.77$, $p = .001$ $\eta_p^2 = .05$ which was qualified by a group x self-esteem interaction effect $F_{HF}(1.62, 403.73) = 6.16$, $p<.01$ $\eta_p^2 = .02$. Post-hoc t-tests showed that HI children had lower self-esteem than NH controls on two domains: the peers' domain ($\Delta = .20$, $p<.002$) and the parents' domain ($\Delta = .20$, $p<.001$) (Figure 1). For the physical appearance domain, no significant group difference was found. A MANCOVA was performed in which we controlled for several important variables (age, gender, intelligence, and SES). The above-described effects retained their significance, so these results were omitted from the results presented here.

When comparing children wearing HAs with those using CIs, the groups did not significantly differ on their level of global self-esteem ($\Delta = .086$, $p = .18$). A 2 (HA or CI) x 3 (domains of self-esteem) MANOVA also revealed no significant differences between the groups in the different domains of self-esteem $F(1, 121) = .014$, $p = .91$ $\eta_p^2<.001$.

Language development, communication skills and self-esteem

As expected on the basis of past research, t-tests revealed that HI children had lower language and communication skills than NH children (story comprehension, $\Delta = .8$, $p<.038$, general communication composite, $\Delta = 17.4$, $p<.001$, and pragmatic composite, $\Delta = 10.4$, $p<.001$, respectively). Therefore, a 2 (group: HI or NH) x 3 (domains of self-esteem) MANCOVA corrected for language development and communication skills was carried out. Again a main effect for group was detected, which was qualified by a group x self-esteem interaction effect: *Wilks'* $\Lambda = .96$ $F(2, 165) = 3.80$ $p = .024$ $\eta_p^2 = .044$. Post-hoc MANCOVAs showed slightly different results than the MANOVAs: HI children still reported lower self-esteem with respect to the parents' domain $F(1, 216) = 4.89$ $p = .028$, whereas differences in the peers' domain were no longer statistically significant $F(1, 216) = .03$ $p = .86$.

Type of education and self-esteem

In order to properly examine levels of self-esteem between HI children in special education (for the HI or deaf) and in mainstream education, these two groups were compared on several factors: age, gender, intelligence, SES, and language and communication skills. HI children attending mainstream education had significantly better language skills ($\Delta = 3.17$, $p<.001$), higher intelligence scores ($\Delta = 2.22$, $p<.001$), and higher communication skills ($\Delta = -22.69$, $p<.001$) than children attending special education.

Regarding global self-esteem, the scores of HI children attending mainstream education did not significantly differ from those attending special education ($\Delta = .10$, $p = .14$). A 2 (type of school: special or mainstream) x 3 (domains of self-esteem) MANCOVA which corrected for language development, communication skills and intelligence revealed a significant difference in the parents' domain only, with children in mainstream education scoring higher then children attending special education: *Wilks'* $\Lambda = .82$ $F(3, 67) = 4.87$ $p = .004$ $\eta_p^2 = .18$.

Audiological factors

Finally, a series of Pearson's correlations were carried out to see which continuous audiological factors were associated with the specific domains of self-esteem (Table 3). For the peers' and physical appearance domains and for global self-esteem, no significant associations were detected. However, for the parents' domain, younger age at implantation, and consequent longer duration of having CIs, were related to higher self-esteem: $r (47) = -.359$ $p = .006$ and $r (47) = .376$ $p = .004$ respectively. These correlations remained significant when a correction for age and language development was performed, using partial correlation analyses: $r (41) = -.28$ $p = .035$ and $r (41) = .28$ $p = .034$ respectively. To analyze differences within the CI group between two nominal variables (i.e. uni- or bilateral implantation, and pre- or perilingual detection of hearing loss), a MANOVA was carried out for each variable. The independent variables were uni- or bilateral implantation and pre- or perilingual onset of hearing loss, and the dependent variables were the 3 specific domains of self-esteem. No differences between the groups were found: *Wilks'* $\Lambda = 1.0$ $F(3, 49) = .06$ $p = .98$ $\eta_p^2 = .004$ and *Wilks'* $\Lambda = .94$ $F(3, 112) = 2.37$ $p = .075$ $\eta_p^2 = .06$ respectively.

Discussion

Self-esteem is a principal prerequisite for healthy psychosocial development and enables children to adjust to stress or burdens [40]. HI children often face demanding situations, so it might be even more important for them to have sufficient levels of self-esteem. By tapping into self-esteem across a number of domains, a differentiated picture of self-esteem was obtained. First, we found that the levels of global self-esteem and perceived physical appearance of HI children did not significantly differ from those of NH controls, despite the former group wearing external amplification devices visible to those around them. This suggests that HI children do not feel more insecure about their looks than other teenagers around this age, which is a positive finding. However, HI children reported lower self-esteem in the domains of perceived social acceptance by peers and perceived parental attention when compared to NH peers. Adequate language development and communication skills can increase self-esteem in the peers' domain, but not in the parental domain.

The fact that HI children reported lower levels of self-esteem than NH children in the social domains indicates that HI children feel less liked and appreciated by parents and peers. This is in line with other studies with HI children [15,16,25]. The reasons for lower self-esteem involving parents could be subjective or objective. Children might perceive that their parents spend less time with them, while in fact parents might spend equal time with them as with their NH children. The quality of contact received by NH versus HI children could be different. Parents usually experience more stress and worries raising a HI than a NH child, because they have to adapt to a new situation which necessitates the investment of time, effort, and resources [41–44]. For example, an HI child requires frequent hospitals visits and involvement in

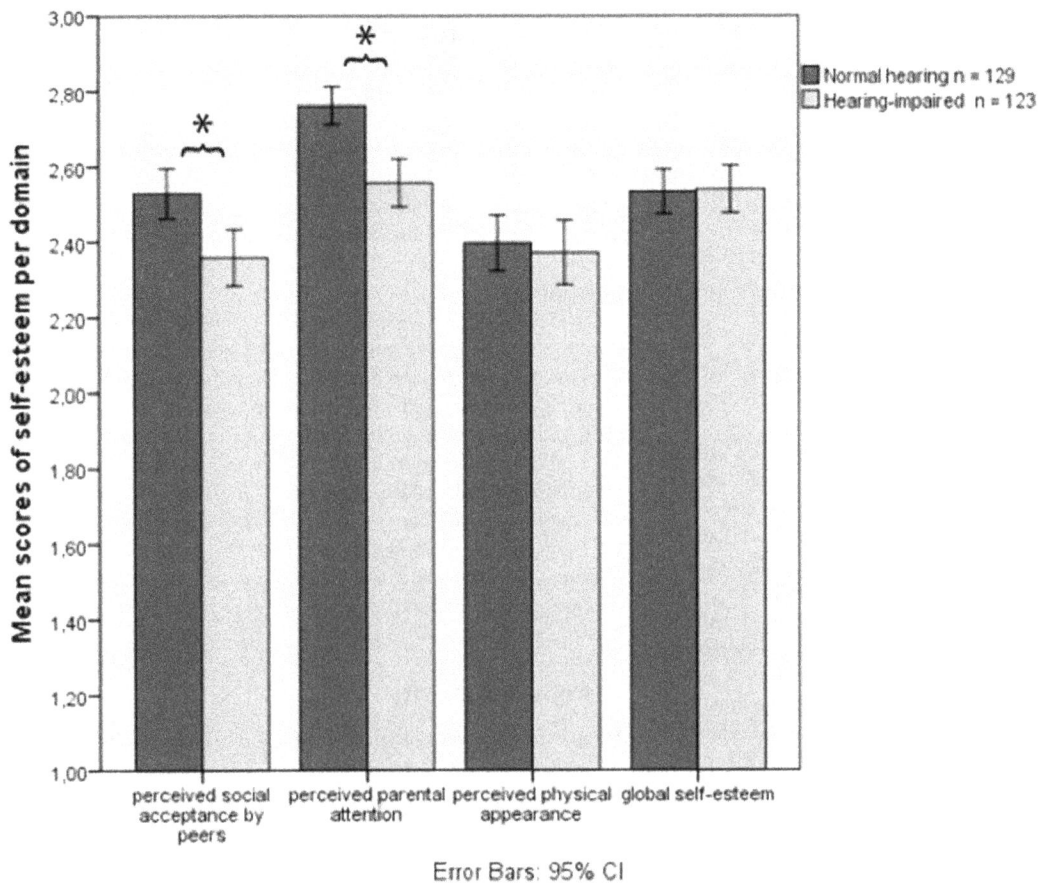

Figure 1. Mean scores of self-esteem per domain. *$p<.05$.

intensive rehabilitation programs. Chronic parental stress can influence the child's functioning and development in a negative way (e.g., more behavioral problems and impaired psychological functioning) [8,45]. First of all, parents are a role model for their children. When parents have difficulties coping with stressful events, children will learn and apply these reactions as well. Secondly, more parental stress will also bring about a less positive atmosphere in the home, creating a less optimal environment for healthy development in children. Thirdly, parents might be focused on the impact of the hearing loss and medical site of this, overlooking the child's emotional need for support and guidance. Possibly, parents try hard to support their HI child by speaking

slowly, helping with homework, or explaining difficult words [46]. Yet, HI children might interpret this extra attention as if they are failing or falling behind.

On the other hand, language development and communication skills influenced self-esteem in the peers' domain. This means that HI children's self-esteem regarding peers equals that of NH children when their language and communication skills are well-developed. Still, HI children are born into a sound-dominated world, where the focus lies on spoken language, resulting in less satisfactory communication. For example, making friends can be harder for HI children and they are also more neglected and less accepted by NH peers [16,47–50]. The communication barrier

Table 3. Pearson's correlations between the four domains of self-esteem and associated variables.

| | Domains of self-esteem | | | |
	Perceived social acceptance by peers	Perceived parental attention	Perceived physical appearance	Global self-esteem
Age of onset hearing loss	−.02	−.04	.06	−.04
Age at first hearing aid	−.02	.09	.04	−.10
Age at CI implantation	.16	−.36*	.20	−.08
Duration of CI use	−.21	.38**	−.07	−.07

*$p<.05$;
**$p<.01$ (two-tailed).

between HI and NH children can function as an obstacle for successful interpersonal relationships and may hamper these children in developing solid social networks [51,52]. This process may pave the way for social isolation and loneliness, with consequences for the child's self-esteem [53,54]. Hence, by improving language development and communication skills, the HI child might experience better contact with peers, which in turn would likely improve their self-esteem in this domain. In this respect, it has to be mentioned that language development and communication skills did not differ between hearing aided children and CI recipients in our sample. Though the literature often showed that CI recipients have better skills in this regard [10,55], most of the literature reports on early-implanted children, while our sample is mainly late-implanted. Therefore, we think that the next generation of CI recipients, with better language and communication will, in turn, have higher self-esteem.

Moreover, this research has revealed that children who attend special education for the HI or deaf have lower self-esteem concerning parents when compared to HI children attending mainstream education. Although we have to bear in mind that HI children with good language skills and/or higher intelligence are more easily referred to mainstream education [20,56–58], this study is the first to show that even after correcting for these variables, children in special education still have lower levels of self-esteem. It could be hypothesized that this stems from reasons related to discrimination or stigma. HI children often have to travel far to attend special education, which results in different environments: they have friends at school and different friends at home. Less contact with peers could hinder bonding and attachment, possibly resulting in lower self-esteem [59]. However, longitudinal studies are needed to reproduce these findings, because a cross-sectional study rules out drawing conclusions about causal relations. Additionally, such longitudinal studies must include larger samples in order to examine the influence of parental and friends' hearing statuses on the level of self-esteem.

A limitation of this study was missing data, especially concerning communication, intelligence and language development. It is possible that this missing data did not occur at random. For example, children who read slowly might not have had enough time to complete all the tests. Yet, comparison showed that the group for which information on these measures was missing did not differ from the group with no missing values on important other variables, including age, gender, SES, and the different domains for self-esteem. This seems to strengthen the basis for our conclusions, but future studies are needed to confirm these outcomes.

To conclude, self-esteem in HI children differs from NH children in the social domains only; the levels of perceived physical appearance and global self-esteem do not differ from those of NH children. Improving language development and communication skills could help to build up higher levels of self-esteem regarding peers. Unfortunately, irrespective of their language and communication skills, HI children in special education show lower levels of self-esteem in the parental domain. The aim of this research was to create more awareness concerning this vulnerable group of children, resulting in increased attention and monitoring by professionals, in order to promote good mental health in each HI child.

Acknowledgments

We gratefully acknowledge all children and their parents for participation in this study.

Author Contributions

Conceived and designed the experiments: ST, AN, CR, MK, WS, JB, JF. Performed the experiments: ST, MK. Analyzed the data: ST, AN, CR. Wrote the paper: ST, AN, CR, MK, WS, JB, JF.

References

1. Rosenberg M (1965) Society and the adolescent self-image. Princeton, NJ: Princeton University Press.
2. Baumeister RF, Campbell JD, Krueger JI, Vohs KD (2003) Does High Self-Esteem Cause Better Performance, Interpersonal Success, Happiness, or Healthier Lifestyles? Psychological science 4: 1–44.
3. Harter S (2006) Self-processes and developmental psychopathology. In: Cicchietti D, Cohen DJ, Developmental Psychopathology. Hoboken, NJ: Wiley & Sons. pp. 370–418.
4. Orth U, Robins RW, Roberts BW (2008) Low self-esteem prospectively predicts depression in adolescence and young adulthood. Journal of Personality and Social Psychology 95: 695–708.
5. Harper JF, Marshall E (1991) Adolescents' problems and their relationship to self-esteem. Adolescence 26: 799–807.
6. Donnellan MB, Trzesniewski KH, Robins RW, Moffitt TE, Caspi A (2005) Low self-esteem is related to aggression, antisocial behavior, and delinquency. Psychological Science 16: 328–335.
7. Polat F (2003) Factors Affecting Psychosocial Adjustment of Deaf Students. Journal of Deaf Studies and Deaf Education 8: 325–339.
8. Kouwenberg M, Rieffe C, Theunissen SCPM, de Rooij M (2012) Peer victimization experienced by Children and Adolescents who are Deaf or Hard of Hearing. PLoS ONE 7.
9. Hintermair M (2008) Self-esteem and satisfaction with life of deaf and hard-of-hearing people - a resource-oriented approach to identity work. Journal of Deaf Studies and Deaf Education 13: 278–300.
10. Tomblin JB, Spencer L, Flock S, Tyler R, Gantz B (1999) A comparison of language achievement in children with cochlear implants and children using hearing aids. J Speech Lang Hear Res 42: 497–509.
11. Theunissen SC, Rieffe C, Kouwenberg M, De Raeve LJ, Soede W, et al. (2013) Behavioral problems in school-aged hearing-impaired children: the influence of sociodemographic, linguistic, and medical factors. Eur Child Adolesc Psychiatry.
12. Percy-Smith L, Cay-Thomasen P, Gudman M, Jensen J, Thomsen J (2008) Self-esteem and social well-being of children with cochlear implant compared to normal-hearing children. International Journal of Pediatric Otorhinolaryngology 72: 1113–1120.
13. Sahli S, Belgin E (2006) Comparison of self-esteem level of adolescents with cochlear implant and normal hearing. International Journal of Pediatric Otorhinolaryngology 70: 1601–1608.
14. Bess FH, Dodd-Murphy J, Parker RA (1998) Children with minimal sensorineural hearing loss: prevalence, educational performance, and functional status. Ear and Hearing 19: 339–354.
15. Van Gent T, Goedhart AW, Knoors HET, Westenberg PM, Treffers PDA (2012) Self-concept and Ego Development in Deaf Adolescents: A Comparative Study. Journal of Deaf Studies and Deaf Education 17: 333–351.
16. Cappelli M, Daniels T, DurieuxSmith A, McGrath PJ, Neuss D (1995) Social development of children with hearing impairments who are integrated into general education classrooms. Volta Review 97: 197–208.
17. Cates JA (1991) Self-Concept in Hearing and Prelingual, Profoundly Deaf Students - a Comparison of Teachers Perceptions. American Annals of the Deaf 136: 354–359.
18. Eriks-Brophy A, Durieux-Smith A, Olds J, Fitzpatrick EM, Duquette C, et al. (2012) Communication, Academic, and Social Skills of Young Adults with Hearing Loss. Volta Review 112: 5–35.
19. Leigh IW, Maxwell-McCaw D, Bat-Chava Y, Christiansen JB (2009) Correlates of psychosocial adjustment in deaf adolescents with and without cochlear implants: a preliminary investigation. Journal of Deaf Studies and Deaf Education 14: 244–259.
20. Keilmann A, Limberger A, Mann W (2007) Psychological and physical well-being in hearing-impaired children. International Journal of Pediatric Otorhinolaryngology 71: 1747–1752.
21. Van Gurp S (2001) Self-concept of deaf secondary school students in different educational settings. Journal of Deaf Studies and Deaf Education 6: 54–69.
22. Blascovich J, Tomaka J (1991) Measures of self-esteem. In: Robinson JP, Shaver PR, Wrightsman LS, Measures of Personality and Social Psychological Attributes. San Diego, SA: Academic Press.
23. Cole DA, Maxwell SE, Martin JM, Peeke LG, Seroczynski AD, et al. (2001) The development of multiple domains of child and adolescent self-concept: A cohort sequential longitudinal design. Child Development 72: 1723–1746.
24. Coleman JS (1981) The adolescent society; Johnstone JWC, editor: Greenwood Press.

25. Loeb RC, Sarigiani P (1986) The impact of hearing impairment on self-perceptions of children. Volta Review 88: 89–100.

26. Rieffe C, Meerum Terwogt M, Bosch JD, Kneepkens CMF, Douwes AC, et al. (2007) Interaction between emotions and somatic complaints in children who did or did not seek medical care. Cognition and Emotion 21: 1630–1646.

27. Van Dijk P, Rieffe C (1999) Somatic complaints in children; a study on the influence of fear, self-esteem and concern on the reporting of physical complaints. Amsterdam: Vrije Universiteit. pp. 23.

28. Veerman JW, Straathof MAE, Treffers DA, Van den Bergh BRH, Brink LT (1997) Competentiebelevingsschaal voor Kinderen: Handleiding [Perceived competence scale for children: manual]. Lisse, The Netherlands: Swets & Zeitlinger.

29. Harter S (1985) Manual for the Self-perception Profile for Children. Denver, CO: University of Denver.

30. Rosenberg M (1979) Conceiving the self: Basic Books.

31. Robins RW, Hendin HM, Trzesniewski KH (2001) Measuring Global Self-Esteem: Construct Validation of a Single-Item Measure and the Rosenberg Self-Esteem Scale. Personality and Social Psychology Bulletin 27: 151–161.

32. Anmyr L, Larsson K, Olsson M, Freijd A (2012) Strengths and difficulties in children with cochlear implants - Comparing self-reports with reports from parents and teachers. International Journal of Pediatric Otorhinolaryngology 76: 1107–1112.

33. Kort W, Schittekatte M, Compaan E (2008) *CELF-4-NL: Clinical Evaluation of Language Fundamentals*: Pearson Assessment and Information B.V., Amsterdam.

34. Semel E, Wiig EH, Secord WA (1987) CELF: Clinical Evaluation of Language Fundamentals - revised; Corp TP, San Antonio, TX.

35. Hermans D, Knoors H, Verhoeven L (2010) Assessment of Sign Language Development: The Case of Deaf Children in the Netherlands. Journal of Deaf Studies and Deaf Education 15: 107–119.

36. Bishop DVM (1998) Development of the Children's Communication Checklist (CCC): A method for assessing qualitative aspects of communicative impairment in children. Journal of Child Psychology and Psychiatry and Allied Disciplines 39: 879–891.

37. Kort W, Schittekatte M, Compaan EL, Bosmans M, Bleichrodt N, et al. (2002) WISC-III NL. Handleiding. Nederlandse bewerking. London: The Psychological Corporation.

38. Wechsler D (1991) The Wechsler intelligence scale for children—third edition. San Antonio, TX: The Psychological Corporation.

39. Tellegen P, Laros J (1993) The Construction and Validation of a Nonverbal Test of Intelligence: the revision of the Snijders-Oomen tests. European Journal of Psychological Assessment 9: 147–157.

40. Dumont M, Provost MA (1999) Resilience in adolescents: Protective role of social support, coping strategies, self-esteem, and social activities on experience of stress and depression. Journal of Youth and Adolescence 28: 343–363.

41. Cohen MS (1999) Families coping with childhood chronic illness: A research review. Families, Systems, & Health 17: 149–164.

42. Quittner AL, Glueckauf RL, Jackson DN (1990) Chronic parenting stress: moderating versus mediating effects of social support. Journal of Personality and Social Psychology 59: 1266–1278.

43. Sach TH, Whynes DK (2005) Paediatric cochlear implantation: The views of parents. International Journal of Audiology 44: 400–407.

44. Quittner AL, Barker DH, Cruz I, Snell C, Grimley ME, et al. (2010) Parenting Stress Among Parents of Deaf and Hearing Children: Associations with Language Delays and Behavior Problems. Parenting: Science & Practice 10: 136–155.

45. Drotar D (1997) Relating parent and family functioning to the psychological adjustment of children with chronic health conditions: What have we learned? What do we need to know? Journal of Pediatric Psychology 22: 149–165.

46. Pinquart M (2013) Do the parent-child relationship and parenting behaviors differ between families with a child with and without chronic illness? A meta-analysis. J Pediatr Psychol 38: 708–721.

47. Nunes T, Pretzlik U, Olsson J (2001) Deaf children's social relationships in mainstream schools. Deafness & Education international 3: 123–136.

48. Wolters N, Knoors HE, Cillessen AH, Verhoeven L (2011) Predicting acceptance and popularity in early adolescence as a function of hearing status, gender, and educational setting. Research in Developmental Disabilities 32: 2553–2565.

49. Kluwin TN, Stinson MS, Colarossi GM (2002) Social processes and outcomes of in-school contact between deaf and hearing peers. Journal of Deaf Studies and Deaf Education 71: 1747–1752.

50. Davis JM, Elfenbein J, Schum R, Bentler RA (1986) Effects of Mild and Moderate Hearing Impairments on Language, Educational, and Psychosocial Behavior of Children. Journal of Speech and Hearing Disorders 51: 53–62.

51. Bat-Chava Y (1993) Antecedents of self-esteem in deaf people: A meta-analytic review. Rehabilitation Psychology 38: 221–234.

52. Calderon R, Greenberg MT (2003) Social and emotional development of deaf children: family, school and program effects. Marschark M, Spencer PE, editors. New York: Oxford University Press.

53. Rubin KH, Mills RSL (1988) The Many Faces of Social-Isolation in Childhood. Journal of Consulting and Clinical Psychology 56: 916–924.

54. Most T, Ingber S, Heled-Ariam E (2012) Social competence, sense of loneliness, and speech intelligibility of young children with hearing loss in individual inclusion and group inclusion. Journal of Deaf Studies and Deaf Education 17: 259–272.

55. Bond M, Mealing S, Anderson R, Elston J, Weiner G, et al. (2009) The effectiveness and cost-effectiveness of cochlear implants for severe to profound deafness in children and adults: a systematic review and economic model. Health Technology Assessment 13: 1–+.

56. Van Eldik T (2005) Mental health problems of Dutch youth with hearing loss as shown on the Youth Self Report. American Annals of the Deaf 150: 11–16.

57. Stinson MS, Whitmire KA (2000) Adolescents who are deaf or hard of hearing: A communication perspective on educational placement. Topics in Language Disorders 20: 58–72.

58. Van Gent T, Goedhart A, Hindley P, Treffers PDA (2007) Prevalence and correlates of psychopathology in a sample of deaf adolescents. Journal of Child Psychology and Psychiatry and Allied Disciplines 48: 950–958.

59. Armsden GC, Greenberg MT (1987) The Inventory of Parent and Peer Attachment - Individual-Differences and Their Relationship to Psychological Well-Being in Adolescence. Journal of Youth and Adolescence 16: 427–454.

16

Age-Related Hearing Impairment (ARHI) Associated with *GJB2* Single Mutation IVS1+1G>A in the Yakut Population Isolate in Eastern Siberia

Nikolay A. Barashkov[1,2*⁹], Fedor M. Teryutin[1,2⁹], Vera G. Pshennikova[1], Aisen V. Solovyev[2], Leonid A. Klarov[3], Natalya A. Solovyeva[1], Andrei A. Kozhevnikov[4], Lena M. Vasilyeva[5], Elvira E. Fedotova[5], Maria V. Pak[6], Sargylana N. Lekhanova[7], Elena V. Zakharova[8], Kyunney E. Savvinova[2,9], Nyurgun N. Gotovtsev[2,9], Adyum M. Rafailo[9], Nikolay V. Luginov[3], Anatoliy N. Alexeev[10], Olga L. Posukh[11,12], Lilya U. Dzhemileva[13], Elza K. Khusnutdinova[13,14], Sardana A. Fedorova[1,2]

1 Department of Molecular Genetics, Yakut Scientific Centre of Complex Medical Problems, Siberian Branch of the Russian Academy of Medical Sciences, Yakutsk, Russian Federation, 2 Laboratory of Molecular Biology, Institute of Natural Sciences, M.K. Ammosov North-Eastern Federal University, Yakutsk, Russian Federation, 3 Department of Radiology, Republican Hospital #2– Center of Emergency Medicine, Ministry of Public Health of the Sakha Republic, Yakutsk, Russian Federation, 4 Republican Centre of Professional Pathology, Republican Hospital #2– Center of Emergency Medicine, Ministry of Public Health of the Sakha Republic, Yakutsk, Russian Federation, 5 Audiology-Logopaedic Center, Republican Hospital #1– National Medical Centre, Ministry of Public Health of the Sakha Republic, Yakutsk, Russian Federation, 6 Department of Pediatric, Medical Institute, M.K. Ammosov North-Eastern Federal University, Yakutsk, Russian Federation, 7 Department of Normal and Abnormal Anatomy, Operative Surgery with Topographic Anatomy and Forensic Medicine, Medical Institute, M.K. Ammosov North-Eastern Federal University, Yakutsk, Russian Federation, 8 Institute of Foreign Philology and Regional Studies, M.K. Ammosov North-Eastern Federal University, Yakutsk, Russian Federation, 9 Institute of Natural Sciences, M.K. Ammosov North-Eastern Federal University, Yakutsk, Russian Federation, 10 Institute of Humanitarian Research and Indigenous Peoples of the North, Siberian Branch of the Russian Academy of Sciences, Yakutsk, Russian Federation, 11 Institute of Cytology and Genetics, Siberian Branch of the Russian Academy of Sciences, Novosibirsk, Russian Federation, 12 Novosibirsk State University, Novosibirsk, Russian Federation, 13 Department of Genomics, Institute of Biochemistry and Genetics, Ufa Scientific Centre, Russian Academy of Sciences, Ufa, Russian Federation, 14 Department of Genetics and Fundamental Medicine, Bashkir State University, Ufa, Russian Federation

Abstract

Age-Related Hearing Impairment (ARHI) is one of the frequent sensory disorders registered in 50% of individuals over 80 years. ARHI is a multifactorial disorder due to environmental and poor-known genetic components. In this study, we present the data on age-related hearing impairment of 48 heterozygous carriers of mutation IVS1+1G>A (*GJB2* gene) and 97 subjects with *GJB2* genotype wt/wt in the Republic of Sakha/Yakutia (Eastern Siberia, Russia). This subarctic territory was found as the region with the most extensive accumulation of mutation IVS1+1G>A in the world as a result of founder effect in the unique Yakut population isolate. The *GJB2* gene resequencing and detailed audiological analysis in the frequency range 0.25, 0.5, 1.0, 2.0, 4.0, 8.0 kHz were performed in all examined subjects that allowed to investigate genotype-phenotype correlations between the presence of single mutation IVS1+1G>A and hearing of subjects from examined groups. We revealed the linear correlation between increase of average hearing thresholds at speech frequencies ($PTA_{0.5,1.0,2.0,4.0 \text{ kHz}}$) and age of individuals with *GJB2* genotype IVS1+1G>A/wt ($r_s = 0.499$, $p = 0.006860$ for males and $r_s = 0.427$, $p = 0.000277$ for females). Moreover, the average hearing thresholds on high frequency (8.0 kHz) in individuals with genotype IVS1+1G>A/wt (both sexes) were significantly worse than in individuals with genotype wt/wt ($p < 0.05$). Age of hearing loss manifestation in individuals with genotype IVS1+1G>A/wt was estimated to be ~40 years ($r_s = 0.504$, $p = 0.003$). These findings demonstrate that the single IVS1+1G>A mutation (*GJB2*) is associated with age-related hearing impairment (ARHI) of the IVS1+1G>A carriers in the Yakuts.

Editor: Francesc Palau, Instituto de Ciencia de Materiales de Madrid – Instituto de Biomedicina de Valencia, Spain

Funding: The authors thank all patients and blood sample donors who have contributed to this study. This study was supported by the Russian Foundation for Basic Research (12-04-00342_a, 12-04-98520_r_vostok_a, 12-04-97004_r_povolzhye_a, 12-04-31230_mol_a, 14-04-01741_A), Federal Program «Scientific and educational staff for innovative Russia» (#16.740.11.0190, #16.740.11.0346), Integration project of SB RAS #92 «Ethnogeny of indigenous peoples in Siberia and North Asia: comparative, historical, ethno-social and genomic analysis», the Sakha Republic President Grant#80 for Young Researchers for 2014 year, Scientific and Educational Foundation for Young Scientists of Republic of Sakha (Yakutia) for 2014 year, Project #656 of Ministry of Education and Science of Russia, by grant #30 (2013–2015) of RAS Program «Fundamental Sciences for Medicine». The funders had no role in study design, data collection and analysis, decision to publish, or preparation of the manuscript.

Competing Interests: The authors have declared that no competing interests exist.

* Email: barashkov2004@mail.ru

⁹ These authors contributed equally to this work.

Introduction

Age-related hearing impairment (ARHI), or presbyacusis, is a common sensory disorder characterized by bilateral sensorineural hearing loss more evident at high frequencies [1], [2]. According to some data, hearing acuity decrease occurs in one out of 25 persons at age older than 45 [3], and about 50% of population over 80 years has a significant hearing impairment [4]. ARHI is a multifactorial disease [1], [5], but the age of disease onset has not been determined. Recently, using a genomewide analysis two loci 8q24.13-q24.22 (ARHI 1, OMIM 612448) [1], [6], 3p26.1-p.25.1 (ARHI 2, OMIM 612976) [1], [7], [8] were linked with this disease.

Genes already known to be associated with hearing impairment are not investigated enough for the presence of genetic associations with ARHI. Mutations in *GJB2* gene coding protein connexin 26 (Cx26) in homozygous and compound-heterozygous states are responsible for a significant part of inherited autosomal recessive forms of hearing loss in different populations [9]. However, several studies suggest that even single mutations in *GJB2* gene (in heterozygous state) have influence on hearing function [10–16]. These studies of hearing thresholds in carriers of recessive mutations in *GJB2* gene – c.35delG, p.Met34Thr, c.167delT (most frequently registered in Europe), and c.235delC single mutation (the study was carried out in China) – had controversial results [10–13], [15], [16].

Splice site mutation IVS1+1G>A in *GJB2* gene is relatively rare, and audiological analysis of hearing threshold in carriers of this single mutation has not been performed previously. High rates of IVS1+1G>A mutation (2–11.7%) were found among some indigenous populations of Eastern Siberia, Russia (Yakuts, Dolgans, Evenks and Evens), with the highest carrier frequency (11.7%) in isolated Yakut population [17]. The genetic data revealed a relatively small size of Yakut ancestor population and the strong bottleneck effect in the Yakut paternal line (80% of Y chromosomes of Yakuts belong to one haplogroup – N1c) [18–21]. Extremely high rate of IVS1+1G>A mutation in relatively genetic homogenous Yakut population gives a unique opportunity to investigate hearing status in individuals heterozygous for this *GJB2* gene mutation.

The purpose of this study is to analyze age-related hearing alteration in *GJB2* mutation IVS1+1G>A carriers versus individuals with normal *GJB2* genotype in Yakut population.

Material and Methods

Sampling design

To form the total sample we invited random volunteers without any complaints on hearing (both in the Yakut Scientific Centre of Complex Medical Problems and during field trips in regions of inhabitance of the Yakutia indigenous population) and informed the potential participants about the aims of upcoming study. We also invited the parents and siblings of deaf children homozygous for the IVS1+1G>A mutation, as they could be the carriers of this mutation. All the volunteers (214 individuals in total) passed otologic-audiological evaluation and genotyping for the *GJB2* gene mutations (spectrum of *GJB2* genotypes is given in Table 1). For the further analysis we selected 145 individuals that matched the following criteria: had *GJB2* genotypes wt/wt or IVS1+1G>A/wt; were older than 20 years old; belonged to Yakut ethnicity (predominantly to the third generation); had no recent history of fever, otitis media, tinnitus; and had no obvious contacts with occupational noise. From those 145 individuals based on genotyping data we formed two groups: Cx26-H – the group included the carriers of single mutation IVS1+1G>A (*GJB2* genotype IVS1+1G>A/wt, 48 individuals or 96 ears); and Cx26-Wt – the group of non-carriers of the IVS1+1G>A mutation (*GJB2* genotype wt/wt, 97 individuals or 194 ears). Subsequently, we stratified these two groups according to age and sex for the purpose of correct comparison (Figure 1).

Audiological examination

Audiological examination was conducted on all 214 individuals (n = 428 ears). Otologic examination was performed with the «Basic-Diagnostik-Set» (KaWe, Germany), tuning fork standard set. Acoustic impedance was measured with impedance meter (Interacoustics AS, Denmark). Air conduction thresholds were measured on frequencies 0.25, 0.5, 1.0, 2.0, 4.0, 8.0 kHz and bone conduction thresholds – on frequencies 0.25, 0.5, 1.0, 2.0, 4.0 kHz with audiometer «MAICO ST20» (MAICO, Germany) in the same conditions for all participants. The results were assessed separately for each ear on air conduction thresholds as on all measured frequencies, and speech range of frequencies – $PTA_{0.5,1.0,2.0,4.0 \text{ kHz}}$ separately.

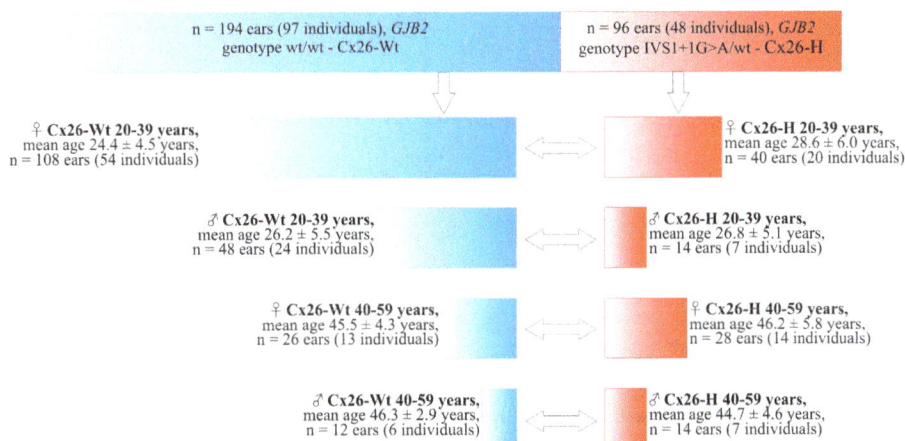

Figure 1. **Design of Cx26-H and Cx26-Wt groups.** Note: Cx26-Wt (IVS1+1G>A non-carriers) is shown in blue, Cx26-H (IVS1+1G>A carriers) is shown in red; bilateral arrows show the compared subgroups; ♀ – female, ♂ – male.

Table 1. Mutation analysis of *GJB2* gene.

№	*GJB2* genotype	Relatives of the deaf children with mutations in *GJB2* gene	Random sample from Yakut population	Frequency of *GJB2* genotypes*, %
1	**wt/wt**	**4**	**113**	**66.47**
2	**IVS1+1G>A/wt**	**35**	**17**	**10.00**
3	IVS1+1G>A/p.Val27Ile	2	2	1.18
4	p.Val27Ile/wt	1	21	12.35
5	p.Val27Ile/p.Val27Ile+p.Thr123Asn	-	1	0.59
6	p.Val27Ile+p.Glu114Gly/wt	-	6	3.53
7	p.Val27Ile+p.Thr123Asn/wt	-	5	2.94
8	p.Met34Thr/wt	-	1	0.59
9	p.Val37Ile/wt	-	3	1.76
10	c.35delG/wt	2	-	-
11	c.360_362delGAG/wt	-	1	0.59
	Total number and percentage of *GJB2*-mutations and polymorphisms	40	57	33.53
	Total number of individuals	44	170	-
	Total number and percentage	214		100

Note: * The frequency of *GJB2* genotypes was calculated in random sample; in bold are *GJB2* genotypes selected for comparative analysis of hearing thresholds.

Mutation analysis of GJB2 gene

A total of 214 genomic DNA samples, which were extracted from leukocytes of peripheral blood, were used for *GJB2* gene mutation analysis. Amplification of the coding (exon 2) and noncoding (exon 1) and flanking intronic regions of *GJB2* gene was conducted with PCR on thermocycler «MJ Mini» (Bio-Rad) using appropriate primers [22–25]. The PCR products were subjected to direct sequencing using the same primers on ABI PRISM 3130XL (Applied Biosystems, USA) («Genomics» Core Facility; Institute of Chemical Biology and Fundamental Medicine, Siberian Branch of the Russian Academy of Sciences, Novosibirsk, Russia). The results of mutation analysis of *GJB2* gene are shown in the Table 1.

Statistical analysis

The results of audiological examination and mutation analysis of *GJB2* gene were summarized in the unified database. Regression and correlation analysis of «age-hearing threshold» association were assessed with Spearman's rank correlation coefficient r_s. Significance of hearing thresholds on measured frequencies was statistically evaluated with the Mann-Whitney U test using software STATISTICA version 8.0. (StatSoft Inc, USA) and Biostatd (McGraw-Hill, Inc.Version 3.03). Differences were statistically significant when $p<0.05$.

Ethical approval

Written informed consent was obtained from all individuals. This study was approved by the local Committee on Biomedical Ethics of Yakut Scientific Center of Complex Medical Problems,

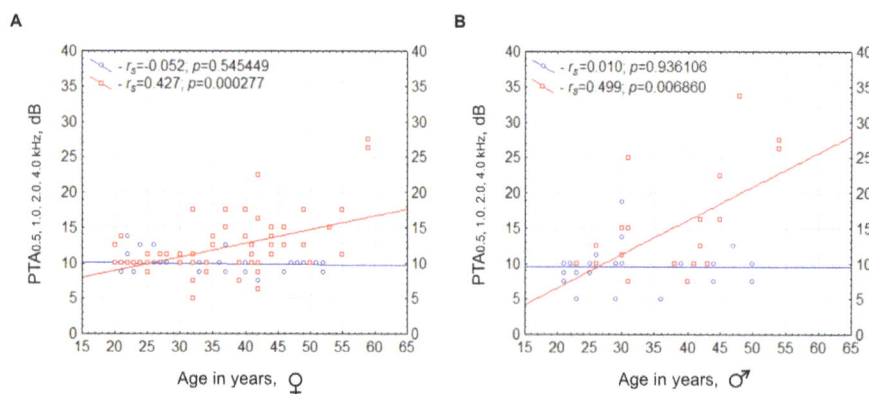

Figure 2. The correlation of increase of hearing thresholds according to age in individuals with genotype IVS1+1G>A/wt. Note: Y-axis – hearing thresholds (dB), X-axis – age in years; r_s – the Spearman's rank correlation coefficient, p – statistical significance of Spearman's rank correlation; blue circles – individuals with *GJB2* genotype wt/wt, red squares – individuals heterozygous for mutation (genotype IVS1+1G>A/wt); blue line shows the absence of hearing thresholds correlation with age in individuals with *GJB2* genotype wt/wt, red line – the linear regression of increase in hearing thresholds according to age in individuals with *GJB2* genotype IVS1+1G>A/wt; A – ♀ female, B – ♂ male.

Table 2. Correlation of increase of hearing thresholds in PTA$_{0.5,1.0,2.0,4.0\ kHz}$ according to age in individuals with *GJB2* genotype wt/wt and IVS1+1G>A/wt.

GJB2 genotype	Parameters	20–29 years	30–39 years	40–49 years	50–59 years
wt/wt	n = ears	128	28	28	10
	r_s	0.036	−0.245	0.159	0.272
	p	0.682	0.208	0.417	0.445
IVS1+1G>A/wt	n = ears	28	26	32	10
	r_s	0.228	−0.125	**0.504**	**0.697**
	p	0.243	0.542	**0.003**	**0.024**

Note: r_s – the Spearman's rank correlation coefficient; values with statistically significant correlation (p<0.05) of increase of hearing thresholds with age are shown in bold.

Siberian Branch of the Russian Academy of Medical Sciences, Yakutsk, Russia (Yakutsk, Protocol No 16, April 16, 2009).

Results

Correlation analysis of hearing thresholds in PTA$_{0.5,1.0,2.0,4.0\ kHz}$ according to age

We conducted correlation analysis of «age-hearing thresholds at PTA$_{0.5,1.0,2.0,4.0\ kHz}$» in IVS1+1G>A single mutation carriers (group Cx26-H) and non-carriers (group Cx26-Wt), for females and males separately. Statistically significant ($p<0.05$) correlation of increase in hearing threshold according to age was detected in IVS1+1G>A carriers (group Cx26-H: $r_s = 0.427$, $p = 0.000277$ in females, $r_s = 0.499$, $p = 0.006860$ in males) and not observed in non-carriers (group Cx26-Wt: $r_s = -0.052$, $p = 0.545449$ in females, $r_s = 0.010$, $p = 0.936106$ in males) (Figure 2 A, B).

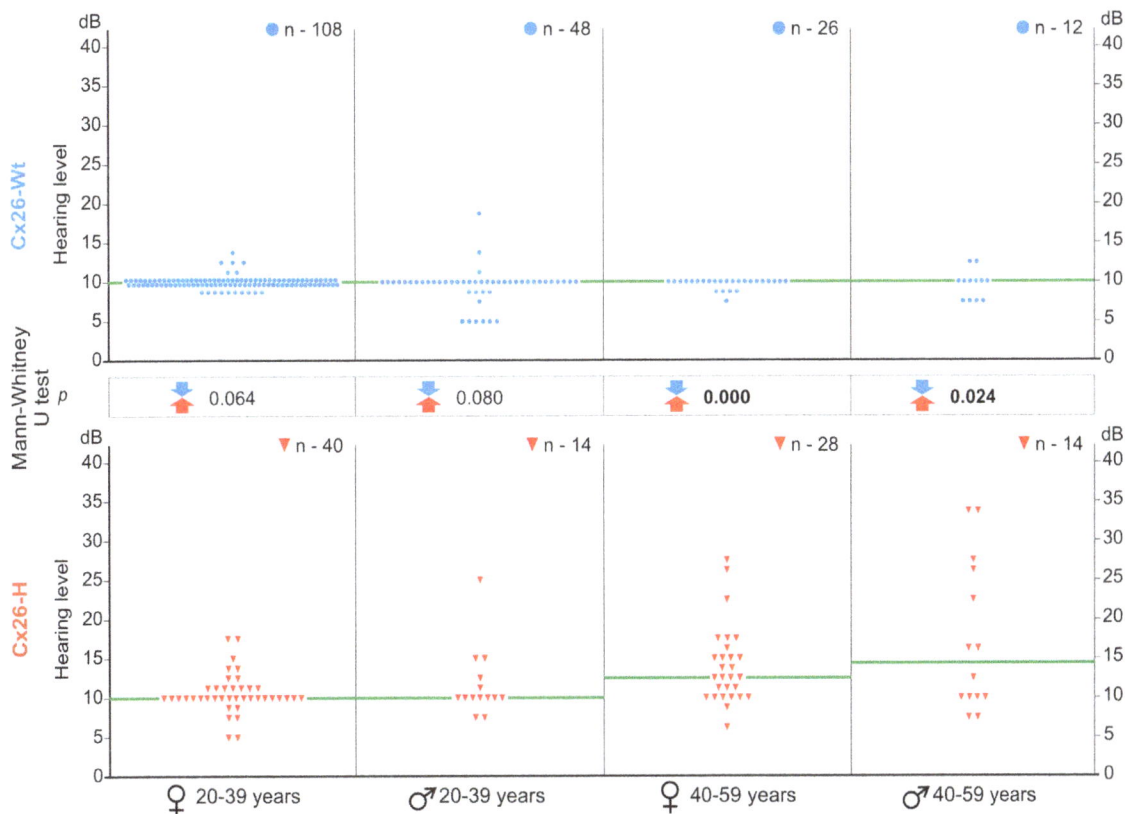

Figure 3. Scatter plots of the hearing thresholds at PTA$_{0.5,\ 1.0,\ 2.0,\ 4.0\ kHz}$ of individuals from compared Cx26-Wt and Cx26-H subgroups according to sex and age. Note: Y-axis – hearing level (hearing threshold, dB). X-axis – audiometric parameters of individuals according to sex and age. Blue circle denotes an individual with *GJB2* genotype wt/wt, red delta denotes an individual with *GJB2* genotype IVS1+1G>A/wt; n – number of ears; statistically significant differences (p<0.05) by the Mann-Whitney U test between the compared subgroups are shown in bold; median hearing thresholds are shown by green line. ♀ – female; ♂ – male.

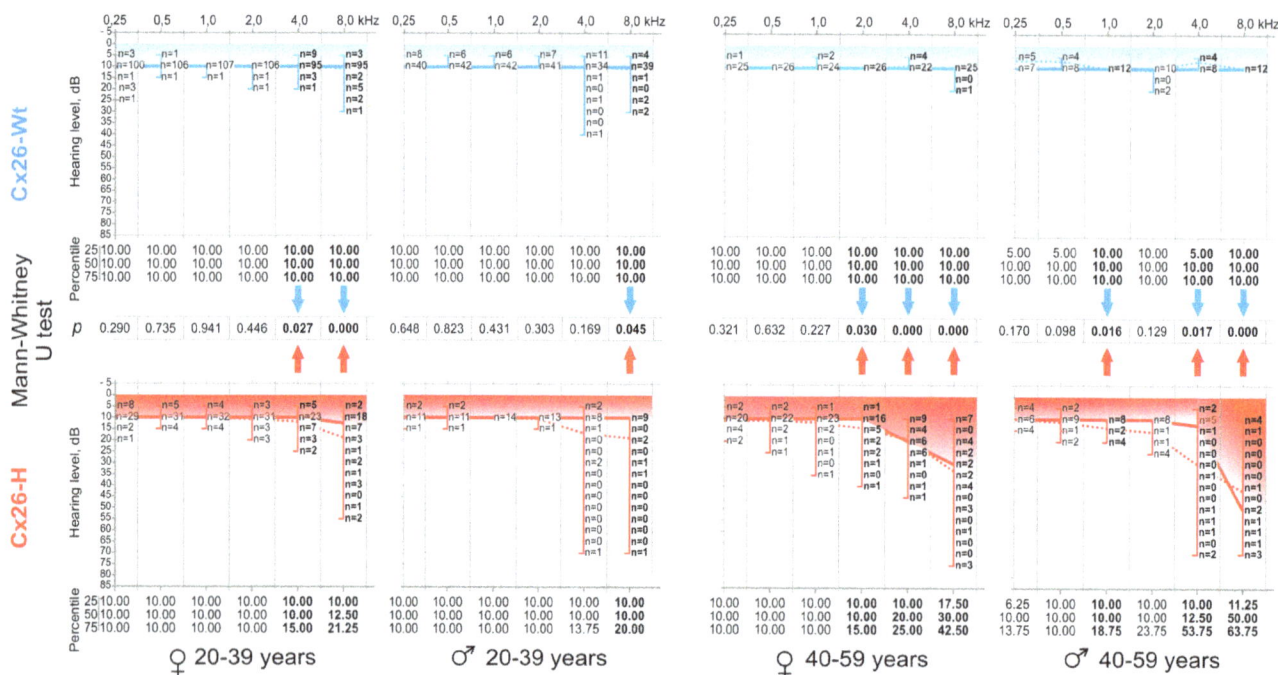

Figure 4. Audiometric parameters at all measured frequencies (0.25, 0.5, 1.0, 2.0, 4.0, 8.0 kHz) of individuals from compared subgroups Cx26-Wt and Cx26-H according to sex and age. Note: Y-axis – hearing thresholds (dB), X-axis – measured frequency (kHz), the audiometric parameters of individuals with *GJB2* genotype wt/wt are shown in blue and of individuals with *GJB2* genotype IVS1+1G>A/wt – in red; n – the number of ears; the frequencies (%) with statistically significant differences (p<0.05) by the Mann-Whitney U test are shown in bold; the arrows show statistically significant differences (p<0.05) by the Mann-Whitney U test; median hearing thresholds are shown by solid line, average hearing thresholds – by dotted line. ♀ – female; ♂ – male.

The age of onset of hearing impairment in single mutation IVS1+1G>A carriers

To determine onset of presbyacusis manifestation, both studied groups Cx26-H and Cx26-Wt were divided into age cohorts 20–29, 30–39, 40–49, and 50–59 years. Correlation analysis of association «age-hearing threshold in PTA$_{0.5,1.0,2.0,4.0 \text{ kHz}}$» was performed in these age cohorts (Table 2). Correlation was not observed in individuals of all age cohorts from group Cx26-Wt and in individuals at ages 20–29 and 30–39 years from group Cx26-H. Statistically significant (*p*<0.05) correlation was observed in hearing thresholds of individuals from group Cx26-H at ages 40–49 years ($r_s = 0.504$, *p* = 0.003), and 50–59 years ($r_s = 0.697$, *p* = 0.024) (Table 2). Thus, hearing impairment onset was identified as approximately 40 years, and further analysis was conducted in two age subgroups: 20–39 and 40–59 years (for females and males, separately).

Detailed audiometric analysis of hearing thresholds in IVS1+1G>A carriers and non-carriers

Comparative analysis of hearing thresholds at frequencies of significant speech range (PTA$_{0.5,1.0,2.0,4.0 \text{ kHz}}$) did not identify differences between groups Cx26-Wt and Cx26-H at age 20–39 years (females *p* = 0.064, males *p* = 0.080). However, statistically significant differences in hearing thresholds were observed at age 40–59 years in both groups Cx26-Wt and Cx26-H (females *p* = 0.000, males *p* = 0.024) (Figure 3).

Following analysis at all measured frequencies (0.25, 0.5, 1.0, 2.0, 4.0, 8.0 kHz) revealed that in group Cx26-Wt averaged audiological profile of females and males aged 20–39 and 40–59 years had a shape of flat curve. Averaged audiological profile of females and males aged 20–39 years in group Cx26-H had a shape

of sloping curve, aged 40–59 years – steep-sloping curve in high-frequent range (4.0–8.0 kHz) (Figure 4).

Hearing threshold median at all measured frequencies did not reach 20.0 dB in males and females aged 20–39 years from both groups (Cx26-Wt and Cx26-H) (Figure 4). However, statistically significant (*p*<0.05) differences were observed at frequency 8.0 kHz in both sexes and at frequency 4.0 kHz – in females (Figure 4).

Statistically significant differences (*p*<0.05) in hearing thresholds at frequencies 4.0–8.0 kHz between groups Cx26-Wt and Cx26-H were observed in females and males aged 40–59 years (differences for females were observed starting from frequency 2.0 kHz, for males – from 1.0 kHz). Moreover, median value of hearing threshold was ≥20.0 dB in single mutation IVS1+1G>A carriers at 4.0–8.0 kHz for females, and at 8.0 kHz – for males (Figure 4).

Discussions

ARHI is multifactorial disorder due to environmental and poor-known genetic components. Studying the contribution of single mutations in *GJB2* gene to ARHI had somewhat controversial results.

Engel-Yeger et al. did not detect difference in mean hearing thresholds between c.35delG mutation – carriers (n = 40 persons) and individuals with normal *GJB2* genotype [11]. However, they found proved differences in otoacoustic emission amplitude between the compared groups [26]. Also, associations between c.35delG heterozygous carrier state and age-related hearing alterations with influence of occupational noise were not shown even on more representative sample (2311 individuals) [13]. It is possible that in these studies the difference in hearing thresholds between carriers and non-carriers was not detected due to the inadequate sample size or due to specific features of the chosen method of analysis.

Moreover, there is a study that detected statistically significant differences in mean hearing thresholds on high frequencies (6.0 and 8.0 kHz) between mutation c.35delG carriers (n = 31) and individuals with normal *GJB2* genotype (n = 29) in Italy, however, this study failed to find a correlation of hearing threshold increase with age [12]. Hearing loss predominantly on high and extra-high frequencies (8.0–16.0 kHz) was found to be significantly more severe in *GJB2* c.35delG heterozygous females in comparison with controls [15]. The recent study of hearing status in carriers of *GJB2* single mutations, c.35delG and p.Met34Thr (c.101T>C), conducted in a UK population from 1991 to 2011 with three-step audiological test of children aged 3, 7 and 11 years (9202 children) showed that hearing thresholds on extra-high frequency (16.0 kHz) in c.35delG and p.Met34Thr (c.101T>C) carriers was significantly worse than in children without *GJB2* gene mutation and tend to increase with age [14].

A recently published study provides the data comparable to our results. The study carried out in China (2011) showed that in c.235delC heterozygous carriers hearing for high-frequency (4.0 and 8.0 kHz) increases at the age of 30–59 years and hearing thresholds in the intermediate frequencies may deteriorate over the age of 40 [16].

Our study provides the first evidence that in a relatively isolated Yakut population the average hearing thresholds at the speech frequencies ($PTA_{0.5,1.0,2.0,4.0 kHz}$) linearly increase (p<0.05) with age in the heterozygous carriers of single site splicing mutation IVS1+1G>A (*GJB2* gene) of both sexes. This correlation is more expressed in males, which probably associated with physiological features and environmental factors. Moreover, audiometric analysis showed that hearing thresholds at high frequency (8.0 kHz) in heterozygous for IVS1+1G>A females and males aged 20–39 years were definitely worse (p<0.05) than in non-carriers. We also found that hearing on lower frequencies (1.0–2.0 kHz) was affected in both heterozygous for IVS1+1G>A females and males aged 40–59 years (Figure 4). At the same time, these parameters in non-carriers do not cause concerns about hearing impairment regardless of age and sex. We determined

onset of hearing worsening in individuals with genotype IVS1+1G>A/wt as ~40 years ($r_s = 0.504$, $p = 0.003$). Thus, we identified that hearing acuity of single mutation IVS1+1G>A carriers on particular frequencies was decreased compared to non-carriers, regardless of sex and age. Splice site mutation IVS1+1G>A, probably leads to a deficiency of normal Cx26 molecules that form intercellular gap junction channels, and this results in impaired recycling of potassium ions in the cochlea with a local organ of Corti intoxication [27]. Thus, carrying the single mutation IVS1+1G>A may cause hearing worsening with ageing.

Conclusion

Despite the controversial results of previous audiological analysis of the c.35delG mutation in heterozygous carriers from Caucasian populations [10–15], the results of this study demonstrate that the single IVS1+1G>A mutation (*GJB2*) is associated with age-related hearing impairment (ARHI) of the IVS1+1G>A carriers among the Yakuts.

Acknowledgments

We thank all patients and blood sample donors who have contributed to this study. This study was supported by the Russian Foundation for Basic Research (12-04-00342_a, 12-04-98520_r_vostok_a, 12-04-97004_r_povolzhye_a, 12-04-31230_mol_a, 14-04-01741_A), Federal Program «Scientific and educational staff for innovative Russia» (#16.740.11.0190, #16.740.11.0346), Integration project of SB RAS #92 «Ethnogeny of indigenous peoples in Siberia and North Asia: comparative, historical, ethno -social and genomic analysis», the Sakha Republic President Grant #80 for Young Researchers for 2014 year, Scientific and Educational Foundation for Young Scientists of Republic of Sakha (Yakutia) for 2014 year, Project #656 of Ministry of Education and Science of Russia, by grant #30 (2013–2015) of RAS Program «Fundamental Sciences for Medicine».

Author Contributions

Conceived and designed the experiments: NB FT SF. Performed the experiments: NB FT VP AS LK NS AK LV EF NL. Analyzed the data: NB FT MP SL EZ KS NG OP LD. Contributed reagents/materials/analysis tools: AR AA OP LD EK SF. Wrote the paper: NB FT OP LD.

References

1. Huyghe JR, Van Laer L, Hendrickx JJ, Fransen E, Demeester K, et al. (2008) Genome-wide SNP-based linkage scan dentifies a locus on 8q24 for an age-related hearing impairment trait. Am. J. Hum. Genet. 83: 401–407.

2. Yamasoba T, Lin FR, Someya S, Kashio A, Sakamoto T, et al. (2013) Current concepts in age-related hearing loss: Epidemiology and mechanistic pathways. Hear. Res. 303: 30–8.

3. Smith RJ, Bale JF Jr, White KR (2005) Sensorineural hearing loss in children. Lancet 365: 879–890.

4. Morton NE, Ann NY (1991) Genetic epidemiology of hearing impairment. Acad. Sci. 630: 16–31.

5. Fransen E, Topsakal V, Hendrickx JJ, Van Laer L, Huyghe JR, et al. (2008) Occupational noise, smoking, and a high body mass index are risk factors for age-related hearing impairment and moderate alcohol consumption is protective: a European population-based multicenter study. J. Assoc. Res. Otolaryngol. 9(3): 264–76.

6. Van Laer L, Van Eyken E, Fransen E, Huyghe JR, Topsakal V, et al. (2008) The grainyhead like 2 gene (GRHL2), alias TFCP2L3, is associated with age-related hearing impairment. Hum. Mol. Genet. 17: 159–169.

7. Friedman RA, Van Laer L, Huentelman MJ, Sheth SS, Van Eyken E, et al. (2009) GRM7 variants confer susceptibility to age-related hearing impairment. Hum. Mol. Genet. 18: 785–796.

8. Van Laer L, Huyghe JR, Hannula S, Van Eyken E, Stephan DA, et al. (2010) A genome-wide association study for age-related hearing impairment in the Saami. European Journal of Human Genetics 18: 685–693.

9. Ballana E, Ventayol M, Rabionet R, Gasparini P, Estivill X Connexins and deafness Homepage. Available: http://www.crg.es/deafness.

10. Morell RJ, Kim HJ, Hood LJ, Goforth L, Friderici K, et al. (1998) Mutations in the connexin 26 gene (GJB2) among Ashkenazi Jews with nonsyndromic recessive deafness. N. Engl. J. Med. 339: 1500–1505.

11. Engel-Yeger B, Zaaroura S, Zlotogora J, Shalev S, Hujeirat Y, et al. (2002) The effects of a connexin 26 mutation 35delG on oto-acoustic emissions and brainstem evoked potentials: homozygotes and carriers. Hearing Research 163: 93–100.

12. Franzé A, Caravelli A, Di Leva F, Marciano E, Auletta G, et al. (2005) Audiometric evaluation of carriers of the connexin 26 mutation 35delG. Eur. Arch. Otorhinolaryngol. 262: 921–924.

13. Van Eyken E, Van Laer L, Fransen E, Topsakal V, Hendrickx JJ, et al. (2007) The contribution of GJB2 (Connexin 26) 35delG to age-related hearing impairment and noise-induced hearing loss. Otol. Neurotol. 28: 970–975.

14. Hall A, Pembrey M, Lutman M, Steer C, Bitner-Glindzicz M (2012) Prevalence and audiological features in carriers of GJB2 mutations, c.35delG and c.101T> C (p.M34T), in a UK population study. BMJ Open 31 2(4): 3–8.

15. Groh D, Seeman P, Jilek M, Popelář J, Kabelka Z, et al. (2013) Hearing function in heterozygous carriers of a pathogenic GJB2 mutation. Phisiol. Res. 62(3): 323–30.

16. Li Q, Fang RP, Wang GJ, Liu F, Dai P (2011) Tonal audiometry of GJB2 235delC single heterozygous mutation carriers. Zhonghua Er Bi Yan Hou Tou Jing Wai Ke Za Zhi 46(7): 543–6. (Article in Chinese).

17. Barashkov NA, Dzhemileva LU, Fedorova SA, Teruytin FM, Posukh OL, et al. (2011) Autosomal recessive deafness 1A (DFNB1A) in Yakut population isolate in Eastern Siberia: extensive accumulation of the splice site mutation IVS1+1G>A in GJB2 gene as a result of founder effect. Journal of Human Genetics 9: 631–639.

18. Zerjal T, Dashnyam B, Pandya A, Kayser M, Roewer L, et al. (1997) Genetic relationships in Asians and Nothern Europeans, revalated by Y-chromosomal analysis. Am. J. Hum. Genet. 60: 1174–1183.
19. Pakendorf B, Novgorodov IN, Osakovskij VL, Danilova AP, Protod'jakonov AP, et al. (2006) Investigating the effects of prehistoric migrations in Siberia: genetic variations and the origins of Yakuts. Hum. Genet. 120: 334–353.
20. Khar'kov VN, Stepanov VA, Medvedev OF, Spiridonova MG, Maksimova NR, et al. (2008) The origin of Yakuts: analysis of Y-chromosome haplotypes. Mol. biol. (Mosk.) 42: 226–237.
21. Fedorova SA, Reidla M, Metspalu E, Metspalu M, Rootsi S, et al. (2013) Autosomal and uniparental portraits of the native populations of Sakha (Yakutia): implications for the peopling of Northeast Eurasia. BMC Evolutionary Biology 13: 127.
22. Kelsell DP, Dunlop J, Stevens HP, Lench NJ, Liang JN, et al. (1997) Connexin 26 mutations in hereditary non-syndromic sensorineural deafness. Nature 387: 80–83.

23. Zelante L, Gasparini P, Estivill X, Melchionda S, D'Agruma L, et al. (1997) Connexin 26 mutations associated with the most common form of non-syndromic neurosensory autosomal recessive deafness (DFNB1) in Mediterra-neans. Hum. Mol. Genet. 6: 1605–1609.
24. Kelley PM, Harris DJ, Comer BC, Askew JW, Fowler T, et al. (1998) Novel mutations in the connexin 26 gene (GJB2) that cause autosomal recessive (DFNB1) hearing loss. Am. J. Hum. Genet. 62: 792–799.
25. Sirmaci A, Akcayoz-Duman D, Tekin M (2006) The c.IVS1+1G>A mutation in the GJB2 gene is prevalent and large deletions involving the GJB6 gene are not present in the Turkish population. J. Genet. 85: 213–216.
26. Engel-Yeger B, Zaaroura S, Zlotogora J, Shalev S, Hujeirat Y, et al. (2003) Otoacoustic emissions and brainstem evoked potentials in compound carriers of connexin 26 mutations. Hearing Research 175 (1–2): 140–51.
27. Lefebvre PP, Van De Water TR (2000) Connexins, hearing and deafness: clinical aspects of mutations in the connexin 26 gene. Brain Res. Brain Res. Rev. 32: 159–162.

17

In Vitro and In Vivo Evaluation of a Hydrogel Reservoir as a Continuous Drug Delivery System for Inner Ear Treatment

Mareike Hütten[1,2◗], **Anandhan Dhanasingh**[3,4◗], **Roland Hessler**[3], **Timo Stöver**[5], **Karl-Heinz Esser**[2], **Martin Möller**[4], **Thomas Lenarz**[1], **Claude Jolly**[3], **Jürgen Groll**[4,6]*, **Verena Scheper**[1,7]*

1 Department of Otolaryngology, Hannover School of Medicine, Hannover, Germany, **2** University of Veterinary Medicine Hannover, Foundation, Institute of Zoology, Hannover, Germany, **3** MED-EL Innsbruck, Research & Development, Innsbruck, Österreich, **4** Interactive Materials Research–DWI e.V. and Institute of Technical and Macromolecular Chemistry, RWTH Aachen University, Aachen, Germany, **5** J.W. Goethe University Hospital and Faculty of Medicine, Department of Otolaryngology, Frankfurt am Main, Germany, **6** University of Würzburg, Department of Functional Materials in Medicine and Dentistry, Würzburg, Germany, **7** Institute of Audioneurotechnology, Hannover School of Medicine, Hannover, Germany

Abstract

Fibrous tissue growth and loss of residual hearing after cochlear implantation can be reduced by application of the glucocorticoid dexamethasone-21-phosphate-disodium-salt (DEX). To date, sustained delivery of this agent to the cochlea using a number of pharmaceutical technologies has not been entirely successful. In this study we examine a novel way of continuous local drug application into the inner ear using a refillable hydrogel functionalized silicone reservoir. A PEG-based hydrogel made of reactive NCO-sP(EO-*stat*-PO) prepolymers was evaluated as a drug conveying and delivery system *in vitro* and *in vivo*. Encapsulating the free form hydrogel into a silicone tube with a small opening for the drug diffusion resulted in delayed drug release but unaffected diffusion of DEX through the gel compared to the free form hydrogel. Additionally, controlled DEX release over several weeks could be demonstrated using the hydrogel filled reservoir. Using a guinea-pig cochlear trauma model the reservoir delivery of DEX significantly protected residual hearing and reduced fibrosis. As well as being used as a device in its own right or in combination with cochlear implants, the hydrogel-filled reservoir represents a new drug delivery system that feasibly could be replenished with therapeutic agents to provide sustained treatment of the inner ear.

Editor: Bernd Sokolowski, University of South Florida, United States of America

Funding: This study was supported by the DFG within the SPP 1259 "Intelligent hydrogels" (RWTH Aachen) and the European Community 6th Framework Programme on Research, Technological Development and Demonstration (Nanotechnology based Drug Delivery. Contract Number: NMP4-CT-2006-026556, Project acronym: NANOEAR; Hannover Medical School, MED-EL, RWTH Aachen). The funders had no role in study design, data collection and analysis, decision to publish, or preparation of the manuscript.

Competing Interests: The data and results presented within this manuscript are in total obtained with MEDEL as a research partner having no financial interest on the outcome of the study. No products exactly comparable to the one used in this study will be released to the market. AD, RH and CJ are employed by MED-EL Corporation. This does not alter the authors' adherence to PLOS ONE policies on sharing data and materials.

* Email: juergen.groll@fmz.uni-wuerzburg.de (JG); scheper.verena@mh-hannover.de (VS)

◗ These authors contributed equally to this work.

Introduction

Hearing loss affects approximately 278 million people worldwide. Next to infectious causes like meningitis, measles, mumps and chronic ear infections, hearing impairment is commonly triggered by exposure to excessive noise, head and ear injury, ageing and the use of ototoxic drugs [1]. Since sensory cells of the inner ear develop exclusively during embryogenesis and are not programmed to regenerate postnatally in mammals [2], in many cases hearing ability can only be regained by the insertion of a cochlear implant (CI) [3].

After CI surgery the acuity of residual hearing and that of CI-mediated hearing are often affected by postoperative intra-cochlear fibroblast growth and a delayed degeneration of neuronal tissue. A histological evaluation of human temporal bones from cochlear implant patients showed fibrous growth formation in 57% of examined cases. The fibrous growth formation were believed to be as a result of intra-cochlear mechanical trauma to the fine structures caused by electrode insertion as well as a foreign body reaction of the host tissue to the implant [4]. As a consequence, increased impedance, reduced speech perception and functional derogation of the device itself may take place [5].

Locally applied glucocorticoid receptor agonists like dexamethasone suppress inflammation in the inner ear and consequently prohibit growth of fibrosis related connective tissue expanse, cell degeneration and loss of residual hearing [6,7]. Due to the relative difficulty in accessing the inner ear, the maintenance of sufficient therapeutic levels of this agent over a prolonged period has been problematic. Available application aids like pump systems and intra-cochlear electrode array loaded with dexamethasone have limited delivery duration, are not rechargeable and/or have to be detached after entirely emitting the drug (reviewed by [8]). Polyethylene glycol (PEG) based hydrogels are one of the widely studied biomaterial as tissue culture scaffold and as drug loading and delivery system [9–11]. Briefly, hydrogels are three dimensionally cross-linked hydrophilic polymer chains that exhibit strong swelling in water and available as degradable or non-degradable depending on the polymer chain chemistry [12]. Non-degradable hydrogel in the free form state loaded with any water soluble low molecular weight drug molecules will be diffused out completely within 24–48 hours depending on how big is the volume of release medium. For the delayed release of drug for at least 4 week time for inner ear treatment, the drug loaded hydrogel has to be physically restricted from release medium which can be achieved by incorporating the drug loaded hydrogel within the thin electrode array. The electrical impedance of the CI which is a hint of fibrous tissue growth is largely taking place in the first 4 weeks of implantation [13].

We have previously shown that six-arm star shaped poly-(ethylene oxide-*stat*-propylene oxide) prepolymers with 80% ethylene oxide (EO) content in the backbone and reactive isocyanate groups at the distal ends of the arms (NCO-sP(EO-stat-PO) can be used to prepare ultra-thin biocompatible coatings that very efficiently minimize unspecific protein adsorption [14]. We have also shown that NCO-sP(EO-stat-PO) may be used to prepare physiologically stable three-dimensional hydrogels [15] and as cross-linker to polysaccharides [16].

In this study, we evaluated the physiologically stable NCO-sP(EO-stat-PO) hydrogel as drug carrier of dexamethasone 21-phosphate disodium salt (referred to as DEX in the manuscript), a hydrophilic modification of dexamethasone with high water solubility, in silicone tubes that connect the inner ear with an external potentially refillable drug reservoir. In order to evaluate the potential use of this hydrogel system together with an implant, we have assessed the processes regarding its filling into silicone tubes, drying for shelf-storage, heat-treatment for sterilization and re-swelling after time to examine tight fit at the inner lumen of the silicone tube. Drug release from the hydrogels was first examined as free gels without outer steric restriction in order to show pure diffusion controlled release. Subsequently, drug release kinetics were examined with the hydrogel filled into a silicone tube with one end open and PBS (pH 7.4) as the release medium. Additionally, the hydrogel was studied as drug diffusion gateway for a drug reservoir made of silicone tubing. In order to understand the drug diffusion behaviour, the hydrogel was primed and replenished with DEX. For *in vivo* evaluation, hydrogel reservoirs were used to deliver DEX into the inner ear in a guinea pig model. Reservoirs primed with PBS only as well as reservoirs being implanted and immediately explanted served as control. The response of the cochlea in terms of foreign body reaction and hearing loss were examined four weeks following the implantation procedure.

Materials and Methods

1. *In vitro* experiments

Star-shaped poly-ethers with a backbone of statistically copolymerized 80% ethylene oxide and 20% propylene oxide, molecular weight of 18000 g/mol (PD = 1.15) with isocyanate (NCO) end groups (NCO-sP(EO-stat-PO) was synthesized as described previously [17]. An overview on the chemical structure of the gel precursor and the cross-linking reaction is shown in Fig. S2. Dexamethasone 21-phosphate disodium salt (DEX; molecular weight 516.4 g/mol) was purchased from Sigma-Aldrich Ger-

many. Silicone tubes of 6 cm length with an internal diameter of 0.31 mm and an outer diameter of 0.64 mm were kindly provided by MED-EL GmbH, Austria.

1.1. Hydrogel preparation and determination of the swelling ratio. Hydrogels were prepared by dissolution of the reactive NCO-sP(EO-*stat*-PO) precursors in water as described before [15]. The cross-linked hydrogels were dried to xerogel condition in triplets in a vacuum chamber overnight and the dry weights were measured. Xerogels were then placed in an excess of phosphate buffered saline (PBS; pH 7.4) at 37°C for studying its swelling kinetics. The weight of the swollen gel was measured at specific time intervals until it reached its equilibrium swelling state. The swelling ratio is determined by the ratio of dry weight of the gel (W_d) to the swollen weight of the gel (W_s): swelling ratio = (W_d/W_s) ×100.

1.2. Drug release studies from free 3D hydrogels. NCO-sP(EO-stat-PO) was dissolved in a 50 mg/mL (w/v) DEX solution in PBS (pH 7.4) to a final concentration of 20% (w/v). Subsequently, 0.5 mL of this solution (containing 25 mg DEX) was placed into a Teflon mould of 15 mm diameter and 3 mm depth and covered airtight for 24 hours. After completed cross-linking, the DEX-loaded hydrogel was dried to zerogel in a vacuum chamber and then placed in PBS at 37°C for swelling and release of the drug molecules. The amount of drug released in to the PBS was measured by CARY 100 Bio UV-visible spectrophotometer at selected time intervals until the minimum detection limits were reached. The wavelength used to detect DEX was 238–242 nm.

1.3. Drug release from hydrogels in silicone tubes. PBS solution containing DEX (50 mg/mL) was used to dissolve homogenously the hydrogel precursor to obtain a 20% w/v concentration. By use of an insulin syringe avoiding air bubbles, the gellifying solution was sucked inside the silicon tubes of length 60 mm and an inner diameter of 0.31 mm with one end open and the other end closed. The silicone tubes were sealed for 24 hours to allow complete gelation and to prevent drying. Subsequently the silicone tubes containing the hydrogel were placed in PBS at 37°C to examine the release of DEX as mentioned in section 1.1.2.

1.4. Hydrogel as diffusion gate in drug reservoir. NCO-sP(EO-*stat*-PO) was dissolved in PBS and sucked inside a silicone tube from the open end for a length of 10, 5 and 2 mm and maintained undisturbed for 24 hours. After cross-linking of the hydrogel, the remaining length of the silicone tube between the closed end and the hydrogel was filled with DEX solution (100 mg/mL) using an insulin syringe. This set-up was again placed in PBS at 37°C to investigate the release profile of DEX as mentioned in section 1.1.2.

2. *In vivo* experiments

Normal hearing Dunkin Hartley guinea pigs (n = 28; Harlan-Winkelmann GmbH, Borchen, Germany) of both sexes, weighing about 400 g were used. All experiments were carried out in accordance with the institutional guidelines for animal welfare of Hannover Medical School following the standards described by both German laws on protecting animals (Tierschutzgesetz) and the European Communities Council Directive 86/609/EEC for the protection of animals used for experimental purposes. The experiments of this study were approved by the regional government (Niedersächsisches Landesamtes für Verbraucherschutz und Lebensmittelsicherheit, LAVES, registration no. 10/0137).

2.1. Hydrogel reservoir. Using a syringe, the NCO-sP(EO-stat-PO) solution was filled into the hollow silicone reservoirs

(4.32 μL total volume). One end of the reservoir was equipped with a silicone septum which could be perforated with a tuberculin syringe with a needle diameter of 0.5 mm for sterile injection of DEX solution. To allow for a less traumatic implantation, each reservoir tip was smoothed down but remained unsealed in order to release DEX from the hydrogel. After being filled the reservoir was sterilized using ethylene oxide. DEX priming was performed during surgery immediately before reservoir insertion into the inner ear.

DEX sodium phosphate (Spectrum chemical MFG. Corp., Gardena, California, USA) was dissolved in PBS (PBS tablets, Invitrogen Corporation, Paisley, Scotland, UK). The DEX concentration in PBS was 50 μg/μL for both HPLC and *in vivo* studies which necessitated a loading of 216 μg DEX per reservoir.

2.2. Acoustically evoked auditory brainstem response measurement. Before surgery (day 0) and subsequently on day 3, 7, 14, 21 and 28, animals were anesthetized (diazepam 2.5 mg/kg p.o., atropine sulfate 0.05 mg/kg s.c., ketamine 30 mg/kg i.m., xylazine 7.5 mg/kg i.m.) in order to perform frequency-specific acoustically evoked auditory brainstem response measurements (AABR). All animals were treated with subcutaneous (s.c.) injections of carprofen (0.5 mg/kg), and atropine (0.05 mg/kg) for analgesia and reduction of secretion respectively.

Four needle electrodes were inserted s.c.: a positive pole at the vertex, a ground electrode in the neck, and negative poles postauricularily on the mastoids. The guinea pigs were placed in a soundproof box positioned on a heating pad with a temperature of 37°C. Speakers were connected to the acoustic meatus by calibrated pipette tips.

For frequency-specific acoustic stimulation and measurement, hardware and software from Tucker-Davis Technologies (Alachua, FL, USA) were used. Stimuli were 10 ms pure tones with a cosine-squared rise-fall time of 1 ms (24-bit Sigma-Delta D/A conversion at 200 kHz sampling rate). Six different frequencies (1, 4, 8, 16, 32, and 40 kHz) generated in 10 dB steps from 20 to 90 dB SPL (decibel sound pressure level) were presented using the TDT software (BioSigRP). The recorded neural signals were digitized at 24 kHz sampling rate (16-bit) and bandpass filtered between 0.3 to 3 kHz. The measurements of every frequency and sound intensity were recorded 270 times and averaged.

For evaluation purposes, data were exported into Microsoft Excel (Microsoft Corporation, Redmond, Washington, Seattle, USA) where the recordings were graphed and the triple standard deviation (SD) of background noise of each measurement, recorded in a phase of non-stimulation was calculated and plotted graphically. Hearing threshold was defined as the lowest stimulus level that generated a visually detected peak 3 exceeding three times SD. In the case where no hearing threshold could be detected at the systems limit of 90 dB SPL, the hearing threshold was set to 100 dB SPL. For every individual, frequency specific hearing thresholds of every measurement were compared to the related hearing threshold determined before surgery on day 0. The difference between the pre-surgical hearing threshold and those following was defined as hearing loss.

2.3. Surgical procedures. Before surgery DEX solution and PBS were prepared freshly and filled into the reservoirs (for details see section 2.1.1).

Anaesthesia was performed similarly to that used for AABR but the dosage of ketamine and xylazine was higher (40 mg/kg i.m., respectively 10 mg/kg i.m.) and animals were supplied with enrofloxacine (10 mg/kg s.c.) for prevention of infection. Following initial AABR measurement on day 0 the postauricular area was bilaterally sheared placed under analgesia (1 ml prilocaine) and disinfected. Under sterile conditions a postauricular approach

was performed to visualize the *Bulla tympanica*. The periosteum was abscised and the middle ear was opened with scalpel and forceps. Using an OP-MI microscope (Carl Zeiss AG, Oberkochen, Germany) the cochlea was identified and ventral to the round window a cochleostomy was drilled in the basal turn of the cochlea (drilling head 600 μm diameter). The reservoir was inserted 3 mm deep into the perilymphathic space of the *Scala tympani* and left in situ. In an additional set of animals, reservoirs were inserted and withdrawn immediately to serve as a control trauma group. In all other groups the implant was fixed and the cochleostomy and fenestration of the middle ear were sealed with carboxylate cement (Durelon Carboxylate Cement, 3 M ESPE AG, 82229 Seefeld, Germany). Thereafter, the protruding part of the reservoir was rolled-up and secured s.c. and the wound was sutured in two layers.

Animals were treated bilaterally but some ears had to be excluded from the study due to e.g. reservoir displacement after tissue harvesting. To summarize the treatments, 11 animals (14 ears used) were treated with DEX administered by the hydrogel reservoir, 10 animals (12 ears used) received PBS released from the hydrogel reservoir and 7 animals (12 ears used) served as trauma group.

2.4. Exploitation of specimens. On day 28 guinea pigs were anesthetised (ketamine 40 mg/kg i.m., xylazine 10 mg/kg i.m., atropine 0.05 mg/kg s.c.), the final AABR measurement was performed after which the sternal area of the animal was placed under analgesia with 4 ml prilocaine (2%). The chest was opened and the animal was perfused intracardially with 200 ml PBS and then fixed with 200 ml of modified Wittmaack fixing solution. The inner ears were extracted while the end section of the reservoirs remained inside the *Scala tympani*.

The *fenestra ovalis* and the apex were pierced with a lancet and the specimens were fixed in advanced Wittmaack fixing solution for up to 24 hours, rinsed for 10 hours with a 4% solution of lithium sulphate (Merck KGaA, Darmstadt, Germany) and dehydrated (2 hours per concentration) in ascending ethanol concentrations (50% v/v, 70% v/v 90% v/v and 100%) or optionally overnight in 70% v/v ethanol. Afterwards they were dried at room temperature and embedded in 5 parts epoxy resin and 2 parts hardening agent (SpeciFix-40 Kit, Struers GmbH, Ballerup, Denmark). Resin was adjusted by the addition of titanium oxide for whitening and reduction of transparency. Specimens and resin were filled into self-made silicone moulds with an inner diameter of 3 cm and a height of 4 cm (silicone source: SORTA Clear 40, Kaupo, Spaichingen, Germany) and placed into vacuum until all spaces in the specimens were filled with epoxy resin. The vaccum was slowly released and the samples were left to harden overnight at room temperature.

2.5. Grinding, Histology. All specimens were grinded with a grinding machine (PowerPro 4000, Bühler, Lake Bluff, Illinois, USA) and abrasive paper. After reaching the cochlea with coarse sand paper (grain size 800) the process was then continued with fine sandpaper (grain size 1200). For every layer of the cochlea, 20 μm were abraded and the section was stained for two minutes with each eosine and toluidine (Merck KGaA, Darmstadt, Germany). The freshly stained surface of the specimen was photographically documented at 30-, 150- and 200-times magnification using a Keyence system (VHX-600 DSO, Osaka, Japan).

For assessment of tissue response inside the *Scala tympani*, Keyence software was used to measure the area occupied with connective tissue in the first and the last mid-modiolar plane section as well as that arithmetically lying in between those two sections. The 7 cross sections of the *Scala tympani* per section were titled as lower basal turn, upper basal turn, first middle turn,

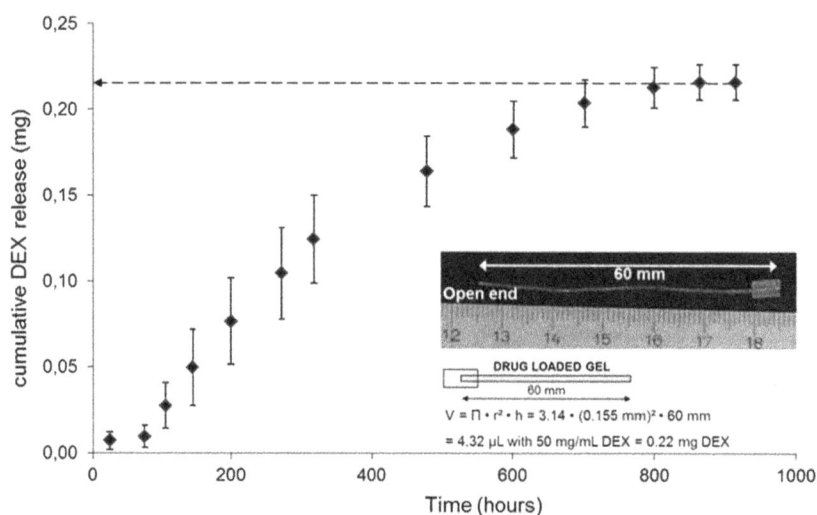

Figure 1. Image of a hydrogel reservoir with one end closed by a silicone septum for fluid injections (right end), while the other end is open in order to release the drug into the area to be addressed (left end) and calculation of the amount of drug inside the hydrogel filled tube. Drug release from this arrangement is shown in the diagram. The data points result from nine experiments from three different NCO-sP(EO-*stat*-PO) batches, each of them used for the preparation of three release setups.

second middle turn, third middle turn, forth middle turn and apical turn [18]. Connective tissue span was set into a ratio to the area of the *Scala tympani* which were measured by tracking the inner outline of the Scala tympani using the Keyence software. Additionally, for every single layer and every part of the *Scala tympani* (lower basal to apical turn) a subjective evaluation using a ranking system was performed in order to monitor the distribution of connective tissue in relation to the point of cochleostomy and the turns of the cochlea. The rationale for subjective ranking was: score 0: no connective tissue; score 1: less than one quarter of the scala tympani is filled with connective tissue; score 2: less than half but more than one quarter of the scala has to be filled with tissue and/or the whole surface of the implants crosscut has to be covered; and score 3: more than half of the scala tympani is filled with connective tissue; see Fig. S1)

In order to correlate results from fibrosis evaluation and AABR measurements, averages of the single values of every group were composed and compared to the averaged results of hearing loss on day 28.

2.6. Statistical Analysis. Statistical analysis was performed using GraphPad Prism 5 (GraphPad Software Inc., La Jolla, California, USA). Since animals were treated bilaterally, the correlation of left and right ears of same individuals were excluded, before using One-way ANOVA in combination with the Tukey post-test to compare mean hearing loss and measurement or ranking of tissue response within the turns for each group or for grouped comparison of tissue formation in the turns. Unpaired students t-test was used to calculate differences between results of mean tissue growth ranking and measurement between groups. Correlation assessment between tissue growth determined by ranking and hearing threshold shift was performed using a nonparametric correlation test (Spearman). Significance was defined as p-values with $* = p < 0.05$, $** = p < 0.01$, $*** = p < 0.001$.

Results

3.1. *In vitro* results - Drug release studies from DEX loaded free form hydrogels

As reported previously [19], the free-form hydrogel reached the EWC state from dry state within 360 minutes and cryo-SEM pictures shows the macro-porous morphology of the hydrogel in the EWC state. (Fig. S2 and S2C). However, the pores are not inter-connected and the molecular mesh size of the hydrogel network remains decisive for diffusion of drug molecules through the hydrogel. The drug release from free standing 3D hydrogels is fully diffusion controlled and almost quantitative within 24 hours (Fig. S3).

3.2. *In vitro* results - Drug release studies from hydrogels in silicone tubes

In this configuration, the release of drug may logically occur only through the open end of the silicone tube. The walls of the silicone tube will restrict the hydrogel to swell to its full equilibrium state, hence at every point of time the hydrogel will exert a swelling force against the inner wall of the silicone tube by which the hydrogel adjusts tightly to the inside wall of the silicone tube. The exact dimension of the silicone tube reservoir with the amount of drug molecule inside the hydrogel and the cumulative release profile is shown in Fig. 1. Reproducibility of the hydrogel packing inside the silicone tube reservoir and the kinetics of the drug release were performed with three batches of separately prepared DEX loaded hydrogels with each of the batches inserted in three different tubes. Although the release of the drug happens by diffusion process, the geometrical constraint result in a time of about 900 hours or 38 days until DEX is quantitatively released. Interestingly, there was only negligible release in the first 50 hours. This may be explained by the initial diffusion of water inside the gel such that maximal water content in the tube is reached allowing the diffusion controlled release to start.

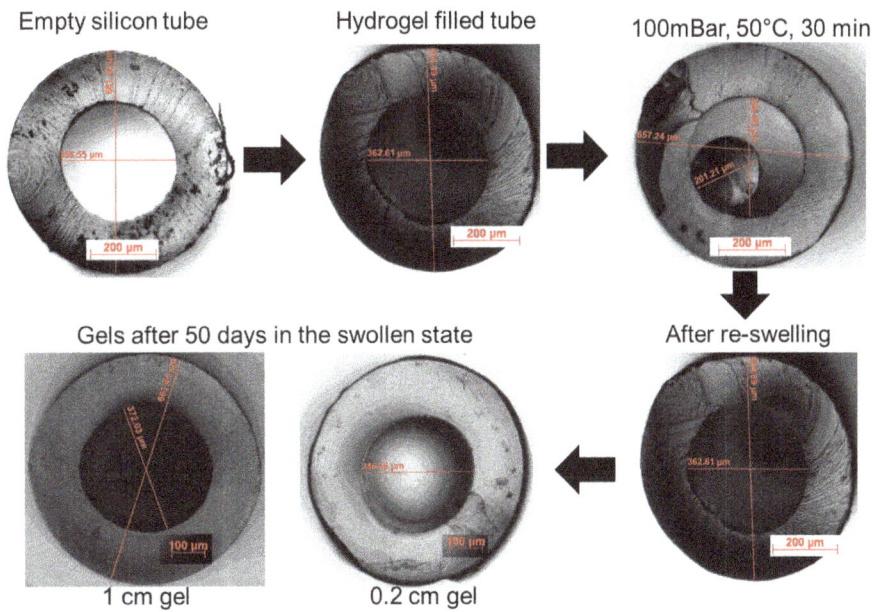

Figure 2. Cross-section images of silicone tubes before and after filling between 2 and 10 mm with with 20% (w/v) NCO-sP(EO-stat-PO) gels (top left and middle), after drying of the gel (top right), re-swelling (bottom right) and after maintaining the gels in a swollen condition for 50 days (bottom left).

3.3. *In vitro* results - Drug release studies from hydrogel as diffusion gate for drug reservoir

In this configuration, the open end of the silicone tube is filled hydrogel for a certain length, so as to create a diffusion gate that could possibly separate the inner ear from an externally accessible drug reservoir. We also evaluated the possibility to dry and re-swell the set-up and whether this would lead to a tight fit of the re-swollen gel inside the tubes. Fig. 2 presents a series of images showing cross-sections of silicone tubes before and after filling with gel. In order to evaluate whether the gels remain in the tubes after drying and re-swelling, the gels in the tubes were warmed to 50°C under reduced pressure (100 mbar) for 30 minutes which resulted in a strong shrinkage of the hydrogel. However, the gels remained at the place in the tubes where they had been placed and after re-swelling the gels tightly closed the inner lumen of the tubes without any visible gaps, this being independent of the hydrogel gate length.

We also checked whether longer incubation times affected the hydrogels within the tubes with regard to signs of degradation or morphological changes. Our results show that at least for 50 days, no changes of the hydrogel within the tubes could be observed.

We then prepared the aforementioned hydrogel gate arrangement in triplets and loaded the free space in the tubes with DEX solutions (100 mg/mL) to study the drug release kinetics. During this procedure (see Fig. S4 for details) it was necessary to create a pinhole at one place in the side wall of the silicone tube. In order to assess whether this pinhole did not result in uncontrolled release during the studies, we checked its tightness by using a dye solution (Fig. S5). This control experiment showed that the pinhole closes tightly after removal of the needle and no uncontrolled release occurs. Fig. S6 shows images of three samples with hydrogel gates of 10, 5 and 2 mm length as well as the calculation of drug loading and the drug release profiles. Again an initial lag-time was observed, however with about 100 hours being twice as long. This results from the need for DEX to diffuse through the hydrogel gates before release can occur. Quantitative release of DEX was

reached in all three gate-length cases after approximately 1200 hours (= 50 days).

Since DEX release started earlier in the completely gel filled tubes and the diffusion time of DEX out of those fully filled tubes remained for 38 days, which covers the critical time period in cochlear implant patients, these results encouraged us to examine whether this system would demonstrate beneficial effects *in vivo*.

3.4. *In vivo* results - AABR measurements

On experimental day 0, prior to surgery, all animals were possessing normal hearing. No significant differences in mean AABR thresholds, given as lowest sound intensity where the brainstem response exceeded the triple standard deviation of the background noise, were observed between experimental groups across all frequencies (data not shown). Postoperatively, all groups suffered from an initial loss of hearing detected in the average of all frequencies measured three days after surgery: the mean $\pm$ SEM difference compared to the day 0 threshold was: 8.33 ± 4.52 dB SPL in the reservoir + DEX group, 16.94 ± 7.04 dB SPL in the reservoir + PBS group and 39.03 ± 7.28 dB SPL in the trauma group (Fig. 3).

This hearing loss stayed statistically stable within every group over the whole experimental time but it significantly differed among the four groups over this time period. Significantly better results in comparison to all other groups from day 3 until day 28 were detected in animals implanted with the reservoir applying DEX (hearing loss on experimental day 28: 14.42 ± 1.54 (mean $\pm$ SEM) dB SPL; $p_{reservoir + DEX \, vs. \, trauma}<0.001$, $p_{reservoir + DEX \, vs. \, reservoir + PBS}<0.01$), whereas the highest hearing loss (43.17 ± 1.08 (mean $\pm$ SEM) dB SPL) was measured in the trauma group ($p_{trauma \, vs. \, reservoir + DEX}<0.001$, $p_{trauma \, vs. \, reservoir + PBS}<0.001$) (Fig. 3)

Concerning the frequency specific hearing loss within each experimental group, differences are only seen between the 1 kHz and 8 kHz spectrum of the trauma group (hearing loss at 1 kHz: 28 ± 4.55; at 8 kHz: 56.5 ± 6.36 dB SPL (mean $\pm$ SD); p<0.05;

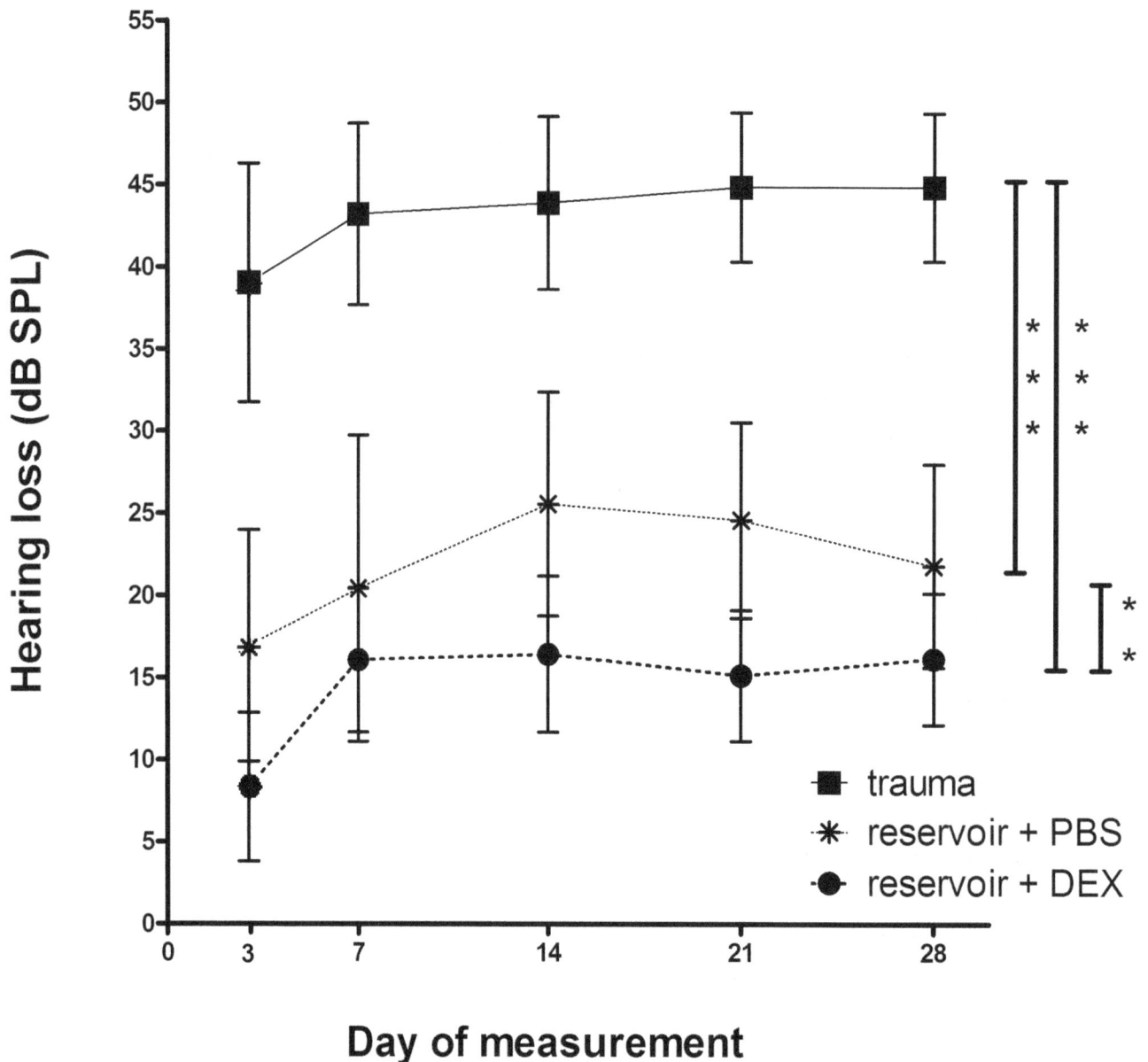

Day of measurement

Figure 3. Mean and SEM of hearing loss (difference between the experimental days hearing threshold and hearing threshold before implantation) development from day 3 to day 28 for all experimental groups. Cochleae of the trauma group (n = 12) suffered from highest hearing loss compared to all other experimental groups. Additionally, individuals implanted with a PBS releasing reservoir (n = 12) lost hearing more significantly compared to the group having been implanted with the DEX filled reservoir (n = 14). The statistical differences using ANOVA test examined on experimental day 28 are plotted at the right side of the graph, demonstrating, that the reservoir + DEX treatment resulted in the significantly best hearing thresholds. (** = p<0.01; *** = p<0.001).

Figure S7), or in the averaged results of all animals of all groups, where the mean hearing loss at 1 kHz was 15.94±3.35 SD dB SPL and thus statistically lower than hearing loss at 8 kHz (36.95±4.02 SD dB SPL, p<0.01), 16 kHz (31.47±4.22 SD, p< 0.05) and 32 kHz (31.45±3.81 SD, p<0.05) (data not shown).

3.5. *In vivo* results - Tissue response

3.5.1. Ranking of tissue growth – whole cochlea length. Using student's t-test the evaluation of fibrotic tissue response in the whole cochlea by use of a subjective scoring system revealed significant differences between the three experimental groups (Fig. 4A). The trauma group suffered from a more intense

tissue response (score: 0.83±0.12 SEM) which can be statistically underscored with a p-value of 0.0133 when compared to the reservoir + PBS group, and p<0.001, when matched with reservoir + DEX. The group treated with the reservoir and PBS (0.47±0.08) also achieved a higher ranking score than the reservoir + DEX treated ones (0.25±0.05 SEM; p<0.05).

3.5.2. Ranking of tissue growth - Distribution across scalae. In all experimental groups tissue growth was significantly worse in the basal half turns of the cochleae (Fig. 5 and S8) compared to the apical region or the middle turns (p<0.001) (Fig. S8). Concerning this characteristic, all groups achieved similar tendencies. In the trauma group basal turns (lower and upper basal turn) achieved a ranking score of 2.04±0.25. Middle turns a score

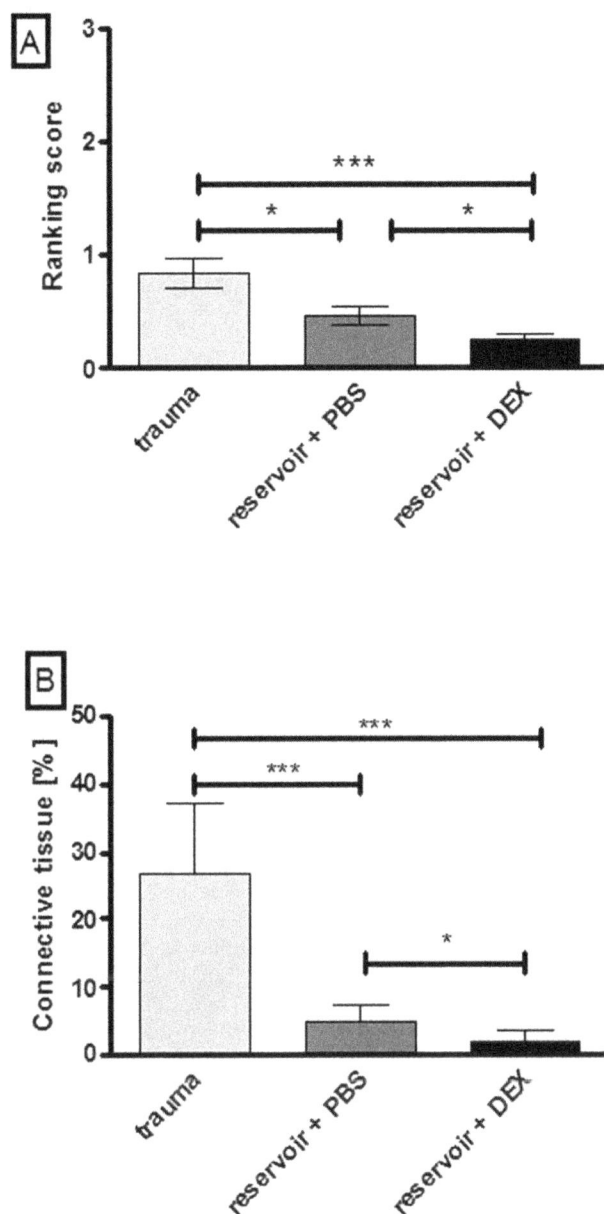

Figure 4. Graphed t-test results of tissue growth ranking (A) and measurement (B) for the whole cochlea length. Using both evaluation methods the tissue growth in the trauma group was significantly increased compared to the reservoir and DEX group with a p value <0.001. When applying the ranking score the difference between reservoir + PBS and trauma or reservoir + DEX was significant with p<0.05 (A). Comparing the tissue growth of the reservoir + PBS group with those of the trauma group or the DEX group using the measuring method, the p value is <0.001 (PBS vs. trauma) and <0.05 (PBS vs. DEX). Error bars: SEM. $*$ = p<0.05, $***$ = p<0.001.

of 0.42 ± 0.19 and apical turns a value of 0.08 ± 0.08 (p<0.001; Fig S8A). Basal turns of the reservoir + PBS group showed tissue growth with a ranking score of 1.45 ± 0.16 (Fig. S8B). Middle turns of 0.09 ± 0.05 and basal turns of the reservoir + DEX group had a score of 0.88 ± 0.11, while middle turns received a score of 0.0004 ± 0.0004 (Fig. S8C). Both of the reservoir groups exhibited no fibrotic tissue response in the apical turns Comparison of fibrotic tissue reaction in middle and apical turns did not show any significant differences (Fig. S8A–C).

Differences between the experimental groups were also demonstrated most clearly in their disparity of tissue growth in the basal regions and the 1st middle turn. Fig. 5, illustrating tissue growth ranking in all turns of all experimental groups, reveals the

trauma group to undergo significantly more tissue growth in the basal turn (2.41 ± 0.23 SEM) than both reservoir groups ($p_{trauma\ vs.\ reservoir+PBS}<0.001$, $p_{trauma\ vs.\ reservoir+DEX}<0.001$). The amount of newly formed tissue in the upper basal turns of all groups did not differ but the tissue in the first middle turn of the trauma group was significantly increased compared to the reservoir + DEX treated ones (p<0.05). In all scales more apical to this, no statistical relevant difference could be demonstrated among the groups and no significant differences were observed between PBS and DEX supported cochleae at all.

3.5.3. Quantitative measurement of tissue growth-whole cochlea length. When measuring the area of fibrotic tissue growth and relating it to the matching area of the *Scala tympani*

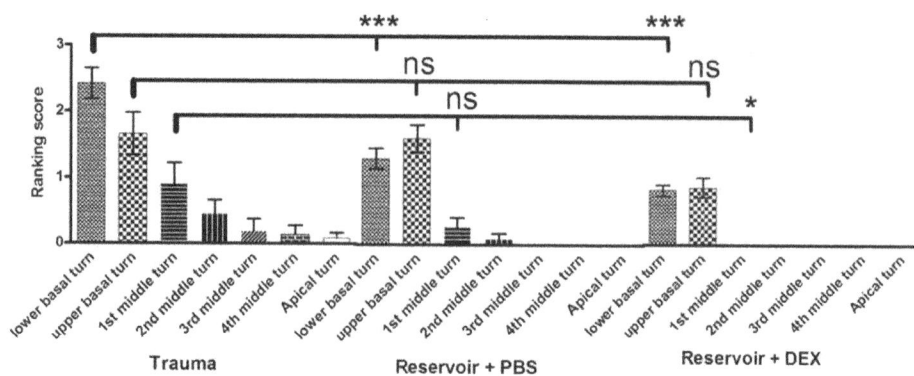

Figure 5. Distribution of fibrosis regarding subjective ranking for all inner ear turns and all experimental groups. In all groups the highest extend of connective tissue growth was detected in the basal turns. Fibroblast growth in more apical turns was only detected in the trauma group and did not take place in reservoir groups at all. Significant differences between the groups were detected (plotted above the SEM bars: * = p< 0.05, *** = p<0.001; reference of the significance is marked by the thick bar) and were most prominent in the lower basal turns (p<0.001). Even though there seems to be a tendency of increased tissue formation in the PBS group compared to the DEX group there is no statistical relevance detectable using One-way ANOVA in combination with the Tukey post-test to compare the means between groups.

we detected the highest tissue formation in the trauma group where 26.78±4.17% (mean ± SEM) of the *Scala tympani* area was covered with fibrotic tissue or bony structures (Fig. 4B). In comparison to cochleae provided with the reservoir + PBS (4.74±1.11%) and reservoir + DEX (2.14±0.55%) the trauma control group suffered from significantly higher tissue proliferation (p<0.001). A relevant difference in tissue formation was detected in reservoir + PBS treated animals compared to DEX treated ones as well (p<0.05).

3.5.4. Quantitative measurement of tissue growth – Distribution across scalae. The significantly most affected location of the cochlea are the basal turns when compared to more apical regions (p between <0.05 and <0.001; Fig. S9A–C). Fig. 6 and Fig. S9 illustrate the decrease of tissue growth from the basal to the apical parts of the cochleae. Comparisons of tissue growth within the turns of each experimental group are plotted in Fig. S9 A–C.

Additionally, the groups showed different amounts of tissue in the individual parts of the cochlea. In the lower basal turn trauma group reached a tissue fraction of mean ± SEM of 65.41±9.32% with a p-value of <0.001 compared to the tissue response found in the lower basal turns of reservoir + PBS group (16.17±4.01%), and reservoir + DEX group (8.25±2.46%) (Fig. 6). Similar findings are seen in the upper basal turn where the trauma group suffered from a tissue growth of 52.36±10.64%, and thus a statistically higher tissue reaction than the reservoir + PBS group (11.86±3.88, p<0.001) and reservoir + DEX group (6.67±1.95%, p<0.001). In the 1st middle turn the differences are found in p-values <0.01 between trauma group with a score of 39.95±12.92%, and reservoir + PBS group with a score of 3.7±2.91% and <0.001 for the reservoir + DEX group with 0.05±0.05%. Evaluation of the 2nd middle turn reveals a p-value of <0.05 for the difference between the trauma group (27.87±12.27%) and reservoir + PBS group (1.43±1.43%) and the reservoir + DEX (0%). In the 3rd middle turn of the trauma group 1.83±1.59% of the scala tympani area was filled with tissue, which was compared to the 3rd middle turns of the PBS or DEX treated groups, where no tissue growth was observed at all, although this tissue reaction was not statistically relevant. In all turns more apical to this point, no statistical distinction was found since no tissue growth was detected apical to the 3rd turn in any of the experimental groups (Fig. 6). Comparing the tissue growth

measured in PBS treated animals to those in DEX treated ones no statistically relevant difference was observed even though the tendency of higher fibrosis rate in PBS treated animals (lower basal: 16.17±4.01%; upper basal 6.67±1.95%; 1st middle 3.70±2.91%; 2nd middle: 1.43±1.43%) compared to DEX treated guinea pigs (lower basal: 8.25±2.46%; upper basal 11.86±3.88%; 1st middle 0.05±0.05%; 2nd middle: 0%) (Fig. 6) was clearly seen.

3.5.5. Differences in ranking and quantitative measurement. Results from subjective ranking of tissue reaction in all images taken from the scala tympani of all experimental animals and the findings from the tissue growth measurement performed in three pictures of each cochlea are very similar but significances differed between both methods when comparing the mean values of the experimental groups. More precisely, ranking showed a p-value of <0.05 for the difference between the trauma and the reservoir + PBS group (Fig. 4A), which is p<0.001 according to the measurement technique (Fig. 4B). Next to this, the statistical results were equal.

3.5.6. Correlation of tissue growth and hearing impairment. Tissue growth concurred with the results of AABR measurements. A profound correlation between mean values of the amount of tissue, determined by subjective ranking, and the averaged hearing loss of all frequencies of the individual animal was ascertained. It was demonstrated that with increasing tissue growth hearing loss increased (Fig. 7A). Using the Spearman-Rho-tests a correlation with r = 0.6338 (p<0.001) was detected.

Correlation between the location of new tissue formation in the scala tympani and hearing loss at specific frequencies was detected as well, that is to say, accumulation of tissue growth in basal parts of the cochlea were associated with loss of hearing in high frequencies, equally, tissue formation in the more apical cochlear turns did accompany loss of hearing in. lower frequencies. For example, the fibrous tissue expanse in the upper basal turn of all evaluated cochleae corresponded significantly (p = 0.0225) to the hearing loss detected at 32 kHz (r = 0.3742). And the other way around, the amount of tissue detected in the 3rd middle turn correlated significantly to the hearing loss at 1 kHz (p = 0.00231; r = 0.3727 (Fig. 7B and C).

The trauma group, which showed almost no residual hearing on day 28 (hearing threshold: 93.75±2.24 dB SPL) and thus the most severe hearing loss (44.86±4.52 dB), was marked by the most

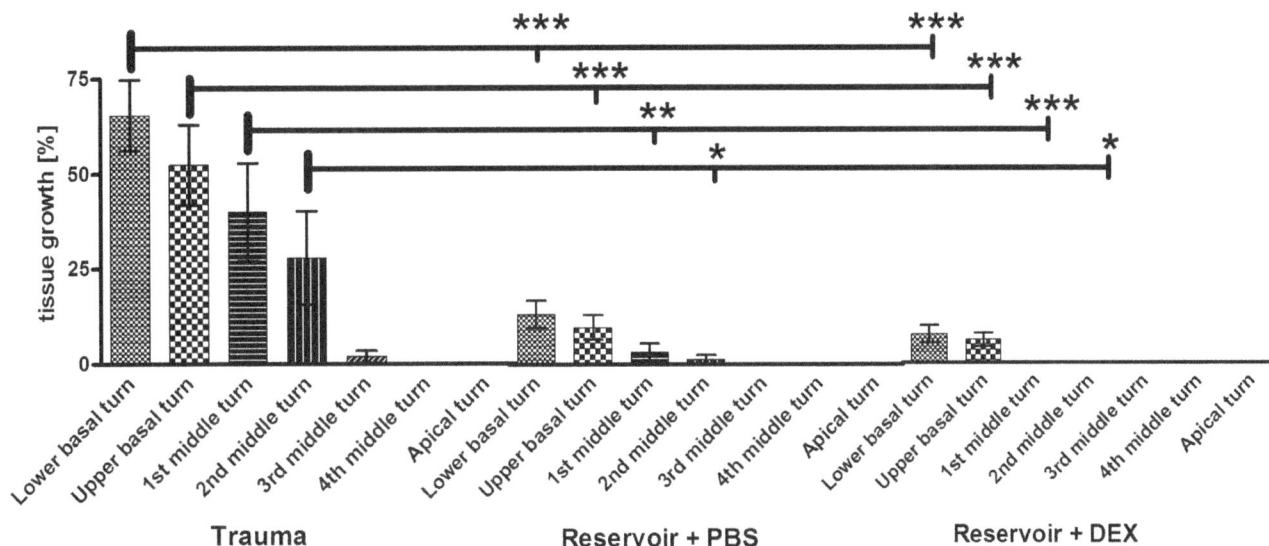

Figure 6. In this graph the mean and SEM percentage of measurement of connective tissue growth in the scala tympani of all experimental groups for each cochlear turn from basal to apical are plotted. The comparison of tissue growth between the groups is illustrated by horizontal lines. Reference of the significance is marked by the thick bar. Highly significant differences were observed between tissue growth in the trauma group and groups receiving PBS or DEX by reservoir. No differences were measured between PBS or DEX treated groups even though a slightly increased connective tissue growth seems to be apparent in the PBS group compared to DEX treated animals. In cochleae implanted with a PBS releasing reservoir tissue growth could be measured from basal up to the 2nd middle turn whereas in the reservoir and DEX treated cochleae connective tissue formation was only visible in the lower and upper basal region. One-way ANOVA in combination with the Tukey post-test was used to compare means between groups: * = p<0.05; ** = p<0.01; *** = p<0.001.

intense new tissue formation especially in the lower basal turn of the cochlea (ranking score for whole cochlea: 0.83±0.12; measurement: 26.78±10.21%). Animals provided with the reservoir plus PBS showed less tissue growth (ranking: 0.47±0.08; measurement: 4.74±2.49%) and reduced hearing loss (21.81±6.18 dB) and cochleae that were treated with the DEX reservoir developed minimal fibrotic outgrowth (ranking score: 0.25±0.05; measurement: 2.14±1.38%) associated with a minimal loss of hearing ability 28 days after implantation (16.15±4 dB).

3.5.7. Angiogenesis and osteogenesis. Additionally to fibrotic tissue growth, an organisation of the tissue in terms of angiogenesis was detected in 5 cochleae of the trauma group and one ear of the reservoir + PBS group. Furthermore, in two cochleae of the trauma group initial signs of osteogenesis were visible (see Fig. S1D).

Discussion

The aim of this study was the evaluation of a novel hydrogel reservoir for inner ear drug delivery *in vitro* and *in vivo*. The hydrogel precursor NCO-sP(EO-*stat*-PO) possesses highly reactive

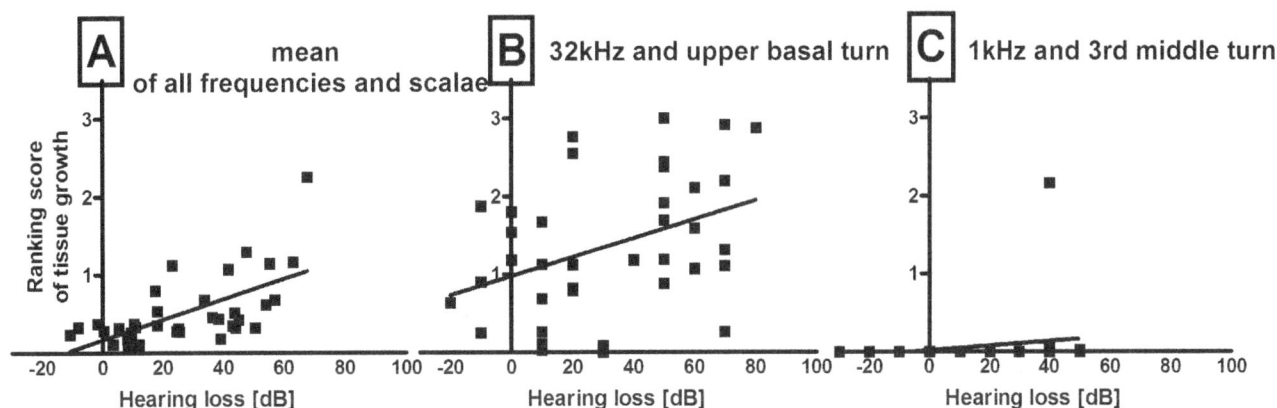

Figure 7. Correlation of hearing loss measured on day 28 and tissue reaction determined by ranking. Graph A illustrates that with the amount of tissue reaction evaluated over the whole cochlea length the loss of residual hearing in all frequencies increases (p<0.001; r = 0.6338). This effect is detectable in lower and higher frequency regions of the cochleae as well. In figure 7B the detected tissue reaction and hearing loss at the upper basal turn and at 32 kHz are plotted as an example for the correlation in higher frequency areas (p<0.05; r = 0.3742). Fig. C is an example for correlation of tissue reaction and hearing loss in lower frequency areas of the cochlea. Here we correlated hearing loss at 1 kHz and tissue growth in the 3rd middle turn (p<0.05; r = 0.3727).

isocyanate (NCO) groups which can potentially react with the alcohol groups of DEX. However, the presence of the phosphate groups and the two sodium counter ions render the molecule extremely hydrophilic while the isocyante groups are placed at relatively hydrophobic iosphorne-rings. Moreover, the hydroxyl groups of the drug molecule are directly attached to the aromatic ring. These various properties prevent permanent covalent binding of DEX to the hydrogel network to any detectable level [19].The free form hydrogels exhibited the fastest release kinetics within 24 hours as the release medium could have access to all the 3D surface of the hydrogels by which the diffusion of entrapped drug molecules in all the direction. The drug release was by swelling controlled diffusion process. The system where the hydrogel was completely filled inside the silicone tube, only the open end of the silicone tube have access to the release medium to the hydrogel. In this configuration, the wall of the silicone tube restricted the swelling kinetics of the hydrogel. In this system, the drug release was purely by diffusion controlled process which took almost 900 hours to release the loaded drug completely. In the other system where, the hydrogel without any drug in it was only acting as the diffusion gate, the drug from the reservoir had to diffuse through the hydrogel gate to reach the release medium; it took almost 1200 hours to release the drug completely. In the 1200 hours, the initial 100 hours was the lag time during which the drug had to diffuse through the gel gate. All these three configurations explain how the release of the drug can be controlled precisely by checking the access of the release medium to the hydrogels. Finally, examination of the hydrogel as a drug delivery matrix in a medical device used for inner ear treatment *in vivo* was carried out.

DEX was chosen for this drug delivery study as model drug because of its well-known anti-inflammatory and hair cell protective effects [6,7,20–22]. DEX suppresses apoptotic activities in response to TNF-α. Studies performed by Messmer and colleagues demonstrate that this effect can be achieved even up to 12 hours after TNF-α application. DEX retards the down-regulation of inhibitors of apoptosis proteins [23], blocks transcription of pro-inflammatory molecules and increases transcription of anti-inflammatory factors and reduces leukocyte migration through decreasing the adherence of these cells to the vascular endothelium [24]. Synthetic glucocorticoids are also able to decrease vascular permeability and vasodilatation, prominent features of the inflammatory reaction and necessary for the emigration of immune cells. Consequently, glucocorticoids reduce oedema and fibrin formation, inhibit capillary and fibroblast proliferation and enhance collagen breakdown [24].

These effects play an essential role in the neutralisation of foreign bodies or bacteria raising the consideration regarding the use of DEX in cases where infection may be likely or is actually present. Conversely, all of these properties are necessary in the suppression of inflammation concerning cochlear implantation. Hence, although a precautious use of DEX is essential, it is a noteworthy ally for offering protection of hearing ability following cochlear implantation [25–27].

The extent of tissue response was determined both by ranking and direct measurement. The results from both the methods were not equal but did tend to deliver the same information. While the measurement of 3 slices per scale per cochlea brought the quality of objective evaluation, the subjective ranking of tissue growth in every single slice covered a quantitative assessment. Since the measurement was performed on 1 mid-modiolar image and the one directly before and one directly after the modiolus, the measured area was identical in all cochleae. This leads to a high comparability between the cochleae but also implies that alteration

could only be detected in this specific region. Although the ranking underlay a subjective assessment, it was exclusively performed by one person who obliterates variation due to diverging assessment criteria of various individuals. In addition, scoring between 0 and 3 only allowed for an unrefined classification although as a positive factor, it involves the whole cochlea. As such, it is considered that the subjective ranking of all slices leads to a more comprehensive and accurate estimate of the level of tissue reaction.

Probably all distinctions between ranking results and measurement results concerning p-values are based on the alteration of modiolus-near or modiolus-distant evaluation and the fact that three images per scale used for objective measurement may not give a synopsis on the status of the whole cochlea. Nevertheless, ranking and measurement methods led to similar results in most cases, indicating that measurement can be used to support the coarser ranking score with more detailed values.

The reservoirs remained inside the *Scala tympani* and interacted with the inner ear in terms of foreign bodies over a time period of four weeks. Nevertheless, AABR results and the distribution of tissue growth along the cochlea length have shown that producing a trauma as performed on animals in the trauma group, has a more devastating influence on the structures of the inner ear. An initial hearing loss after surgery was observed on day 3 which remained stable over time. We consider that this initial hearing loss is brought about by the implantation procedure as well as the physical presence of the implant itself in the *Scala tympani* which may modify the fluid and basilar membrane movement and induce inflammatory reactions. An additional reason may be due to mechanical damage of hair cells although this would occur only in the basal region of the cochlea where the implant is located and would consequently affect only the higher frequency regions. Due to the fact that no differences in hearing loss between lower and higher frequencies were observed, this seems unlikely.

In contrast to Braun and colleagues who reported DEX-dependent hearing preservation without tissue reduction [28], we observed a correlation of hearing ability and fibrosis which has recently been reported by O'Leary [29]. These parameters depend on the same factor, inflammation, which lends to the concept that the tissue growth modifies the influence of the travelling wave towards the basilar membrane which in turn reduces exhibition of hair cells. Reduction of the nutrition requirement of sensory cells in this area may also occur as a consequence. Additionally, tissue proliferation inside the *Scala tympani* may disturb the travelling wave on its way towards the apical turns and consequently prohibit the stimulation of more apical sensory cells. As a result of this, hearing of higher frequencies is reduced as well as the sensation of low frequencies albeit the inflammation bring localised mostly in the basal turns.

All animals of the trauma group suffered from significantly increased hearing loss and tissue reaction compared to the other experimental groups. We believe that the double movement of the reservoir inside the cochlea of trauma group specimens, insertion as the first manipulation and explantation as the second, is a valid reason for this finding. In contrast, cochleae of the other groups had to sustain only one traumatic manipulation.

These results indicate that common application aids that have to be removed after usage may lead to traumatic changes of the inner ear. Consequently we suggest that an application aid, at least if its properties are comparable to the hydrogel reservoirs tested in this study, should be bound to the CI and remain inside the cochlea. Further studies concerning this topic would be necessary to evaluate if the findings from this study are generally representative for removable drug delivery systems. In addition to the different mechanical stimuli, it is important to consider whether more immunologically active cells arrived from the blood into the *Scala tympani* after the necessary rupture of the *Stria vascularis* during cochleostomy in cochleae of the trauma group. Although the opening of the cochleostomy was filled with carboxylate cement, it was not blocked with a close-fitting implant like the silicone reservoir and as a result the blood vessels inside the *Stria* may not have been compressed. Additional irritation by the cement may be assumed with respect to reports concerning pulpa irritation in dental medicine [30,31] and to a newly published study stating that dental cement, applied on guinea pig inner ears, leads to a strong new bone formation [32], even though this method is a widely used [33,34] and other reports have also assessed carboxylate cement to be non-irritating [35,36].

Luttikhuizen and colleagues stated in 2006 that inflammatory processes are related to components of the blood stream; not only immune cells like macrophages but, for example, proteins like fibrinogen, the complement system, antibodies and various inflammatory factors [37]. They are attracted by chemotactic factors that are secreted from injured tissue or by cells stressed by the presence of foreign bodies [4,38]. Although materials of current implants are biologically inert, they still trigger inflammatory responses of the surrounding tissue. This is based upon endogenous proteins that attach to the surface of the implant and attract components of the nonspecific immune system. In the later stages of the inflammatory process, following earlier leucocytic invasion, fibroblasts migrate towards the implant and build a tissue coating around the foreign material in order to protect the healthy tissue. This step is clearly seen in many specimens with implanted reservoirs (see Section 3.2.2).

Angiogenesis, another cardinal sign of inflammation, is seen in cochleae of the trauma and reservoir + PBS group. In cochleae of the trauma group angiogenesis had already progressed into a stage of osteogenesis. Subsequent to fibrotic tissue growth, angiogenesis follows as a consequence of the coagulation cascade and hypoxia and is incited by locally released histamine and fibrin fragment E [37]. Since most of these cells and substances are bound to the blood stream, the correlation between the effluence of blood into the cochlea and higher levels of inflammation must be considered.

Furthermore, the diameter and related rigidity as well as the material composition of the inserted piece of the reservoir, played an accessory role for the severity of the inflammatory reaction. Previous reports by Jolly and colleagues [26] demonstrated that electrode trauma depends on the size and flexibility of the array and that reduction of trauma can be achieved by flexible implants that easily adapt to the angulations of the cochlear turns. This information can be transferred to the implantation of silicone reservoirs that appear to be flexible which according to Jolly [26] should provoke less irritation in the tissue of the cochlea. This depends strongly on the composition of the material. The process of implantation and fixation of the reservoirs explains similarities between the impact administrated by reservoirs with either PBS or DEX. Nevertheless, significant higher fibrosis in PBS treated ears discovered over the whole length of the cochleae and the distinct angiogenesis in these cochleae prove the influence of DEX applied via the reservoir.

Conclusions

In this study, the technical feasibility of incorporating hydrogels prepared from NCO-sP(EO-*stat*-PO) pre-polymers within the silicone tube for sustained release of DEX for several weeks through diffusion process into the inner ear was demonstrated which encouraged the *in vivo* studies.

Animal experiments using normal hearing Dunkin Hartley guinea pigs followed by treatment and regular measurement of hearing loss showed significantly lower fibrosis in case of DEX loaded hydrogel reservoir as compared to a PBS releasing control-reservoir and pure trauma. Most importantly, the hearing loss was significantly lower in case of the DEX loaded hydrogel reservoirs as compared to the other groups. In contrast, considerable functional and morphological changes were detected in the trauma group. We hypothesize that the insertion and immediate explantation of a delivery device is even more destructive to the inner ear than the impact of a foreign body in terms of a reservoir.

Our results strongly suggest that the NCO-sP(EO-*stat*-PO) hydrogel reservoir is a promising drug delivery device to apply water-soluble drugs in therapeutically relevant doses into the inner ear for a sustained treatment period. We conclude that the hydrogel used in combination with a rechargeable design of reservoir is a promising alternative of drug delivery device. This method might be optimized by adapting the reservoir to the cochlear implant in order to combine its insertion with the inevitable implantation of the CI, and thus avoiding additional trauma. This would allow surgeons to decide on the execution of drug application during surgery.

Supporting Information

Figure S1   Representative images of tissue response scores A) representatively depicts the score 0 mainly detected in animals of the reservoir + DEX group. Images B) and C) illustrate score 1 and 2 representative for the reservoir + PBS or trauma groups. Score 3 is shown in D) which is taken from an animal of the trauma group. In this figure the reorganization of fibrotic tissue response (black arrow) in terms of ossification (white arrow) is clearly seen. Asterixes: hydrogel; black arrow head: silicone reservoir, missing in image D), taken from the trauma group, where the tubing was implanted and subsequently explanted.

Figure S2   Relevant chemical structure (A) Hydrogel precursor and the chemical reaction of isocyanates with H_2O, (B) shows the swelling kinetics of the hydrogel from its dry state to its fully swollen state, (C) microporous structure of the swollen hydrogel.

Figure S3   Structure of dexamethasone 21-phosphate disodium salt (DEX) and its complete release profile from the free form hydrogel.

Figure S4   Experimental procedure for sample preparation of the release studies from the silicone tubes with hydrogel gates.

Figure S5   Control experiment using a dye-solution showing that the pin-hole created in the silicone tube during loading of the DEX solution does not result in uncontrolled release.

Figure S6   Picture of hydrogel-gates with three different lengths in silicone tubes (top left), calculation of the amount of DEX in each of the tubes (top right) and result of the release studies (bottom).

Figure S7 Frequency specific hearing loss. The mean and SD of hearing loss of all experimental groups after 28 days of implantation is plotted for each frequency tested. In all groups the hearing loss seems to be less affected in the lower frequencies but statistical evaluation did not show any significant differences between the frequency specific hearing loss in any of the experimental groups.

Figure S8 Tissue growth evaluated by ranking. The mean ± SEM results of subjective ranking of tissue formation in the cochlea turns of each experimental group are plotted. In all groups the tissue reaction is significantly increased in the basal regions compared to the middle and apical regions. Fibrotic tissue response in more apical turns was only detected in the trauma group (A) and did not take place in reservoir groups treated with PBS (B) or DEX (C). One-way ANOVA in combination with the Tukey post-test was used to compare the tissue growth within the different cochlea turns of each experimental group: ** = p<0.01; *** = p<0.001. Reference of the significance is marked by the thick bar.

Figure S9 Tissue growth evaluated by measurement. The mean ± SEM percentage of scala tympani area of each

cochlea turn covered with tissue is plotted for each experimental group. In all groups the tissue reaction is significantly increased in the basal regions compared to the middle and apical regions. Fibroblast growth in more apical turns was only detected in the trauma group (A) and did not take place in reservoir groups treated with PBS (B) or DEX (C). One-way ANOVA in combination with the Tukey post-test was used to compare the fibrous tissue growth within the different cochlea turns of each experimental group: ** = p<0.01; *** = p<0.001. Reference of the significance is marked by the thick bar.

Acknowledgments

We thank Dr. Henning Voigt, Hannover School of Medicine, for his support in quality management, and Peter Erfurt, Hannover School of Medicine, for his technical advice in grinding techniques.

Author Contributions

Conceived and designed the experiments: MH AD RH TS KE MM TL CJ JG VS. Performed the experiments: MH AD RH JG VS. Analyzed the data: MH AD CJ JG VS. Contributed reagents/materials/analysis tools: TS KE MM TL CJ JG VS. Contributed to the writing of the manuscript: MH AD RH CJ JG VS.

References

1. WHO (2014). http://www.who.int/mediacentre/factsheets/fs300/en/.
2. Ruben RJ (1967) Development of the inner ear of the mouse: a radioautographic study of terminal mitoses. Acta Otolaryngol: Suppl 220: 221–244.
3. Lenarz T (1998) Cochlear implants: selection criteria and shifting borders. Acta Otorhinolaryngol Belg 52: 183–199.
4. Nadol JB Jr., Eddington DK (2004) Histologic evaluation of the tissue seal and biologic response around cochlear implant electrodes in the human. Otol Neurotol 25: 257–262.
5. Birman CS, Sanli H, Gibson WP, Elliott EJ (2014) Impedance, Neural Response Telemetry, and Speech Perception Outcomes After Reimplantation of Cochlear Implants in Children. Otol Neurotol.
6. Abi-Hachem RN, Zine A, Van De Water TR (2010) The injured cochlea as a target for inflammatory processes, initiation of cell death pathways and application of related otoprotectives strategies. Recent Pat CNS Drug Discov 5: 147–163.
7. Eshraghi AA, Adil E, He J, Graves R, Balkany TJ, et al. (2007) Local dexamethasone therapy conserves hearing in an animal model of electrode insertion trauma-induced hearing loss. Otol Neurotol 28: 842–849.
8. Borenstein JT (2011) Intracochlear drug delivery systems. Expert Opin Drug Deliv 8: 1161–1174.
9. Merrill EW (1993) Poly(ethylene oxide) star molecules: synthesis, characterization, and applications in medicine and biology. J Biomater Sci Polym Ed 5: 1–11.
10. Peppas NA, Keys KB, Torres-Lugo M, Lowman AM (1999) Poly(ethylene glycol)-containing hydrogels in drug delivery. J Control Release 62: 81–87.
11. Kim P, Kim DH, Kim B, Choi SK, Lee SH, et al. (2005) Fabrication of nanostructures of polyethylene glycol for applications to protein adsorption and cell adhesion. Nanotechnology 16: 2420–2426.
12. Hoffman AS (2002) Hydrogels for biomedical applications. Adv Drug Deliv Rev 54: 3–12.
13. Paasche G, Bockel F, Tasche C, Lesinski-Schiedat A, Lenarz T (2006) Changes of postoperative impedances in cochlear implant patients: the short-term effects of modified electrode surfaces and intracochlear corticosteroids. Otol Neurotol 27: 639–647.
14. Groll J, Amirgoulova EV, Ameringer T, Heyes CD, Rocker C, et al. (2004) Biofunctionalized, ultrathin coatings of cross-linked star-shaped poly(ethylene oxide) allow reversible folding of immobilized proteins. J Am Chem Soc 126: 4234–4239.
15. Dalton PD, Hostert C, Albrecht K, Moeller M, Groll J (2008) Structure and properties of urea-crosslinked star poly[(ethylene oxide)-ran-(propylene oxide)] hydrogels. Macromol Biosci 8: 923–931.
16. Dhanasingh A, Salber J, Möller M,Groll J (2010) Tailored hyaluronic acid hydrogel through hydrophilic prepolymer cross-linkers. Soft Matter 6: 618–629.
17. Goetz H, Beginn U, Bartelink C F, Gruenbauer H J M, Möller M (2002) Preparation of isphorone diisocyanate terminated star polyethers. Macromol Mater Eng 287: 223–230.
18. Scheper V, Paasche G, Miller JM, Warnecke A, Berkingali N, et al. (2009) Effects of delayed treatment with combined GDNF and continuous electrical

19. Dhanasingh A, Groll J (2012) Polysaccharide based covalently linked multi-membrane hydrogels. Soft Matters Advance article.
20. James DP, Eastwood H, Richardson RT, O'Leary SJ (2008) Effects of round window dexamethasone on residual hearing in a Guinea pig model of cochlear implantation. Audiol Neurootol 13: 86–96.
21. Kim HH, Addison J, Suh E, Trune DR, Richter CP (2007) Otoprotective effects of dexamethasone in the management of pneumococcal meningitis: an animal study. Laryngoscope 117: 1209–1215.
22. Takemura K, Komeda M, Yagi M, Himeno C, Izumikawa M, et al. (2004) Direct inner ear infusion of dexamethasone attenuates noise-induced trauma in guinea pig. Hear Res 196: 58–68.
23. Messmer UK, Pereda-Fernandez C, Manderscheid M, Pfeilschifter J (2001) Dexamethasone inhibits TNF-alpha-induced apoptosis and IAP protein downregulation in MCF-7 cells. Br J Pharmacol 133: 467–476.
24. Tizard IR (2004) Veterinary Immunology: An Introduction. Saunders.
25. Chandrasekhar SS, Rubinstein RY, Kwartler JA, Gatz M, Connelly PE, et al. (2000) Dexamethasone pharmacokinetics in the inner ear: comparison of route of administration and use of facilitating agents. Otolaryngol Head Neck Surg 122: 521–528.
26. Jolly C, Garnham C, Mirzadeh H, Truy E, Martini A, et al. (2010) Electrode features for hearing preservation and drug delivery strategies. Adv Otorhinolaryngol 67: 28–42.
27. Meltser I, Canlon B (2011) Protecting the auditory system with glucocorticoids. Hear Res 281: 47–55.
28. Braun S, Ye Q, Radeloff A, Kiefer J, Gstoettner W, et al. (2011) Protection of inner ear function after cochlear implantation: compound action potential measurements after local application of glucocorticoids in the guinea pig cochlea. ORL J Otorhinolaryngol Relat Spec 73: 219–228.
29. O'Leary SJ, Monksfield P, Kel G, Connolly T, Souter MA, et al. (2013) Relations between cochlear histopathology and hearing loss in experimental cochlear implantation. Hear Res 298: 27–35.
30. Ito M, Yagasaki H (2001) Bone substitute product and method of producing the same. United States Patent US 6,214,048 B1.
31. Seltzer S, Maggio J, Wollard RR, Brough SO, Barnett A (1976) Tissue reactions to polycarboxylate cements. J Endod 2: 208–214.
32. Burghard A, Lenarz T, Kral A, Paasche G (2014) Insertion site and sealing technique affect residual hearing and tissue formation after cochlear implantation. Hear Res 312C: 21–27.
33. Scheper V, Wolf M, Scholl M, Kadlecova Z, Perrier T, et al. (2009) Potential novel drug carriers for inner ear treatment: hyperbranched polylysine and lipid nanocapsules. Nanomedicine (Lond) 4: 623–635.
34. Vivero RJ, Joseph DE, Angeli S, He J, Chen S, et al. (2008) Dexamethasone base conserves hearing from electrode trauma-induced hearing loss. Laryngoscope 118: 2028–2035.
35. el-Kafrawy AH, Dickey DM, Mitchell DF, Phillips RW (1974) Pulp reaction to a polycarboxylate cement in monkeys. J Dent Res 53: 15–19.

36. Lervik T (1978) The effect of zinc phosphate and carboxylate cements on the healing of experimentally induced pulpitis. Oral Surg Oral Med Oral Pathol 45: 123–130.

37. Luttikhuizen DT, Harmsen MC, Van Luyn MJ (2006) Cellular and molecular dynamics in the foreign body reaction. Tissue Eng 12: 1955–1970.

38. Nadol JB, Jr., Hsu WC (1991) Histopathologic correlation of spiral ganglion cell count and new bone formation in the cochlea following meningogenic labyrinthitis and deafness. Ann Otol Rhinol Laryngol 100: 712–716.

18

Unilateral Tinnitus: Changes in Connectivity and Response Lateralization Measured with fMRI

Cornelis P. Lanting[1,2]*, Emile de Kleine[1,2], Dave R. M. Langers[1,3], Pim van Dijk[1,2]

1 Department of Otorhinolaryngology/Head and Neck Surgery, University Medical Center Groningen, University of Groningen, Groningen, Netherlands, **2** Graduate School of Medical Sciences (Research School of Behavioural and Cognitive Neurosciences), University of Groningen, Groningen, Netherlands, **3** National Institute for Health Research, Nottingham Hearing Biomedical Research Unit, School of Clinical Sciences, University of Nottingham, Queen's Medical Centre, Nottingham, United Kingdom

Abstract

Tinnitus is a percept of sound that is not related to an acoustic source outside the body. For many forms of tinnitus, mechanisms in the central nervous system are believed to play a role in the pathology. In this work we specifically assessed possible neural correlates of unilateral tinnitus. Functional magnetic resonance imaging (fMRI) was used to investigate differences in sound-evoked neural activity between controls, subjects with left-sided tinnitus, and subjects with right-sided tinnitus. We assessed connectivity patterns between auditory nuclei and the lateralization of the sound-evoked responses. Interestingly, these response characteristics did not relate to the laterality of tinnitus. The lateralization for left- or right ear stimuli, as expressed in a lateralization index, was considerably smaller in subjects with tinnitus compared to that in controls, reaching significance in the right primary auditory cortex (PAC) and the right inferior colliculus (IC). Reduced functional connectivity between the brainstem and the cortex was observed in subjects with tinnitus. These differences are consistent with two existing models that relate tinnitus to i) changes in the corticothalamic feedback loops or ii) reduced inhibitory effectiveness between the limbic system and the thalamus. The vermis of the cerebellum also responded to monaural sound in subjects with unilateral tinnitus. In contrast, no cerebellar response was observed in control subjects. This suggests the involvement of the vermis of the cerebellum in unilateral tinnitus.

Editor: Berthold Langguth, University of Regensburg, Germany

Funding: This work was financially supported by the Heinsius Houbolt Foundation and the Netherlands Organization for Scientific Research (NWO VENI research grant 016.096.011 awarded to DL), and the COST action TINNET (Tinnitus Research Network: New Treatments for Tinnitus). The funders had no role in study design, data collection and analysis, decision to publish, or preparation of the manuscript.

Competing Interests: The authors have declared that no competing interests exist.

* Email: c.p.lanting@umcg.nl

Introduction

Subjective tinnitus is a prevalent hearing disorder that is characterized by an auditory sensation in the absence of an external acoustic stimulus. Presumably, hearing loss results in the sensory deprivation of neurons that are tuned to the affected frequencies. In an effort to restore their reduced activity back to normal levels, neurons may change the strength, or gain, of the existing connections or initiate new connections [1]. As a result, spontaneous firing rates (SFR) of neurons in the auditory system may increase [2,3].

In addition, neural synchrony may also increase as a consequence of neurons responding to the same limited amount of sensory input [2,4]. Normally a driving stimulus, i.e. a sound source, causes a time-locked elevated firing rate that is synchronous across many neurons. Therefore, when as a consequence of hearing loss and corresponding homeostatic changes in the firing pattern of neurons, both spontaneous activity and synchrony are elevated, it can be perceived as the presence of a sound in the absence of a true sound source [5,6].

Since spontaneous activity elevation and synchrony cannot be measured using fMRI, other paradigms have been used to study tinnitus [7,8]. Measuring changes in hemodynamics following the response to a sound in patients with unilateral tinnitus showed an increased sound-evoked response in the inferior colliculus (IC) in

patients compared to controls [9,10]. Recently, however, is was shown that this increased response may have been associated with hyperacusis - a reduced tolerance to loud sounds and commonly described by tinnitus sufferers - rather than with tinnitus [11].

In addition to the changes in firing rate, synchrony, and increased sound-evoked responses, there may be other, more subtle changes. One of these changes may relate to the perceived lateralization of tinnitus. It is conceivable that if tinnitus is perceived strongly lateralized, differences in the sound-evoked activity to monaural stimuli can be observed. Normally, the lateralization to monaural sound is mostly contralateral; evoked responses in the auditory pathway tend to be stronger to contralateral than to ipsilateral stimuli, with a notable exception being the cochlear nucleus, which receives only input from the ipsilateral auditory nerve. If unilateral tinnitus corresponds to reduced or increased lateralized activity along the auditory pathway, it could thus affect the normal lateralization to sound. The hypothesis here is that in patients with unilateral tinnitus the normal lateralization to sound has changed. By using monaural stimuli and measuring the lateralization to sound stimuli, we are able to assess changes related to unilateral tinnitus.

Further, it may be the case that tinnitus corresponds to changes in connectivity patterns between nuclei in the auditory pathway and other non-auditory systems. The auditory part of the thalamus seems to play a specific role in the perception of tinnitus. In a recent model, tinnitus results from impaired inhibitory connections from limbic regions to the auditory thalamus [12,13]. In this model, tinnitus (originating from e.g. homeostatic changes) would be inhibited after a short while due to feedback connections from limbic areas. If however limbic regions are compromised, this inhibition mechanism that would normally 'tune out the tinnitus' breaks down, and chronic tinnitus results. It might thus be the case that due to changes in this corticothalamic feedback-loop the thalamus receives less inhibition, which in turn may results in changes in the functional connectivity between the auditory brainstem and auditory cortex.

In a different model of tinnitus generation the thalamus also plays a major role. Specifically, thalamocortical rhythms that naturally occur in the brain, relating to e.g. sleep and consciousness [14], may be affected by deafferentation due to e.g. hearing loss in the case of tinnitus. It is thought that, as a consequence of such reduced input to the thalamus or a protracted functioning of the thalamus, the normal rhythms of the thalamocortical loop change to an increased large-scale, slow-rate oscillatory coherent theta (4–8 Hz) activity, in turn reducing lateral inhibition and disinhibiting more high-frequent gamma (30–70 Hz) oscillations [15]. As a consequence, we hypothesize that both models lead to changes in the normal connectivity-patterns between the brainstem, the thalamus, and the cortex.

In a recent study of tinnitus in subjects with moderate sensory hearing loss, indeed a reduction in functional connectivity was observed between the brainstem and cortex [16]. The goal of this study was to measure this in a group of participants with near-normal hearing. We therefore I) measure sound-evoked response levels in the auditory pathway, II) determine the corresponding preferred lateralization of sound in nuclei of the auditory pathway, and III) study the functional connectivity levels between these nuclei. We measured these three parameters in subjects without tinnitus and compared those to findings in subjects with unilateral tinnitus and near-normal hearing thresholds.

Parts of the data were presented previously [9], describing increased sound-evoked activity in the inferior colliculi (IC), but not in auditory cortex, of patients with unilateral tinnitus. Data of new subjects (four more controls, four more patients with unilateral tinnitus) were acquired and analyzed. In addition to sound-evoked activity, the current study focuses on the lateralization and connectivity patterns.

Materials and Methods

Subjects

Fourteen subjects with unilateral tinnitus were recruited at the University Medical Center Groningen, all without neurological and psychiatric history. Additionally, sixteen subjects without tinnitus were recruited. Hearing thresholds were obtained using standard pure-tone audiometry at the octave frequencies from 250 to 8000 Hz. All subjects were selected to have near-normal hearing. Compared to the previous study [9], four more controls and four more patients were included (one with right-sided tinnitus, three with left-sided tinnitus).

Subjects were selected to have a maximum averaged difference in hearing thresholds between the left ear and right ear of 10 dB in the range of 250–2000 Hz. A trained audiologist assessed all participants and the subjects with tinnitus were asked about various tinnitus characteristics such as etiology, tinnitus laterality, type, and severity. The following measures were determined in each tinnitus patient: (1) the frequency of a tone contralateral to the tinnitus ear, best matching the pitch of the tinnitus, (2) the level of a contralateral tone (in dB SL) at this frequency, best matching

the tinnitus loudness, (3) the minimum masking level (MML) defined as the lowest level of an ipsilateral, narrowband noise centered at the tinnitus matching frequency, that fully masked the tinnitus. Eleven out of 14 subjects completed a Tinnitus Reaction Questionnaire, TRQ [17]. Finally, the handedness of each subject was determined using a translated version of the Edinburgh inventory [18]. General subject characteristics are summarized in Table 1 and a more detailed description of the tinnitus subjects can be found in Table 2. The study was approved by the local medical ethics committee (Medical Ethics Committee (METc) of the University Medical Center Groningen). All subjects were informed about the purpose of the study before giving written informed consent prior to testing.

Imaging paradigm

All imaging experiments were performed on a 3 T MRI system (Philips Intera, Philips Medical Systems, Best, The Netherlands) with an eight-channel phased-array head coil (SENSE head coil). A T1-weighted fast-field echo scan was acquired for anatomical orientation (TR 11.1 ms; TE 4.6 ms; flip-angle 15°; matrix 256×256×9; voxel-size 1.0×1.0×2.0 mm^3). The functional imaging session included three 8-min runs, each consisting of a dynamic series of 51 identical 2200-ms single-shot T2*-sensitive echo planar imaging (EPI) volume acquisitions (TR 10 s; TE 22 ms; flip-angle 80°; matrix 128×128×41; voxel-size 1.0×1.0×2.0 mm^3; interleaved slice order, no slice gap; SENSE reduction factor 2.7), and were acquired using a coronal orientation, aligned to the brainstem when viewed on a midsagittal cross-section. The influence of acoustic scanner noise was reduced by using a sparse sampling strategy [19,20] in which auditory stimuli were presented during a 7.8-s gap of scanner silence between the end of each acquisition and the onset of the successive one. An additional 3D T1-weighted fast-field echo scan (TR 25 ms; TE 4.6 ms; flip-angle 30°; matrix 256×256×160; voxel-size 0.94×0.94×1.0 mm^3) was acquired with the same orientation as the functional scans to serve as anatomical reference.

Sound stimuli

Auditory stimuli were delivered by an MR compatible electrodynamic system (MR Confon GmbH) [21]. This system was driven by a PC setup equipped with a digital-to-analog converter (National Instruments 6052E, National Instruments Corporation, Austin, TX) controlled by Labview 6.1 (National Instruments Corporation, Austin, TX). The auditory stimuli consisted of temporally and spectrally modulated broadband 'dynamically rippled' noise [22]. The stimuli had a frequency range of 125–8000 Hz with a spectral modulation density of 1 cycle per octave, a temporal modulation frequency of 2 cycles per second and a modulation amplitude of 80%. The rippled noise stimuli were presented immediately when an MR acquisition started and ended 0.5 s before the next acquisition. All stimuli were 9.5 s in duration. Stimuli were presented at 40 or 70 dB (SPL) either at the left or the right ear. The stimuli were presented in a pseudo-randomized order. Each condition (four in total) was presented ten times per functional run. An additional 'silent' condition (i.e., no stimulus) was presented eleven times. Subjects were instructed to respond by left or right button presses with the right thumb whenever they perceived an audible stimulus in the left or right ear, respectively. This was done to monitor the subjects' attention to sound stimuli during acquisition.

Data analysis

MR images were analyzed using Matlab 7.1 (R14) (The Mathworks Inc., Natick, MA) and SPM8 (Functional Imaging

Table 1. General subject characteristics.

Characteristics	Controls (n = 16)	Left-sided tinnitus (n = 8)	Right-sided tinnitus (n = 6)
Age (years)			
average	39.1	46.5	52.8
standard deviation	16.6	8.1	13.1
range	23–76	40–62	31–76
Gender			
male	8 (50%)	4 (50%)	4 (67%)
Tinnitus			
average pitch (kHz)	-	8.0	7.4
range (kHz)	-	0.8–14.0	3.0–11.0
average loudness (dB SL)	-	23	21
range(dB SL)	-	5–38	5–45
average MML (dB SL)	-	46	41
range (dB SL)	-	19–69	16–65
Handedness			
right handed	14 (88%)	6 (86%)	5 (83%)

Laboratory, The Wellcome Department of Imaging Neuroscience, London, UK, http://www.fil.ion.ucl.ac.uk/spm/). The functional images were corrected for motion and spatially coregistered with the T1-weighted high-resolution anatomical image. The high-resolution anatomical image was segmented in grey matter, white matter and cerebrospinal fluid segments. The gray-matter segment of the anatomical image was normalized to a custom normalization template (for more details, see [9]) and the resulting transformation parameters were also applied to the functional data. The normalized functional data were spatially smoothed using an isotropic Gaussian kernel with a full width at half maximum of 4 mm, to improve signal-to-noise ratio characteristics while retaining the ability to discern small auditory structures (i.e., the brainstem nuclei). Functional images were interpolated to voxel dimensions of $2.0 \times 2.0 \times 2.0$ mm^3.

A general linear model (GLM) was set up for each subject to analyze the relative contribution of each stimulus condition to the measured response. The GLM included four covariates of interest, one for each condition, one constant factor to model the baseline signal or the signal during the silent condition and a linear term to correct for linear drift in the scanner signal. The GLM was applied to the data of all voxels and four contrast images were created, one for each condition (i.e., left 40 dB vs. baseline (L40), left 70 dB vs. baseline (L70), right 40 dB vs. baseline (R40) and right 70 dB vs. baseline (R70)). An omnibus F-test, including all four conditions, was assessed to detect the combined effect of all sound stimuli.

The four contrast images (per subject) were entered in a second-level random-effects analysis based on a flexible factorial design with factors for group (i.e., controls, subjects with tinnitus perceived on the left side and subjects with tinnitus perceived on the right side), subject, and stimulus condition.

In addition to the random-effects analysis, a non-parametric permutation test was performed to assess potential differences in the responses between the two patient groups. We used SnPM (http://www.sph.umich.edu/ni-stat/SnPM/) and permuted the labels of the two patient groups (i.e., right-sided tinnitus and left-sided tinnitus) and assessed whether the actual differences between

groups were significant based on both the t-statistic and cluster size [23].

Region of interest analysis

Following the voxel-wise analyses, we performed a region of interest (ROI) analysis, determining sound-evoked responses in 10 anatomical areas comprising (parts of) the auditory pathway and one area in the vermis of the cerebellum that was included based on previous findings [24]. The left and right primary auditory cortices were defined as the combination of the TE1.0, TE 1.1 and TE 1.2 areas defined by the SPM Anatomy toolbox [25–27]. For the left and right auditory association cortices (AAC) we used the left and right superior temporal gyrus as defined by Brodmann (BA 22) based on the AAL template in MRIcron (http://www.sph.sc.edu/comd/rorden/mricron/). Both of the ROIs of the primary and association cortices were normalized to match our anatomical template in order to have a corresponding image space. The left and right medial geniculate body of the thalamus (MGB), the left and right inferior colliculi (IC), the left and right cochlear nuclei (CN), and the ROI consisting of the vermis of the cerebellum were manually drawn based on an anatomical atlas [28,29]. We used the xjView (http://www.alivelearn.net/xjview8) Matlab toolbox to select a relatively large volume around these nuclei, thus allowing for small differences between subjects that remain after normalization. Table 3 shows the size of each ROI, measured in voxels (of $2 \times 2 \times 2$ mm^3), and the location of their center of mass (given in MNI coordinates).

Based on the single-subject F-test (sound vs. baseline), the 10% most active voxels in each ROI were used (i.e., those exceeding the 90th percentile of the distribution of F-values).

A percentage signal change was calculated for each of these ROIs. First, the regression coefficients of the selected voxels within the region of interest were averaged for each condition separately. Next, these values were divided by the average baseline level of activity for the same voxels in order to get a percentage signal change.

Table 2. Tinnitus characteristics.

Sub	Age	Sex	Tinnitus laterality	Tinnitus duration (y)	Incident triggering tinnitus	Tinnitus quality	Tinnitus Pitch (kHz)	Tinnitus Loudness (dB SL)	MML (dB SL)	Severity	TRQ
10	55	m	right ear	2	unknown	pure-tone	3	5	16	mild	32
13	50	m	right ear	4	noise trauma	n/a	6	16	30	n/a	29
16	65	f	right ear	3	unknown	pure-tone	11	18	43	mild	33
18	67	f	right ear	5	unknown	ringing/pulse	6	20	n/a	mild	3
19	31	m	right ear	14	noise trauma	ringing	10	45	53	mild	25
29 (*)	49	m	right ear	1	blow on the ear	pure-tone	8	23	65	mild	32
Avg	52.8	-	-	4.8	-	-	7.4	21	41	-	24
7*	49	m	left ear	6	car accident	pure-tone	8	35	70	mild	26
9	53	m	left ear	4	unknown	ringing	8	23	40	mild	9
11	62	f	left ear	6	flushing the ear	buzzing	8	15	48	severe	74
14	42	f	left ear	12	unknown	cricket	14	20	68	mild	61
17	37	f	left ear	9	unknown	hissing	8	25	43	severe	89
27 (*)	43	f	left ear	1	unknown	ringing	0.75	12	n/a	mild	n/a
28 (*)	40	m	left ear	0.5	unknown	pure-tone	8	13	19	severe	n/a
30 (*)	46	m	left ear	2	unknown	pure-tone	9	38	38	mild	n/a
Avg	46.5	-	-	5.1	-	-	8.0	23	46	-	52

n/a: not available; n: no; y: yes;
*one subject (subject #7) was excluded from analyses due to gross motion artefacts that occurred during the imaging sessions; MML: minimum masking level; TRQ: Tinnitus reaction Questionnaire.
(*) indicate new subjects with respect to Lanting et al., (2008) [9].

Table 3. Volume and center of mass of each ROI.

ROI	left hemisphere		right hemishpere	
	voxels	location	voxels	location
Auditory association cortex (AAC)	1339	(−58, −28,6)	1569	(60, −30,6)
Primary auditory cortex (PAC)	469	(−46, −16,4)	563	(48, −14,0)
Medial geniculate body (MGB)	53	(−16, −26, −8)	63	(16, −26, −8)
Inferior colliculus (IC)	29	(−6, −36, −12)	33	(4, −36, −12)
Cochlear nucleus (CN)	63	(−8, −37, −44)	52	(8, −38, −42)
Cerebellum vermis	287	(0, −54, −4)	-	-

The volume is measured in number of voxels ($2 \times 2 \times 2$ mm^3) and the center of mass is given in MNI coordinates.

To test for differences between the subject groups and potential interactions between the groups and the experimental conditions, repeated measures ANOVAs were performed for each ROI separately, using the percentages signal change obtained earlier. Two main factors were defined: (I) stimulus condition (L40, L70, R40, and R70) as repeated measure (within subject) and (II) subject group (controls, left-sided tinnitus and right-sided tinnitus). In addition, the interaction between the two main factors was assessed (group × stimulus). A Bonferroni correction for multiple comparisons (i.e., over the number of tested ROIs) was applied. To rule out any influence of potential confounding variables we performed regression analyses of the activation levels in each of the ROIs with hearing thresholds (pure tone average for left and right ear separately), and age.

Response lateralization

Since monaural stimuli were used, it was possible to determine the preferred stimulus lateralization. From the ROI analysis we obtained for each subject the mean response for each condition. The mean responses to left (L) and right ear (R) stimuli were calculated by averaging the response to the 40 and 70 dB (SPL) stimuli at each ear. A lateralization index (LI) was obtained for each of the regions of interest separately, defined as $LI = L-R/(|L|+|R|)$, with possible outcomes ranging from −1 to +1 for unilateral positive responses to right and left ear stimulation, respectively.

Connectivity analysis

For our connectivity analysis, we used the Pearson correlation coefficient [30,31]. Our model consisted of ten auditory regions: the left and right CN, IC, MGB, PAC and AAC. In addition, the vermis of the cerebellum was included as an eleventh ROI. The mean signal of the 10% most active voxels within each ROI (i.e., those exceeding the 90th percentile of the distribution of F-values) was calculated for each point in time (i.e., for each scan). The obtained fMRI time courses of these ROIs were transformed to zero mean and unit variance for each subject. These arrays were concatenated over subjects resulting in a matrix containing 11 time courses of 2448 elements (16 subjects×153 time points) for the control group and a matrix containing 11 time courses of 1989 elements (13 subjects×153 time points) for the patient group. For each group, the covariance matrix Σ was calculated, which contains the Pearson cross-correlation for all possible ROI pairs, respectively.

To assess whether observed differences between the groups were significant, the Jensen-Bregman LogDet Divergence (JBLD), a dissimilarity measure for differences between covariance matrices,

was used [32]. First, the observed JBLD (or dissimilarity) value was calculated using the two groups' covariance matrices Σ. Next, we randomly permuted the assignment of subjects to the two groups (retaining the original group sizes), obtained new time courses and the resulting covariance matrices, and calculated the JBLD value for each of the permutations. This was repeated 50000 times and a reference distribution of similarity values was obtained. To assess whether the observed difference exceeded the significance level of $p = 0.05$, we calculated the proportion p of sampled permutations where the absolute difference was greater than, or equal to, the observed difference.

Second, we calculated the observed differences in correlation coefficients between the subject groups for the connection between each pair of ROIs separately. Similar to the permutation testing on the JBLD dissimilarity value, both the observed correlations and the reference distributions were obtained using the same set of permutations as before. Finally, the observed values were compared against the reference distributions and a p-value was obtained for each of the ROIs.

Potential confounding variables, such as age, average hearing thresholds, and average left-right differences in hearing thresholds were accounted for by analyzing the relation (or correlation) of the JBLD dissimilarity value with each of the variables for each of the permutations. The assumption here is that if any of the variables has a confounding effect on the JBLD dissimilarity values, these values would be correlated with the confounding variables. Conversely, it would be expected that in a subset of permutations with the same degree of e.g., hearing loss, its (confounding) effect on the dissimilarity value would be accounted for.

Results

Audiometry and tinnitus assessment

The mean audiogram of each group is displayed in Fig. 1. There were no significant differences between the average thresholds of the groups for the frequency range 0.25–2 kHz. At 4 and 8 kHz, the tinnitus subjects showed thresholds that were significantly elevated ($p < 0.01$) relative to those of the controls whereas there was no significant difference ($p > 0.1$) between the two groups of subjects with tinnitus. These two groups of subjects with tinnitus were reasonably well matched (see Tables 1 and 2) concerning the average values of the duration of the tinnitus (4.8 and 5.1 years) tinnitus pitch (7.4 and 7.9 kHz), the average loudness of the tinnitus (21 and 23 dB SL) and the average MML (41 and 46 dB SL). Thirteen of the 14 patients were asked to categorize the severity of their tinnitus as mild, moderate, or severe. Ten patients considered their tinnitus as mild whereas the

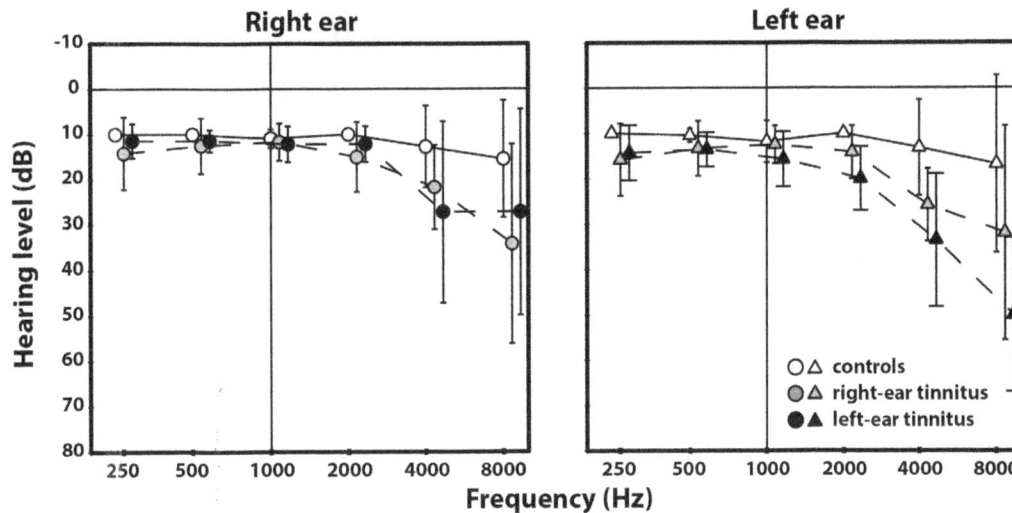

Figure 1. Mean pure-tone hearing thresholds for the right and the left ear for the three subject groups. The solid line represents the hearing thresholds of the control group and the two dashed lines represent the hearing thresholds of the two groups with unilateral tinnitus. The error bars indicate the standard deviation around the mean.

other three reported their tinnitus as severe. This closely corresponded to the obtained TRQ scores, where available (severe: TRQ scores of 74 and 89; mild: TRQ scores between 9 and 61). For further details see Table 2.

Sound evoked activation

The group-level significance of the sound-evoked hemodynamic responses is displayed in Fig. 2 ($n = 29$; one subject (subject 7) in the group with right-sided tinnitus was excluded from further analyses due to motion artifacts). It clearly shows significant sound-evoked responses in the left and right CN, IC, MGB, and the bilateral auditory cortices (see table 4 for the location and F-value of the responses). When contrasting the whole patient group against the controls, no significant differences were observed, with the exception of the vermis of the cerebellum as shown in Fig. 3.

The dissimilarity between the two patient groups was investigated by performing a non-parametric permutation test based on both the t-statistic and cluster size. Neither of these two measures showed any significant differences ($p = 0.05$ FWE) between the subject groups, indicating that responses were neither different in strength nor in extent. Because the lateralization of the tinnitus did not influence the strength or location of sound-evoked activation, we decided to pool the data from the two patient groups in a number of the analyses that followed.

Region of interest analysis

We performed ROI analyses, averaging the 10% most active voxels within each ROI, using ten ROIs in the auditory pathway and the vermis of the cerebellum. The box plots in figure 4 show the responses to the four experimental conditions, L40, L70, R40 and R70, for controls and subjects with tinnitus for the various ROIs. In addition, it shows the mean value per condition for each subject group. For the size and location of each of the ROIs please refer to Table 3.

With the exception of the CN, activation in the auditory pathway is strongest in response to the contralateral ear. For the CN we observe a weak ipsilateral preference. In addition, with the exception of the MGB, there is a clear sound intensity dependency, i.e., the 70 dB (SPL) stimuli yielded a larger response than the 40 dB (SPL) stimuli. The only ROI that showed a

significant difference between controls and patients with tinnitus was the vermis of the cerebellum ($p<0.05$, corrected for multiple comparisons). For all conditions, both patient groups clearly showed a larger response in the vermis of the cerebellum than controls (see Fig. 4). Finally, the right PAC and right IC showed a significant interaction of group × condition ($p<0.05$, corrected for multiple comparisons). Patients, on average, showed a smaller difference between the ipsilateral (right-ear) stimuli and the contralateral (left-ear) stimuli than the controls in these ROIs (see Fig. 4).

To rule out any influence of hearing loss in the left and right ear, age, and the TRQ value, we performed regression analyses on the percentage signal change with each of these factors as explanatory variables. These showed that these potential confounds could not account for the differences between controls and tinnitus patients ($p>0.1$ in all ROIs).

Response lateralization

Fig. 5 shows the preferred stimulus lateralization index for each nucleus for the controls and for the pooled patient groups. Post-hoc analysis using permutation testing revealed that the two patient groups did not differ significantly ($p>0.1$). The ipsilateral lateralization of the CN and the contralateral lateralization of the IC, MGB, PAC, and AAC are clearly visible. The PAC showed the strongest contralateral lateralization, followed by the AAC, and the IC each with a contralateral lateralization, whereas the MGB shows a weaker lateralization. The vermis of the cerebellum, in contrast, did not show a clear lateralization (which can also be observed from Fig. 4). Significant group differences were observed in the right PAC ($p<0.05$) and right IC ($p<0.001$). In these nuclei, the lateralization index was significantly lower in subjects with tinnitus than in controls. Overall, the lateralization index was closer to zero in patients than in controls (repeated measures ANOVA, $p<0.01$) regardless of the lateralization of the tinnitus. Since differences between left- and right ear hearing thresholds might have an influence on the observed lateralization, we calculated the for each subject the root-mean-square (RMS) difference in hearing thresholds, taking into account differences between the left- and right ear thresholds across all frequencies.

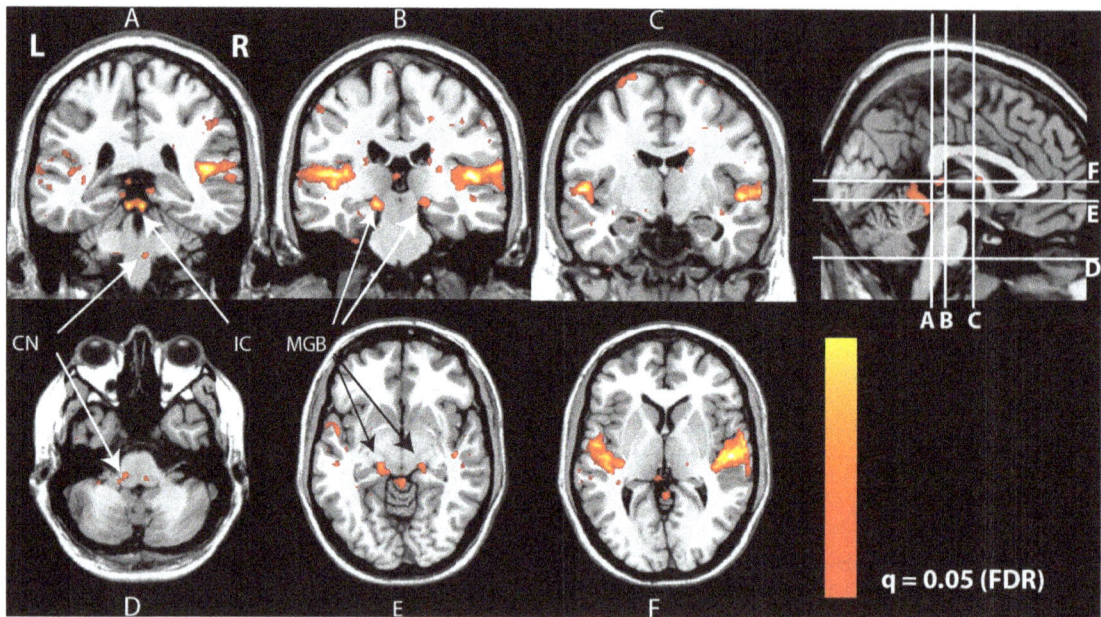

Figure 2. Sound-evoked responses. Coronal and transversal cross-sections of the human brain in grey-scale with a red-yellow color-coded overlay showing significant responses to sound. The colored areas show a significant response to sound stimuli (omnibus F-test, $F>8.34$, $q<0.05$ FDR, pooled over all subjects). Evident from this figure is the auditory pathway, showing the cochlear nuclei (CN; panel A and D), the inferior colliculi (IC; panel A and E), the medial geniculate bodies (MGB; panel B and E) and the auditory cortices (panels A–C and F).

This analysis showed that, although the variability of this left-right ear asymmetry is smaller in the control group than in the patient group (5.9 and 7.4 dB, respectively), they do not differ significantly (p = 0.34, based on permutation testing, randomly assigning the group label and calculating the difference between the groups).

Connectivity analysis

We calculated the Pearson correlation coefficients (see Fig. 6) between all nuclei that were included in the ROI analysis. The strongest Pearson correlations in the control group were observed between the ipsilateral PAC and AAC (0.78, 0.79 for left and right, respectively), and the left and right homologous nuclei at each level of the auditory pathway, varying between 0.25 (IC) and 0.53 (MGB). The ipsilateral connections between the IC and PAC and IC and AAC were also relatively strong (range: 0.27–0.40), whereas the contralateral connections were less strong (range: 0.07–0.14). The connections of both the bilateral IC and CN with the bilateral MGB nuclei were also notable (0.18–0.47), but without a clear lateralization.

The pattern of connectivity of the patient group was similar to that in controls in the sense that the strongest Pearson correlations

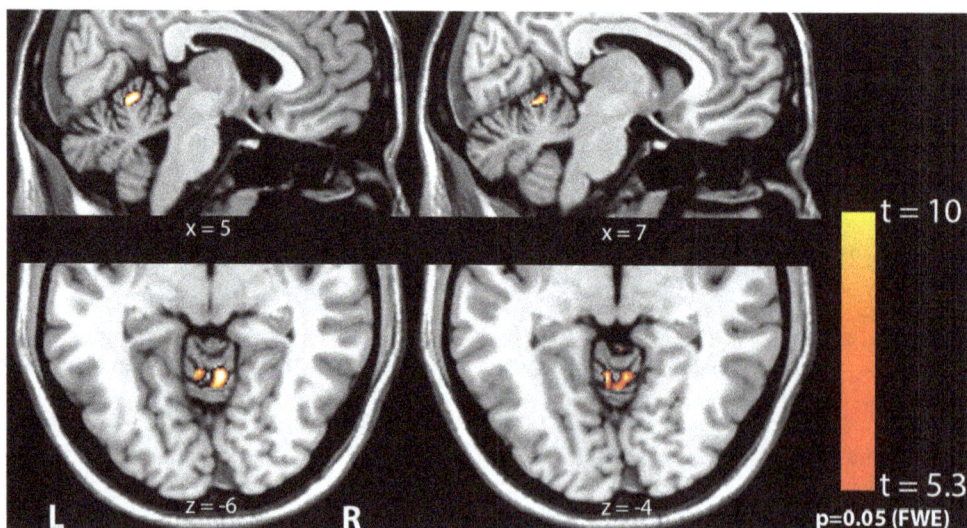

Figure 3. Coronal and sagittal cross-sections of the human brain in grey-scale with a red-yellow color-coded overlay showing voxels in the vermis of the cerebellum that show a significantly larger response to sound in patients compared to controls ($t>5.34$, $p<0.05$ FWE).

Table 4. Location of the maxima as in figure 2, one for each ROI (MNI coordinates) and their F-values (auditory ROIs) or t-value (vermis of cerebellum).

ROI	left hemisphere		right hemishpere	
	location	*statistical value (F)*	*location*	*statistical value (F)*
Auditory association cortex (AAC)	(−44, −28,10)	19.3	(54,−18,4)	19.0
Primary auditory cortex (PAC)	(−36, −22,6)	16.1	(40, −22,6)	20.4
Medial geniculate body (MGB)	(−14, −26, −6)	4.5	(16, −26, −6)	11.0
Inferior colliculus (IC)	(−6, −34, −12)	13.7	(2, −36, −10)	13.6
Cochlear nucleus (CN)	(−10, −36, −44)	4.0	(5, −34, −44)	4.0
Cerebellum vermis	(−2, −52,0)	14.5 (*t-value*)	-	-

were observed between left and right homologous nuclei at each level of the auditory pathway, varying between 0.38 (PAC) and 0.66 (AAC), and between the ipsilateral PAC and AAC (0.85, 0.74 for left and right, respectively). The connectivity pattern in the patient group, however, was distinctly dissimilar in two ways. First, there was a strong connection of the cerebellum with the PAC and AAC (range: 0.22–0.43) in the patients, compared to lower values in the controls (0.08–0.15). Second, the pattern of the correlation coefficients between the cortical areas (PAC and AAC) on the one hand, and the subcortical areas (MGB, IC and CN) on the other hand, was qualitatively different than that in the controls (see the white dotted outline in figure 6). Expressed as an average correlation coefficient, this value is lower in patients (0.11) than in controls (0.21). The same holds for the average correlation between the thalamus and the cortical areas: the patients show a lower value than in control (resp. 0.20 and 0.31).

To assess the statistical significance of these differences, they were also expressed in the Jensen-Bregman LogDet Divergence (JBLD). Compared to all the possible permutations, the actual dissimilarity was significantly higher ($p = 0.002$). The covariance matrices thus detectably differed between the groups. Permutation testing was also used to assess which of the connections was driving this difference, or in other words, which of the individual connections was significantly different between the groups. This is visualized in the rightmost panel of Fig. 6 as a significance map for the differences between the controls and patients for the Pearson correlation. The most prominent differences in Pearson correlation between the controls and patients related to the connections between the left and right IC, between the right IC and right PAC, and between the right IC and the right AAC.

To assess the influence of potential confounding variables, such as differences in hearing loss and age, and differences between left and right ear hearing thresholds, we analyzed the correlation of these variables with the JBLD dissimilarity values for all permutations. For example, if the dissimilarity was driven by differences in age between the subject groups, one would expect the JBLD dissimilarity value to be correlated with the group age-difference. In other words, plotting the dissimilarity value versus age for all possible permutations of age-difference between the groups would show a correlation between the two variables.

However, age only weakly correlated ($r = -0.05$) with the dissimilarity values (Fig. S1); Moreover, when looking in a range of 2 years around the actual measured difference between the groups,

the permutation analysis showed that the measured dissimilarity is significantly larger than expected ($p = 0.002$ based on $n = 3320$ permutations within the selected age-bin), indicating that age cannot account for the dissimilarity between groups.

The same applies to differences in hearing loss, taken as the difference in average hearing thresholds at 4 and 8 kHz between the groups, where a small correlation coefficient of $r = -0.02$ was found between the dissimilarity index and hearing loss (Fig. S2). As with age, a significantly dissimilarity was found ($p = 0.006$ based on $n = 2336$ permutation within the selected bin; actual HL difference ± 5 dB), indicating that differences of the hearing thresholds between the groups are not likely to have had a strong influence on the dissimilarity index.

Finally, we assessed whether differences in hearing thresholds between the left and right ear between the groups were of influence. This seems not the case as there is no strong correlation with the left-right differences in thresholds and the dissimilarity index ($r = 0.03$), and the dissimilarity is significantly larger than expected in a subset of the permutations (Fig. S3).

Discussion

Tinnitus is an auditory phenomenon that in many patients is related to peripheral hearing loss. Yet, its pathogenesis is believed to be based on mechanisms in the central auditory system [7,33–35]. If auditory processing by the brain is indeed different between subjects with and without tinnitus, this may result in differences in the way the brain responds to sound. Hence, we measured the response to sound in subjects with unilateral tinnitus en controls without tinnitus, all having normal or near-normal hearing.

Our findings are summarized as follows: (1) the amplitude of the sound-evoked brain responses was similar in all auditory brain areas of subjects with vs. without tinnitus; (2) tinnitus subjects displayed an enlarged response to sound in the cerebellum; (3) the lateralization of the response was less pronounced in tinnitus subjects than in controls; (4) there was no correspondence between lateralization of the sound-evoked responses and the lateralization of the tinnitus percept; (5) connectivity measures differed between tinnitus subjects and controls and showed decreased subcortical-cortical connectivity patterns in patients compared to controls.

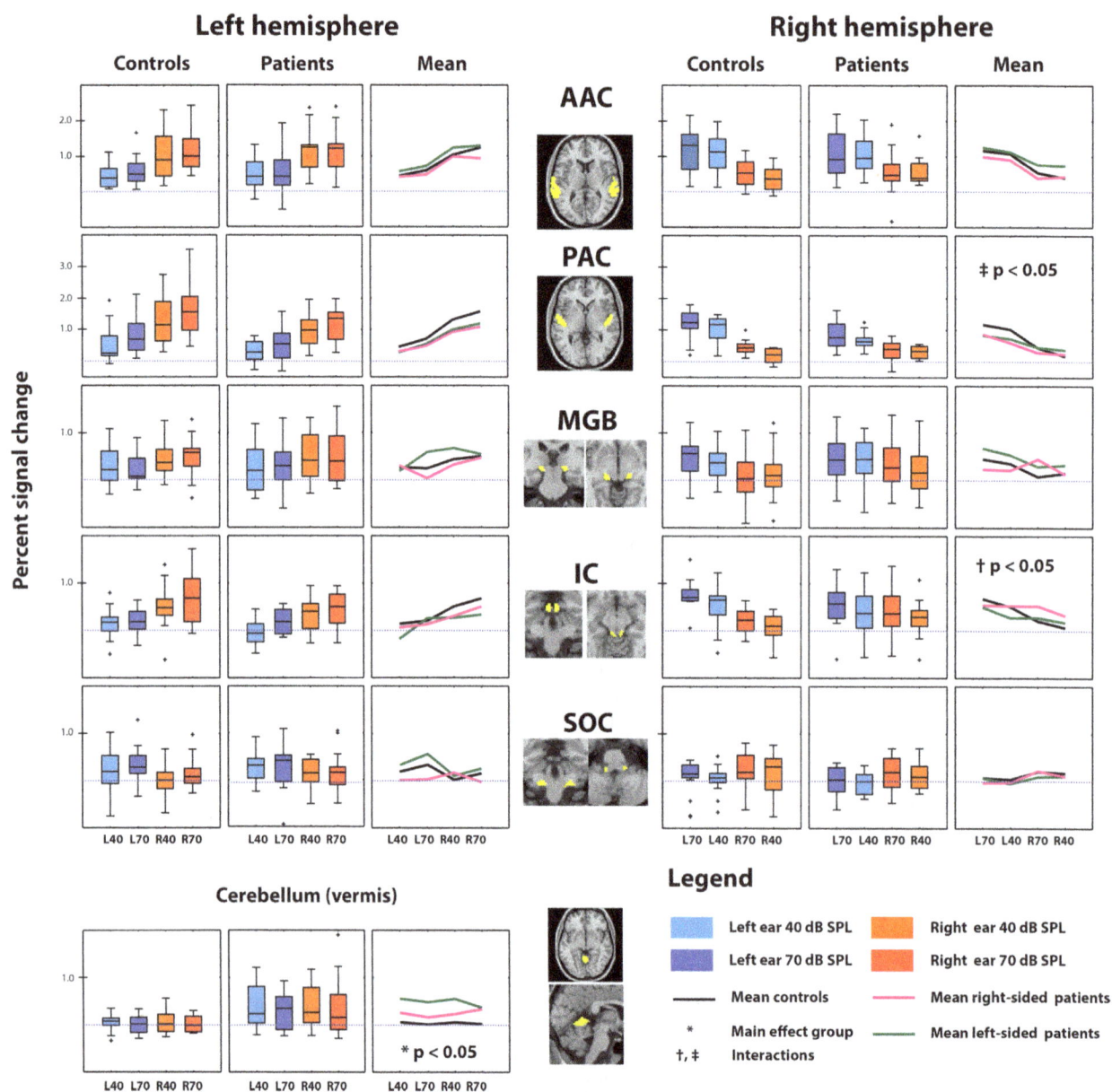

Figure 4. Region of interest analysis. The percentage signal changes measured in each ROI of the left and right hemisphere (AAC, PAC, MGB, IC and CN) and the vermis of the cerebellum for both subject groups. The location of each ROI is indicated in yellow on cross-sections of the brain. The responses to the four experimental conditions are shown as box plots for each group separately. For each group, the mean per condition is visualized in the line plot next to the box plots.

Sound-evoked responses in the auditory pathway

Changes in the sound-evoked responses in the auditory pathway have been previously linked to tinnitus, most notably with changes in the response characteristics of the inferior colliculus (IC) in subjects with tinnitus compared to controls [9–11,36]. As mentioned, parts of the data of the current paper have been described earlier [9]. The current study added four controls and four tinnitus patients to the subject groups. In contrast to the earlier analysis [9], the current analysis did not show increased sound-evoked activity in the tinnitus patients (see Fig. 4).

In order to explain the apparent discrepancies, we highlight the effect of adding new subjects as well as the effect of methodological differences. Performing the old analysis on the full subject group included in the current work (see Fig. S4.) confirms previous

results: sound-evoked responses as measured with this method are increased in the IC of patients with tinnitus compared to controls [9]. However, for our current analysis the voxel selection-criterion changed in two ways with respect to earlier [9]. Previously, IC ROIs were drawn manually for each subject. In contrast, we now used an objective method, in which a standard anatomical atlas was used to determine the location of the IC. A probability map, showing the overlap between ROIs across subject shows that the old and new ROI overlap nicely, but that the individual (old) ROIs are bigger in size (see the inset in Fig. S4).

The second difference is that previously the 10% of the voxels with the highest t-values were selected for each stimulus condition separately. Consequently, the voxels considered were not necessarily identical across conditions. However, the connectivity

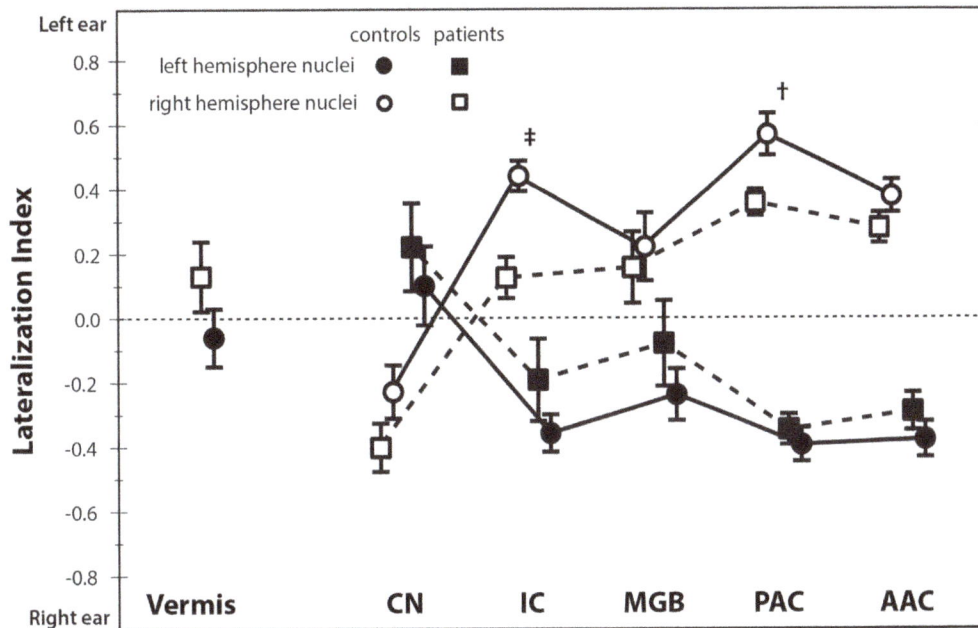

Figure 5. Sound lateralization in the auditory pathway. The lateralization indices for the left hemisphere nuclei (filled symbols) and the right hemisphere nuclei (open symbols) of the auditory pathway (AAC, PAC, MGB, IC and CN) and the cerebellum. A lateralization index of +1 indicates a response to left-ear stimuli only, whereas a value of −1 indicates a response to right-ear stimuli only. The error bars indicate the standard error of the mean. The symbols indicate the two nuclei (†: PAC and ‡: IC) where the difference in lateralization index is significantly different between the two patients and controls.

analysis employed in the current study requires the selection of a fixed set of voxels across conditions. Therefore, an omnibus F-test was used, selecting a fixed set of voxels for all stimulus conditions. As is evident in Fig. 4 and Fig. S4, with the new voxel selection criterion, there are no differences between tinnitus subjects and controls in the response amplitudes of the inferior colliculus.

It is of interest that the method used by Lanting et al. (2008) does show a difference between tinnitus subjects and controls, while the current method does not. At present we have no clear interpretation of this effect, but it warrants further investigation in future research.

Apart from these differences there is a more fundamental issue with increased sound-evoked responses and tinnitus. That is

because it has been shown that subjects without clinical hyperacusis but with decreased loudness discomfort levels (LDLs) show increased sound-evoked responses in the IC [11]. Increased sound-evoked responses thus seem a proxy for hyperacusis but not necessarily for tinnitus, at least at the level of the IC. Unfortunately, since neither previously [9] nor in this work we have measured LDLs, it may be the case that some of the patients that show increased sound-evoked responses do so because of hyperacusis rather than their tinnitus.

The results presented here show that we did not find increased sound-evoked responses in patients with tinnitus but that it depends –at least partly- on the ROI definition, The analysis also revealed a clear level dependency in the cortex, thalamus and

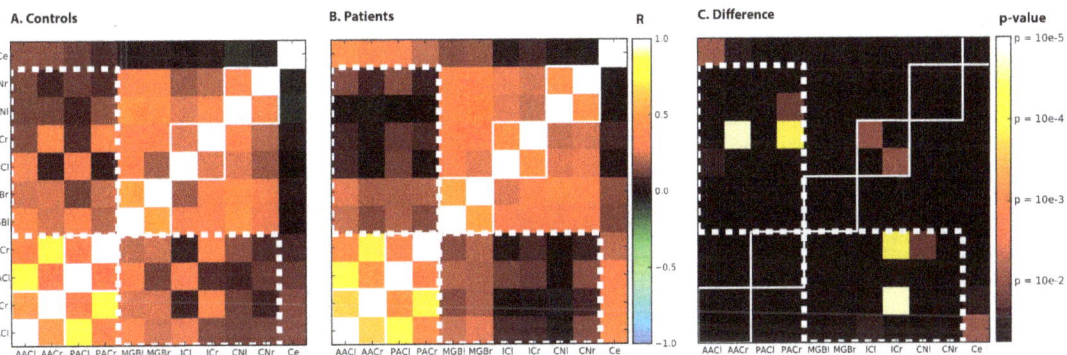

Figure 6. Connectivity patterns. Observed functional connectivity patterns in controls (**panel A. Controls**) and subjects with tinnitus (**panel B - Patients**). Pearson cross-correlation coefficients were calculated and color-coded based on the value of the coefficient. **Panel C. Differences** shows the differences in connectivity measures between subject groups for the different ROIs. Significance maps are associated with the observed difference between controls and patients for the Pearson correlation coefficients for each connection. The solid white lines represent homologue auditory nuclei at each level and the white dotted lines indicate the set of connections where on average the connectivity between subcortical and cortical areas is decreased in patients.

midbrain (Fig. 4). The response in each of the auditory nuclei increased with increasing level, which is in agreement with earlier findings [9,37–40]. Moreover, the ROI analysis shows that the AAC, PAC, IC, and -to a lesser degree- the MGB show response lateralization; activation occurred most strongly in response to stimulation of the contralateral ear. The CN shows strongest activation in response to stimulation of the ipsilateral ear, as would be expected.

The cerebellum and tinnitus

The only brain region where the response to sound significantly differed between subjects with tinnitus and controls was the vermis of the cerebellum (see figure 3) Although the role of the cerebellum in auditory processing is largely unknown, there are a few studies that show a cerebellar association with sound processing. For example, connections between the CN and the cerebellum indicate that the cerebellum receives auditory input [41–43]. In addition, the vermis is thought to play a specific role in binaural processing, where auditory cues are used to control, for example, neck muscles to move the head towards a sound source [44,45]. Finally, in humans and other animals alike, lesions in the medial part of the cerebellum are associated with a lack of long-term habituation of the acoustic startle response [46–48].

There is also some evidence for the role of the cerebellum in tinnitus. Brozoski and colleagues found that, in addition to elevated levels of activity in the auditory brainstem, there was also increased activity in the paraflocculus of cerebellum of rats with behavioral tinnitus [49]. In subjects with gaze-evoked tinnitus, the vermis seems to be more activated compared to controls [50]. Finally, as previously reported, a cerebellar response to sound was found in normal hearing controls but not in tinnitus subjects that were able to modulate their tinnitus by jaw protrusion [24]. On the whole, the evidence suggests a role of the cerebellum in tinnitus. The exact nature of this role, however, remains unclear at the moment.

Reduced lateralization and tinnitus

The lateralization index (see Fig. 5) is a quantity that summarizes the relative response of a brain area (e.g. a ROI) to stimulation of the right and left ear, respectively. The index was significantly lower in the right primary auditory cortex and the right inferior colliculus in patients than in controls, indicating a less pronounced preference for responding to the contralateral ear. Moreover, the lateralization was far less pronounced in subjects with tinnitus than in controls. The reduced lateralization, at least at the level of the IC, in combination with the significant interaction (group x condition; see Fig. 4), is in line with previous work that showed no clear response lateralization in the IC in patients with unilateral tinnitus [9]. Importantly, analyses showed that this reduced lateralization is not due to inherent differences between left- and right ear hearing-thresholds.

This decreased lateralization might relate to a diminished efficiency in the inhibitory ipsilateral input to the IC. Where the contralateral pathway receives mainly excitatory input, the ipsilateral pathway receives both inhibitory and excitatory input [51]. A reduction in the inhibitory pathway could thus lead to a more equal input from both ears via normal contralateral excitatory input and, through normal excitatory and reduced inhibitory input, relatively more excitatory input from the ipsilateral ear. This, in turn would lead to a decrease in the lateralization index.

Remarkably, the preferred stimulus lateralization indices show no relation to the lateralization of the tinnitus both in this work and previous papers [9,10]. Normally, sound from one ear is

predominantly represented in the contralateral hemisphere [52]. Thus, tinnitus in e.g. the left ear would be expected to correspond to aberrant neural activity in the right cortex. Yet, we find a bilateral diminished lateralization. Apparently there is no clear relation between the lateralization to sound in subjects with tinnitus with the lateralization of the tinnitus. Note, however, that the absence of a clear difference in lateralization between the two patient groups may be due to the relative small sample-size of patients with eight and six patient for respectively the left- and right-sided tinnitus patient group. This point makes that the conclusion may not be easy to generalize and that there may be more subtle differences in lateralization.

Changes in connectivity patterns

Finally, we studied the connectivity patterns between nuclei of the auditory pathway in a similar fashion as was previously done in subjects with unilateral hearing loss [52] and recently in subjects with mild to severe hearing loss and tinnitus [16]. In functional MR imaging, functional connectivity measures express the degree of similarity of the measured signals in time in various areas of the brain. Activity that co-varies suggests that the neural processes underlying this activity are related. Simple (Pearson) cross-correlations between ROI responses were computed, a measure that is usually referred to as functional connectivity [31]. Yet, the connectivity patterns reported here do not necessarily match direct anatomical connectivity patterns obtained using e.g. anterograde and retrograde labeling techniques in animals [53], or non-invasive diffusion tensor imaging in humans [54]. The functional connection between two nuclei may be related to shared input that both receive, or mediated via a third nucleus using an indirect path. The connection between e.g. the left and right MGB is an example of a connection that is likely to involve shared input from the IC, rather than an actual direct connection. Functional connectivity therefore has its limitations in terms of anatomical connections and the direction of information from one area to another.

Thus, two studies in patient populations that differ in their degree of hearing loss, respectively mild to moderate sensorineural hearing loss [16] and no hearing loss to mild high-frequency hearing loss (this study), show consistent differences in the connectivity patterns of patients compared to controls. The connectivity pattern was found to differ significantly between groups. More specifically, we showed a decreased (average) correlation between the cortical and subcortical clusters in tinnitus patients compared to controls. Importantly, these differences do not seem related with confounding variables such as age and hearing loss (figures S1–S3). Since the connection between both clusters comprises the thalamus, conveying information from the brainstem to the auditory cortex, it is possible that the difference in functional connectivity is related to a thalamic dysfunction.

According to one of the models of chronic tinnitus, the nucleus accumbens and associated paralimbic areas in the ventromedial prefrontal cortex (vmPFC) play an important role in long-term habituation to continuous unpleasant sounds [12]. Sound-evoked neural activity is normally relayed from the auditory periphery via the brainstem and thalamus to the auditory cortex for conscious perception. The same signal is also directed via the amygdala to the nucleus accumbens for evaluation of the sound's emotional content [55]. From the nucleus accumbens, projections feed back to the thalamic reticular nucleus (TRN), which in turn selectively inhibits the sections of the thalamus corresponding to the irrelevant sound frequencies. This gain-control mechanism leads to filtering of unwanted sounds, which then do not reach conscious perception in the auditory cortex. As long as this feedback system is intact, the tinnitus signal is filtered out. If, however, parts of the feedback system have become compromised, such as lesions that translate in decreased gray matter volumes in (parts of) the vmPFC [55–57], the abnormal sound may be passed on to the cortex causing the conscious perception of tinnitus.

In a different model, tinnitus seems to be related to changes in thalamocortical rhythms that naturally occur in the brain [14]. As a consequence of hearing loss and reduced input to the thalamus, normal rhythms of the thalamocortical loop change to increased large-scale, slow-rate oscillatory coherent theta (4–8 Hz) activity, in turn reducing lateral inhibition and disinhibiting more high-frequent gamma (30–70 Hz) oscillations [15]. Tinnitus-related increases in the low-frequency delta-band (0.5–4 Hz) and decreases in the alpha-band (8–13 Hz) was previously shown [58].

For both models, it could be argued that tinnitus leads to reduced connectivity between thalamus and cortex, or even brainstem and cortex. If the thalamus is disinhibited (by e.g. reduced inhibitory input from the TRN) more excitatory activity reaches the cortex [12], ultimately leading to tinnitus. Due to this increased cortical (tinnitus-related) activity, there is little room for activity relating to other (non-tinnitus) sound stimuli, which may lead to a reduction in connectivity patterns.

Decreased connectivity also applies to the model by Llinas et al., (1999). Here deafferentation leads to reduced thalamic activity, like for example in patients with gaze-evoked tinnitus [59]. The decrease of thalamic activity may affect the normal flow of auditory processing from brainstem to cortex, possibly resulting in reduced connectivity as observed in this study. Thus the data observed show abnormal patterns of connectivity, compatible with both models, although the precise nature of the changes, and the exact role of the thalamus remain unknown.

In conclusion, the connectivity and lateralization results show that tinnitus involves the interplay between multiple brain regions, both along and beyond the classical auditory pathway. Although the conscious perception of tinnitus is ultimately based on patterns of neural activity in the auditory cortex, this work indicates that tinnitus seems related to abnormal connectivity patterns between subcortical nuclei and cortical brain areas.

Supporting Information

Figure S1 Dissimilarity as a function of the age-difference between controls and patients. Each of the points corresponds to one permutation. For each of the 50000 permutations the dissimilarity index and difference in age between the groups were determined. Their marginal distributions are displayed on top or at the right side, respectively. The red lines indicate the actual dissimilarity index (horizontal red line) and the actual difference in age (vertical red line). The blue lines indicate the 95-percentile range of the distributions.

Figure S2 Dissimilarity as a function of the difference in hearing-level (HL) between controls and patients. For each of the 50000 permutations the dissimilarity index and difference in HL between the groups were determined. Their marginal distributions are displayed on top or at the right side, respectively. The red lines indicate the actual dissimilarity index (horizontal red line) and the actual difference in age (vertical red line). The blue lines indicate the 95-percentile range of the distributions.

Figure S3 Dissimilarity as a function of the difference in left-right hearing-levels between controls and patients. For each of the 50000 permutations the dissimilarity index and difference in left-right hearing-levels between the groups were determined. Their marginal distributions are displayed on top or at the right side, respectively. The red lines indicate the actual dissimilarity index (horizontal red line) and the actual difference in age (vertical red line). The blue lines indicate the 95-percentile range of the distributions.

Figure S4 Sound-evoked responses in the left IC in controls (panel A), subjects with right-sided tinnitus (panel B) and subjects with left-sided tinnitus. The panels show four box plots per condition (left 40 dB, left 70 dB, right 40 dB, right 70 dB). The dark red bars show the average responses determined over the 10% most active voxels according to a (condition-wise) t-test in a manually drawn ROI. These results are identical to those reported by Lanting et al, (2008). The orange box plots represent results from identical analyses performed on the same subjects combined with the subjects that were added for this study (four controls, one patient with right-sided tinnitus and three with left-sided tinnitus; indicated with (*) in table 2). The dark blue box plots represent the analysis of the complete data-set with the identical t-test procedure again selecting the 10% most active voxel but using a ROI definition that was based on an anatomical template (MNI) and identical for each subject. The light blue box plots represent the results when an F-test (including all conditions) was used instead of the (condition-wise) t-test. The ROI selection has arguably the biggest effect on the size of the sound-evoked responses, especially in the patients groups. This effect is less dramatic in the controls. The insets (D–F) show the location and extent of the left IC ROIs. It shows a probability map, indicating the amount of overlap between subjects' ROIs as used in the Lanting et al., 2008 study, thresholded at 80% overlap between all subjects in red-yellow colours. In blue is shown the template ROI as defined on the MNI template.

Author Contributions

Conceived and designed the experiments: CL EDK PVD. Performed the experiments: CL. Analyzed the data: CL. Contributed reagents/materials/analysis tools: CL EDK DL PVD. Wrote the paper: CL EDK DL PVD.

References

1. Noreña AJ (2011) An integrative model of tinnitus based on a central gain controlling neural sensitivity. Neurosci Biobehav Rev 35: 1089–1109. doi:10.1016/j.neubiorev.2010.11.003.

2. Noreña AJ, Eggermont JJ (2003) Changes in spontaneous neural activity immediately after an acoustic trauma: implications for neural correlates of tinnitus. Hear Res 183: 137–153.

3. Kaltenbach JA, Zacharek MA, Zhang J, Frederick S (2004) Activity in the dorsal cochlear nucleus of hamsters previously tested for tinnitus following intense tone exposure. Neurosci Lett 355: 121–125.

4. Seki S, Eggermont JJ (2003) Changes in spontaneous firing rate and neural synchrony in cat primary auditory cortex after localized tone-induced hearing loss. Hear Res 180: 28–38.

5. Dominguez M, Becker S, Bruce I, Read H (2006) A spiking neuron model of cortical correlates of sensorineural hearing loss: Spontaneous firing, synchrony, and tinnitus. Neural Comput 18: 2942–2958. doi:10.1162/neco.2006.18.12.2942.

6. Chrostowski M, Yang L, Wilson HR, Bruce IC, Becker S (2011) Can homeostatic plasticity in deafferented primary auditory cortex lead to travelling waves of excitation? J Comput Neurosci 30: 279–299. doi:10.1007/s10827-010-0256-1.

7. Lanting CP, de Kleine E, van Dijk P (2009) Neural activity underlying tinnitus generation: results from PET and fMRI. Hear Res 255: 1–13. doi:10.1016/j.heares.2009.06.009.

8. Adjamian P, Sereda M, Hall DA (2009) The mechanisms of tinnitus: perspectives from human functional neuroimaging. Hear Res 253: 15–31. doi:10.1016/j.heares.2009.04.001.

9. Lanting CP, De Kleine E, Bartels H, Van Dijk P (2008) Functional imaging of unilateral tinnitus using fMRI. Acta Otolaryngol 128: 415–421. doi:10.1080/00016480701793743.

10. Melcher JR, Levine RA, Bergevin C, Norris B (2009) The auditory midbrain of people with tinnitus: abnormal sound-evoked activity revisited. Hear Res 257: 63–74. doi:10.1016/j.heares.2009.08.005.

11. Gu JW, Halpin CF, Nam E-C, Levine R a, Melcher JR (2010) Tinnitus, diminished sound-level tolerance, and elevated auditory activity in humans with clinically normal hearing sensitivity. J Neurophysiol 104: 3361–3370. doi:10.1152/jn.00226.2010.

12. Rauschecker JP, Leaver AM, Mühlau M (2010) Tuning out the noise: limbic-auditory interactions in tinnitus. Neuron 66: 819–826. doi:10.1016/j.neuron.2010.04.032.

13. Zhang J (2013) Auditory cortex stimulation to suppress tinnitus: mechanisms and strategies. Hear Res 295: 38–57. doi:10.1016/j.heares.2012.05.007.

14. Llinás R, Ribary U (1993) Coherent 40-Hz oscillation characterizes dream state in humans. Proc Natl Acad Sci U S A 90: 2078–2081.

15. Llinás RR, Ribary U, Jeanmonod D, Kronberg E, Mitra PP (1999) Thalamocortical dysrhythmia: A neurological and neuropsychiatric syndrome characterized by magnetoencephalography. Proc Natl Acad Sci U S A 96: 15222–15227. doi:10.1073/pnas.96.26.15222.

16. Boyen K, de Kleine E, van Dijk P, Langers DRM (2014) Tinnitus-related dissociation between cortical and subcortical neural activity in humans with mild to moderate sensorineural hearing loss. Hear Res 312: 48–59. doi:10.1016/j.heares.2014.03.001.

17. Wilson PH, Henry J, Bowen M, Haralambous G (1991) Tinnitus reaction questionnaire: psychometric properties of a measure of distress associated with tinnitus. J Speech Hear Res 34: 197–201.

18. Oldfield RC (1971) The assessment and analysis of handedness: the Edinburgh inventory. Neuropsychologia 9: 97–113.

19. Hall DA, Haggard MP, Akeroyd MA, Palmer AR, Summerfield AQ, et al. (1999) "Sparse" temporal sampling in auditory fMRI. Hum Brain Mapp 7: 213–223.

20. Langers DRM, van Dijk P, Backes WH (2005) Interactions between hemodynamic responses to scanner acoustic noise and auditory stimuli in functional magnetic resonance imaging. Magn Reson Med 53: 49–60. doi:10.1002/mrm.20315.

21. Baumgart F, Kaulisch T, Tempelmann C, Gaschler-Markefski B, Tegeler C, et al. (1998) Electrodynamic headphones and woofers for application in magnetic resonance imaging scanners. Med Phys 25: 2068–2070.

22. Langers DRM, Backes WH, van Dijk P (2003) Spectrotemporal features of the auditory cortex: the activation in response to dynamic ripples. Neuroimage 20: 265–275. doi:10.1016/S1053-8119(03)00258-1.

23. Nichols TE, Holmes AP (2002) Nonparametric permutation tests for functional neuroimaging: a primer with examples. Hum Brain Mapp 15: 1–25.

24. Lanting CP, de Kleine E, Eppinga RN, van Dijk P (2010) Neural correlates of human somatosensory integration in tinnitus. Hear Res 267: 78–88. doi:10.1016/j.heares.2010.04.006.

25. Morosan P, Rademacher J, Schleicher A, Amunts K, Schormann T, et al. (2001) Human primary auditory cortex: cytoarchitectonic subdivisions and mapping into a spatial reference system. Neuroimage 13: 684–701. doi:10.1006/nimg.2000.0715.

26. Rademacher J, Morosan P, Schormann T, Schleicher A, Werner C, et al. (2001) Probabilistic mapping and volume measurement of human primary auditory cortex. Neuroimage 13: 669–683. doi:10.1006/nimg.2000.0714.

27. Eickhoff SB, Stephan KE, Mohlberg H, Grefkes C, Fink GR, et al. (2005) A new SPM toolbox for combining probabilistic cytoarchitectonic maps and functional imaging data. Neuroimage 25: 1325–1335. doi:10.1016/j.neuroimage.2004.12.034.

28. Woolsey TA, Hanaway J, Gado MH (2003) The Brain Atlas; a visual guide to the human central nervous system. second edi. John Wiley & Sons.

29. Martin JH (2003) Neuroanatomy; text and atlas. third edit. McGraw-Hill.

30. Horwitz B (2003) The elusive concept of brain connectivity. Neuroimage 19: 466–470.

31. Friston KJ (1994) Functional and effective connectivity in neuroimaging: A synthesis. Hum Brain Mapp 2: 56–78. doi:10.1002/hbm.460020107.

32. Cherian A, Sra S, Banerjee A, Papanikolopoulos N (2013) Jensen-Bregman LogDet divergence with application to efficient similarity search for covariance matrices. IEEE Trans Pattern Anal Mach Intell 35: 2161–2174. doi:10.1109/TPAMI.2012.259.

33. Jastreboff PJ (1990) Phantom auditory perception (tinnitus): mechanisms of generation and perception. Neurosci Res 8: 221–254.

34. Eggermont JJ, Roberts LE (2004) The neuroscience of tinnitus. Trends Neurosci 27: 676–682. doi:10.1016/j.tins.2004.08.010.

35. Kaltenbach JA, Zhang J, Finlayson P (2005) Tinnitus as a plastic phenomenon and its possible neural underpinnings in the dorsal cochlear nucleus. Hear Res 206: 200–226. doi:10.1016/j.heares.2005.02.013.

36. Melcher JR, Sigalovsky IS, Guinan JJ, Levine RA (2000) Lateralized tinnitus studied with functional magnetic resonance imaging: abnormal inferior colliculus activation. J Neurophysiol 83: 1058–1072.

37. Hall DA, Haggard MP, Summerfield AQ, Akeroyd MA, Palmer AR, et al. (2001) Functional magnetic resonance imaging measurements of sound-level encoding in the absence of background scanner noise. J Acoust Soc Am 109: 1559–1570.

38. Sigalovsky IS, Melcher JR (2006) Effects of sound level on fMRI activation in human brainstem, thalamic and cortical centers. Hear Res 215: 67–76. doi:10.1016/j.heares.2006.03.002.

39. Langers DRM, Backes WH, van Dijk P (2007) Representation of lateralization and tonotopy in primary versus secondary human auditory cortex. Neuroimage 34: 264–273. doi:10.1016/j.neuroimage.2006.09.002.

40. Röhl M, Uppenkamp S (2012) Neural coding of sound intensity and loudness in the human auditory system. J Assoc Res Otolaryngol 13: 369–379. doi:10.1007/s10162-012-0315-6.

41. Petacchi A, Laird AR, Fox PT, Bower JM (2005) Cerebellum and auditory function: an ALE meta-analysis of functional neuroimaging studies. Hum Brain Mapp 25: 118–128. doi:10.1002/hbm.20137.

42. Huang CM, Liu G, Huang R (1982) Projections from the cochlear nucleus to the cerebellum. Brain Res 244: 1–8.

43. Huang C, Liu G (1990) Organization of the auditory area in the posterior cerebellar vermis of the cat. Exp Brain Res 81: 377–383.

44. Huang CM, Liu L, Pettavel P, Huang RH (1990) Target areas of presumed auditory projections from lateral and dorsolateral pontine nuclei to posterior cerebellar vermis in rat. Brain Res 536: 327–330.

45. Aitkin LM, Boyd J (1975) Responses of single units in cerebellar vermis of the cat to monaural and binaural stimuli. J Neurophysiol 38: 418–429.

46. Leaton RN, Supple WF (1991) Medial cerebellum and long-term habituation of acoustic startle in rats. Behav Neurosci 105: 804–816.

47. Maschke M, Drepper J, Kindsvater K, Kolb FP, Diener HC, et al. (2000) Involvement of the human medial cerebellum in long-term habituation of the acoustic startle response. Exp Brain Res 133: 359–367.

48. Timmann D, Musso C, Kolb FP, Rijntjes M, Jüptner M, et al. (1998) Involvement of the human cerebellum during habituation of the acoustic startle response: a PET study. J Neurol Neurosurg Psychiatry 65: 771–773.

49. Brozoski TJ, Ciobanu L, Bauer CA (2007) Central neural activity in rats with tinnitus evaluated with manganese-enhanced magnetic resonance imaging (MEMRI). Hear Res 228: 168–179. doi:10.1016/j.heares.2007.02.003.

50. Coad ML, Lockwood A, Salvi R, Burkard R (2001) Characteristics of patients with gaze-evoked tinnitus. Otol Neurotol 22: 650–654.

51. Ehret G, Romand R (1997) The Central Auditory System. Oxford University Press.

52. Langers DRM, van Dijk P, Backes WH (2005) Lateralization, connectivity and plasticity in the human central auditory system. Neuroimage 28: 490–499. doi:10.1016/j.neuroimage.2005.06.024.

53. Lee CC, Winer J a (2005) Principles governing auditory cortex connections. Cereb Cortex 15: 1804–1814. doi:10.1093/cercor/bhi057.

54. Crippa A, Lanting CP, van Dijk P, Roerdink JBTM (2010) A diffusion tensor imaging study on the auditory system and tinnitus. Open Neuroimag J 4: 16–25. doi:10.2174/1874440001004010016.

55. Leaver AM, Renier L, Chevillet MA, Morgan S, Kim HJ, et al. (2011) Dysregulation of limbic and auditory networks in tinnitus. Neuron 69: 33–43. doi:10.1016/j.neuron.2010.12.002.

56. Leaver AM, Seydell-Greenwald A, Turesky TK, Morgan S, Kim HJ, et al. (2012) Cortico-limbic morphology separates tinnitus from tinnitus distress. Front Syst Neurosci 6: 21. doi:10.3389/fnsys.2012.00021.

57. Mühlau M, Rauschecker JP, Oestreicher E, Gaser C, Röttinger M, et al. (2006) Structural brain changes in tinnitus. Cereb Cortex 16: 1283–1288. doi:10.1093/cercor/bhj070.

58. Weisz N, Moratti S, Meinzer M, Dohrmann K, Elbert T (2005) Tinnitus perception and distress is related to abnormal spontaneous brain activity as measured by magnetoencephalography. PLoS Med 2: e153. doi:10.1371/journal.pmed.0020153.

59. Van Gendt MJ, Boyen K, de Kleine E, Langers DRM, van Dijk P (2012) The relation between perception and brain activity in gaze-evoked tinnitus. J Neurosci 32: 17528–17539. doi:10.1523/JNEUROSCI.2791-12.2012.

19

Relation between Speech-in-Noise Threshold, Hearing Loss and Cognition from 40–69 Years of Age

David R. Moore[1,2,3]*, Mark Edmondson-Jones[1,4], Piers Dawes[5], Heather Fortnum[1,4],
Abby McCormack[1,2,4], Robert H. Pierzycki[1,4], Kevin J. Munro[5,6]

1 NIHR Nottingham Hearing Biomedical Research Unit, Nottingham, United Kingdom, 2 MRC Institute of Hearing Research, University Park, Nottingham, United Kingdom, 3 Cincinnati Children's Hospital Medical Center and Department of Otolaryngology, University of Cincinnati College of Medicine, Cincinnati, Ohio, United States of America, 4 Otology and Hearing Group, Division of Clinical Neuroscience, School of Medicine, University of Nottingham, Nottingham, United Kingdom, 5 School of Psychological Sciences, University of Manchester, Manchester, United Kingdom, 6 Central Manchester University Hospitals NHS Foundation Trust, Manchester Academic Health Science Centre, Manchester, United Kingdom

Abstract

Background: Healthy hearing depends on sensitive ears and adequate brain processing. Essential aspects of both hearing and cognition decline with advancing age, but it is largely unknown how one influences the other. The current standard measure of hearing, the pure-tone audiogram is not very cognitively demanding and does not predict well the most important yet challenging use of hearing, listening to speech in noisy environments. We analysed data from UK Biobank that asked 40–69 year olds about their hearing, and assessed their ability on tests of speech-in-noise hearing and cognition.

Methods and Findings: About half a million volunteers were recruited through NHS registers. Respondents completed 'whole-body' testing in purpose-designed, community-based test centres across the UK. Objective hearing (spoken digit recognition in noise) and cognitive (reasoning, memory, processing speed) data were analysed using logistic and multiple regression methods. Speech hearing in noise declined exponentially with age for both sexes from about 50 years, differing from previous audiogram data that showed a more linear decline from <40 years for men, and consistently less hearing loss for women. The decline in speech-in-noise hearing was especially dramatic among those with lower cognitive scores. Decreasing cognitive ability and increasing age were both independently associated with decreasing ability to hear speech-in-noise (0.70 and 0.89 dB, respectively) among the population studied. Men subjectively reported up to 60% higher rates of difficulty hearing than women. Workplace noise history associated with difficulty in both subjective hearing and objective speech hearing in noise. Leisure noise history was associated with subjective, but not with objective difficulty hearing.

Conclusions: Older people have declining cognitive processing ability associated with reduced ability to hear speech in noise, measured by recognition of recorded spoken digits. Subjective reports of hearing difficulty generally show a higher prevalence than objective measures, suggesting that current objective methods could be extended further.

Editor: Joel Snyder, UNLV, United States of America

Funding: DRM was supported by the Intramural Programme of the Medical Research Council [Grant U135097130] and by Cincinnati Children's Hospital. The Nottingham Hearing Biomedical Research Unit is funded by the National Institute for Health Research. This paper presents independent research funded in part by the National Institute for Health Research (NIHR). The views expressed are those of the authors and not necessarily those of the NHS, the NIHR or the Department of Health. This research was facilitated by the NIHR Manchester Biomedical Research Centre. The funders had no role in study design, data collection and analysis, decision to publish, or preparation of the manuscript.

Competing Interests: The authors have declared that no competing interests exist.

* Email: david.moore2@cchmc.org

Introduction

The detection of quiet tones of varying frequency, has for >70 years been the gold standard test of hearing [1]. However, the most frequent complaint expressed by people about their hearing is inability to follow speech in noisy environments [2]. Pure-tone audiograms, measures of tone detection threshold across frequency [2], and speech perception measured in the quiet [3], do not predict well the handicap produced by hearing loss. These principles were first recognized long ago [4–7], as was the finding that speech-in-noise (SiN) hearing ability decreases with age [3], even while the audiogram may remain relatively stable [4]. SiN measures that use familiar speech correlate with the average level

of hearing based on the pure-tone audiogram (the 'pure tone average', PTA [8–10]) and may offer an alternative gold standard more relevant to everyday hearing. Despite much research, SiN hearing has until recently received little attention in large population studies and limited clinical application. However, the development of the Digit Triplets Test (DTT [11]), a measure of SiN hearing that can be administered without specialist supervision and in any quiet room (go to actiononhearingloss.org.uk for a demonstration and test), enabled inclusion in UK Biobank [12,13]. UK Biobank is an internationally accessible data resource based on a very large-scale, ongoing, longitudinal study across England, Scotland and Wales of many aspects of health, starting in middle age (40–69 year olds; www.ukbiobank.ac.uk).

We report here on the baseline UK Biobank DTT data, compared in the same participants with other UK Biobank data on cognitive ability and self-reported hearing, and with other large, audiogram-based studies [14–18]. Paraphrasing Neisser [19], cognition is the transformation of sensory information into meaning. It may refer to a broad range of constructs relevant to hearing including attention, memory, intelligence, learning, processing speed and language. Language skills were not tested directly in UK Biobank, but they undoubtedly contributed to some extent to the self-report questions on hearing, the DTT, and all the cognitive tests, especially some items in the test of Fluid Intelligence (Fig. S3 in Results S1).

We first asked whether the increase in tone threshold with age, previously measured by the audiogram and by sentences in noise [20], is paralleled by an increase in DTT speech reception threshold (DTT SRT). Given the presumed greater cognitive demand of DTT, involving speech recognition and working memory, we predicted that an increase in DTT SRT with age would be greater than the relative increase in PTA because of a combination of reduced audibility and reduced cognition [21]. This prediction bears on a fundamental clinical issue, how best to measure and treat hearing impairment. This is a timely issue because of the increase of hearing-related problems in an aging population [21] and the large proportion of middle age people with significant and treatable hearing loss who currently remain untreated [22].

Sensitivity to high frequency tones begins to decline in most people by 30–40 years old [16,18] then spreads to lower frequencies from 40 years onwards (Fig. 1B, C). Overall, 21% of UK 40–69 year olds had clinical hearing loss (PTA>20 dB hearing level, HL, 0.5–4.0 kHz in better ear) in the mid-1980s [14], the last time it was measured in a large UK population. The version of the DTT used in UK Biobank, like the original telephone test, has a high frequency limit of 4.0 kHz, so is a suitable test for comparison with those historical data. Cognitive function is most commonly measured using IQ, processing speed and working memory tests [23]. In UK Biobank, cognition is assessed using visually delivered measures of fluid intelligence, processing speed, executive function, number storage (digit span), and visuospatial working memory (shape pairs matching). It is not currently known which aspects of cognition are most closely related to hearing but the broad cognitive categories tested in UK Biobank have all been implicated [24,25]. We report here the relationships between those categories and DTT SRT in middle age.

SiN hearing varies significantly in difficulty, and everyday relevance, with the nature of both the speech (typically syllables, words or sentences) and the noise (e.g. 'white', speech-shaped, modulated, or real, competing speakers). The DTT choice of single digit words promotes easy understanding and the opportunity to 'fill-in' missed acoustic information, while steady-state, speech-shaped noise enables masking across the speech range, but does not allow the 'glimpsing' that can reduce masking in more complex noise. Overall, DTT performance correlates more closely with PTA than do some other SiN tests [10]. The DTT is reproducible, easy to standardize, available in several languages, does not require a sound booth, and may be delivered through the internet. However, it has been suggested [9,10] that it may not be as sensitive to cognitive function as some other SiN tests.

Self-report of hearing difficulties, using questionnaire instruments or often only one or two questions, has commonly been used to assess the prevalence of hearing loss in large epidemiological studies [14,26]. Some studies [14,27] have reported the relationship of self-report with audiometric measures but only

rarely have self-report data been validated against standard audiometric measures [28–30]. Self-report assessed by a single question ('Do you feel you have a hearing loss?') has been reported to demonstrate high sensitivity and specificity. A multi-question hearing handicap inventory had lower sensitivity but higher specificity and a positive predictive value. Both question and inventory were recommended for assessing burden but could not measure hearing loss [28].

In this study we investigated the relation between DTT SRT and cognitive ability as a function of age, sex, socioeconomic status, and noise exposure. The results were compared with self-report of hearing difficulties and findings from other studies, including some previously unpublished data from the NIH Toolbox [18,23], of age-related changes in tone sensitivity and cognitive performance. It was predicted that DTT SRT would decline with age more rapidly than tone sensitivity and that the decline in DTT SRT would be more closely associated with increased self-reported hearing difficulty.

Methods

Complete details of all UK Biobank procedures are available at www.ukbiobank.ac.uk.

Ethics statement

This research was covered by the UK Biobank ethics agreement. Within England, UK Biobank has approval from the North West Multi-centre Research Ethics Committee (MREC). All participants provided written informed consent.

Population and setting

Participants (n = 502,642; Table 1) volunteered between March 2007 and July 2010 following invitation letters to 9.2 million eligible UK residents [12]. Data were gathered at 22 assessment centres in England, Scotland and Wales. Participants attended a two-hour appointment during which they answered, via a touch-screen, questions about their life history, lifestyle and health, including their hearing. They also completed a hearing test and several tests of cognitive ability. Participants were free to opt out of the study at any time, either during the assessment or subsequently. Further details of UK Biobank recruitment, the DTT, and prevalence of hearing loss are presented elsewhere [31].

Hearing tests

All participants (Table 1) were asked "Do you have any difficulty with your hearing?" and "Do you find it difficult to follow a conversation if there is background noise (such as TV, radio, children playing)?" Possible answers were 'Yes'; 'No'; 'Do not know'; 'Prefer not to answer'. About one third of the participants were also asked "Have you ever worked in a noisy place where you had to shout to be heard?" and "Have you ever listened to music for more than 3 hours per week at a volume which you would need to shout to be heard or, if wearing headphones, someone else would need to shout for you to hear them?" Possible answers for these noise and music exposure questions were 'Yes, for more than 5 years'; 'Yes, for around 1–5 years'; 'Yes, for less than a year'; 'No'; 'Do not know'; 'Prefer not to answer'.

Guided by a video demonstration (see http://biobank.ctsu.ox.ac.uk/crystal/videos/hearing.swf), about one third of the participants (Table 1) completed a truncated DTT with fifteen (monosyllabic single digit) triplets (e.g. 5-0-8) presented separately to each ear via circumaural headphones (Sennheiser D25 [31]). A noise, shaped spectrally to the complete set of 9 digits, was played

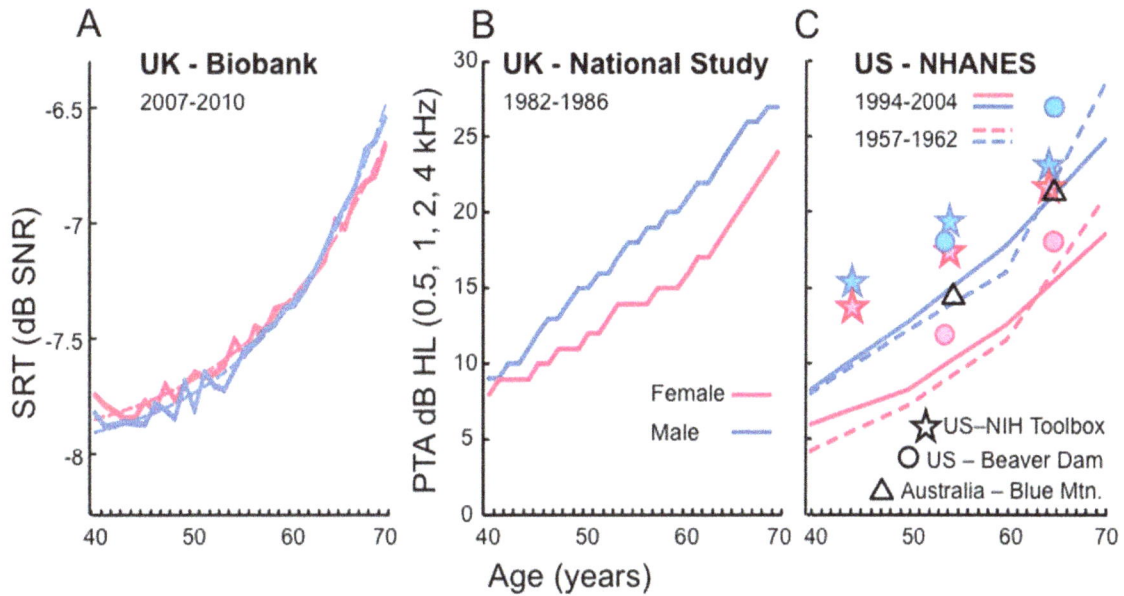

*US – NHANES: Unilateral loss counted as unaffected

Figure 1. Hearing declines from 40–69 years of age. (A) UK Biobank: Mean DTT speech reception threshold (SRT; better ear) data, corrected for differences in socio-economic between samples. Exponential functions with an additive constant are fitted to the data. (B) National Study of Hearing (UK [14]): Mean pure tone average (PTA) thresholds (0.5, 1, 2, 4 kHz; better ear). (C) National Health and Nutrition Examination Survey (NHANES, US [16]): Mean PTA thresholds (0.5–4 kHz). Other data points from NIH Toolbox (US, 2011 [18]), Beaver Dam Epidemiology of Hearing Loss Study (US, 1993 [15]), Blue Mountains Hearing Study (Australia, 1997–2000 [17]).

Table 1. Characteristics of UK Biobank participants.

Demographics	Female		Male		All	
	N (%)	mean±sd % +ve	N (%)	mean±sd % +ve	N (%)	mean±sd % +ve
Gender	273,448 (54%)	-	229,194 (46%)	-	502,642 (100%)	-
Age	273,448 (100%)	56.3±8.0 yrs	229,194 (100%)	56.7±8.2 yrs	502,642 (100%)	56.5±8.1 yrs
Auditory tests/questions						
SRT (better ear; dB)	87,650 (32%)	−7.4±1.6 dB	73,305 (32%)	−7.4±1.8 dB	160,955 (32%)	−7.4±1.7 dB
Hearing difficulty	258,576 (95%)	21%	219,120 (96%)	31%	477,696 (95%)	26%
Hearing in noise	266,966 (98%)	33%	224,032 (98%)	43%	490,998 (98%)	38%
Noisy workplace exposure	92,881 (34%)	11%	77,501 (34%)	37%	170,382 (34%)	23%
Loud music exposure	92,424 (34%)	9%	77,109 (34%)	17%	169,533 (34%)	12%
Cognitive tests						
Fluid Intelligence	90,202 (33%)	5.9±2.1 correct	75,306 (33%)	6.1±2.2 correct	165,508 (33%)	6.0±2.2 correct
Prospective Memory	93,382 (34%)	76%	78,219 (34%)	77%	171,601 (34%)	76%
Visual Memory	270,996 (99%)	4.7±3.7 pairs	227,054 (99%)	4.7±3.9 pairs	498,050 (99%)	4.7±3.8 pairs
Reaction Time	270,470 (99%)	567±117 ms	226,412 (99%)	551±116 ms	496,882 (99%)	560±117 ms
Digit Span	28,179 (10%)	6.4±1.8 digits	23,637 (10%)	6.6±1.9 digits	51,816 (10%)	6.5±1.8 digits

Number and performance of participants completing each auditory and cognitive measure. Percentages for each N other than gender are corrected for missing data. Mean ± sd: descriptive statistics for age, SRT, cognitive tests. % +ve: percent positive responses to each question. Cognitive test performance shows number of questions correctly answered (FI), % correct responses (PM), and number of incorrectly chosen pairs (VM).

simultaneously. Both noise and (suprathreshold) speech levels were initially adjusted together to a comfortable level. The speech level was then fixed and noise level was varied adaptively after each triplet, dependent on the listener's correct touchscreen response to all three digits, to obtain criterion performance of 50% correct. The measure of hearing, the DTT SRT, was the mean signal-to-noise ratio from the last eight triplets. Testing of each ear took ~4 minutes.

Participants were asked about several other aspects of hearing, including their use of hearing aids or cochlear implants. If they used hearing aids they were asked to remove them prior to completing the DTT. If they used cochlear implants they were asked not to attempt the test. Further studies using the UK Biobank resource and dealing in detail with associations and predictions between hearing and hearing aids [32], tinnitus [33], visual impairment and dual sensory problems [34], cigarette smoking and alcohol consumption [35], have or will be published elsewhere.

Cognitive tests

Variable numbers of participants completed each test (Table 1), primarily due to the introduction of different tests at different stages during the UK Biobank project. The Fluid Intelligence test comprised thirteen questions designed to test logic and reasoning ability (e.g. If Truda's mother's brother is Tim's sister's father, what relation is Truda to Tim?; Fig. S3 in Results S1). The Prospective (long-term) Memory test presented the following instruction early in the cognitive test battery: "At the end of the games we will show you four coloured shapes and ask you to touch the Blue Square. However, to test your memory, we want you to actually touch the Orange Circle instead." In two rounds, the Visual (short-term) Memory ('Pairs matching') test presented a matrix (1st round: 2×3; 2nd round: 3×4) of cards showing 3 and 6 pairs of shapes, respectively. The shapes were concealed and the participant was required to recall locations of matching shape pairs. Correct responses were confirmed. The Reaction Time test of processing speed sequentially presented twelve pairs of shapes. The participant pressed a button as quickly as possible if a pair of shapes matched. Finally, in the Digit Span ('Numeric memory') test of verbal working memory participants were initially presented on the screen with two digits and were required to key in the digits in reverse order. After each correct response the digit sequence was increased by one. The task ended after two incorrect responses. Raw score was the maximum number of correctly recalled and ordered digits. Performance on the Prospective Memory, Reaction Time and Digit Span tests additionally depended on executive function and all tests depended on alerting and orienting attention.

Analysis and reporting

Analysis of self-report measures used binary logistic regression. Standardised scores, which each maximised the variability within the sampled population, were derived for each cognitive test using principal components analysis. A composite score was defined as a simple sum of the five standardised scores. Both individual and composite cognitive scores were standardised to have zero mean and unit standard deviation, such that higher values corresponded to higher ability. Scores were grouped into deciles for analysis. Regression modelling techniques accounting for sex, socio-economic deprivation (Townsend score, a proxy measure of socioeconomic status [31]), noise exposure (work and music), and interaction of socio-economic deprivation and noise with sex, were used to dissociate decline in hearing from decline in cognition with increasing age. Age at which full-time education was completed

was not accounted for in these models but varied little between women (mean = 16.68, s.d. = 2.17) and men (mean = 16.76 years; s.d. = 2.52). Modelling that included cognitive scores was restricted to the 40,655 participants who completed all auditory and cognitive tests and questions. Data were assumed to be missing completely at random, as the primary reason for absent responses was the phased introduction of test components.

Results

Hearing

Age-related decline of hearing differs between test measures (Fig. 1). DTT SRT, averaged across participants, declined exponentially with age, starting from a low (sensitive) level in the 40 s (Fig. 1A). Both the absolute level and the rate of age-related decline of DTT SRT in men and women advanced in close parallel as individuals in the population became older, although SRT was slightly better in younger men than in younger women, and slightly better in older women than in older men. Tone sensitivity (indexed by the PTA, [9]) has also been shown in several studies across a 50 year time span to decline with age (Figs. 1B,C). However, in contrast to DTT SRT, tone sensitivity has previously been shown to decline rapidly through the 40 s, at least among men. Men had markedly poorer sensitivity than women at all ages >40, but women's sensitivity started to deteriorate in parallel with that of men when they reached their 60 s. A reduction in the rate of declining tone sensitivity with advancing age has been noted in some more recent studies (Fig. 1C [16,18,36]), but high frequency sensitivity remains much more susceptible to aging and clearly poorer in men (Fig. S1 in Results S1).

In UK Biobank, more men reported having problems with their hearing than did women (Fig. 2). Reported problems for both sexes grew linearly with age. By 69 y.o., men were reporting hearing difficulties, and difficulties in noise, at 40–60% higher prevalence than women. This increasing difference between men and women with age was not paralleled by objective measures of either speech or tone hearing (Fig. 1), nor by direct comparison between the prevalence of reported difficulty and DTT hearing (Fig. S2 in Results S1). Responses to questions about workplace noise (Table 2) showed the same relationship for women and men between increasing duration of noise exposure and the objective measure of decreased DTT SRT. Note, however, that the maximum effect size (mean 0.19 dB loss of SRT for >5 years exposure) was relatively small compared with age-related hearing loss (Fig. 1A; Table 3). No difference was found between the sexes for the effect of workplace noise on DTT SRT, and no significant effect of music exposure on DTT SRT was found. In contrast, both workplace noise and music exposure were significantly related to subjective reports of 'difficulty hearing' (Table 2) and 'hearing in noise' (Table S1 in Results S1). But while a far higher proportion of men than women reported exposure both to a noisy workplace and to loud music (Table 1), there was not a consistent dose-response difference between the sexes (Table 2). Men who experienced shorter noisy workplace exposure were less likely than women to report difficulty with their hearing, whereas men who experienced longer exposure were more likely than women to report difficulty. For music, there was no significant difference between the sexes.

Cognition

Cognitive performance, like hearing, decreased with advancing age on all tests (Fig. 3, Table 3). For four tests, the pattern of decline was relatively simple and monotonic. However, Fluid Intelligence did not begin to decline until 60 y.o., then declined

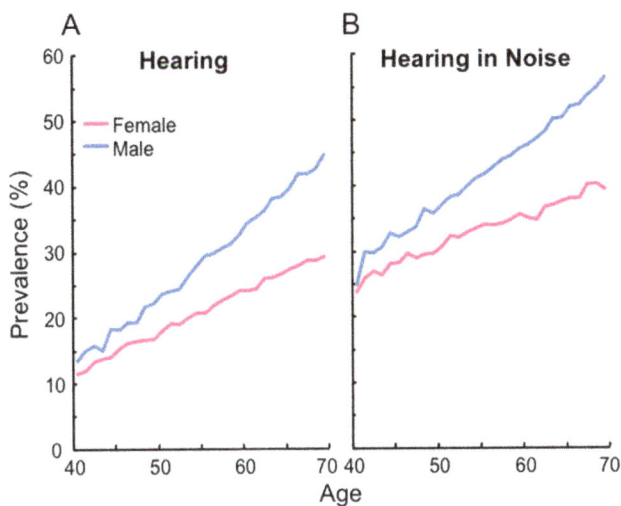

Figure 2. Men report greater difficulty hearing than women.
Prevalence of self-report of (A) hearing difficulty and (B) difficulty hearing speech-in-noise in women and men from 40–70 y.o., corrected for socio-economic.

linearly for ages >60. Responses to individual Fluid Intelligence questions suggested this was due to a decline in both verbal and non-verbal performance from about this age (Fig. S3 in Results S1). Men performed better than women on all tests except prospective memory. The mean gap between the sexes increased with age on Reaction Time and Digit Span. Correlation between scores on individual tests varied from r = 0.19–0.38 (Table S2 in Results S1).

Relation between hearing and cognition

Better DTT SRT was associated with better cognitive ability. Fig. 4 shows cognitive ability on each test, plotted as deciles from 1 (lowest) to 10 (highest), as a function of DTT SRT. DTT SRT decreased by about 0.7 dB across the range of ability (i.e. from decile 1 to 10) on each cognitive test. This was similar in size to the increase in average DTT SRT across the 40–69 year age range (women: 0.75 dB, men: 1.05 dB; Table 3). DTT SRT differences were greatest at the lower end of cognitive ability. These results suggested that the ability to compensate for impaired DTT SRT depended strongly on cognitive performance, especially at the lower end of the spectrum. However, DTT SRT declined with age across the cognitive spectrum (Fig. S5 in Results S1).

Discussion

Hearing in quiet and in noise

We found that, on average, DTT SRT declines substantially during late middle age, confirming earlier studies [11,20]. However, we also found little decline in DTT SRT until the 50 s, whereas declining PTA, based on the same frequency range used in the DTT, begins in the 30 s [14,16,18]. These differences may be due to the high 'redundancy' of the DTT speech signal relative to a single tone. Digits are a closed set of overlearned words. A listener can access many auditory tone channels, only some of which need be fully functional, to gain cues to digit identity. For example, many English digits can be distinguished using only vowels. Small changes in sensitivity to higher frequency tones in the 30 s and 40 s can therefore over-estimate real-life

difficulty with speech, even when there is little or no contextual information, as in the DTT. At later ages, deficits in DTT SRT escalate rapidly and, by the early 60 s, are advancing relatively more rapidly than loss of tone sensitivity, presumably due to both more widespread loss of tone sensitivity and reduced auditory processing in the brain. Historically, tone sensitivity studies have also reported that men's hearing begins to deteriorate before that of women, particularly at high sound frequencies, and that the difference is maintained into old age. Some recent evidence [18] suggests that disparity may be declining, at least in the main speech range of hearing. Nevertheless, the UK Biobank data are notable in showing a close similarity between the DTT hearing of men and women across most of the age range studied, but with men showing a slightly greater decline in the late 60 s.

The different patterns of age-related hearing loss revealed by the two measures is evidence that DTT SRT utilizes different or additional mechanisms to those revealed by audiometry. One candidate mechanism may be an age-related loss of inner hair cell afferent synapses, as recently reported in mice [37]. In that example of supra-threshold hearing loss, mid-frequency pure tone thresholds measured by wave 1 of the auditory brainstem response were still normal in older (64–80 week old) mice when supra-threshold response amplitude was reduced relative to younger (4–16 week old) mice. The results suggest a loss of the number and synchrony of functional cochlear nerve fibres. In a human parallel of these findings, cochlear nerve neuron (spiral ganglion) cell bodies appear to be lost continually from a young age (<20 years [38]) when, again, auditory thresholds and otoacoustic emissions are normal, signifying intact hair cells. However, no differences in this process were seen between the sexes or across the length of the cochlea. Because aging men typically have poorer high frequency, but may not have poorer low frequency hearing than women (Fig. 1B; Fig. S1 in Results S1 [39]), we also suggest that the high redundancy of the speech signals enables men to identify the digits used in the current study based on the lower frequency cues (e.g. vowels) they can hear.

Subjective reports of hearing difficulty were predictable from DTT SRT, but did not match the pattern of decline in DTT SRT (or PTA [14–18]) with increasing age. A surprisingly high proportion of 40–50 y.o. people with normal DTT SRT indicated that they had difficulty hearing. That proportion rose with age and reduced DTT SRT, as expected, but the proportion of men reporting difficulty was markedly higher than that of women at nearly all ages. Two explanations for these phenomena are that the tests did not capture the handicap experienced, or that people misperceived their hearing to be worse than it really was. We think both these factors contributed to the results. Challenges to making realistic measures of speech hearing include the variety of situations encountered in everyday life and the variety of speech hearing to which individual brains are 'tuned'. For example, we do most of our listening in reverberant rooms having a wide range of acoustic characteristics known to affect speech intelligibility [40]. Accents can be remarkably variable both between older, established communities and within modern, multi-ethnic urban centres, making calibration difficult, both for the audiologist and for the listener. The band-limited (<4 kHz) UK Biobank DTT probably captures some, but not all hearing loss that affects suprathreshold listening. Newly-developed, internet-deliverable SiN hearing tests that have shown greater sensitivity to high frequency hearing loss than the UK Biobank DTT [41,42], may help further in meeting these challenges, and other SiN tests may capture additional relevant properties of the acoustic environment. For example, a modified version of the widely used QuickSIN [43] sentence-in-noise test incorporates separately measurable audiovi-

Table 2. Noisy workplace and music exposure: objective and subjective effects on hearing.

Objective (SRT)	Female (dB)	p	Male (dB)	p	All (dB)	p	Factor (p)	Sex (p)
Noisy workplace	-	-	-	-	-	-	<0.001	0.572
<1year					0.05	0.10		
1–5 years					0.08	0.01		
>5 years					0.19	<0.001		
Music exposure	-	-	-	-	-	-	0.24	0.79

Subjective ('Difficulty')	Female (OR)	p	Male (OR)	p	All (OR)	p	Factor (p)	Sex (p)
Noisy workplace	-	-	-	-	-	-	<0.001	<0.001
<1year	1.72	<0.001	1.33	<0.001	-	-		
1–5 years	1.76	<0.001	1.84	<0.001	-	-		
>5 years	2.19	<0.001	2.89	<0.001	-	-		
Music exposure	-	-	-	-	-	-	<0.001	0.11
<1year					1.50	<0.001		
1–5 years					1.87	<0.001		
>5 years					1.98	<0.001		

Objective (SRT): General linear modelling of better ear speech reception threshold (dB) based on number of years workplace noise exposure relative to no exposure. Factor: Main effect for noise/music exposure. Sex: Interaction with gender. The model also includes terms for age, sex and cognition (Table 3).
Subjective ('Difficulty hearing'): Logistic modelling of question association yielding odds ratios (OR) between no exposure and number of years indicated. Other details as for objective test. Similar results were obtained for 'Difficulty hearing in noise' (Table S1 in Results S1).

Table 3. Modelling speech-in-noise.

	Female		Male		All		Factor	Sex
	dB	p	dB	p	dB	p	p	p
Gender (Female)								
Male	-	-	-	-	-0.16	<0.001	<0.001	<0.001
Age (40–44)	-	-	-	-	-	-	<0.001	<0.001
45–49	0.03	0.48	0.02	0.60	-	-		
50–54	0.12	0.001	0.16	<0.001	-	-		
55–59	0.31	<0.001	0.39	<0.001	-	-		
60–64	0.52	<0.001	0.66	<0.001	-	-		
65–69	0.75	<0.001	1.05	<0.001	-	-		
Deprivation	-	-	-	-	-	-	0.37	0.47
Cognition (1 = poor)	-	-	-	-	0	-	<0.001	0.39
2	-	-	-	-	-0.31	<0.001		
3	-	-	-	-	-0.43	<0.001		
4	-	-	-	-	-0.45	<0.001		
5	-	-	-	-	-0.51	<0.001		
6	-	-	-	-	-0.59	<0.001		
7	-	-	-	-	-0.59	<0.001		
8	-	-	-	-	-0.63	<0.001		
9	-	-	-	-	-0.63	<0.001		
10 = good	-	-	-	-	-0.70	<0.001		

General linear modelling of better ear speech reception threshold (dB) based on gender, age, socio-economic, and cognition. Gender, Age and Cognition reference levels were females, the youngest quintile, and the poorest performers, respectively. Factor: Main effect for Age/Deprivation/Cognition. Sex: Interaction with gender.

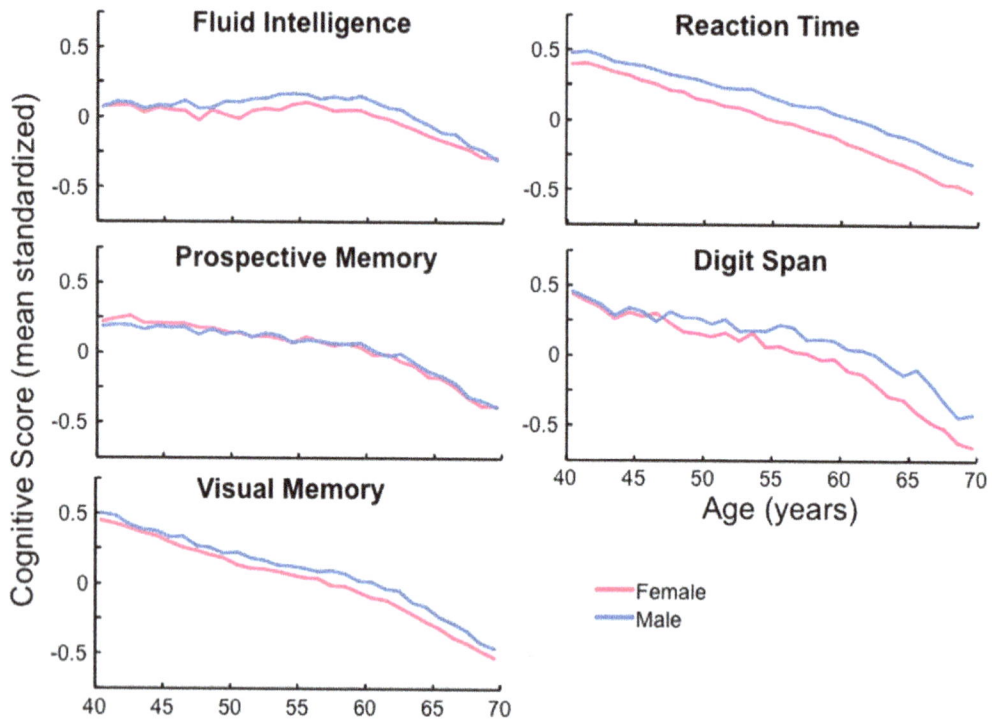

Figure 3. Cognitive performance declines with age. Cognitive performance of men and women in the UK Biobank study expressed as a mean standardized (z) score for ease of comparison between different tests.

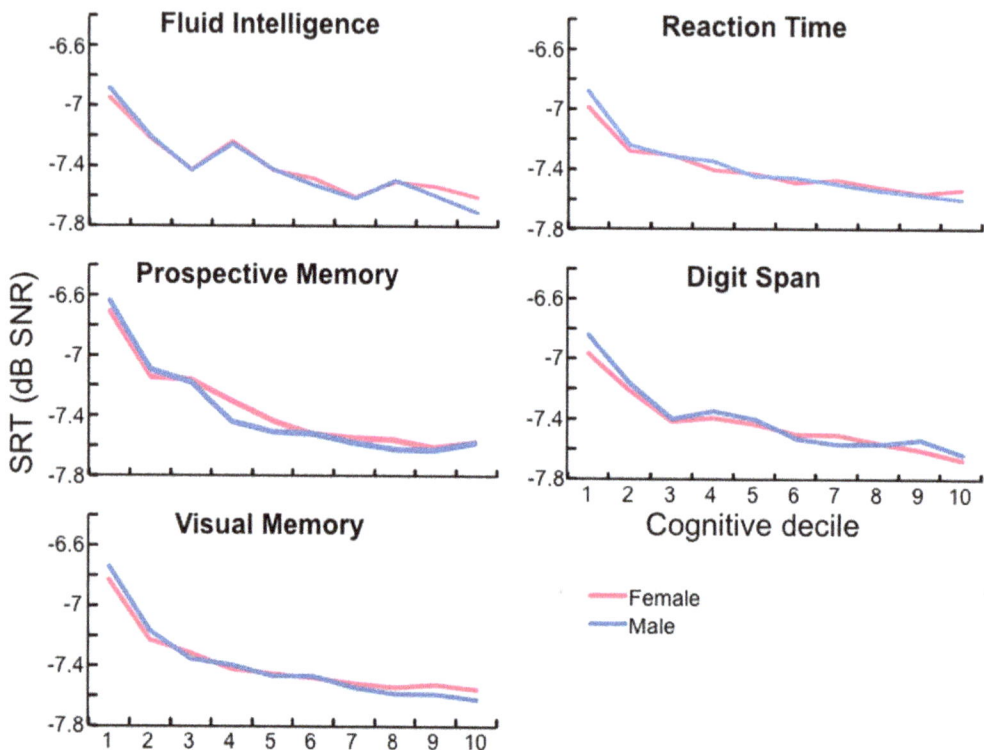

Figure 4. Better cognition is associated with better hearing. Relation between mean SRT and mean performance on each cognitive test (by decile of standardized score from 1 = low to 10 = high), all ages (40–69 y.o.) combined.

sual, reverberation, and spatial cues, and a speeded speech condition [44] (see [45] for a review of SiN tests). Nevertheless, self-report remains an important 'reality check' on the usefulness of any measure of hearing.

This raises the second possibility, that people misperceive their degree of handicap. Everyone has difficulty hearing in some circumstances, and those circumstances are typically in a busy, noisy, reverberant room, such as a bar [40]. The UK Biobank data suggest this 'baseline' rate for perceived difficulty hearing in noise is around 25% for women and 35% for men (Fig. S2 in Results S1). There are many possible reasons why men may both have high estimates of their degree of handicap and have poorer tone sensitivity. One is that they may operate in noisier environments than women. In fact, more men than women reported spending time in noisy environments, both at work and at leisure, and men having longer exposure to noise also reported more difficulty hearing. Nevertheless, the DTT SRT of men did not differ significantly from exposure-matched women who made fewer reports of hearing difficulties, possibly because the men had an increased prevalence of auditory pathology that was not captured by the DTT SRT. Self-reported difficulty in relation to music exposure, which was significant, had quite high odds ratios, and did not differ between the sexes, was similarly not matched by any significant change in DTT SRT.

Cognition and hearing

DTT SRT was found to decline with decreasing cognitive ability, consistent with previous reports using other SiN tests [46,47]. If some aspect(s) of cognition (e.g. long-term memory [48]) was more important than others for speech-in-noise hearing and listening, that aspect should associate more strongly than others with DTT SRT. However, the decline was seen on each cognitive test used, to about the same extent, suggesting that some general cognitive factor may have been responsible. It has been suggested that reduced tone sensitivity is the 'primary predictor' of speech intelligibility with advancing age [49] and that age-related changes in cognitive function are mediated by age-related changes in 'global sensory processing' (hearing, vision, touch composite [47]). The current data suggest a much more prominent role for cognition in hearing, at least for the DTT. Other data from the NIH Toolbox, reported here for the first time, even suggest that poor cognitive function plays a role, albeit a relatively minor one, in reduced PTA (Fig. S4 in Results S1; [18]).

A critical question is whether decreasing tone sensitivity, decreasing cognitive function, both, or another factor (e.g. 'common cause' [50]) is primarily responsible for age-related decline of DTT SRT. Our analysis showed that, across the ages examined, better cognitive function was associated independently with a 0.7 dB reduction in DDT SRT. The effect of increasing age was additive to that effect, leading to a 0.7 (female) to 1.0 dB (male) increase in DDT SRT. In auditory terms, the decline in DTT SRT with age could be due to both peripheral and central factors. Peripheral hearing loss certainly contributes, since we know that tone sensitivity declines with age, even in the most cognitively able [50]. But declining central function may also contribute. For example, there is recent evidence that age-related decline in the maximum speed of auditory temporal processing includes a specifically central mechanism [51]. It is currently unknown whether this is operative within the central auditory system, which includes extensive sub-cortical networks, or within higher level processing areas that include those with multimodal

cognitive functions. In either case, such a mechanism could have a marked effect on speech perception, since reduced temporal fine structure can reduce consonant discrimination [52]. Because of the high reliance of auditory processing on precise timing, auditory processing may prove a sensitive model for testing the 'Processing speed theory' of cognitive decline [53], according to which declining processing speed is the common cause of cognitive decline.

Clinical significance

It is clear that cognitive factors play a major role in speech perception. Although even tone sensitivity is influenced by cognition (e.g. motivation, learning [54]), that influence is not strong, so there is an argument for the addition of tests of speech perception to routine audiometric assessment. Among the older population, differences in the cognitive abilities of the most and least able become more extreme [55] and reports of difficulties hearing speech in noisy environments become more common, as shown here and elsewhere [2]. SiN assessment may help identify those individuals who are likely to benefit from different interventions. Among middle-aged people, who do not typically seek assistance for their hearing loss [22], poorer SiN ability could be a first warning of a need for intervention. Unlike the audiogram, the DTT and some other SiN hearing tests can be delivered remotely for unsupervised, user-based testing via the internet, and are already being used for widespread hearing screening (e.g. visit actiononhearingloss.org.uk). A DTT (the Dutch Digits-in-Noise, DIN, test) has recently been suggested as a clinical diagnostic test [9]. Despite the close association with cognition demonstrated here, DTTs that use steady noise masking have been suggested to be less cognitively demanding than other SiN tests (e.g. using speech maskers [7]). However, this view has been questioned by DTT data [9] showing an extremely high correlation (r = 0.96, following level correction) with performance on Plomp and Mimpen [20] sentences. In contrast to other SiN tests, DTTs are also readily transferrable across cultural and even language groups (www.HearCom.eu [42], [10]). Together, these findings suggest the possibility of a DTT as an international standard for SiN testing.

Supporting Information

Results S1 This file contains Table S1, Table S2, and Figure S1–Figure S5. Table S1, Noisy workplace and music exposure: Relation to 'Hearing in noise' question. Table S2, Pairwise Pearson correlation coefficients between cognitive test measures. Figure S1. Average (PTA) tone detection thresholds declined from 18–85 years (NIH Toolbox data [13]). Figure S2, Reported difficulty hearing increased with declining DTT hearing. Figure S3, Fluid intelligence varied with question, age and gender. Figure S4, PTA did not vary substantially with cognitive ability. Figure S5, Hearing declined with both cognitive ability and age.

Acknowledgments

Disclaimer: This paper presents independent research funded in part by the National Institute for Health Research (NIHR). The views expressed are those of the authors and not necessarily those of the NHS, the NIHR or the Department of Health.

This research has been conducted using the UK Biobank resource. Funding to support the present research was provided by the National Institute of Health Research, the Medical Research Council, the University of Manchester, the Central Manchester University Hospitals NHS Foundation Trust, and Cincinnati Children's Hospital. Additional data were obtained from the NIH Toolbox standardization project [18]. We thank the participants of the UK Biobank resource and NIH Toolbox project for donating their time.

Author Contributions

Conceived and designed the experiments: DRM. Analyzed the data: DRM MEJ PD KJM. Contributed reagents/materials/analysis tools: DRM MEJ PD. Wrote the paper: DRM MEJ PD HF AMC RHP KJM. Liaised with UK Biobank: DRM MEJ PD HF AMC RHP KJM.

References

1. Johnson EW (1970) Tuning forks to audiometers and back again. Laryngoscope 80: 49–68.
2. Vermiglio AJ, Soli SD, Freed DJ, Fisher LM (2012) The relationship between high-frequency pure-tone hearing loss, hearing in noise test (HINT) thresholds, and the articulation index. J Am Acad Audiol 23: 779–788.
3. Plomp R (1986) A signal-to-noise ratio model for the speech-reception threshold of the hearing impaired. J Speech Hear Res 29: 146–154.
4. Bergman M (1971) Hearing and aging. Implications of recent research findings. Audiology 10: 164–171.
5. CHBBC (1988) Speech understanding and aging. Working Group on Speech Understanding and Aging. Committee on Hearing, Bioacoustics, and Biomechanics, Commission on Behavioral and Social Sciences and Education, National Research Council. J Acoust Soc Am 83: 859–895.
6. Gordon-Salant S, Frisina RD, Fay RR, Popper AN, editor (2009) The Aging Auditory System. New Yor: Springer.
7. Humes LE, Kidd GR, Lentz JJ (2013) Auditory and cognitive factors underlying individual differences in aided speech-understanding among older adults. Front Syst Neurosci 7: 55.
8. Smits C, Kapteyn TS, Houtgast T (2004) Development and validation of an automatic speech-in-noise screening test by telephone. Int J Audiol 43: 15–28.
9. Smits C, Theo Goverts S, Festen JM (2013) The digits-in-noise test: assessing auditory speech recognition abilities in noise. J Acoust Soc Am 133: 1693–1706.
10. Jansen S, Luts H, Dejonckere P, van Wieringen A, Wouters J (2013) Efficient Hearing Screening in Noise-Exposed Listeners Using the Digit Triplet Test. Ear Hear 34: 773–778.
11. Smits C, Houtgast T (2005) Results from the Dutch speech-in-noise screening test by telephone. Ear Hear 26: 89–95.
12. Allen N, Sudlow C, Downey P, Peakman T (2012) UK Biobank: Current status and what it means for epidemiology. Health Policy and Technology 1: 123–126.
13. Collins R (2012) What makes UK Biobank special? Lancet 379: 1173–1174.
14. Davis A (1995) Hearing in Adults: Whurr Publishers limited. 1011 p.
15. Cruickshanks KJ, Wiley TL, Tweed TS, Klein BE, Klein R, et al. (1998) Prevalence of hearing loss in older adults in Beaver Dam, Wisconsin. The Epidemiology of Hearing Loss Study. Am J Epidemiol 148: 879–886.
16. Hoffman HJ, Dobie RA, Ko CW, Themann CL, Murphy WJ (2010) Americans hear as well or better today compared with 40 years ago: hearing threshold levels in the unscreened adult population of the United States, 1959–1962 and 1999–2004. Ear Hear 31: 725–734.
17. Chia EM, Wang JJ, Rochtchina E, Cumming RR, Newall P, et al. (2007) Hearing impairment and health-related quality of life: the Blue Mountains Hearing Study. Ear Hear 28: 187–195.
18. Gershon R, Beaumont J (2012) NIH Toolbox norming study data set: Sensation [data file] Version 1.0. Chicago, IL: Northwestern University and National Institutes of Health.
19. Neisser U (1967) Cognitive Psychology. New York: Appleton-Century-Crofts.
20. Plomp R, Mimpen AM (1979) Speech-reception threshold for sentences as a function of age and noise level. J Acoust Soc Am 66: 1333–1342.
21. Moore DR, Fullgrabe C (2012) Cognitive contributions to hearing in older people. J Hear Sci 2: 58–60.
22. Davis A, Smith P, Ferguson M, Stephens D, Gianopoulos I (2007) Acceptability, benefit and costs of early screening for hearing disability: a study of potential screening tests and models. Health Technol Assess 11: 1–294.
23. Weintraub S, Dikmen SS, Heaton RK, Tulsky DS, Zelazo PD, et al. (2013) Cognition assessment using the NIH Toolbox. Neurology 80: S54–64.
24. Moore DR, Ferguson MA, Edmondson-Jones AM, Ratib S, Riley A (2010) Nature of auditory processing disorder in children. Pediatrics 126: e382–390.
25. Sorqvist P, Stenfelt S, Ronnberg J (2012) Working memory capacity and visual-verbal cognitive load modulate auditory-sensory gating in the brainstem: toward a unified view of attention. J Cogn Neurosci 24: 2147–2154.
26. Rosenhall U, Pedersen K, Moller MB (1987) Self-assessment of hearing problems in an elderly population. A longitudinal study. Scand Audiol 16: 211–217.
27. Wilson DH, Walsh PG, Sanchez L, Davis AC, Taylor AW, et al. (1999) The epidemiology of hearing impairment in an Australian adult population. Int J Epidemiol 28: 247–252.
28. Sindhusake D, Mitchell P, Smith W, Golding M, Newall P, et al. (2001) Validation of self-reported hearing loss. The Blue Mountains Hearing Study. Int J Epidemiol 30: 1371–1378.
29. Clark K, Sowers M, Wallace RB, Anderson C (1991) The accuracy of self-reported hearing loss in women aged 60–85 years. Am J Epidemiol 134: 704–708.
30. Nondahl DM, Cruickshanks KJ, Wiley TL, Tweed TS, Klein R, et al. (1998) Accuracy of self-reported hearing loss. Audiology 37: 295–301.

31. Dawes P, Fortnum H, Moore DR, Emsley R, Norman P, et al. (2014) Hearing in middle age: a population snapshot of 40- to 69-year olds in the United Kingdom. Ear Hear 35: e44–51.
32. Dawes P, Emsley R, Cruickshanks KJ, Moore DR, Fortnum H, et al. (In revision) Hearing loss and cognitive decline: the role of hearing aids, social isolation and depression.
33. McCormack A, Edmondson-Jones M, Fortnum H, Dawes P, Middleton H, et al. (2014) The prevalence of tinnitus and the relationship with neuroticism in a middle-aged UK population. J Psychosom Res 76: 56–60.
34. Dawes P, Dickinson C, Emsley R, Bishop P, Cruickshanks K, et al. (2014) Vision impairment and dual sensory problems in middle age. Ophthalmic Physiol Opt 34: 479–488.
35. Dawes P, Cruickshanks K, Moore DR, Edmondson-Jones M, McCormack A, et al. (2014) Cigarette smoking, passive smoking, alcohol consumption and hearing loss. J Assoc Res Otolaryngol 15: 663–674.
36. Zhan W, Cruickshanks KJ, Klein BE, Klein R, Huang GH, et al. (2010) Generational differences in the prevalence of hearing impairment in older adults. Am J Epidemiol 171: 260–266.
37. Sergeyenko Y, Lall K, Liberman MC, Kujawa SG (2013) Age-related cochlear synaptopathy: an early-onset contributor to auditory functional decline. J Neurosci 33: 13686–13694.
38. Makary CA, Shin J, Kujawa SG, Liberman MC, Merchant SN (2011) Age-related primary cochlear neuronal degeneration in human temporal bones. J Assoc Res Otolaryngol 12: 711–717.
39. Dubno JR, Eckert MA, Lee FS, Matthews LJ, Schmiedt RA (2013) Classifying human audiometric phenotypes of age-related hearing loss from animal models. J Assoc Res Otolaryngol 14: 687–701.
40. Bronkhorst AW (2000) The cocktail party phenomenon: A review of research on speech intelligibility in multiple-talker conditions. Acta Acustica united with Acustica 86: 117–128.
41. Leensen MC, de Laat JA, Snik AF, Dreschler WA (2011) Speech-in-noise screening tests by internet, part 2: improving test sensitivity for noise-induced hearing loss. Int J Audiol 50: 835–848.
42. Vlaming MSMG, MacKinnon RC, Jansen M, Moore DR (2014) Automated screening for high-frequency hearing loss. Ear Hear 35 epub ahead of print.
43. Killion MC, Niquette PA, Gudmundsen GI, Revit LJ, Banerjee S (2004) Development of a quick speech-in-noise test for measuring signal-to-noise ratio loss in normal-hearing and hearing-impaired listeners. J Acoust Soc Am 116: 2395–2405.
44. Brungart DS, Sheffield BM, Kubli LR (2014) Development of a test battery for evaluating speech perception in complex listening environments. J Acoust Soc Am in the press.
45. Houtgast T, Festen JM (2008) On the auditory and cognitive functions that may explain an individual's elevation of the speech reception threshold in noise. Int J Audiol 47: 287–295.
46. Pichora-Fuller MK, Schneider BA, Daneman M (1995) How young and old adults listen to and remember speech in noise. J Acoust Soc Am 97: 593–608.
47. Humes LE, Busey TA, Craig J, Kewley-Port D (2013) Are age-related changes in cognitive function driven by age-related changes in sensory processing? Atten Percept Psychophys 75: 508–524.
48. Ronnberg J, Lunner T, Zekveld A, Sorqvist P, Danielsson H, et al. (2013) The Ease of Language Understanding (ELU) model: theoretical, empirical, and clinical advances. Front Syst Neurosci 7: 31.
49. Akeroyd MA (2008) Are individual differences in speech reception related to individual differences in cognitive ability? A survey of twenty experimental studies with normal and hearing-impaired adults. Int J Audiol 47 Suppl 2: S53–71.
50. Baltes PB, Lindenberger U (1997) Emergence of a powerful connection between sensory and cognitive functions across the adult life span: a new window to the study of cognitive aging. Psychol Aging 12: 12–21.
51. Dobreva MS, O'Neill WE, Paige GD (2011) Influence of aging on human sound localization. J Neurophysiol 105: 2471–2486.
52. Rosen S (1992) Temporal information in speech: acoustic, auditory and linguistic aspects. Philos Trans R Soc Lond B Biol Sci 336: 367–373.
53. Salthouse TA (1996) The processing-speed theory of adult age differences in cognition. Psychol Rev 103: 403–428.
54. Zwislocki J, Maire F, Feldman AS, Rubin H (1958) On the effect of practice and motivation on the threshold of audibility. Journal of the Acoustical Society of America 30: 254–262.
55. Rabbitt P (1993) Does it all go together when it goes? The Nineteenth Bartlett Memorial Lecture. Q J Exp Psychol A 46: 385–434.

20

Both Central and Peripheral Auditory Systems Are Involved in Salicylate-Induced Tinnitus in Rats

Guanyin Chen[1,9], **Lining Feng**[2,9], **Zhi Liu**[1], **Yongzhu Sun**[1], **Haifeng Chang**[3], **Pengcheng Cui**[1]*

1 Department of Otolaryngology Head and Neck Surgery, Tangdu Hospital, the Fourth Military Medical University, Xi'an, China, **2** Department of Clinical Medicine, Faculty of Aerospace medicine, the Fourth Military Medical University, Xi'an, China, **3** Department of Radiology, Tangdu Hospital, the Fourth Military Medical University, Xi'an, China

Abstract

Objective: This study was designed to establish a low dose salicylate-induced tinnitus rat model and to investigate whether central or peripheral auditory system is involved in tinnitus.

Methods: Lick suppression ratio (R), lick count and lick latency of conditioned rats in salicylate group (120 mg/kg, intraperitoneally) and saline group were first compared. Bilateral auditory nerves were ablated in unconditioned rats and lick count and lick latency were compared before and after ablation. The ablation was then performed in conditioned rats and lick count and lick latency were compared between salicylate group and saline group and between ablated and unablated salicylate groups.

Results: Both the R value and the lick count in salicylate group were significantly higher than those in saline group and lick latency in salicylate group was significantly shorter than that in saline group. No significant changes were observed in lick count and lick latency before and after ablation. After ablation, lick count and lick latency in salicylate group were significantly higher and shorter respectively than those in saline group, but they were significantly lower and longer respectively than those in unablated salicylate group.

Conclusion: A low dose of salicylate (120 mg/kg) can induce tinnitus in rats and both central and peripheral auditory systems participate in the generation of salicylate-induced tinnitus.

Editor: Manuel S. Malmierca, University of Salamanca- Institute for Neuroscience of Castille and Leon and Medical School, Spain

Funding: The authors have no support or funding to report.

Competing Interests: The authors have declared that no competing interests exist.

* Email: cuipc@fmmu.edu.cn

9 These authors contributed equally to this work.

Introduction

Tinnitus, a disorder experienced by a significant proportion of the general population [1,2], is a phantom auditory perception that cannot be attributed to any external sound. The subjective property of tinnitus makes the establishment of an appropriate animal model difficult. Among the medicines that can induce tinnitus in humans as a side-effect, salicylate, an active ingredient of aspirin, is the most prevalently used drug [3,4]. In establishing a salicylate-induced tinnitus rat model, the rats were conditioned to associate silence and sound respectively with danger and safety in licking water. When salicylate was administrated intraperitoneally (i.p.), a high lick ratio in the silence period would be produced and this high lick ratio is the manifestation of the subjective appearance of sound (tinnitus) [5,6,7,8,9,10].

With the prevalent use of the salicylate-induced tinnitus animal models, the process of tinnitus generation induced by salicylate

should be explored. Although much progress has been made in understanding the pathophysiological changes of salicylate-induced tinnitus, the mechanisms by which tinnitus is generated are incompletely understood and recent findings are inconsistent. Salicylate can penetrate the blood–brain barrier, thereby providing an opportunity to directly act on the central auditory system [11]. By superfusing central auditory nuclei slices, some studies have reported that salicylate can reduce inhibitory post-synaptic currents [12,13,14] and increase the spontaneous activity [15,16] and these findings are consistent to the results obtained from the systemic application of salicylate [17]. In addition to the in vitro effects salicylate exerts on the central auditory system, several studies have identified that the mechanisms underlying salicylate-induced tinnitus may also involve a peripheral component of the auditory system. The activation of N-methyl-D-aspartate (NMDA) receptors in the spiral ganglion neurons may play an essential role in salicylate-induced tinnitus. Behavioral evidence suggested that the local application of the NMDA antagonist MK-801 to the cochlea could strongly reduce tinnitus generation [7,18]. Salicylate may inhibit cochlear cyclooxygenase and enable cochlear NMDA receptors, thus leading to elevated activity in the central auditory system. This elevated activity in the central auditory system may be perceived as tinnitus [19]. Salicylate-induced changes in the gene expression in spiral ganglion neurons and in the auditory cortex were reversed by the local application of γ-aminobutyric acid receptor modulator to the cochlea [20]. Moreover, some studies have found that the rate of spontaneous discharge of auditory nerve fibers, a main indicator of the influence of salicylate, was increased after salicylate administration [21,22]. The findings of all these studies indicate that both central and peripheral auditory systems play a key role in the generation of salicylate-induced tinnitus.

Ablating a possible "tinnitus generator" along the auditory pathway is an important approach to investigating its role in tinnitus generation. Some previous researches have found that in guinea pigs central neuronal activities whose increase levels are correlated to tinnitus reduced immediately after ablation of ispilateral auditory nerve and would not increase before a latency period of at least 3 days [23,24], indicating that auditory nerve ablation could not produce tinnitus within 3 days after ablation.

This study was designed to establish a tinnitus rat model using a low dose of salicylate and to investigate whether central or peripheral auditory system is involved in salicylate-induced tinnitus by bilateral ablation of auditory nerves in vivo and behavior observation. To discuss the problems, a tinnitus model in conditioned rats was first established using a low dose of salicylate in Experiment One, and the practicability of the lick count and the lick latency, that is, the start time of licking water, during the first 30 s of the first trial was also examined as competent indicators to observe tinnitus performances. The bilateral auditory nerves of unconditioned rats were ablated, and the effect of the ablation itself on rats was observed in Experiment Two. Finally, the effect of salicylate on conditioned rats with bilateral auditory nerves ablation was studied in Experiment Three. We hypothesized that the central auditory system may be involved in salicylate-induced tinnitus because of the possible appearance of tinnitus evidences in the salicylate group compared with the saline group in the ablated rats and the peripheral auditory system may be also involved in salicylate-induced tinnitus because of the probably difficult appearance of tinnitus evidences in the ablated rats compared with the unablated rats in the salicylate groups.

Materials and Methods

Animals

Thirty-two male albino Sprague–Dawley rats (280 g to 500 g) were used. Each rat had free access to food but was water-restricted to ~90% of their pre-deprivation weight. The rats were individually housed on a 12 h/12 h dark/light schedule to maintain their normal biorhythms. The experimental protocol was approved by the Animal Care and Use Committee of the Four Military Medical University. Every effort was made to minimize the use and the discomfort of the rats.

Measurement of auditory brainstem response

Using a clinical auditory-evoked potential system (Madson Electronics, Copenhagen, Denmark), the threshold recordings of auditory brainstem response (ABR) to click and tone bursts were measured in a sound isolation room. The vertex, bilateral retroauricular areas and snout were depilated using 10% Na_2S (Sinopharm Chemical Reagent) under anesthesia [30 mg/kg body

weight (b. w.) sodium pentobarbital (Merck KGaA, Darmstadt, Germany), i.p.] before the measurement. Rats were fixed in the prone position. ABR signals were detected using three electrodes placed in the vertex, the retroauricular area and the snout respectively for the active electrode, reference electrode and ground electrode. Acoustic stimuli were delivered by a headphone 2 cm away from each ear hole and were averaged 256 times at the rate of 21.1/s. ABR signals were band-pass filtered (100 Hz to 3000 Hz) and were amplified (×10,000). ABR measurement was made in a 10-ms recording window. The threshold recordings of ABR to click and tone bursts started from 90 db sound pressure level (SPL) and 68 db SPL, respectively, and were 5 db SPL steps down to the threshold below which a repeated waveform III was not detected. Rats whose thresholds of click and tone bursts were both <20 db SPL (inclusion criteria) were used in this study.

Conditioning equipment

The operant behavioral system (AniLab Software and Instrument Company Limited, Ningbo, China) was used in the experiment (Fig. 1). The software of the system worked under a Windows operating system [25]. A metal spout of a water bottle was placed through a hole (1 cm diameter) in the wall of the conditioning chamber (0.29 m×0.29 m×0.26 m) and was connected to the anode of an electrical stimulator. The hole was 12 cm away from a stainless steel grid floor which was connected to the cathode of the electrical stimulator. Sound stimuli calibrated with a sound level meter (AR824; Smart Sensor, Hong Kong, China) were generated with the soundcard (SoundMAX) of a computer (Lenovo R60e; Beijing, China), and were delivered to a loudspeaker vertically mounted 10 cm above the hole inside the conditioning chamber. The sampling rate and the bit depth of the soundcard and the loudspeaker are 48 kHz and 16 bit, respectively. Whenever rats licked water, the behavioral system automatically recorded the licking responses and/or delivered a mouth shock (0.2 mA to 0.5 mA; duration, 1 s). The average amount of water delivered on an individual lick was 4 mg-5 mg.

All rats were trained and tested in the same conditioning chamber housed in a sound-attenuating box (0.6 m×0.5 m×0.6 m) lined with sound-absorbing foam. A top-

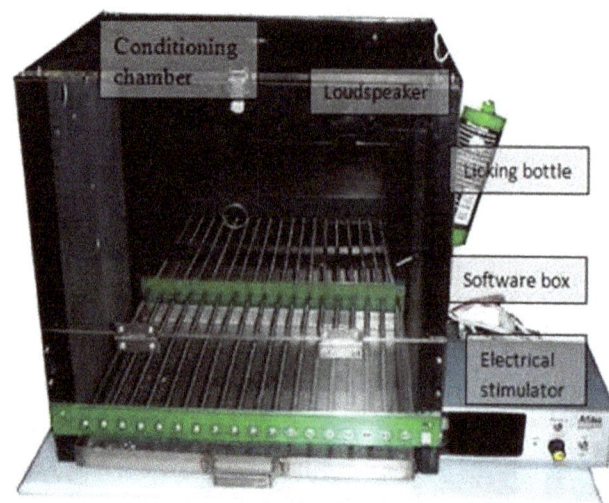

Figure 1. The operant behavioral system used in the study. It includes a conditioning chamber, a licking bottle, an electrical stimulator, and a behavioral software box. The loudspeaker is not shown in the picture.

mounted light was used to illuminate the inside of the box, and a USB camera next to the light sent pictures to the computer screen.

Behavioral protocol

The protocol was based on a classical lick suppression model [5] and was modified for the purpose of this study.

All rats were trained every day in a 15 min session, in which a pure tone (8 kHz, 50 db SPL) was turned off at the first 30 s of the 1st, 5th, 9th and 13th minute. The suspension of the pure tone was paired with a mouth shock whenever rats licked water in the silence period. The lick count recorded in the silence period was indicated by A, whereas the lick count in the subsequent 30 s (the sound period) was signified by B. The suppression ratio R = A/(A+ B) in the silence period was thus obtained. Each session was composed of the above four trials and produced 4 Rs. R between 0.4 and 0.6 indicated no difference in the licking responses between the silence and the sound periods, whereas R = 0 indicated the complete suppression of licking water in the silence period. Rats were considered to be conditioned if R<0.2. Before training, rats underwent an acclimation period of 2 days, in which the mouth shock was not used. The purpose of the acclimation was to make rats familiar with the new position of the licking water and to examine whether the pure tone itself had an effect on the licking responses. After acclimation, rats underwent a behavioral training period and then a test period, which lasted 7 and 4 days, respectively. The aim of the behavioral training was to condition the rats to distinguish sound from silence in an approach to associating the sound with licking water (high R in the sound period) and the silence with stopping licking (low R in the silence period). After training, R was not only a running index by which the extent of the behavioral training was obtained, but also an indicator to determine whether the rats had heard sound because high/low R can be explained only by more/less likelihood to hear sound. In the test period, rats in the salicylate group and saline group were injected respectively with 120 mg/kg salicylate (i.p.) and an equivalent volume of saline for 2 consecutive days and then were tested 2 h after injection. No mouth shock was applied in the test period.

Bilateral auditory nerves ablation

Rats were anesthetized (as described above). Subsequently, auditory nerves were bilaterally ablated, based on the methods described in previous studies [23,24]. The surgical procedure was applied under aseptic conditions and was carried out visually for ~1 h at 5× to 10× magnification of a dissecting microscope (Zhenjiang Xin Tian Medical Devices Company, Limited, Nanjing, China). An incision (1.5 cm) was made in the retro-auricular area, about 1 cm away from the bottom of the ear. The lateral wall of the bulla was exposed and opened. After puncturing the lateral cochlear wall at the basal turn of the modiolus near the internal auditory canal, the auditory nerve was ablated. The cochlea was packed with absorbable gelatin foam (Jinling Pharmaceutical Company, Limited, Nanjing, China) and the scalp incision was sutured. The auditory nerve on the other side was ablated in the same way. ABR measurement was immediately made after the ablation to ensure that the auditory nerves were fully ablated. Rats were injected with saline (i.p.) after the operation to restore its original body weight (7±0.6 mL) and were allowed 24 h to recover before the test period.

Experiment One: Effects of salicylate on conditioned rats

To establish a low dose salicylate-induced tinnitus model, fourteen rats underwent acclimation period and training period and ten of them were considered to be conditioned steadily after

the training period. They were randomly divided into the salicylate group and the saline group in the test period. The rats were injected respectively with 120 mg/kg salicylate (i.p.) and an equivalent volume of saline for 2 consecutive days and then were tested 2 h after injection for 4 consecutive days in the test period. The lick count and the lick latency during the first 30 s of the first trial and the average R of the four trials in each session were collected during the test period. The weight of water consumption was acquired by recording the increase of the body weight after the test period. In addition, ABR measurement was made after the test period in salicylate group.

Experiment Two: Effects of bilateral auditory nerves ablation on unconditioned rats

To observe the effects of bilateral auditory nerves ablation on the behaviors of rats, four rats undergoing acclimation period, training period (no mouth shock), ablation surgery, and test period were subjected to Experiment Two. One of them died of bleeding during the surgery. Rats were unconditioned in the training period because no mouth shock existed when rats licked water in the silence period. ABR measurement was made immediately after the ablation. Salicylate or saline was not applied in the test period. The lick count and the lick latency during the first 30 s of the first trial before ablation and for 2 consecutive days after ablation were recorded and compared.

Experiment Three: Effects of salicylate on conditioned rats with bilateral auditory nerves ablation

To determine the involvement of central auditory system in salicylate-induced tinnitus, sixteen rats underwent acclimation period, training period and ablation surgery. Six of them were excluded either because of unconditioned performance or die of bleeding or anesthesia during the surgery. Ten of them went through the experiment and were randomly divided into the salicylate group and the saline group in the test period after the ablation and ABR was measured. The rats were injected respectively with 120 mg/kg salicylate (i.p.) and an equivalent volume of saline 24 h after the surgery for 2 consecutive days and they were tested in the test period 2 h after injection. The lick count and the lick latency during the first 30 s of the first trial were detected for 2 consecutive days after ablation in the test period. To determine the involvement of peripheral auditory system in salicylate-induced tinnitus, the lick count and the lick latency between the ablated rats in the salicylate group in Experiment Three and the unablated rats in the salicylate group in Experiment One were compared.

Statistical analysis

SPSS 16.0 version was used in the study. Data were considered to be normal distribution and homogenous variances when $P>0.1$ in Shapiro-Wilk test and Levene's test. Suppression ratio (R) and the water consumption were compared using one-way ANOVA and these data are shown in mean ± standard error (SEM). The lick count and the lick latency were compared using Mann-Whitney U test and these data are shown in median ± quartile range (QR). $P<0.05$ was considered significant.

Results

Experiment One: Effects of salicylate on conditioned rats

As shown in Fig. 2, both the R values of the salicylate group and the saline group were between 0.4 and 0.6 in the acclimation period. R<0.2 was acquired in the training period. On each of the first 3 test days, the R in the salicylate group was significantly higher than that in the saline group [1st: $F(1, 8) = 20.59$, $P<0.01$; 2nd: $F(1, 8) = 35.84$, $P<0.01$; 3rd: $F(1, 8) = 5.69$, $P<0.05$], but no significant difference was found on the 4th test day [$F(1, 8) = 1.05$, $P>0.05$]. On each of the first 2 test days, the lick count and the lick latency during the first 30 s of the first trial in the salicylate group was significantly higher [1st: $T = 15$, $P<0.01$; 2nd: $T = 15$, $P<0.01$] (Fig. 3) and shorter [1st: $T = 15$, $P<0.01$; 2nd: $T = 16$, $P<0.01$] (Fig. 4) respectively than those in the saline group.

No statistically significant differences in the water consumption were found between the saline group and the salicylate group during the test period [1st: $F(1, 8) = 0.113$, $P = 0.745$; 2nd: $F(1, 8) = 0.056$, $P = 0.819$; 3rd: $F(1, 8) = 0.147$, $P = 0.711$; 4th: $F(1, 8) = 0.007$, $P = 0.936$] (Fig. 5). ABR thresholds to click and tone bursts did not change before and 2 h after the salicylate administration as shown in Table 1.

Experiment 2: Effects of bilateral auditory nerves ablation on unconditioned rats

ABR thresholds to click and tone bursts in the bilateral ears of all the rats under study were respectively more than 90 db SPL and 68 db SPL after the ablation as shown in Table 1. During the first 30 s of the first trial on each of the first 2 test days after the ablation, no significant changes compared with those before the ablation were observed in the lick count [1st: $T = 10$, $P = 0.827$; 2nd: $T = 7$, $P = 0.127$] (Fig. 6) and in the lick latency [1st: $T = 9$, $P = 0.513$; 2nd: $T = 10$, $P = 0.827$] (Fig. 7).

Experiment 3: Effects of salicylate on conditioned rats with bilateral auditory nerves ablation

ABR thresholds to click and tone bursts after the ablation were respectively more than 90 db SPL and 68 db SPL in Experiment Three as shown in Table 1. The lick count in the salicylate group during the first 30 s of the first trial was significantly higher than that in the saline group on the 2nd test day [$T = 18$, $P<0.05$]. No significant changes were found on the 1st test days [1st: $T = 21$, $P = 0.1$] (Fig. 6). The lick latency in the salicylate group during the first 30 s of the first trial was significantly shorter than that in the saline group on the first 2 test days [1st: $T = 18$, $P<0.05$; 2nd: $T = 17$, $P<0.05$] (Fig. 7). On the first 2 test days, no significant

changes were observed in the lick count during the first 30 s of the first trial in the saline groups between Experiment One and Experiment Three [1st: $T = 26$, $P = 0.7$; 2nd: $T = 23$, $P = 0.331$]. However, the lick count during the first 30 s of the first trial in the salicylate group in Experiment Three was almost significantly lower than that in the salicylate group in Experiment One [$T = 19$, $P = 0.07$] (Fig. 6) on the 1st test day. On the first 2 test days, no significant changes were found in the lick latency during the first 30 s of the first trial in the saline groups between Experiment One and Experiment Three [1st: $T = 25.5$, $P = 0.675$; 2nd: $T = 24$, $P = 0.465$]. However, on the 1st test day, the lick latency during the first 30 s of the first trial in the salicylate group in Experiment Three was significantly longer than that in the salicylate group in Experiment One [$T = 15$, $P<0.01$] (Fig. 7).

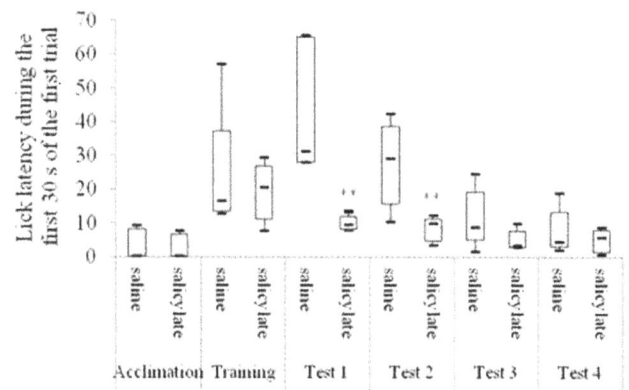

Figure 3. Lick count during the first 30 s of the first trials in different behavioral periods. "Acclimation" shows the average of the lick count of all rats in the saline or the salicylate group in the 2-day acclimation period; "Training" shows the average of the lick count of all rats in the saline or the salicylate group in the 7-day training period; Tests 1–4 show the 1st, 2nd, 3rd, and 4th day in the test period, respectively. **$P<0.01$ is compared with the saline group.

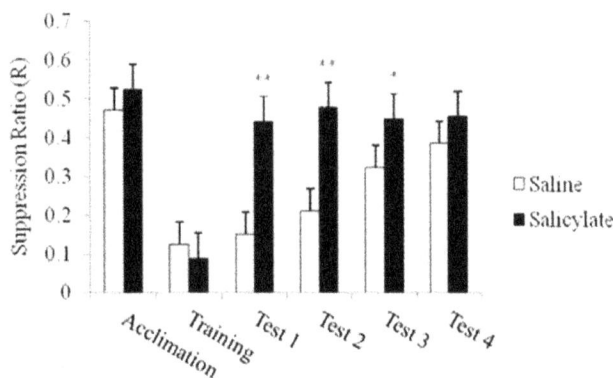

Figure 2. Changes of the suppression ratio (R) in different periods in the saline group and the salicylate group: "Acclimation" shows the average R of all rats in the saline or the salicylate group in the 2-day acclimation period; "Training" shows the average R of all rats in the saline or the salicylate group in the 7-day training period; Tests 1–4 show the 1st, 2nd, 3rd, and 4th day in the test period, respectively. Vertical bars represent mean ± standard error (SEM). **$P<0.01$ and *$P<0.05$ are compared with the saline group.

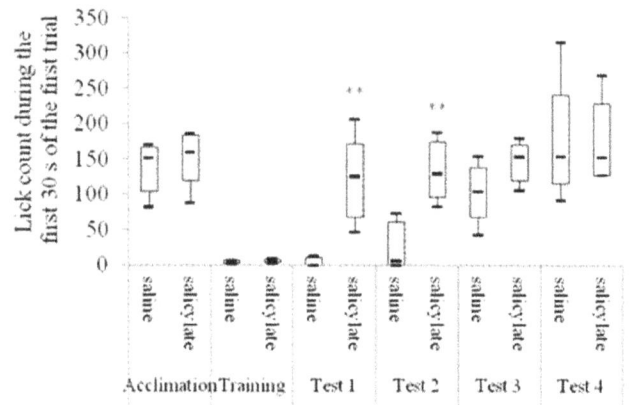

Figure 4. Lick latency (i.e. the start time of licking water) during the first 30 s of the first trials in different behavioral periods. "Acclimation" shows the average of the lick latency of all rats in the saline or the salicylate group in the 2-day acclimation period; "Training" shows the average of the lick latency of all rats in the saline or the salicylate group in the 7-day training period;. Tests 1–4 show the 1st, 2nd, 3rd, and 4th day in the test period, respectively. **$P<0.01$ is compared with the saline group.

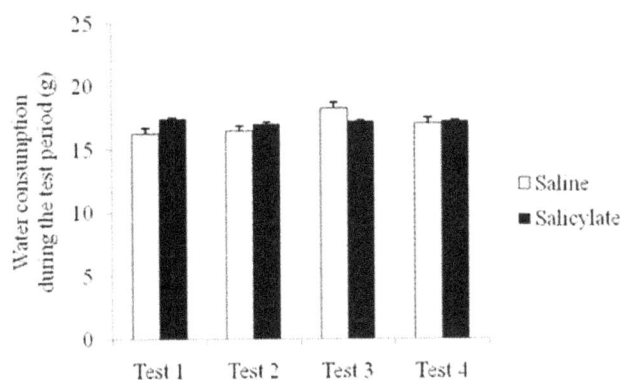

Figure 5. Water consumption during the 4 days in the test period. Tests 1–4 show the 1st, 2nd, 3rd, and 4th day, respectively. Vertical bars represent mean ± standard error (SEM).

Discussion

Experiment 1: Effects of salicylate administration on conditioned rats

In our study, we used 120 mg/kg salicylate to induce tinnitus in rats. The background sound had no effect on the licking responses in the acclimation period and a stable and qualified R value was produced in the training period. The significantly higher R values in salicylate group indicate that the rats have heard sound (tinnitus) in the silence period and the intensity of tinnitus may be similar to the background sound which was 50 db SPL. Studies have found that salicylate could induce hearing loss and thirst which may result in the high R in the salicylate group [8]. However, no change of the ABR thresholds after salicylate application was observed in our study, indicating no hearing loss existed in the rats of the salicyate group. In addition, no significant difference in the water consumption between the saline group and the salicylate group further shows that subjective sound (tinnitus) is responsible for the high R in the salicylate group. The significantly higher lick count and significantly shorter lick latency during the first 30 s of the first trial suggest that the two indicators could be used in observing salicylate-induced tinnitus.

Many studies have reported that tinnitus can be reliably induced by at least 150 mg/kg salicylate [5,6,7,8,9,26]. However, in our experiment we found that 120 mg/kg salicylate can also produce tinnitus in rats. Our finding is consistent with a previous study which found that the minimum dose of salicylate in tinnitus generation was between 75 mg/kg and 150 mg/kg and a 52 db SPL tone may be induced by 150 mg/kg salicylate [27].

Experiment 2: Effects of bilateral auditory nerves ablation on unconditioned rats

Auditory nerve ablation is a traumatic procedure for rats and may influence their behaviors. ABR measurement showed that the bilateral auditory nerves were completely ablated. No significant changes were found after the ablation in the lick count and the lick latency during the first 30 s of the first trial on the first 2 test days compared with those before the ablation, indicating that the ablation did not significantly affect the behavioral performance of the rats.

It was verified that the metabolic activity marker [14C] 2-deoxyglucose (2DG) was immediately reduced after the ipilateral auditory nerve ablation, and was increased at least 3 days after ablation. The spontaneous increase of metabolic activity was consistent with the findings seen after salicylate administration [24]. Therefore, they suggested that the increased activities may reflect a tinnitus-like phenomenon in guinea pigs. In order to get rid of the interference of the spontaneous increase activities in the auditory pathway after auditory nerve ablation in our study, we recorded and compared the data in 2 days after the ablation.

Experiment 3: Effects of salicylate on conditioned rats with bilateral auditory nerves ablation

In this experiment, the conditioned rats with bilateral auditory nerves ablation were afraid to lick water at the beginning of the test period but they would be consistent with licking when they started to lick water. This may be explained that there was no external alternative appearance of silence and sound and only silence period was left for the rats with bilateral auditory nerves ablation. Moreover, the rats were conditioned to associate silence with stopping licking water in the training period and no mouth shock existed in the following test period. Therefore, the conditioned rats with permanent hearing loss (similar with the permanent silence period) underwent long lick latency before they started to lick water in the test period and they would lick water continuously when they started to lick. This made their conditioned behavior washed out quickly. Therefore, the data collected from the first 30 s of the first trial was the most meaningful in this experiment and we compared them with those in Experiment One.

The R values in Experiment One were calculated from the lick count under the condition of normal hearing, while the R values after bilateral auditory nerves ablation in Experiment Two and Three were derived from the lick count under the condition of hearing loss. The findings that the lick count and the lick latency during the first 30 s of the first trial in the salicylate group were significantly higher and shorter respectively than those in the saline group in Experiment Three are similar to those in Experiment One. These results suggest that tinnitus can be induced in rats with bilateral auditory nerves ablation in the salicylate group and that a direct pharmacological effect of salicylate on central auditory structures which are unique for the generation of salicylate-induced tinnitus in ablated rats. It has been reported that salicylate may suppress GABAergic and inhibitory neurons and raise excitability in the central system and thus produce tinnitus in in vitro studies by salicylate perfusion of the pyramidal neurons and interneurons of auditory cortex [12,14]. In addition, salicylate perfusion can increase the spontaneous activities of inferior colliculus and the hyperexcitability may be related to tinnitus [15,16]. Our in vivo result is the first time to confirm the direct central effect of salicylate in tinnitus generation by behavioral evidences and is similar with these in vitro findings which all reported that the central auditory system may be involved in salicylate-induced tinnitus generation.

Given that the ablation itself had exerted no significant effect on the lick count and the lick latency, the significantly longer lick latency and nearly significant lower lick count in the salicylate group during the first 30 s of the first trial in Experiment Three compared with those in the salicylate group in Experiment One indicate that the peripheral auditory system promotes the generation of salicylate-induced tinnitus in normal hearing rats. It has been conformed that salicylate and mefenamate inhibited cochlear cyclooxygenase and increased levels of arachidonate which potentiated NMDA receptor currents. The increased currents were closely related to the occurrence of tinnitus according to the behavioral evidences of rats [17,19]. Local cochlear application of the GABA^{A} receptor modulator midazolam reduced the perception of salicylate-induced tinnitus in a

Table 1. Auditory brainstem response thresholds (db SPL) in different experimental conditions.

Animal number	Left ear						Right ear					
	Before experiment		After salicylate		After surgery		Before experiment		After salicylate		After surgery	
	click	tone	click	tone	click	tone	click	tone	click	tone	click	tone
1-1-1(V)	included©						included					
1-1-3(V)	included						included					
1-2-2(V)	included						included					
1-2-8(V)	included						included					
1-2-9(V)	included						included					
1-1-6(S)	5	5	5	5			5	5	5	5		
1-1-8(S)	10	5	10	5			10	5	10	5		
1-1-9(S)	15	5	15	5			10	5	10	5		
1-2-4(S)	5	5	5	5			5	5	5	5		
1-2-6(S)	10	5	10	5			10	5	10	5		
2-5-5(A)	included				>90	>68	included				>90	>68
2-5-6(A)	included				>90	>68	included				>90	>68
2-5-7(A)	included				>90	>68	included				>90	>68
3-1-2(VA)	10	5			>90	>68	10	5			>90	>68
3-1-5(VA)	included				>90	>68	included				>90	>68
3-2-1(VA)	10	5			>90	>68	10	5			>90	>68
3-2-2(VA)	included				>90	>68	included				>90	>68
3-2-5(VA)	included				>90	>68	included				>90	>68
3-1-0(SA)	10	5			>90	>68	10	5			>90	>68
3-2-0(SA)	included				>90	>68	included				>90	>68
3-2-4(SA)	5	5			>90	>68	5	5			>90	>68
3-3-3(SA)	included				>90	>68	included				>90	>68
3-5-1(SA)	included				>90	>68	included				>90	>68

In the column of animal number, the first number stands for Experiment One, Two, and Three, respectively. The last two numbers stand for the serial number of rats used in the study. The following letters "V", "S", "A", "VA", "SA" in the parentheses stand for the saline group, salicylate group, ablated group, saline+ablated group and salicylate+ablated group, respectively.
©The threshold of click and tone meet the inclusion criteria.

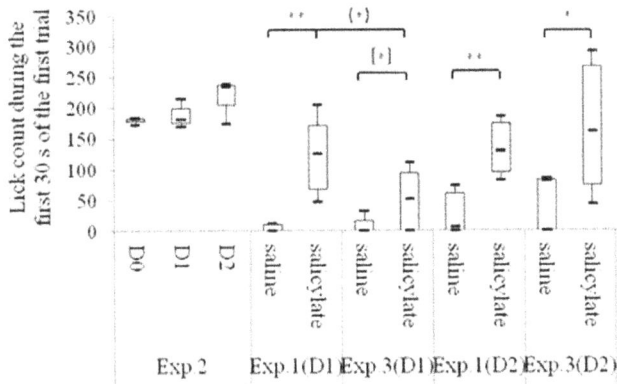

Figure 6. Lick count during the first 30 s of the first trials of Experiment 1, Experiment 2 and Experiment 3. D 0 to D 2 in Experiment 2 indicate the day before operation, the 1st day, and the 2nd day after operation, respectively. D 1 and D 2 in Experiment 1 and Experiment 3 indicate the 1st test day and the 2nd test day, respectively. (*) P = 0.07 for comparison of the salicylate groups between Experiment 1 and Experiment 3. [*] P = 0.1 for comparison between the salicylate group and the saline group in Experiment 3. **P<0.01. *P<0.05.

rat behavioral modal [20]. In addition, a recent study has found that an altered profile of input from the cochlea could determine the expanded cortical representation of the tinnitus induced by salicylate [28]. Our behavioral finding is supported by these previous reports which observed that salicylate may result in tinnitus by acting on the peripheral auditory system.

There are several limitations in this study. The first limitation is that bilateral auditory nerves ablation is a traumatic procedure for rats although no significant difference existed in lick performance after surgery compared with that before surgery. The second limitation is that the present study has no data concerning the perfusion of brain slices or local cochlear application to show the specific auditory structures of salicylate, although we showed that both the central and peripheral auditory systems are involved into the salicylate-induced tinnitus. The third limitation of the present study is that the number of specimens is not high enough for perfect statistical analyses, although the data showed that the lick

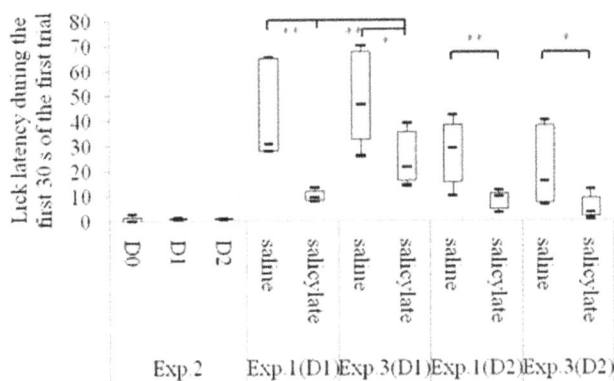

Figure 7. Lick latency (i.e. the start time of licking water) during the first 30 s of the first trials of Experiment 1, Experiment 2 and Experiment 3. D 0 to D 2 in Experiment 2 indicate the day before operation, the 1st day, and the 2nd day after operation, respectively. D 1 and D 2 in Experiment 1 and Experiment 3 indicate the 1st test day and the 2nd test day, respectively. **P<0.01. *P<0.05.

latency had significant difference and the similar tendency of lick account. Before our study, we refer to these previous studies in which the number of specimens was similar with us [9,10,26].

In conclusion, a tinnitus rat model using a low dose of salicylate (120 mg/kg) is established and the behavioral performances of rats with bilateral auditory nerves ablation show that both the central and peripheral auditory systems participate in salicylate-induced tinnitus. Further studies should be conducted to investigate the specific central auditory structures involved in salicylate-induced tinnitus generation.

Supporting Information

File S1 Figure S1. Auditory brainstem response (ABR) recording of No. 16 rat after salicylate injection in salicylate group in Experiment One. "L" stands for left ear; "R" stands for right ear; "I" stands for intensity of click or tone; "8K" stands for the frequency of tone is 8000 Hz; "[a. b]": "a" represents the chronological number of the test and "b" refers to the channel number collected. Figure S2. Auditory brainstem response (ABR) recording of No. 18 rat after salicylate injection in salicylate group in Experiment One. Figure S3. Auditory brainstem response (ABR) recording of No. 19 rat after salicylate injection in salicylate group in Experiment One. Figure S4. Auditory brainstem response (ABR) recording of No. 24 rat after salicylate injection in salicylate group in Experiment One. Figure S5. Auditory brainstem response (ABR) recording of No. 26 rat after salicylate injection in salicylate group in Experiment One. Figure S6. Auditory brainstem response (ABR) recording of No. 16 rat before experiment in salicylate group in Experiment One. Figure S7. Auditory brainstem response (ABR) recording of No. 18 rat before experiment in salicylate group in Experiment One. Figure S8. Auditory brainstem response (ABR) recording of No. 19 rat before experiment in salicylate group in Experiment One. Figure S9. Auditory brainstem response (ABR) recording of No. 24 rat before experiment in salicylate group in Experiment One. Figure S10. Auditory brainstem response (ABR) recording of No. 26 rat before experiment in salicylate group in Experiment One. Figure S11. Auditory brainstem response (ABR) recording of No. 11 rat in saline group in Experiment One. Figure S12. Auditory brainstem response (ABR) recording of No. 13 rat in saline group in Experiment One. Figure S13. Auditory brainstem response (ABR) recording of No. 22 rat in saline group in Experiment One. Figure S14. Auditory brainstem response (ABR) recording of No. 28 rat in saline group in Experiment One. Figure S15. Auditory brainstem response (ABR) recording of No. 29 rat in saline group in Experiment One.

File S2 Figure S1. Auditory brainstem response (ABR) recording of No. 55 rat after surgery in Experiment Two. Figure S2. Auditory brainstem response (ABR) recording of No. 56 rat after surgery in Experiment Two. Figure S3. Auditory brainstem response (ABR) recording of No. 57 rat after surgery in Experiment Two. Figure S4. Auditory brainstem response (ABR) recording of No. 55 rat before experiment in Experiment Two. Figure S5. Auditory brainstem response (ABR) recording of No. 56 rat before experiment in Experiment Two. Figure S6. Auditory brainstem response (ABR) recording of No. 57 rat before experiment in Experiment Two.

File S3 Figure S1. Auditory brainstem response (ABR) recording of No. 10 rat after surgery in salicylate group in Experiment Three. Figure S2. Auditory brainstem response (ABR) recording of

No. 20 rat after surgery in salicylate group in Experiment Three. Figure S3. Auditory brainstem response (ABR) recording of No. 24 rat after surgery in salicylate group in Experiment Three. Figure S4. Auditory brainstem response (ABR) recording of No. 33 rat after surgery in salicylate group in Experiment Three. Figure S5. Auditory brainstem response (ABR) recording of No. 51 rat after surgery in salicylate group in Experiment Three. Figure S6. Auditory brainstem response (ABR) recording of No. 10 rat before experiment in salicylate group in Experiment Three. Figure S7. Auditory brainstem response (ABR) recording of No. 20 rat before experiment in salicylate group in Experiment Three. Figure S8. Auditory brainstem response (ABR) recording of No. 24 rat before experiment in salicylate group in Experiment Three. Figure S9. Auditory brainstem response (ABR) recording of No. 33 rat before experiment in salicylate group in Experiment Three. Figure S10. Auditory brainstem response (ABR) recording of No. 51 rat before experiment in salicylate group in Experiment Three. Figure S11. Auditory brainstem response (ABR) recording of No. 12 rat after surgery in saline group in Experiment Three. Figure S12. Auditory brainstem response (ABR) recording of No. 15 rat after surgery in saline group in Experiment Three. Figure S13. Auditory brainstem response (ABR) recording of No. 21 rat after surgery in saline group in Experiment Three. Figure S14. Auditory brainstem response (ABR) recording of No. 22 rat after surgery in saline group in Experiment Three. Figure S15. Auditory brainstem response (ABR) recording of No. 25 rat after surgery in saline group in Experiment Three.

Figure S16. Auditory brainstem response (ABR) recording of No. 12 rat before experiment in saline group in Experiment Three. Figure S17. Auditory brainstem response (ABR) recording of No. 15 rat before experiment in saline group in Experiment Three. Figure S18. Auditory brainstem response (ABR) recording of No. 21 rat before experiment in saline group in Experiment Three. Figure S19. Auditory brainstem response (ABR) recording of No. 22 rat before experiment in saline group in Experiment Three. Figure S20. Auditory brainstem response (ABR) recording of No. 25 rat before experiment in saline group in Experiment Three.

Data S1 Raw data of suppression ratio (R), water consumption, lick count and lick latency of Experiment One, Experiment Two and Experiment Three.
(XLSX)

Acknowledgments

We are grateful to Mrs. Juan Sun and Mr. Xiaocheng Wang for their technical assistance.

Author Contributions

Conceived and designed the experiments: GC LF PC. Performed the experiments: GC. Analyzed the data: GC. Contributed reagents/materials/analysis tools: ZL YS HC. Wrote the paper: GC.

References

1. Axelsson A, Ringdahl A (1989) Tinnitus–a study of its prevalence and characteristics. Br J Audiol 23: 53–62.
2. Henry JA, Dennis KC, Schechter MA (2005) General review of tinnitus: prevalence, mechanisms, effects, and management. J Speech Lang Hear Res 48: 1204–1235.
3. Day RO, Graham GG, Bieri D, Brown M, Cairns D, et al. (1989) Concentration-response relationships for salicylate-induced ototoxicity in normal volunteers. Br J Clin Pharmacol 28: 695–702.
4. Halla JT, Atchison SL, Hardin JG (1991) Symptomatic salicylate ototoxicity: a useful indicator of serum salicylate concentration? Ann Rheum Dis 50: 682–684.
5. Jastreboff PJ, Brennan JF, Coleman JK, Sasaki CT (1988) Phantom auditory sensation in rats: an animal model for tinnitus. Behav Neurosci 102: 811–822.
6. Bauer CA, Brozoski TJ, Rojas R, Boley J, Wyder M (1999) Behavioral model of chronic tinnitus in rats. Otolaryngol Head Neck Surg 121: 457–462.
7. Guitton MJ, Caston J, Ruel J, Johnson RM, Pujol R, et al. (2003) Salicylate induces tinnitus through activation of cochlear NMDA receptors. J Neurosci 23: 3944–3952.
8. Ruttiger L, Ciuffani J, Zenner HP, Knipper M (2003) A behavioral paradigm to judge acute sodium salicylate-induced sound experience in rats: a new approach for an animal model on tinnitus. Hear Res 180: 39–50.
9. Lobarinas E, Sun W, Cushing R, Salvi R (2004) A novel behavioral paradigm for assessing tinnitus using schedule-induced polydipsia avoidance conditioning (SIP-AC). Hear Res 190: 109–114.
10. Turner JG, Brozoski TJ, Bauer CA, Parrish JL, Myers K, et al. (2006) Gap detection deficits in rats with tinnitus: a potential novel screening tool. Behav Neurosci 120: 188–195.
11. Jastreboff PJ, Hansen R, Sasaki PG, Sasaki CT (1986) Differential uptake of salicylate in serum, cerebrospinal fluid, and perilymph. Arch Otolaryngol Head Neck Surg 112: 1050–1053.
12. Wang HT, Luo B, Zhou KQ, Xu TL, Chen L (2006) Sodium salicylate reduces inhibitory postsynaptic currents in neurons of rat auditory cortex. Hear Res 215: 77–83.
13. Wang HT, Luo B, Huang YN, Zhou KQ, Chen L (2008) Sodium salicylate suppresses serotonin-induced enhancement of GABAergic spontaneous inhibitory postsynaptic currents in rat inferior colliculus in vitro. Hear Res 236: 42–51.
14. Su YY, Luo B, Wang HT, Chen L (2009) Differential effects of sodium salicylate on current-evoked firing of pyramidal neurons and fast-spiking interneurons in slices of rat auditory cortex. Hear Res 253: 60–66.
15. Basta D, Ernst A (2004) Effects of salicylate on spontaneous activity in inferior colliculus brain slices. Neurosci Res 50: 237–243.
16. Basta D, Goetze R, Ernst A (2008) Effects of salicylate application on the spontaneous activity in brain slices of the mouse cochlear nucleus, medial geniculate body and primary auditory cortex. Hear Res 240: 42–51.
17. Sun W, Lu J, Stolzberg D, Gray L, Deng A, et al. (2009) Salicylate increases the gain of the central auditory system. Neuroscience 159: 325–334.
18. Peng BG, Chen S, Lin X (2003) Aspirin selectively augmented N-methyl-D-aspartate types of glutamate responses in cultured spiral ganglion neurons of mice. Neurosci Lett 343: 21–24.
19. Ruel J, Chabbert C, Nouvian R, Bendris R, Eybalin M, et al. (2008) Salicylate enables cochlear arachidonic-acid-sensitive NMDA receptor responses. J Neurosci 28: 7313–7323.
20. Panford-Walsh R, Singer W, Ruttiger L, Hadjab S, Tan J, et al. (2008) Midazolam reverses salicylate-induced changes in brain-derived neurotrophic factor and arg3.1 expression: implications for tinnitus perception and auditory plasticity. Mol Pharmacol 74: 595–604.
21. Evans EF, Borerwe TA (1982) Ototoxic effects of salicylates on the responses of single cochlear nerve fibres and on cochlear potentials. Br J Audiol 16: 101–108.
22. Kumagai M (1992) [Effect of intravenous injection of aspirin on the cochlea]. Hokkaido Igaku Zasshi 67: 216–233.
23. Sasaki CT, Babitz L, Kauer JS (1981) Tinnitus: development of a neurophysiologic correlate. Laryngoscope 91: 2018–2024.
24. Kauer JS, Nemitz JW, Sasaki CT (1982) Tinnitus aurium: fact... or fancy. Laryngoscope 92: 1401–1407.
25. Zhang F (2006) SuperState: a computer program for the control of operant behavioral experimentation. J Neurosci Methods 155: 194–201.
26. Lobarinas E, Sun W, Stolzberg D, Lu J, Salvi R (2008) Human Brain Imaging of Tinnitus and Animal Models. Semin Hear 29: 333–349.
27. Jastreboff PJ, Brennan JF (1994) Evaluating the loudness of phantom auditory perception (tinnitus) in rats. Audiology 33: 202–217.
28. Stolzberg D, Chen GD, Allman BL, Salvi RJ (2011) Salicylate-induced peripheral auditory changes and tonotopic reorganization of auditory cortex. Neuroscience 180: 157–164.

21

Carina® and Esteem®: A Systematic Review of Fully Implantable Hearing Devices

Janaina Oliveira Bentivi Pulcherio[1], Aline Gomes Bittencourt[2]*, Patrick Rademaker Burke[2], Rafael da Costa Monsanto[3], Rubens de Brito[2], Robinson Koji Tsuji[2], Ricardo Ferreira Bento[2]

1 Department of Otolaryngology, Hospital Central da Polícia Militar, Rio de Janeiro, Brazil, **2** Department of Otolaryngology, University of São Paulo School of Medicine, São Paulo, Brazil, **3** Department of Otolaryngology, Banco de Olhos de Sorocaba Hospital, São Paulo, Brazil

Abstract

Objective: To review the outcomes of the fully implantable middle ear devices Carina and Esteem regarding the treatment of hearing loss.

Data Sources: PubMed, Embase, Scielo, and Cochrane Library databases were searched.

Study Selection: Abstracts of 77 citations were screened, and 43 articles were selected for full review. From those, 22 studies and two literature reviews in English directly demonstrating the results of Carina and Esteem were included.

Data Extraction: There were a total of 244 patients ranging from 18 to 88 years. One hundred and 10 patients were implanted with Carina and with 134 Esteem. There were registered 92 males and 67 females. Five studies provided no information about patients' age or gender. From the data available, the follow-up ranged from 2 to 29.4 months.

Data Synthesis: The comparison of the results about word recognition is difficult as there was no standardization of measurement. The results were obtained from various sound intensities and different frequencies. The outcomes comparing to conventional HAs were conflicting. Nevertheless, all results comparing to unaided condition showed improvement and showed a subjective improvement of quality of life.

Conclusion: There are still some problems to be solved, mainly related to device functioning and price. Due to the relatively few publications available and small sample sizes, we must be careful in extrapolating these results to a broader population. Additionally, none of all these studies represented level high levels of evidence (i.e. randomized controlled trials).

Editor: Yeur-Hur Lai, College of Medicine, Taiwan

Funding: The authors have no support or funding to report.

Competing Interests: The authors have declared that no competing interests exist.

* Email: alinebittencourt@hotmail.com

Introduction

Hearing aids (HAs) are external listening devices that provide amplification and are traditionally used to treat hearing loss. Nevertheless, conventional HAs can lead to technical problems like feedback, requirement of regular maintenance, insufficient high-frequency gain for individuals with "ski-slope" hearing loss, inability to participate in water activities, sound distortion, effect of the ambient noise reaching the microphones and occlusion effect [1–5]. Clinical conditions like skin problems, malformation of the external ear and otitis can also limit their use [1,2,4,5]. In addition, social factors (social stigma and cosmetic issues) may be mentioned [1,3,4].

The implantable devices are alternatives developed to promote greater comfort to patients with hearing loss bypassing the limitations of sound transmission through the external auditory meatus while keeping an external microphone, as it resides completely underneath the skin behind the ear.

The field of fully implantable middle ear devices (MEDs) is promising. Few studies are now available and they lack high level of evidence. This review aims to analyze the indications, the pre-operative assessment and mainly the effectiveness of the Carina system (Otologics LLC of Boulder, Colorado, USA) and the Esteem device (Envoy Medical Corporation, USA).

Materials and Methods

A literature search was performed regarding the fully implantable hearing devices Carina and Esteem on July, 2014, using Pubmed, Embase, Scielo and Cochrane databases. The keywords used were "carina" AND "ear", "esteem" AND "ear", "fully implantable hearing aid", "esteem" AND "Envoy". Additional filters were used: English language, human subjects; the period of publication was set to 2000–2014. Duplicates were excluded at this point. The abstract of all the resulting studies were read, and after removing studies that did not comply with the inclusion/exclusion criteria, the remaining studies were read in full.

The criteria for study selection were as follows:

a) Inclusion criteria:

– Case reports, prospective and retrospective studies referring to the outcomes of CARINA and ESTEEM implants.

b) Exclusion criteria:

– Studies that did not review the results after the implantation of the device.

The results obtained in the different studies selected for appraisal were then gathered.

A flowchart of the decision process involved into the studies selection can be viewed below (Figure 1).

Results

The search resulted on 77 citations. Titles and abstracts of 43 papers were screened as potentially relevant articles and selected for full review. Twenty-two original articles and two literature reviews met the study's eligibility criteria and were included in this review.

There were a total of 244 patients ranging from 18 to 88 years. One hundred and 10 patients were implanted with Carina and 134 with Esteem. There were registered 92 males and 67 females. Five studies provided no information about patients' age or gender. From the data available, the follow-up ranged from 2 to 29.4 months (Table 1).

1. History

The use of MEDs for treatment of hearing loss became part of the clinical practice in Europe and United States. The Vibrant Soundbridge (Med-El Corporation, Innsbruck, Austria), which has an external auditory processor, was the first device routinely used in the last 90's [6,7]. The first fully implantable MEDs was developed in 1999 by Implex GmbH from Germany, but was withdrawn from the market because of technical and economic problems [3].

Two fully implantable MEDs are currently available for use: the Esteem used in Europe and in the United States and the fourth generation of the Carina, approved for use in all European Community countries and on phase II efficacy studies for the Food and Drug Administration (FDA) approval.

2. Mechanisms

The mechanism of MEDs is correct hearing loss by stimulating the ossicular chain or the round window directly [6–10]. The Esteem is the first totally implanted MEDs based on piezoelectric technology. It consists of a titanium dual-channel sound processor housed in a temporal bone niche, a nonrechargeable battery and 2 piezoelectric transducers (a "sensor" and a "driver"). The "sensor" is placed on the body of the incus where it can detect tympanic membrane vibration, converts it to electrical signal and sends it to the sound processor. The sound processor, on the other hand, amplifiers, filters, and sends the stimulus to the piezoelectric transducers (the "driver") that modifies the electrical sign back to mechanical energy and causes vibration to the stapes. Therefore, the device is microphone free and the sound is received directly by the eardrum/ossicular chain [4,11,12].

Piezoelectric crystals are more efficient than electromagnets, once the power consumption is reduced because there is no need

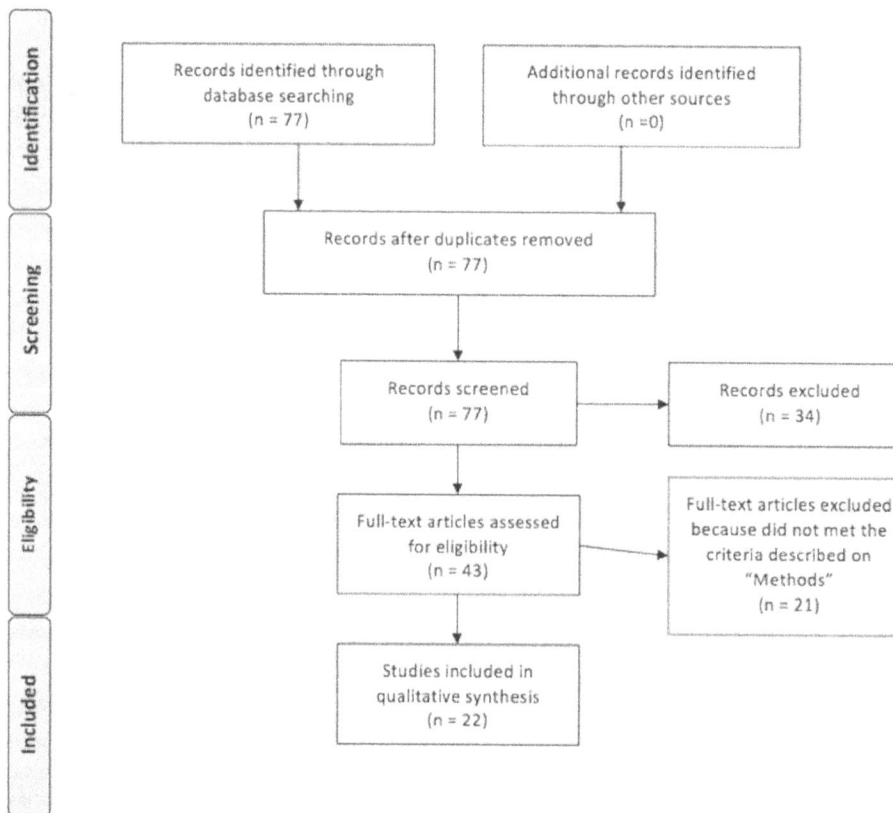

Figure 1. Decision process of the selection of the studies included in this review. Adapted from: Moher D, Liberati A, Tetzlaff J, Altman DG, The PRISMA Group (2009). Preferred Reporting Items for Systematic Reviews and Meta-Analyses: The PRISMA Statement. PLoS Med 6(6): e1000098.

Table 1. Demographic characteristics of the studies.

Study	Year	Patients (n)	MED	Gender	Mean Age	Side	Mean Follow-up (mths)
Barbara et al.	2009	6	Esteem	NR	NR	NR	NR
Barbara et al.	2011	18	Esteem	NR	NR	NR	NR
Bruschini et al.	2009 and 2010	8	Carina	7 M, 1F	46.6	6R, 2L	16.9
Chen et al.	2004	7	Esteem	2F, 5 M	64.4	4R, 3L	10
Deveze et al.	2010	1	Carina	1F	63	1R	6
Gerard et al.	2012	13	Esteem	9F, 4 M	NR	9R, 4L	4
Jenkins et al.	2007 and 2008	20	Carina	10F, 10 M	62.8	9R, 11L	2
Kam et al.	2012	6	Carina	3F, 3 M	48.5	4R, 2L	12
Kraus et al.	2011	57	Esteem	19F, 38 M	52.9	35R, 22L	12
Lachowska et al.	2012	1	Carina	1F	18	1R, 1L	9
Lefebvre et al.	2009	6	Carina	NR	NR	NR	12
Martin et al.	2009	11	Carina	7F, 4 M	50.8	5R, 6L	24
Memari et al.	2011	10	Esteem	7 M, 3F	32.7	6L, 4R	29.4
Monini et al.	2013	15	Esteem	8F, 7 M	NR	NR	NR
Murali	2009	3	Esteem	2 M, 1F	28,6	2R, 1L	NR
Shohet	2011	5	Esteem	NR	NR	NR	12
Siegert	2007	5	Carina	4 M, 1F	31,4	NR	3
Tringali et al.	2008	1	Carina	1 M	14	1R	2
Tringali et al.	2009	1	Carina	1F	48	1R	15
Zenner and Rodriguez	2010	50	Carina	NR	NR	NR	NR

n – number; MED – middle ear device; mths – months; M – male; F – female; NR – not reported.

to create a magnetic field[1]. Consequently the lithium battery life is now compatible with total implantability [1]. The expected battery life is 4.5 years with continuous use (24 hours per day/7 days per week) to 9 years (if only used for 8 hours per day) [3,11–14]. The battery changing may be performed as a surgical procedure under local anesthesia [1,13].

To prevent feedback phenomenon from the device, implantation requires separation of the incustapedial joint and resection of a segment (about 2 millimeters) of the long process of the incus [1,14]. Some studies have demonstrated that the Esteem device may provide effective bandwidth output that exceeds 8 kHz [15]. Low distortion permits increasing acoustic gain (can reach up to + 55 dB) without compromising audibility [11,14]. An open ear canal eliminates the occlusion effect [4]. Natural directionality and auricular filtering (at high frequencies) are preserved [13].

The Carina system is the successor of the semi-implantable MET (*Middle Ear Transducer*) system [3,8]. It consists on a microphone, battery, magnet, digital signal processor, transducer and a connector. Sounds are captured by the microphone and relayed to the sound processor within the implant capsule. The sound processor analyses the sound information, amplifies it according to the programmed settings, and converts it into electrical signals that are relayed to the transducer attached to the incus. This transducer translates electrical signals into a mechanic motion that directly stimulates the ossicular chain or the round window. Ossicles are not disarticulated [3,9,13,16–18].

The battery is charged by a coil placed on the skin over the implant, using a belt or waistband. It may be performed daily during 1 to 1.5 hours and each charge lasts 32 hours [3,10,16,17]. As stated by the manufacturer, the battery lifetime is at least 10 years, after which the entire electronic capsule must be surgically removed for replacement. The middle ear transducer is not removed.

3. Implantation technique
3.1. Carina system. The usual Carina system implantation is performed through a post-auricular incision with a posterior small atticotomy (about 2 cm wide) [18] to expose the body of the incus and the head of the malleus. The arm of the mounting bracket of the device can be modified to place the device on the incus and is fitted to the mastoid cortex using bone screws. Bone beds for the device and the microphone must be drilled so that the electronics capsule and the microphone can be positioned and secured [9,19].

There are 3 convenient microphone placement locations: anterior and superior to the external auditory canal (temporalis region), posterior to the external auditory canal (retro-auricular region), and on the mastoid tip. It is noteworthy that the microphone is very sensitive to changes in the tissue thickness over time, resulting in feedback. Thus, it may be placed in a region of minimal tissue thickening changes during head and neck movements, which is not the case of the mastoid tip. It is also necessary to avoid the contraction effects of the sternocleidomastoid muscle [19]. Moreover, there is no consensus regarding the optimal placement of the microphone [9].

The tip of the transducer is advanced into the hole on the incus and the positioning is evaluated using software specifically developed by Otologics (Transducer Loading Assistant) to ensure correct placement of the device [17].

The tip of Carinas transducer can be crimped to different tips such as stapes head, stapes superstructure, stapes footplate or round window [9]. The round window may be used in patients for whom multiple ossiculoplasty procedures have been unsuccessful and particularly when the stapes footplate is fixed or no longer

accessible [9,17]. This transducer tip can also be extended by applying a small titanium ball and placed on the body of the incus [9].

The implantation of Carina to stimulate the round window is performed through a post-auricular incision with a posterior tympanotomy to expose the round window niche. The round window membrane movement is checked by the mobilization of the stapes or the long process of the incus. The transducer is placed on the round window with or without placement of the incus. The tip of transducer is adapted by clipping modified total ossicular replacement prosthesis (TORP) to the end of the transducer or can be put in contact with the staples footplate or even coupled to a stapedotomy piston. The other end of the TORP is placed on a fascia graft protecting the round window membrane. This surgical technique allows the implantation of device despite of a nonfunctioning ossicular chain and an abnormal middle ear anatomy as long as round window membrane is present to receive the tip of the transducer [6,9].

3.2. Esteem Device. The ear with the poorest functional hearing is selected for implantation. If both ears are equal in performance, the candidate can choose the side to be implanted. The procedure is performed under general anesthesia [1].

A post-auricular incision is made and a bone recess is fashioned posterior to the mastoid to house the sound processor. A tympanomastoidectomy is performed widely exposing the facial recess to accommodate the driver. The chorda tympani nerve is sacrificed in about 60% of the cases [13.14]. The intact ossicular motion can be measured using a laser doppler vibrometer. The incus and stapes are disarticulated and the distal 1 to 3 mm of the long process of the incus is gently removed using either malleus nipper or a cutting laser to prevent a mechanic feedback. Transducers are contained in the mastoid cavity with hydroxyapatite cement so their piezoelectric crystals are positioned. The sensor is interfaced with the incus using glass ionomeric cement and the driver is cemented to the stapes [1,13].

In a study to detect the site of maximum ossicular motion that would be optimal for attachment of the sensor portion of the protesis, Chung et al. [2] used a laser doppler vibrometer to measure the vibrational responses at 7 locations on the middle ear ossicles. They observed that maximum vibrational motion of the middle ear is deliverable to the piezoelectric transducer of Esteem through the superior part of the malleus head, on the lateral part of the incus body, and on the superior part of the incus body near the incudomalleal joint.

After implant placement, the entire system is tested and postoperative functional gain is estimated. If gain is deemed inadequate, the implant is repositioned to improve performance.

Both devices, Carina and Esteem are turned on in about 6 to 8 weeks after implantation [6,11,14,19–21]. There is an implant programming called "commander" that is used by audiologist for follow-up to program each patient's device. The patient himself can also modify the filtering of background noise levels, adjust volume, and place the device on stand-by mode using a remote control component called "personal programmer" [1,22,23].

4. Indications
The fully implantable hearing devices are indicated mainly as an alternative treatment for moderate to severe hearing loss in patients with normal and abnormal middle ears who either do not benefit from conventional HAs or choose not to wear them [1,4,5,10,13]. Patients with low tegmen mastoideum or tympani, anteriorly displaced sigmoid sinus, small facial recess, or laterally displaced facial nerve are not candidates [13,14,19,20].

Recently, Carinas indications has been extended to patients with ossicular defects in whom conventional ossiculoplasty itself would not restore sufficient hearing function. The Carina device can be deployed in several places permitting the contact with the ossicular chain. Round window implantation is also a possibility and bypasses the normal conductive pathway to the cochlea and apart from the condition of ossicular chain or external ears such as congenital auricular atresia [7,8,9,22].

5. Outcomes

The advantages of fully implantable HAs led to greater patient satisfaction. The good performance of them is due to several factors as absence of occlusion effect or feedback, cosmetic advantage, and the possibility of use the device every day [11]. These factors were considered although some of the performance outcome measures with the Carina were lower than those pre-operatively with HAs in the study of Bruschini et al. [17].

Listening to body sounds (muscle movement, heartbeat, breathing, hair noise, local stimulating noise) was not a complaint of 13 patients implanted with Esteem studied by Gerard et al. [14] but was related by the patient bilaterally implanted with Carina by Lachowska et al. [16] and was cited by Martin et al. [9].

The Hearing in Noise Test (HINT) is a more reliable test for the evaluation of daily conditions. The ability to understand in quiet was 88% and in noise was 62% for the 7 patients implanted with Esteem studied by Chen et al. [1] Shohet et al. [15] reported improvement in 4 of 5 patients over HAs. None of these two studies showed statistical significance. The HINT for the 57 patients (also implanted with Esteem) studied by Kraus et al. [13] was not worse than in quit conditions. For the Carina device, Jenkins et al. [19] reported a deterioration of HINT after 6 months of implantation but had dramatically improved after refitting and remained better than the patients' own hearing aid until 1-year follow up.

The Esteem Questionnaire was designed by St. Croix Medical to evaluate subjective questions specifically about the Esteem device. Kraus et al. [13] used this tool to assess the quality of life of 57 patients at 12 months. The majority of subjects considered their device to be equal to or much better than their own HA in all subcales (clarity of sound, speech in noise, natural voices, understanding conversation, self-confidence and active lifestyle).

The Client oriented scale improvement (COSI) questionnaire is used to document a patient's goals/needs and to measure improvements in hearing ability [4,11]. Before the application of this test, every patient selects 5 major listening situations that he/she would like to improve and assign a maximum score of 5 for each situation. Monini et al. [4] applied this test to the 2 groups of their study 3 months after implantation. In the goup A (moderate to severe SNHL) the mean COSI final score was 13.5 for conventional HA and 22.7 for the Esteem (p = 0.00001). In the group B (severe to profound SNHL) there was no statistical significance (p = 0.270) for the benefit. The mean COSI scores in the study of Barbara et al. [11] changed from 17.7 (in itinere) to 20.6 (final score) for moderate SNHL and from 18.1 (in itinere) to 18.2 (final score) for severe SNHL.

The Glasgow Benefit Inventory (GBI) is an 18-item questionnaire, with scores ranging from −100 to +100, developed especially to measure patients' benefit after otorhinolaryngological interventions [11]. This test was used in Barbara et al. [11] study and showed only a slightly better score in the moderate hearing loss population.

5.1. Fully implantable devices compared with hearing aids. Chen et al. [1] reported that the functional gain for the Esteem implanted in was similar to HAs at 0.5, 1, 2 and 3 KHz

and this gain decreased at 3 kHz. Monini et al. [4] found that a mean gain difference of 13 dB favorable to the Esteem device, compared to HAs in both groups moderate-to-severe and severe-to-profound sensorineural hearing loss (SNHL), but with no statistical significance. Otherwise, Memari et al. [20] (n = 10) showed that average gain in 5 frequencies ranged from no gain in 1 patient to 20 dB in another 1. Barbara et al. [11] referred improvement from 70 dB to 48 dB in the whole sample. Shohet et al. [15] reported a functional gain of 22 dB with this same device.

In the study by Lefebvre et al. [6], the 6 patients who underwent implantation of Carina transducing sound via the round window showed essentially the same thresholds for frequencies above 3 kHz comparing to conventional HAs.

The average functional gain at 500, 1 k and 2 k Hz was found to be 35.6 dB and 35.0 dB in 6 patients with Carina and the conventional HA, respectively, revealing an insignificant difference according to Kam et al. [22] Gain on frequencies above 3 kHz is generally limited but residual hearing at such frequencies can still be maintained or slightly improved [14].

Zenner and Rodriguez [24] (n = 50) reported that the average functional gain varied by frequency between 25 and 30 dB for audiometric test frequencies of 5 and 6 KHz.

The word recognition (WR) improvement for Esteem comparing to conventional HA's varied among the studies. While Chen et al. [1] found an index of improvement with Esteem of 17% compared to HAs, Kraus et al. [13] found that 62% of their subjects (n = 52) had improvement, 27% were the same, and 11% were worse. Neither studies presented information of statistical significance. Monini et al. [4], showed that WR raised to 55% with conventional HA and to 66% with the Esteem in the group with moderate-to-severe SNHL. In the group with severe-to-profound SNHL the improvement was to 46% with conventional HA and to 57% with the Esteem. However the difference was not statistically significant. Carina results in WR were conflicting in all articles studied. Zenner and Rodriguez [24] (n = 50) reported that a significant improvement, up to 82% correct, in speech discrimination scores was obtained. The case report of Deveze et al. [26] showed improvement from 40% to 80% with Carina device at 65 dB, comparing to the patient's own HAs. Nevertheless, Kam et al. [22] found insignificant difference between conventional HAs and the Carina in terms of WR both in quiet and in noise.

The APHAB (Abbreviated Profile of Hearing Aid Benefit) scale was applied before and after implantation in some studies [1,10,11,13,18,19], and it consists of questionnaires in four areas: EC (Ease of Communication), BN (Background Noise), RV (Reverberation) and AV (Aversiveness) [1,10,19]. According to *Instruction for Manual Scoring of the APHAB*, a significant benefit has occurred if a difference of 22% is obtained for the EC, RV, or BN score [1]. Jenkins et al. [19] found that patients preferred the Carina over their own HAs for all questionnaires. According to Kam et al. [22], the APHAB scale for Carina and HA were 84.9 and 37.2, respectively.

5.2. Fully implantable devices compared with unaided. Comparing the outcomes of Carina implantation to unaided patients, the mean functional gain was 29 dB and 24 dB (p = 0.0004) in Martin et al. [9] and Bruschini et al. [17] respectively. Tringali et al. [7] showed a mean improvement of 39 dB with no information about statistical significance. Bruschini et al. [18] reported a mean functional gain of 26.4 dB (p = 0.0000001).

Five patients suffering from congenital auricular atresia submitted to Carina had functional gain of 36 dBHL in 4 frequencies by pure tone audiometry (1, 2, 3 e 4 kHz) as shown by Siegert et al. [8].

Kraus et al. [13] (n = 57) studied the 12-month results of the Esteem and found that the functional gain was 27 dB for 48 patients and 4 of them were stable at ±10 dB. Gerard et al. [14] found that the mean gain was 25±11 dB and the best results were obtained at frequencies between 500 and 3 k Hz.

According to Gerard et al. [14], the Esteem device, when compared to unaidaded, showed a mean WR gain of 64±33% at 50 dB SPL. At 50 dB, the WR improved from 10% at unaided condition and 23% with HA to 78% with Esteem according to Shohet et al. [15] A great improvement was reported by Barbara et al. [11] (42% to 79% in a group with moderate hearing loss and 30% to 72% in a group with severe hearing loss). Murali et al. [22] showed that postoperative WR on an average for all their 3 patients for closed set and open set were 100% and 95% respectively. All Carina results in WR comparing to unaided condition showed improvement. WR mean melioration according to the studies of Bruschini et al.[17,18] were 18% to 58% [17] and from 32.5% to 68.75% [18].

When the APHAB scale was applied, Martin et al. [9] showed significant benefit for Carina over unaided conditions for EC (from 49.8 to 19.9%) and RV (from 57.7 to 44.8%). AV increased (25.8 to 38.6%). Chen et al. [1] found that the average score for AV was −33 and −6 for HAs and Esteem compared to unaided condition, respectively, what means a 27% improvement of Esteem over the HAs. On this same comparison, Kraus et al. [13] showed that the mean difference on the global scale was 8.9±2.6 (p<0.01). The APHAB questionnaire revealed 85% of satisfaction improvement with Esteem compared to HAs in the 4 subscales in the study of Gerard et al. [14] Their 2 dissatisfied patients underwent revision surgery for poor functional results.

5.3. Fully implantable devices activated and inactivated. The middle and inner ear conditions were evaluated by some authors. Tringali et al. [21], Martin et al. [9] and Bruschini et al. [18] found no significant changes postoperatively, indicating minimal surgical trauma during Carina implantation. Jenkins et al. [19] observed no pre- nor post implantation differences for bone conduction and slight differences in pre- and post implant for air conduction.

As Esteem implantation induces an additional conductive hearing loss, Monini et al. [4] observed a conductive threshold shift of 35 dB on average over the whole frequency range. Barbara et al. [11,25] showed a bone conduction threshold worsening from baseline after Esteem implantation. For Kraus et al. [13] the average change was mean −0.8±1.1 dB. At 12 months only one patient had a threshold shift from 55 to 75 dB at 4 kHz. In the other hand, Chen et al. [1] and Gerard et al. [14] showed no significant changes of cochlear function by comparing bone conduction threshold before and after implantation of Esteem.

6. Complications and adverse events

Occasional feedback for the Carina device was cited by Kam et al. [22] and Bruschini et al. [18], but it was resolved through the fine-tuning of the fitting and gain reduction (Table 2). Bruschini et al. [18] reported a case of a patient who had the microphone implanted in the tip of mastoid and complained of too much feedback noise, especially when turning the head. It was necessary to reposition the implant.

Martin et al. [9] reported 2 cases of postoperative infection after Carina implantation and the need of reoperation in both. Another patient from their study had a decide failure but the patient declined revision surgery.

Jenkins et al. [19] (n = 20) cited fullness or pressure sensation in 10% of the subjects using Carina, middle ear effusion and partial device extrusion in 15%, vertigo and tinnitus in 5% and

conductive hearing loss in 20%. Three of the 20 have not been reached until 1-year follow-up of and 16 patients have asked to be explanted and reimplanted with a device modification. Lefebvre et al. [6], on the other hand, showed no complication up to 12-month follow-up of Carina.

For 57 patients with Esteem, Kraus et al. [13] reported 133 adverse events in 52 patients. There were 5.2% of revision surgeries, 3.5% developed wound infection (one them required explantation), 5.2% evolved with facial paresis (1 patient maintained House-Brackmann level II). Still about Esteem, Chen et al.[1] reported temporary swelling of the lower eyelid, sore jaw, nausea, diarrhea, elbow pain, arm and hand pain, and numbness. A device-related wound complication occurred that ultimately required implant removal in one subject.

The minor complications reported by Gerard et al. [14] with the Esteem device were: temporary partial facial palsy (7.6%), disruption of chorda tympani nerve (61.5%), revision surgery because of healing difficulty (7.6%) and 23% of revision surgeries for poor functional results. The major complication was the implant removal because of wound infection (15.3%).

Discussion

This systematic review evaluated the outcomes of Carina and Esteem implantation, devices currently available for use. The fully implantable MED is an alternative for many patients with limited benefits using conventional HAs, even those with only cosmetic issues. The indications are now not only for SNHL. Some authors had shown great outcomes using these devices for patients with external ear and ossicular chain defects, extending the indication for conductive and mixed hearing losses.

All the studies showed improvement of sound field threshold from unaided to aided conditions with fully implantable MED. About gain, there are conflicting results among the different studies. Some of them have no statistical significance. Some studies reported a functional gain but with a limited benefit on frequencies above 3 kHz [1,6,14].

The concern about middle ear conditions and cochlear function after implantation of some authors lies in the issues of surgical procedure. No changes in bone conduction before and after implantation were observed in most of the studies for the Carina. As Esteem implantation induces an additional conductive hearing loss, 2 studies showed a conductive threshold [4,11].

The comparison of the results about word recognition is difficult to make because there was no standardization of measurement. The results were obtained from various sound intensities and different frequencies. Also, some studies reported only the improvement; some showed the pre- and post-operative results; some offered only the graphics. All results comparing to unaided condition showed improvement. The results comparing to conventional HAs were conflicting.

For APHAB scale, all studies that evaluated the comparison between unaided and aided conditions and between the middle-ear device and conventional HAs for both Esteem and Carina showed benefit [1]. It means a subjective improvement of quality of life.

The complications involved in Carina and Esteem implantation were also studied. The main complications related to Esteem implantation were related to the surgical procedure. It should be kept in mind that the need for explantation will demand reconstruction of the ossicular chain. Otherwise, the hearing threshold will increase due to the overlapping of conductive hearing loss on a preexisting SNHL.

Table 2. Complications related to the fully implantable middle ear devices.

Study	Year	MED	Patients (n)	Adverse Effects (n)	Surgical Complications (n)	Device Adverse Effects (n)	Revisions (n)
Bruschini et al.	2009	Carina	5	NR	None	Feedback (5)	1
Bruschini et al.	2010	Carina	8	Extrusion of the cable of microphone (1), Psychological problems and explantation (1)	NR	Feedback (1), Device failure (1)	2
Chen et al.	2004	Esteem	7	Wound complication (1)	Temporary swelling of the lower eyelid, sore jaw, nausea, diarrhea, elbow pain, arm and hand pain, and numbness (2)	No benefit (3), Low gain (3)	3
Gerard et al.	2012	Esteem	13	Secondary healing difficulty (1), recurrent tissue edema (1), S aureus wound infection (2)	Temporary partial facial palsy (1), rupture of chorda tympani nerve (8),	Poor and deteriorating functional results (4)	4
Jenkins	2007 and 208	Carina	20	fullness or pressure sensation (2), conductive hearing loss (4), lightheadedness (1), tinnitus (1), partial device extrusion (3), and middle ear effusion (3)		partial device extrusion (3), inability to charge or establish communication (2),increased charging times beyond 1.5 hours	
Kam et al.	2012	6	None	None	feedback		1
Kraus et al.	2011	Esteem	57	Taste disturbance (24), middle ear effusion (18), pain (8), dizziness (9), tinnitus (7), headache (3), infection (2)	Facial paresis/paralysis (4)	Limited benefit (4)	3
Martin et al.	2009	Carina	11	Infection (2), vertigo (1), tinnitus (1)	NR	Hearing loss (1), poor sound transmission (1)	1
Memari et al.	2011	Esteem	10	NR	Temporary facial weakness (1)	No benefit (2)	NR
Murali et al.	2009	Esteem	3	None	transient facial paresis (1)	NR	0

n – number; MED – middle ear device; NR – not reported.

For Carina device, despite of the events related to surgical procedure, many studies showed device malfunction or failure with a need for revision surgery or explantations. This fact may be due to charging issues.

Conclusion

The use of fully implantable MED is now part of otology practice all around the world and this field is promising for those dissatisfied with their current conventional air-conduction hearing aids. Although there are still some problems yet to be solved mainly related to device functioning and price.

Due to the relatively few publications available and small sample sizes, we must be careful in extrapolating these results to a broader population. Additionally, none of all these studies represented level high levels of evidence (i.e. randomized controlled trials).

Author Contributions

Wrote the paper: JOBP AGB PRB RM RB RKT RFB.

References

1. Chen DA, Backous DD, Arriaga MA, Garvin R, Kobylek D, et al. (2004) Phase 1 clinical trial results of the Envoy System: a totally implantable middle ear device for sensorineural hearing loss. Otolaryngol Head Neck Surg 131: 904–916.
2. Chung J, Song WJ, Sim JH, Kim W, Oh SH (2013) Optimal ossicular site for maximal vibration transmissions to coupled transducers. Hear Res 301: 137–145.
3. Klein K, Nardelli A, Stafinski T (2012) A systematic review of the safety and effectiveness of fully implantable middle ear hearing devices: the carina and esteem systems. Otol Neurotol 33: 916–921.
4. Monini S, Biagini M, Atturo F, Barbara M (2013) Esteem middle ear device versus conventional hearing aids for rehabilitation of bilateral sensorineural hearing loss. Eur Arch Otorhinolaryngol 270: 2027–2033.
5. Butler CL, Thavaneswaran P, Lee IH (2013) Efficacy of the active middle-ear implant in patients with sensorineural hearing loss. J Laryngol Otol 127 Suppl 2: S8–16.
6. Lefebvre PP, Martin C, Dubreuil C, Decat M, Yazbeck A, et al. (2009) A pilot study of the safety and performance of the Otologics fully implantable hearing device: transducing sounds via the round window membrane to the inner ear. Audiol Neurotol 14: 172–180.
7. Tringali S, Pergola N, Ferber-Viart C, Truy E, Berger P, et al. (2008) Fully implantable hearing device as a new treatment of conductive hearing loss in Franceschetti syndrome. Int J Pediatr Otorhinolaryngol 72: 513–517.
8. Siegert R, Mattheis S, Kasic J (2007) Fully implantable hearing aids in patients with congenital auricular atresia. Laryngoscope. 117: 336–340.
9. Martin C, Deveze A, Richard C, Lefebvre PP, Decat M, et al. (2009) European results with totally implantable carina placed on the round window: 2-year follow-up. Otol Neurotol 30: 1196–1203.
10. Jenkins HA, Atkins JS, Horlbeck D, Hoffer ME, Balough B, et al. (2007) U.S. Phase I preliminary results of use of the Otologics MET Fully-Implantable Ossicular Stimulator. Otolaryngol Head Neck Surg 137: 206–212.
11. Barbara M, Biagini M, Monini S (2011) The totally implantable middle ear device 'Esteem' for rehabilitation of severe sensorineuralhearing loss. Acta Otolaryngol 131: 399–404.
12. Leuwer R, Müller J (2005) Restoration of hearing by hearing aids: conventional hearing aids - implantable hearing aids - cochlear implants - auditory brainstem implants. GMS Curr Top Otorhinolaryngol Head Neck Surg. 4: Doc03.
13. Kraus EM, Shohet JA, Catalano PJ (2011) Envoy Esteem Totally Implantable Hearing System: phase 2 trial, 1-year hearing results. Otolaryngol Head Neck Surg 145: 100–109.
14. Gerard JM, Thill MP, Chantrain G, Gersdorff M, Deggouj N (2012) Esteem 2 middle ear implant: our experience. Audiol Neurotol 17: 267–274.
15. Shohet JA, Kraus EM, Catalano PJ (2011) Profound high-frequency sensorineural hearing loss treatment with a totally implantable hearing system. Otol Neurotol 32: 1428–1431.
16. Lachowska M, Niemczyk K, Yazbeck A, Morawski K, Bruzgielewicz A (2012) First bilateral simultaneous implantation with fully implantable middle ear hearing device. Arch Med Sci 8: 736–742.
17. Bruschini L, Forli F, Santoro A, Bruschini P, Berrettini S (2009) Fully implantable Otologics MET Carina device for the treatment of sensorineural hearing loss. Preliminary surgical and clinical results. Acta Otorhinolaryngol Ital 29: 79–85.
18. Bruschini L, Forli F, Passetti S, Bruschini P, Berrettini S (2010) Fully implantable Otologics MET Carina device for the treatment of sensorineural and mixed hearing loss: Audio-otological results. Acta Otolaryngol 130: 1147–1153.
19. Jenkins HA, Atkins JS, Horlbeck D, Hoffer ME, Balough B, et al. (2008) Otologics fully implantable hearing system: Phase I trial 1-year results. Otol Neurotol 29: 534–541.
20. Memari F, Asghari A, Daneshi A, Jalali A (2011) Safety and patient selection of totally implantable hearing aid surgery: Envoy system, Esteem. Eur Arch Otorhinolaryngol 268: 1421–1425.
21. Tringali S, Pergola N, Berger P, Dubreuil C (2009) Fully implantable hearing device with transducer on the round window as a treatment of mixed hearing loss. Auris Nasus Larynx 36: 353–358.
22. Kam AC, Sung JK, Yu JK, Tong MC (2012) Clinical evaluation of a fully implantable hearing device in six patients with mixed and sensorineural hearing loss: our experience. Clin Otolaryngol. 37: 240–244.
23. Murali S, Krishnan PV, Bansal T, Karthikeyan K, Natarajan K, et al. (2009) Totally implantable hearing aid surgical technique and the first Indian experience with Envoy Esteem. Indian J Otolaryngol Head Neck Surg 61: 245–251.
24. Zenner HP, Rodriguez JJ (2010) Totally implantable active middle ear implants: ten years' experience at the University of Tübingen. Adv Otorhinolaryngol 69: 72–84.
25. Barbara M, Manni V, Monini S (2009) Totally implantable middle ear device for rehabilitation of sensorineural hearing loss: preliminary experience with the Esteem, Envoy. Acta Otolaryngol 129: 429–432.
26. Deveze A, Rameh C, Sanjuan M, Lavieille JP, Magnan J (2010) A middle ear implant with a titanium canal wall prosthesis for a case of an open mastoid cavity. Auris Nasus Larynx 37: 631–635.

22

Epigenome-Wide DNA Methylation in Hearing Ability: New Mechanisms for an Old Problem

Lisa E. Wolber[1], Claire J. Steves[1], Pei-Chien Tsai[1], Panos Deloukas[2,3,4], Tim D. Spector[1], Jordana T. Bell[1⁹], Frances M. K. Williams[1*⁹]

1 Department of Twin Research and Genetic Epidemiology, King's College London, London, United Kingdom, 2 William Harvey Research Institute, Barts and The London School of Medicine and Dentistry, Queen Mary University of London, London, United Kingdom, 3 King Abdulaziz University, Jeddah, Saudi Arabia, 4 Wellcome Trust Sanger Institute, Hinxton, Cambridge, United Kingdom

Abstract

Epigenetic regulation of gene expression has been shown to change over time and may be associated with environmental exposures in common complex traits. Age-related hearing impairment is a complex disorder, known to be heritable, with heritability estimates of 57–70%. Epigenetic regulation might explain the observed difference in age of onset and magnitude of hearing impairment with age. Epigenetic epidemiology studies using unrelated samples can be limited in their ability to detect small effects, and recent epigenetic findings in twins underscore the power of this well matched study design. We investigated the association between venous blood DNA methylation epigenome-wide and hearing ability. Pure-tone audiometry (PTA) and Illumina HumanMethylation array data were obtained from female twin volunteers enrolled in the TwinsUK register. Two study groups were explored: first, an epigenome-wide association scan (EWAS) was performed in a discovery sample (n = 115 subjects, age range: 47–83 years, Illumina 27 k array), then replication of the top ten associated probes from the discovery EWAS was attempted in a second unrelated sample (n = 203, age range: 41–86 years, Illumina 450 k array). Finally, a set of monozygotic (MZ) twin pairs (n = 21 pairs) within the discovery sample (Illumina 27 k array) was investigated in more detail in an MZ discordance analysis. Hearing ability was strongly associated with DNA methylation levels in the promoter regions of several genes, including *TCF25* (cg01161216, p = 6.6×10^{-6}), *FGFR1* (cg15791248, p = 5.7×10^{-5}) and *POLE* (cg18877514, p = 6.3×10^{-5}). Replication of these results in a second sample confirmed the presence of differential methylation at *TCF25* (p(replication) = 6×10^{-5}) and *POLE* (p(replication) = 0.016). In the MZ discordance analysis, twins' intrapair difference in hearing ability correlated with DNA methylation differences at *ACP6* (cg01377755, r = −0.75, p = 1.2×10^{-4}) and *MEF2D* (cg08156349, r = −0.75, p = 1.4×10^{-4}). Examination of gene expression in skin, suggests an influence of differential methylation on expression, which may account for the variation in hearing ability with age.

Editor: Martina Paulsen, Universität des Saarlandes, Germany

Funding: This work was funded by Action on Hearing Loss and AgeUK. The authors would like to thank all volunteers from the TwinsUK register, who contributed to this study and acknowledge the work of all researchers who helped in the completion of this work. The study was funded by the Wellcome Trust; European Community's Seventh Framework Programme (FP7/2007–2013). The study also receives support from the National Institute for Health Research (NIHR) BioResource Clinical Research Facility and Biomedical Research Centre based at Guy's and St Thomas' NHS Foundation Trust and King's College London. Tim Spector is holder of an ERC Advanced Principal Investigator award. The funders had no role in study design, data and analysis, decision to publish, or preparation of the manuscript.

Competing Interests: The authors have declared that no competing interests exist.

* Email: frances.williams@kcl.ac.uk

⁹ These authors contributed equally to this work.

Introduction

The term epigenetics [1] refers to the regulation of gene expression primarily by DNA methylation and changes to DNA folding. Epigenetics plays an important role in gene expression regulation and cell differentiation in the developing organism [2,3]. While the genetic code is fixed, epigenetic changes may be dynamic and have been shown to change during a lifetime [4]. DNA methylation is one of the most commonly studied epigenetic changes and involves the addition of a methyl-group to the 5th carbon molecule of a cytosine base, generating 5-methyl-cytosine. This stable modification occurs primarily at the CpG dinucleotide, but has also been detected at CpH sides, where H can stand for C, A or T. Each diploid human genome contains on average 10^8

cytosines, of which about 10^7 are combined with guanine as CpG dinucleotide [5]. CpG dinucleotides often cluster in CpG-islands in the promoter region of genes. The majority of CpG islands in promoters are unmethylated. DNA methyl-transferases are responsible for *de novo* methylation of DNA [6] and facilitating stable transmission of epigenetic marks during cell division [7].

Epigenetic changes can be influenced by both environmental exposure [4,8] and genetic variation [9]. Therefore, samples for studying the association of methylation with any given trait should ideally be matched for genetic and environmental variation. This could best be achieved by using family data or monozygotic twins, which are assumed to be genetically identical and well matched for environmental exposures [10]. Family and twin studies have identified differentially methylated regions associated with age [11] and multiple complex traits [4,12] and have further been used to estimate rates of heritability in DNA methylation [8,11]. Current advances in technology allow for high-resolution screening of DNA methylation profiles across the genome. Multiple platforms exists, but to date the majority of studies have successfully used the Illumina Infinium HumanMethylation 27 k and HumanMethylation 450 k Bead Chips to assay genome-wide DNA methylation profiles across individuals [11,13].

Age-related hearing impairment (ARHI) is a common complex trait affecting 46% of the population over the age of 48 [14]. Epigenetic changes in the ageing ear have been proposed to account for age-related changes to hearing ability and syndromic forms of hearing loss [15,16]. Changes in DNA methylation are influenced by environmental exposure and could therefore provide the essential link between the environment and changes in gene expression. Furthermore, epigenetic changes with age could explain how a previously healthy individual develops hearing loss with age. Several forms of syndromic hearing loss, such as Rett and Stickler syndrome, have been associated with epigenetic change [17,18,19]. Here, an epigenome-wide association study (EWAS) of hearing ability was performed, the first EWAS of ARHI to our knowledge. This research aimed to determine significant associations of differentially methylated regions with hearing ability in subjects from the TwinsUK cohort. The most significantly associated CpG sites were replicated in an independent sample and gene expression profiles were investigated at the genes identified.

Materials and Methods

Ethics statement

The study was approved by the National Research Ethics service London-Westminster (REC reference number: 07/H0802/84). Fully informed written consent was obtained from all participants prior to study conduction. All research described was conducted according to the rules described in the Declaration of Helsinki.

Subjects

Hearing data in form of air-conduction PTA was collected from participants of the TwinsUK cohort between 2009 and 2013. Hearing thresholds were determined at frequencies 0.125–8 kHz for each ear according to the recommendations of the British Society of Audiology [20]. Pure-tone audiometry information was summarised by principal component analysis (PCA) [23]. All participants completed a questionnaire covering exposure to environmental risk factors for ARHI and previous ear diseases. Subjects reporting a family history of hereditary hearing loss or signs of conductive hearing loss were excluded from the analysis.

DNA methylation profiles

Whole blood samples for DNA methylation screening were profiled using two different DNA methylation assays, the Infinium HumanMethylation 27 k BeadChip (26,690 CpG sites) and the Infinium HumanMethylation 450 k BeadChip Kit. In both arrays, the DNA methylation level at a specific CpG site is expressed as the β value, which represents the ratio of the methylated probe signal over the methylated and unmethylated probe signals. The β score ranges from 0 to 1, where 0 indicates absence of methylation and 1 represents a fully methylated CpG site.

The Illumina Infinium HumanMethylation 27 k array measures methylation at 27,578 CpG sites, covering 14,495 genes. This array covers primarily CpG sites located in promoter regions of genes with on average two CpG sites per consensus coding sequence and three to twenty assays per cancer gene [21]. The

Illumina Infinium HumanMethylation450 k array covers 485,577 methylation sites in 99% of RefSeq genes (21,231 genes) with an average of 17.2 CpG sites per gene region. [22].

To identify potential confounders of the Illumina Infinium HumanMethylation 27 k array, principal component analysis (PCA) was performed using the normalised DNA methylation values. The first five principal components resulting from this analysis were correlated with following covariates: chronological age, methylation chip and position of sample on the chip. Both methylation chip and position of sample on the chip were significantly correlated with the first two principal components from this analysis and therefore included as fixed effects in further analysis [11]. The same procedure was performed for the Illumina Infinium HumanMethylation 450 k array with covariates age, chip, position of sample on the chip and bisulfite converted DNA concentration levels. Chip, position on the chip and bisulfite converted DNA concentration levels were significantly associated with the first 3 principal components and were therefore included as fixed effects in the linear mixed effects models.

Epigenome-wide association study

The discovery EWAS of hearing was performed in 115 adult female subjects with available PTA data and Illumina Infinium HumanMethylation 27 k profiles [11]. The DNA methylation profiles used in the EWAS were obtained from 26,690 DNA methylation probes, which mapped uniquely to the human genome (hg18) [9]. After further exclusion of probes mapping to the X-chromosome and probes with missing data, 24,641 autosomal probes remained for the EWAS [11]. The Illumina Infinium HumanMethylation 27 k profiles have been published previously [11]. DNA methylation was transformed to a standard normal distribution per probe using quantile normalisation. To determine the association between hearing ability and DNA methylation a linear mixed effect model was applied. DNA methylation levels at each CpG site were regressed against hearing ability (PC1), with adjustment for age, methylation chip, order of samples on the chip and twin relatedness. To exclude associations with DNA methylation due to covariates other than hearing, the full model was compared to a null model, excluding hearing as a predictor variable. The null and the full model were compared for model fit in an analysis of variance (ANOVA). Only associations where the full model fitted the data significantly better ($p < 0.05$) than the null model were reported. For each significantly associated probe, the effect size (beta), standard error of effect (se) and the p-value from the analysis of variance comparing full and null model were reported. To confirm that the regions of association were not age-dependent differentially methylated regions (age DMRs), models including and excluding age as a fixed effect were compared. Furthermore, associated probes were checked against previously reported age DMRs [11]. In addition, to exclude an underlying association between genetic (rather then epigenetic) variation and PC1, genetic variants in the DMR genomic loci were tested for association with PC1, in a PC1 genome-wide association scan from the TwinsUK cohort (n = 1028). To adjust for multiple testing in the EWAS initially a Bonferroni corrected significance threshold assuming 24,641 independent tests ($p = 0.05/24641 = 2.03 \times 10^{-6}$) was assumed epigenome-wide significant. Furthermore, since the Illumina Infinium HumanMethylation 27 k array contains on average 2 probes per promoter and high levels of co-methylation between nearby probes have previously been reported [9], we also considered 2 additional Bonferroni corrected thresholds: a genome-wide significant threshold correcting for 14,495 independent genes ($p = 0.05/14495 = 3.45 \times 10^{-6}$) and a genome-wide suggestive threshold correcting for 14,495 independent genes ($p = 0.1/14495 = 6.90 \times 10^{-6}$).

Replication study

The replication sample consisted of 203 females from the TwinsUK registry. For the replication study only the 10 probes most highly associated in the discovery EWAS were investigated, while the remaining 485567 probes from the 450 k array were neglected. The 10 selected probes were examined for replication in the second sample using a linear mixed effect model. DNA methylation was transformed to standard normal per probe using a quantile normalisation. DNA methylation at each CpG site was regressed against hearing ability (PC1) with adjustment for age, methylation chip, order of samples on the chip, bisulfite conversion levels and twin relatedness. To exclude association with DNA methylation due to covariates, the full model was compared to a null model, in which hearing was excluded as a predictor variable. The null and the full models were compared for model fit in an analysis of variance. For each of the 10 probes, the effect size (beta), standard error of effect (se) and the p-value from the analysis of variance comparing full and null model were reported. Replication of association was considered if association was in the same direction and nominally significant ($p \leq 0.05$). To confirm that replicating probes were not age-dependent DMRs, models including and excluding age as a fixed effect were compared. To determine the significance and effect of joint association signals in the discovery (27 k) and replication (450 k) samples, a meta-analysis was conducted for the ten most highly associated probes using METAL [23] based on the inverse-variance option.

DMR validation using methylated DNA immunoprecipitation sequencing (MeDIPseq)

To further validate the findings from the EWAS (27 k) and replication study (450 k) using an alternative technique, the top ranked DMR was also explored using methylated DNA immuno-precipitation followed by high throughput sequencing (MeDIPseq) data. The MeDIPseq validation sample consisted of 46 unrelated healthy females with PTA scores and previously published MeDIPseq profiles [24]. MeDIPseq DNA methylation levels were generated and quantified as previously described [24], and relative methylation scores in a 1 kb region on chr 16 (chr16: 88466501–88467500 on hg 18) overlapping probe cg01161216 (chr16: 88466949 on hg 18) were explored for association with PTA. A linear fixed effect model was applied, where the DNA methylation signal at the locus surrounding the chromosomal position of probe cg01161216 was regressed on hearing ability (PC1), adjusted for age. To exclude an association of DNA methylation with age, the full model was compared to a null model, excluding hearing as a predictor variable. The null and full models were compared for model fit using analysis of variance (ANOVA).

Whole blood cell subtype heterogeneity

Previous studies have reported that association with DNA methylation measured in whole blood samples can be driven by blood cell subtype heterogeneity [25]. To adjust for this, eosinophil, lymphocyte, neutrophil and monocyte cell counts in the blood samples were included (as fixed effects) in the full and null models for the ten most highly associated probes. 106 out of 115 subjects had complete blood cell counts available and were included in this analysis.

Exploring methylation changes in monozygotic twins

Monozygotic twin pairs with PTA and Illumina HumanMethylation 27 k data were selected for the MZ discordance analysis (n = 21 pairs). Intra-pair DNA methylation difference per probe was calculated as the difference in DNA methylation residuals (adjusted for chip and position on the chip) between co-twins. DNA methylation residuals were calculated from quantile normalised β values per probe. Differences in DNA methylation were compared to differences in PC1 were using Spearman rank correlation.

Effect of DNA methylation on gene expression

To investigate the influence of DNA methylation on gene expression, expression levels in skin tissue collected as part of the Multiple Tissue Human Expression Resource (MuTHER) (http://www.muther.ac.uk) were examined [26]. Quantile normalised gene expression in skin was adjusted for experimental batch effect and RNA concentration in the tissue sample and residuals correlated with DNA methylation residuals (adjusted for chip and position on the chip) at the corresponding probes using Pearson correlation. Furthermore, skin expression residuals were correlated with PC1 values, to test for an effect of gene expression on the phenotype.

Results

Subjects and phenotypes

Two independent samples with hearing data and DNA methylation profiles were selected from the TwinsUK registry to perform the discovery EWAS (n = 115) using Illumina HumanMethylation 27 k profiles, and the replication EWAS (n = 203) using Illumina HumanMethylation 450 k profiles. Subjects included in the discovery EWAS had a mean age of 56.7 years (± 7.9 years of standard deviation from the mean, age range 33–80 years) and included 25 dizygotic twin (DZs) pairs, 21 monozygotic twin (MZs) pairs and 23 singletons. The replication sample included 203 females, comprising 61 MZ twin pairs, 22 DZ twin pairs and 37 unpaired twins (singletons), with a mean age of 63.21 (± 8.87 years of standard deviation from the mean, age range 41–82 years). The discovery and replication samples are summarised in Table 1. Variance in PTA was summarised using principal component analysis, where PC1 represented the threshold shift over all frequencies (0.125–8.0 kHz) and captured 54.25% of the variance. A high PC1 score thus corresponded to reduced hearing ability [27].

DNA methylation profiles

Genome-wide DNA methylation levels were obtained in the set of 115 female twins using the Illumina 27 k array. The majority of autosomal CpG sites included in this analysis were unmethylated (β<0.3, 68.9% of probes), few probes were hemi-methylated (β: 0.3–0.7, 11.2% of probes) or fully methylated (β>0.7, 19.9% of probes).

Discovery EWAS

Genome-wide DNA methylation levels at 24,461 autosomal probes were previously obtained in the set of 115 discovery female twins using the Illumina 27 k array [11] and compared to hearing ability. DNA methylation at 2,519 (out of 24,641) probes was nominally associated (ANOVA p-value≤0.05) with hearing ability for PC1. A Manhattan plot of the EWAS for hearing PC1 is shown in Figure 1 and the strongest signal reached Bonferroni adjusted genome-wide suggestive evidence for association ($p = 6.9 \times 10^{-6}$).

Table 1. Characteristics of the female TwinsUK samples.

sample	zygosity	n	age at DNA extraction		age at hearing test		PC 1 ±sd
			mean ±sd	range	mean ±sd	range	
discovery (27 k)	MZ	42	55.43±6.93	45-68	62.00±6.60	50-72	-0.28±1.47
	DZ	50	57.68±8.88	33-80	64.32±7.68	47-83	0.72±1.53
	singleton	23	56.91±7.35	43-70	64.83±6.12	50-75	0.29±1.78
	Total	115	56.70±7.91	33-80	63.57±7.05	47-83	0.27±1.61
replication (450 k)	MZ	122	55.64±8.83	37-73	63.82±8.79	46-82	0.60±2.13
	DZ	44	52.88±10.59	33-78	60.86±10.58	41-86	0.21±2.48
	singleton	37	55.87±6.20	42-66	63.97±6.28	49-75	0.21±1.74
	Total	203	55.09±8.87	33-78	63.21±8.87	41-86	0.45±2.15
validation (MeDIPseq)	singleton	46	60.02±7.85	41-83	62.28±7.86	43-86	-0.10±2.08

Demographic characteristics of the discovery (27 k DNA methylation bead chip), replication (450 k DNA methylation bead chip) and validation (methylated DNA immunoprecipitation and high throughput sequencing (MeDIPseq) samples are listed. Samples zygosity is shown (monozygotic (MZ) and dizygotic (DZ) twins) as well as unpaired twins (singletons). Demographic measures include number of subjects (n), mean chronological age at DNA extraction in years and age range, as well as mean chronological age at hearing assessment in years. Mean and standard deviation (sd) of hearing principal component 1 (PC1), representing the overall threshold shift in the audiogram, are given.

The most highly associated probe was cg01161216 which maps to the promoter region of transcription factor 25 (*TCF25*)(beta±se = −0.245±0.05, p = 6.6×10^{-6}). Further associations were observed for CpG sites in the promoter regions of the phosphoglucomutase 3 (*PGM3*) gene (beta±se = −0.26±0.06, p = 4.5×10^{-5}), the cysteine dioxygenase type 1 (*CDO1*) gene (beta±se = −0.24±0.06, p = 4.7×10^{-5}), the nucleolar complex associated 2 homolog (*NOC2L*) gene (beta±se = −0.20±0.05, p = 5.4×10^{-5}), the myosin binding protein C (*MYBPC3*) gene (beta±se = −0.19±0.05, p = 5.4×10^{-5}), the fibroblast growth factor receptor 1 (*FGFR1*) gene (beta±se = −0.24±0.06, p = 5.7×10^{-5}), the DNA polymerase epsilon catalytic subunit (*POLE*) gene (beta±se = −0.16±0.04, p = 6.3×10^{-5}), vacuolar protein sorting 4 homolog B (*VPS4B*) gene (beta±se = 0.20±0.05, p = 6.5×10^{-5}), the heterogeneous nuclear ribonucleoprotein A0 (*HNRNPA0*) gene (beta±se = 0.14±0.03, p = 6.9×10^{-5}), and probe cg25017250 (beta±se = −0.23±0.06, p = 7.0×10^{-5}) mapping to the apolipoprotein C-4 (*APOC4*) gene. The ten most highly associated EWAS probes are listed in Table 2.

After exclusion of chronological age as a fixed effect, association of DNA methylation with hearing PC1 remained significant for all of the ten most highly associated probes (Table 2).

Replication of highly associated EWAS probes

The ten most highly associated CpG probes from the discovery sample were examined in the replication sample (Table 1). Association between DNA methylation and PC1 was replicated at 2 probes - in the promoter regions of genes *TCF25* and *POLE* (Table 2 and depicted in Figure 2). Figure 2 depicts the association between raw methylation betas with hearing PC1 at *TCF25* and *POLE* in the discovery and replication samples. While probe cg01161216 (*TCF25*) was hypomethylated (ß<0.3) in all subjects, probe cg18877514 (*POLE*) was hypermethylated (ß>0.7) (Figure 2). The association between adjusted DNA methylation residuals and PC1 at *TCF25* and *POLE* in the discovery and replication samples can be found in Figure S1. None of the replicating DMRs showed an underlying association of single nuclear polymorphisms with PC1 200 kb up- and downstream of the respective genes (*TCF25*, *POLE*) in a genome-wide association study.

After exclusion of chronological age as a fixed effect, association of DNA methylation with PC1 remained significant at *TCF25* and *POLE* (cg01161216: p(no age) = 1.06×10^{-8}; cg18877514 p(no age) = 2.83×10^{-2})(Table 2).

To assess the behaviour of additional probes mapping to the *TCF25* and *POLE* loci with respect to hearing, the association between DNA methylation and hearing PC1 was explored for all probes mapping to *TCF25* and *POLE* according to hg19 (Figure 3). According to the locus plots, 3 further nominally significant associated DMRs (p<0.05) mapped to each *TCF25* and *POLE*.

Although DNA methylation was not found significantly associated at 8 out of 10 probes in the replication sample, DNA methylation at five further probes (cg25383093, cg19923810, cg21370143, cg15791248 and cg25017250) showed the same direction of effect as in the discovery sample (Table 2). In the meta-analysis of results from the 27 k and 450 k chips, DNA methylation at 7 out of 10 probes was nominally significantly associated with PC1 (Table 2), with differential DNA methylation at *TCF25* showing the most significant association (cg01161216, p = 4.89×10^{-9})(Table 2).

PC1 EWAS

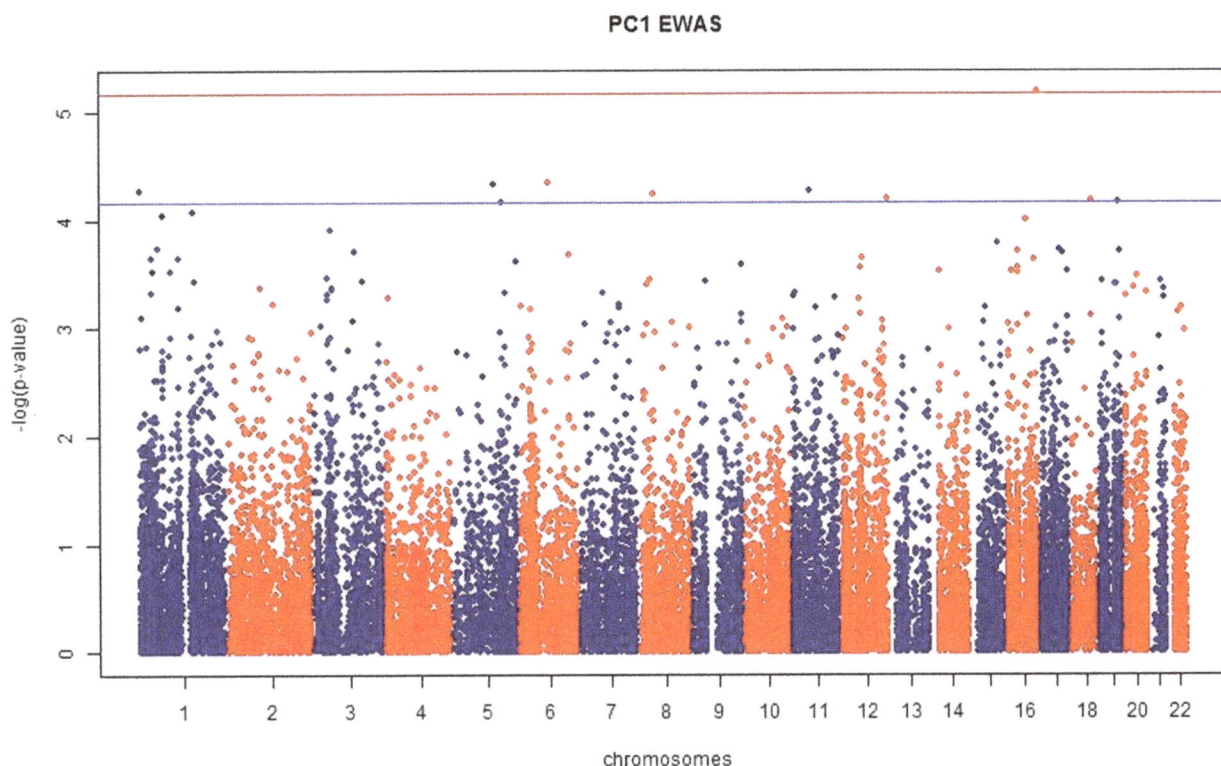

Figure 1. Manhattan Plot of PC1 EWAS results. The manhattan plot depicts the significance of association with PC1 as the negative logarithm of the p-value (-log(p-value)) versus the chromosomal location (chromosomes) for each of the 24,641 tested DNA-methylation probes. The red line defines a Bonferroni adjusted genome-wide suggestive significance threshold of $p = 6.9 \times 10^{-6}$. The ten most highly associated probes are located above the horizontal blue line corresponding to $p < 6.985 \times 10^{-5}$.

Validation of TCF25 using MeDIPseq

To validate the peak EWAS DMR using a different technology, TCF25 DNA methylation levels based on MeDIPseq data were also explored for association with hearing in 46 unrelated females from TwinsUK [24]. The mean age of subjects in the validation sample was 62.28 (± 7.86 years of standard deviation from the mean, age range 43–86 years) (Table 1). MeDIPseq DNA methylation levels at a 1 kb locus overlapping probe cg01161216 were selected and compared to PC1. DNA methylation at this locus was significantly associated with hearing PC1 ($p = 4.09 \times 10^{-2}$) and showed the same direction of effect (beta$\pm$se $= -8.72 \times 10^{-6} \pm 4.13 \times 10^{-6}$) as both the discovery EWAS and replication datasets.

Blood cell heterogeneity

To account for potential effects of blood cell heterogeneity, the peak DMRs were also explored for association with proportion of eosinophils, lymphocytes, neutrophils and monocytes in a subset of 106 subjects from the discovery sample. The ten most highly associated probes in the discovery EWAS remained significantly associated ($p > 0.005$) with PC1 after adjustment for blood cell heterogeneity.

Monozygotic co-twin study

MZ discordance analyses were performed in 21 female MZ twin pairs ($n = 42$) selected from the discovery sample with a mean age of 55.43 years (± 6.93 years of standard deviation, age range: 45–68 years) (Table 1). Mean intrapair difference in PC1 was -0.42 (± 1.34 sd, range: 3.47 and -2.86). The intra-pair differences in PC1 were compared with intra-pair differences in DNA methylation at 24,641 autosomal CpG sites. Of these, 794 CpG sites were nominally significant ($p < 0.05$). PC1 discordance was most strongly associated with differential methylation at lysophosphatidic acid phosphatase 6 (*ACP6*, cg01377755, r = -0.75, $p = 1.2 \times 10^{-4}$). Further strongly correlated differentially methylated genes included myocyte enhancer factor 2D (MEF2D, cg08156349, r = -0.75, $p = 1.4 \times 10^{-4}$), tachykinin precursor 1 (*TAC1*, cg07550362, r = -0.72, $p = 3.3 \times 10^{-4}$), ATPase family AAA domain-containing 3C (*ATAD3C*, cg27383362, r = -0.70, $p = 5.5 \times 10^{-4}$), brain-specific serine protease 3 (*PRSS12*, cg21208104, r = 0.70, $p = 6.3 \times 10^{-4}$), ADAM metallopeptidase domain 18 (*ADAM18*, cg23566335, r = 0.70, $p = 6.5 \times 10^{-4}$), chromobox homolog 2 (*CBX2*, cg22892904, r = -0.69, $p = 7.8 \times 10^{-4}$), septin 3 (*SEPT3*, cg04283938, r = -0.68, $p = 8.6 \times 10^{-4}$), transmembrane protein 121 (*TMEM121*, cg23886551, r = -0.68, $p = 8.6 \times 10^{-4}$) and torsin family 1 member B (*TOR1B*, cg14299800, r = -0.68, $p = 9.1 \times 10^{-4}$) (Table 3).

Influence of DNA methylation on gene expression in skin

To investigate the influence of DNA methylation on gene expression, expression profiles in skin were explored because skin originates from the same embryonic tissues as the inner ear, and expression profiles were not available for the cochlea. For 172 individuals with 27 k array data, DNA methylation at the two replicating probes (cg01161216 and cg18877514) was examined for association with gene expression (*TCF25* and *POLE*, respectively). After adjustment of both DNA methylation and skin expression for batch effects, DNA methylation residuals and gene

Table 2. Results of epigenome wide association of hearing PC1 for discovery and replication samples and their meta-analysis.

probe	gene	27 k (n = 115)				450 k (n = 203)				meta-analysis (n = 318)			
		beta	se	p-value	p-value (no age)	beta	se	p-value	p-value (no age)	dir	beta	se	p-value
cg01161216	**TCF25**	**-0.24454**	**0.05189**	**6.60E-06**	**4.98E-04**	**-0.12362**	**0.03087**	**8.55E-05**	**1.06E-08**	**- -**	**-0.1552**	**0.0265**	**4.89E-09**
cg25383093	PGM3	-0.26056	0.05631	4.46E-05	7.46E-05	-0.00816	0.03367	8.08E-01	7.66E-02	- -	-0.0746	0.0289	9.80E-03
cg07644368	CDO1	-0.23819	0.05639	4.67E-05	2.06E-03	0.02340	0.03877	5.50E-01	4.40E-01	- +	-0.0606	0.0319	5.80E-02
cg19923810	NOC2L	-0.20035	0.04784	5.38E-05	3.24E-05	-0.02523	0.03111	4.26E-01	8.16E-01	- -	-0.0773	0.0261	3.05E-03
cg21370143	MYBPC3	-0.19031	0.04546	5.44E-05	1.03E-05	-0.05170	0.03407	1.30E-01	1.62E-01	- -	-0.1016	0.0273	1.95E-04
cg15791248	FGFR1	-0.24243	0.05799	5.73E-05	5.01E-05	-0.01488	0.03846	6.96E-01	5.13E-01	- -	-0.0844	0.0321	8.46E-03
cg18877514	**POLE**	**-0.16287**	**0.03931**	**6.33E-05**	**9.08E-04**	**-0.06827**	**0.02839**	**1.70E-02**	**2.83E-02**	**- -**	**-0.1007**	**0.0230**	**1.20E-05**
cg05934874	VPS4B	0.19644	0.04751	6.55E-05	8.98E-04	-0.08786	0.02993	3.67E-03	1.88E-02	+ -	-0.0071	0.0253	7.80E-01
cg12241297	HNRNPA0	0.13623	0.03269	6.90E-05	4.52E-04	-0.06433	0.02882	2.65E-02	3.18E-02	+ -	0.0234	0.0216	2.80E-01
cg25017250	APOC4	-0.23167	0.05495	6.98E-05	1.06E-03	-0.03949	0.03585	2.71E-01	1.71E-02	- -	-0.0969	0.0300	1.25E-03

The ten most highly associated differentially methylated regions in the discovery EWAS (27 k) are shown. Probes are characterised by the nearest gene, the association effect (beta), standard error of the effect (se) and significance of model fit (p-value). Significance of model fit excluding age as a model parameter (p-value (no age)) is reported for both the discovery (27 k) and replication (450 k) sample. The ten most highly associated probes were taken forward for replication (450 k) with effect (beta) standard error of the effect and significance of model fit (p-value) listed. Results of the meta-analysis are presented as direction of effect (dir, discovery and replication direction shown), combined effect (beta), standard error of the combined effect (se) and significance of the combined association (p-value). Association of DNA methylation and hearing PC1 was replicated for probes cg01161216 and cg18877514 (highlighted in bold).

A

PC1 versus raw DNA methylation at cg01161216

B

PC1 versus raw DNA methylation at cg18877514

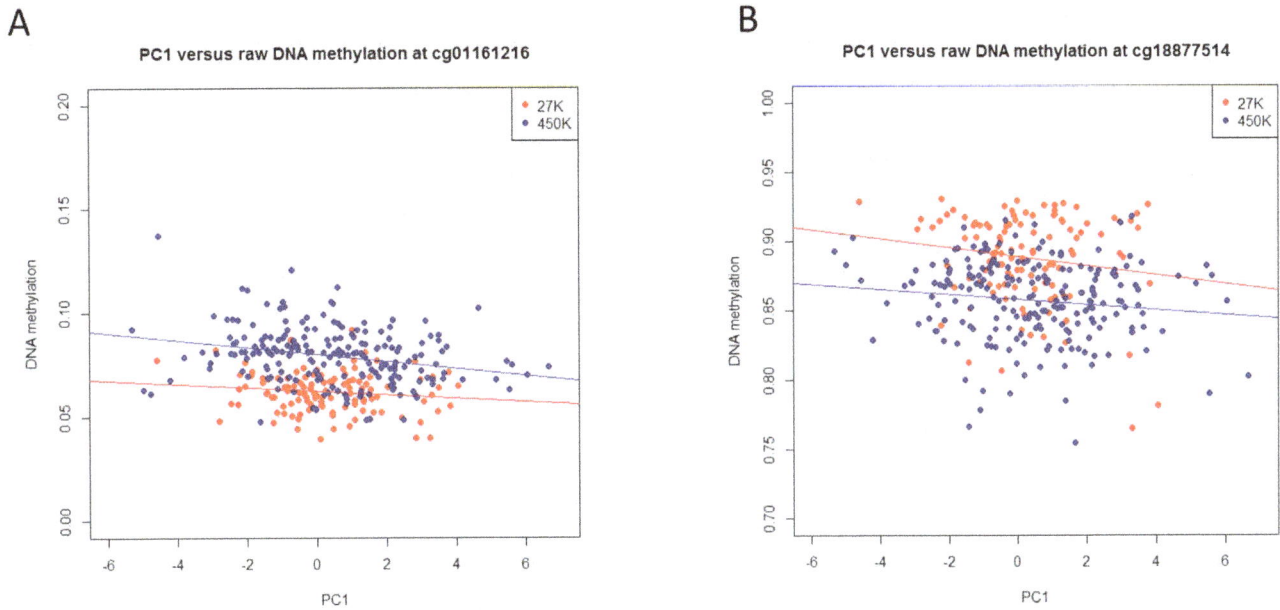

Figure 2. Association of hearing PC1 values and raw DNA methylation at *TCF25* (cg01161216) and *POLE* (cg18877514). A, B Hearing PC1 values were plotted versus raw DNA methylation betas for both the discovery (27 k, red dots) and the replication (450 k, blue dots) samples. Linear regression lines were fitted for both datasets (27 k:red line, 450 k:blue line).

expression residuals showed a weak negative correlation for *TCF25* (r = −0.02) (Figure 4, A) and *POLE* (r = −0.06) (Figure 4, B). In general, DNA methylation in whole blood was only weakly correlated with gene expression in skin tissue. Furthermore, the effect of gene expression levels of *TCF25* and *POLE* on hearing ability was explored. Gene expression showed a weak positive correlation with PC1 values (*TCF25*: r = 0.12; *POLE*: r = 0.16)(Figure 4, Panel C and D).

Discussion

Changes in DNA methylation have been associated with increasing age and age-related disorders [11]. Here, for the first time the effect of genome-wide DNA methylation on hearing ability was investigated. Genome-wide association and candidate gene studies of hearing ability with age have yet to explain much of the estimated variance in this phenotype. Our approach identified

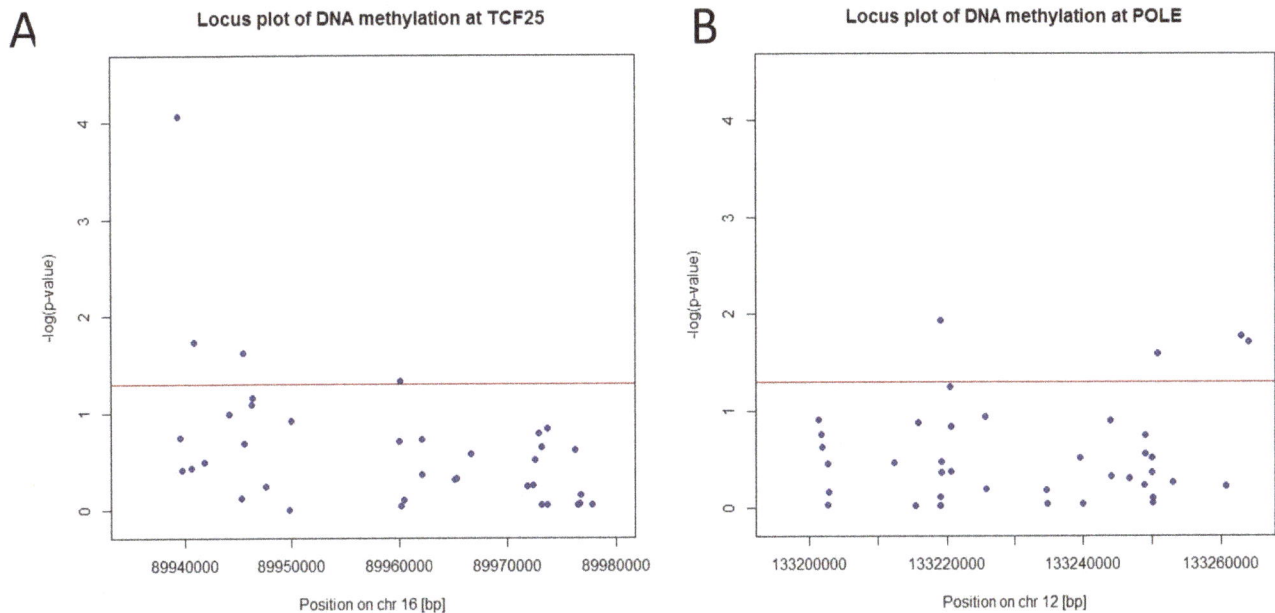

A

Locus plot of DNA methylation at TCF25

B

Locus plot of DNA methylation at POLE

Figure 3. DNA methylation association with hearing PC1 at *TCF25* and *POLE*. Hearing PC1 association with all available Illumina 450 k DNA methylation probes annotated to *TCF25* (A) and *POLE* (B) gene regions according to hg19. Significance of association with hearing PC1 expressed as the negative logarithm of the p-value was plotted against base pair [bp] location for chromosomes 16 and 12, respectively. The red horizontal lines represent the significance threshold for nominal significance (p = 0.05).

Table 3. Results of the MZ intra-pair difference association analysis.

MZ pair difference analysis (n = 42)

probe	gene	rho	p-value
cg01377755	ACP6	−0.753	1.24E-04
cg08156349	MEF2D	−0.749	1.41E-04
cg07550362	TAC1	−0.722	3.25E-04
cg27383362	ATAD3C	−0.703	5.49E-04
cg21208104	PRSS12	0.697	6.26E-04
cg23566335	ADAM18	0.696	6.47E-04
cg22892904	CBX2	−0.688	7.82E-04
cg04283938	SEPT3	−0.684	8.59E-04
cg23886551	TMEM121	−0.684	8.59E-04
cg14299800	TOR1B	−0.682	9.13E-04

This table shows the results for the MZ discordance analysis. Results are listed for the ten most highly correlated probes with corresponding gene, Spearman rank correlation coefficient (rho) and significance of correlation (p-value).

epigenetic changes at a number of genes that were associated with hearing ability, and two of these changes in genes *TCF25* and *POLE* replicated in an independent sample. DNA methylation levels at the strongest signal in *TCF25* validated using an alternative method (MeDIPseq). Hearing PC1 was also strongly associated with DNA methylation at *FGFR1*, a gene known to be essential for maintenance of glial cells and cochlear neurons in the spiral ganglion [28]. These findings suggest that epigenetic changes may account for the variance in severity and age of onset of ARHI.

Nominally significant associations (p<0.05) with PC1, which represents the overall threshold shift in the pure-tone audiogram and hence impaired hearing ability, were identified at 2,519 CpG sites. The ten most highly associated probes remained nominally significant after exclusion of chronological age as a fixed effect in the model, showing that none of these associated probes are age-related differentially methylated probes. Furthermore association remained significant after adjustment for blood cell heterogeneity, indicating that blood cell subtypes were not driving these association signals. Two of the ten signals were replicated in a second independent sample. Changes in DNA methylation in the promoter region of *TCF25* were highly associated with PC1 in both the discovery EWAS and the replication cohort, with meta-analysis p = 4.89×10^{-9}. The meta-analysis of the discovery and replication sample was conducted to determine the joint effect of both samples; nevertheless the results of this analysis were driven primarily by the discovery EWAS findings.

As both the discovery and replication data used the same array design from Illumina based on DNA hybridisation an alternative technique, MeDIPseq, was used to validate our findings. MeDIPseq in venous blood from 46 unrelated samples confirmed the association between hearing PC1 and DNA methylation levels at *TCF25* (p = 0.04). This transcription factor belongs to the family of basic helix-loop-helix transcription factors, which is widely expressed in many organs including dorsal root ganglia in mouse embryos [29]; however mouse models of Tcf25 deficiency are not yet available. Over-expression of Tcf25 leads to increased cell death and binding to the X-linked inhibitor of apoptosis protein [30]. Using the ENCODE database [31], probe cg01161216 maps to an area with enhancer and promoter associated histone marks and transcription factor binding sites. Differential expression of *TCF25* might be involved in increased

cell death of sensory cells and neurons of the cochlea, resulting in ARHI.

We also identified a differentially methylated DNA methylation probe mapping to the promoter of the *POLE* gene. *POLE* is a DNA polymerase essential for elongation of the leading strand in cell division. In addition, *POLE* is involved in cell cycle regulation and therefore regulates a variety of cellular processes. According to UCSC browser and the ENCODE database [31], probe cg18877514 maps to an area rich in repeating elements with enhancer and promoter associated histone marks and transcription factor binding sites. *Pole* knockout mice with a random gene disruption are embryonic lethal, while *Pole* targeted knock-in mice present with premature death due to cancer and increased tumourigenesis in general [32].

Among the top associations in the discovery EWAS was a DMR in the promoter of *FGFR1*, a gene known to be essential for maintenance of glial cells and cochlear neurons in the spiral ganglion [28]. However, our replication study did not confirm the differential methylation in the promoter of *FGFR1* identified in the discovery EWAS, but the DMR did manifest the same direction of effect. This gene is of particular interest, having been associated with hearing ability in mice [28]. *FGFR1* encodes a fibroblast growth factor receptor, reported to be essential for healthy development of the organ of Corti [33]. Conditional knockout of fibroblast growth factor receptors (*FGFR1* and *FGFR2*) in glial cells in the spiral ganglion resulted in loss of spiral ganglion neurons and age-related hearing loss in mice [28]. Our results show a negative association between DNA methylation at the promoter of *FGFR1* and hearing PC1 (beta = -0.24 ± 0.06 se), indicating that greater methylation (and expected reduced gene expression) of *FGFR1* showed good hearing ability. This direction of effect is not consistent with that observed in mouse cochlea [28].

DNA methylation in the promoter of genes has been associated with repression of gene expression. At our peak DMR in *TCF25*, DNA methylation was found minimally negatively correlated with gene expression in skin (r = −0.02; *POLE*: r = −0.06) – the tissue with the most embryologic similarity to cochlea. However, DNA methylation may be highly tissue specific [34,35] and in this study DNA methylation was determined from whole blood samples. That gene expression in skin showed a weak positive correlation with hearing PC1 for both *TCF25* (r = 0.12) and *POLE* (r = 0.16),

A

DNA methylation at cg01161216 versus TCF25 expression in skin

B

DNA methylation at cg18877514 versus POLE expression in skin

C

TCF25 expression in skin versus PC1

D

POLE expression in skin versus PC1

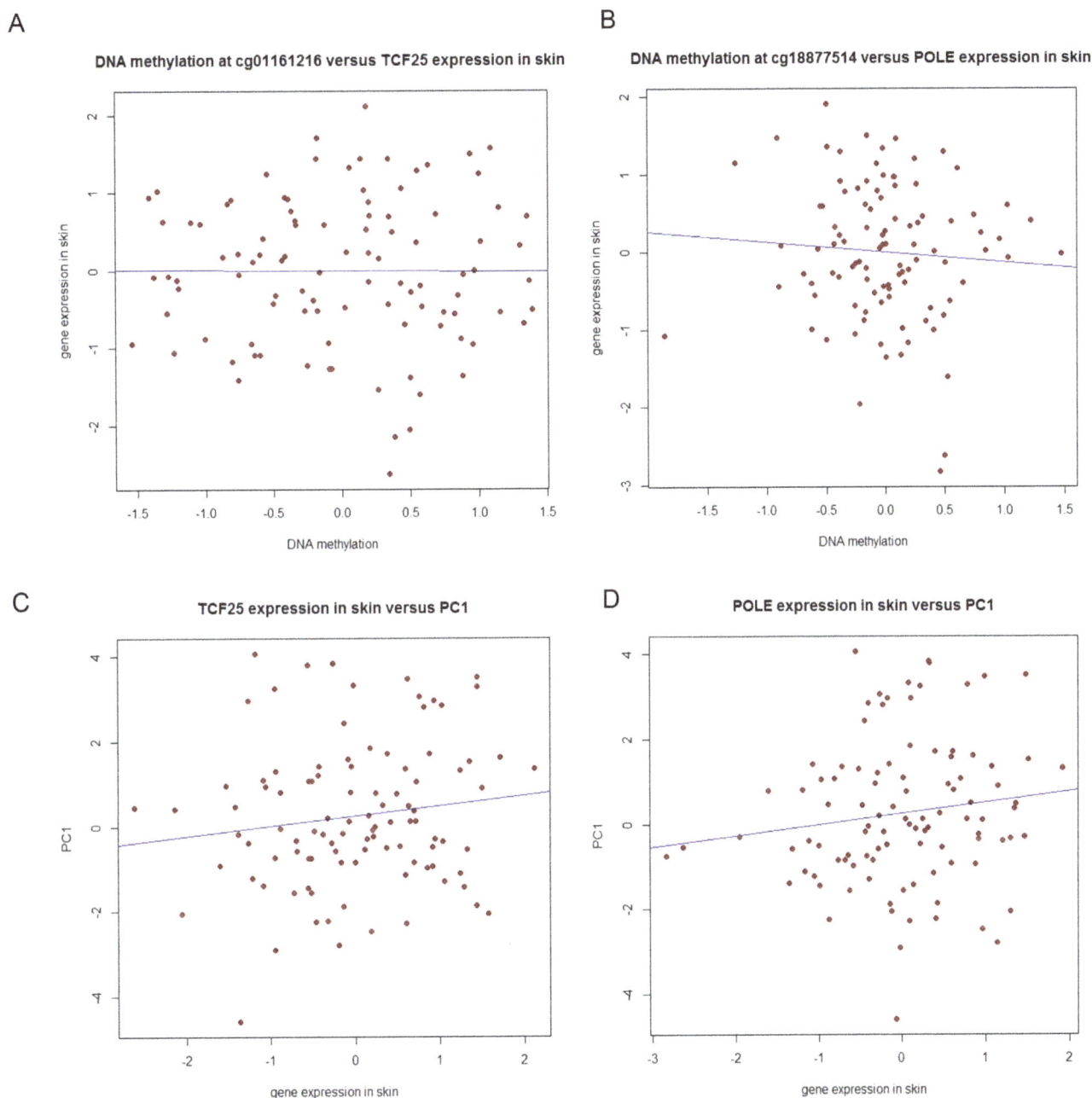

Figure 4. Effect of DNA methylation on gene expression in skin and effect of gene expression on PC1. A. DNA methylation residuals showed a weak negative correlation ($r = -0.02$) with expression residuals of TCF25 in skin samples. Both quantile normalised DNA methylation betas and quantile normalised gene expression values were adjusted for experimental batch effects (chip and position on the chip for methylation betas and experimental batch and RNA concentration for gene expression profiles) previous to analysis. The regression line (blue line) depicts the linear association between DNA methylation residuals and gene expression residuals. **B**. DNA methylation residuals at probe cg18877514 were weakly negatively correlated ($r = -0.06$) with *POLE* expression residuals in skin tissue. Both quantile normalised DNA methylation betas and quantile normalised gene expression values were adjusted for experimental batch effects (chip and position on the chip for methylation betas and experimental batch and RNA concentration for gene expression profiles) prior to analysis. The regression line (blue line) depicts the linear association between DNA methylation residuals and gene expression residuals. **C**. *TCF25* expression residuals in skin showed a weak positive correlation ($r = 0.12$) with PC1. Quantile normalised gene expression values were adjusted for experimental batch effects and RNA concentration. The regression line (blue line) depicts the linear association between gene expression residuals and PC1 values. **D**. *POLE* expression residuals in skin showed a weak positive correlation ($r = 0.16$) with PC1. Quantile normalised gene expression values were adjusted for experimental batch effects and RNA concentration. The regression line (blue line) depicts the linear association between gene expression residuals and PC1 values.

indicates that individuals with decreased hearing ability (high PC1 value) show higher RNA levels of *TCF25* and *POLE* in skin. Whether these findings pertain to RNA expression in the inner ear remains to be determined.

Monozygotic twin pairs are a preferred study sample for epigenetic studies as they are assumed to be genetically identical. In addition, both dizygotic and monozygotic twin pairs show an increased proportion of shared environment due to the nature of their time shared in uterus and upbringing. The MZ discordance analysis was performed to best utilise the unique study sample presented here and for completeness. Nevertheless, the relatively low sample size and restricted discordance within the twin pairs limited the statistical power to detect strong epigenetic effects. Association was examined between intra-pair discordance for PC1 and intra-pair differences in DNA methylation at CpG sites genome-wide. The most highly associated probes were found in the promoters of *ACP6* and *MEF2D*. The function of acid phosphatase 6 is yet unknown and *Acp6* knockout mice are described as phenotypically normal [32]. In contrast, myocyte enhancer factor 2D is a member of the myocyte enhancer factor family of transcription factors, which are involved in neuronal development and differentiation under regulation of class 2 histone deacetylases. *MEF2D* is expressed in mouse cochlear neurons and sensory cells at P15 and was diminished in IGF knockout mice, which show sensorineural hearing loss [36]. The data indicate that *MEF2D* is a plausible candidate gene for ARHI and may be under epigenetic control.

Our study has several strengths and limitations. DNA methylation is likely to play an important role in gene expression contributing to important phenotypic differences between tissues, between individuals and with age. Methods of analysis of methylation data are in their infancy: there are many important covariates to be considered. We elected to remove one of these, gender, by confining our studies to females, which predominate in the TwinsUK database. Thus our results pertain to women and may not extrapolate to men. Strengths included ability to exclude age and blood cell heterogeneity as potential confounders. The high proportion of related individuals in this sample reduced both the genetic and environmental variance compared to a population sample of unrelated individuals. Although the discovery and replication datasets were well matched for gender, ethnicity, age and hearing ability, the replication sample included by chance a higher proportion of monozygotic twin pairs (450 k sample: 60% MZs) compared to the discovery sample (27 k sample: 37% MZs), which might have resulted in the reduced significance of associations obtained in the replication sample. Association in the EWAS did not reach epigenome-wide significance by Bonferroni corrected significance levels (considering 24,641 independent tests: $p \leq 2.03 \times 10^{-6}$). However, DNA methylation of neighbouring CpG sites is unlikely to be independent thus a Bonferroni correction may be considered overly stringent. Taking co-methylation into account by correcting for the number of genes, the peak DMR in *TCF25* surpassed genome-wide suggestive evidence for association. Further limitations of the study included the choice of tissue: although DNA methylation is tissue specific, whole blood samples were used as an initial approach to this investigation because they were readily available and inner ear tissue from humans was not. In addition, discordance in hearing ability within TwinsUK monozygotic twin pairs was relatively limited. Finally, it should be noted that this study makes no assumptions about causal relationships between DNA methylation and ARHI. A longitudinal study design would

be required to confirm that the methylation changes inferred by these results predated the onset of hearing impairment.

In conclusion, this is the first study investigating the association between hearing ability with age and DNA methylation genome-wide in humans. Strong associations with DNA methylation in the promoters of 10 genes were identified, of which two (*TCF25* and *POLE*) were replicated in an independent cohort. Functional studies will be required to explore further the effect of epigenetic regulation of these genes in ARHI. Proof of epigenetic regulation in the development of ARHI would highlight the impact of changes in DNA methylation with age and therefore be of fundamental importance not only for hearing loss but also other age-related disorders.

Supporting Information

Data S1 Replication study dataset (450 k). The replication study dataset shows DNA methylation betas at the 10 probes selected for replication from the Illumina HumanMethylation 450 k Beadchip for all subjects of the replication study (n = 203). Each subject has been allocated an anonymous identification number (PUBLIC.ID) and is presented by a family-identification number to identify twin siblings (family_zygosity), the age at hearing test (Age_pta), their hearing PC1 value (PC1_unadjusted), gender (SEX), age at DNA extraction (DNA_age), bisulfite conversion values (BSCng_ul), DNA methylation chip and order on the chip (chip and chipo, respectively).

Figure S1 Association of hearing PC1 values and DNA methylation residuals at *TCF25* (cg01161216) and *POLE* (cg18877514). **A, B** Hearing PC1 values were plotted versus DNA methylation beta residuals (adjusted for age, batch effects and relatedness) for both the discovery (27 k, red dots) and the replication (450 k, blue dots) samples. A linear regression lines was fitted for both datasets (27 k:red line, 450 k:blue line).

Acknowledgments

This work was funded by Action on Hearing Loss and AgeUK.

The authors would like to thank all volunteers from the TwinsUK register, who contributed to this study and acknowledge the work of all researchers who helped in the completion of this work. The study was funded by the Wellcome Trust; European Community's Seventh Framework Programme (FP7/2007–2013). The study also receives support from the National Institute for Health Research (NIHR) BioResource Clinical Research Facility and Biomedical Research Centre based at Guy's and St Thomas' NHS Foundation Trust and King's College London. Tim Spector is holder of an ERC Advanced Principal Investigator award.

Author Contributions

Conceived and designed the experiments: LEW JTB FMKW PT CJS. Performed the experiments: LEW PT CJS. Analyzed the data: LEW. Contributed reagents/materials/analysis tools: PD TDS CJS. Wrote the paper: LEW.

References

1. Waddington CH (2012) The Epigenotype. International Journal of Epidemiology 41: 10–13.
2. Bird AP (1986) CpG-rich islands and the function of DNA methylation. Nature 321: 209.
3. Holliday R (1990) MECHANISMS FOR THE CONTROL OF GENE ACTIVITY DURING DEVELOPMENT. Biological Reviews 65: 431–471.
4. Fraga MF, Ballestar E, Paz MF, Ropero S, Setien F, et al. (2005) Epigenetic differences arise during the lifetime of monozygotic twins. Proceedings of the National Academy of Sciences of the United States of America 102: 10604–10609.
5. Rakyan VK, Down TA, Balding DJ, Beck S (2011) Epigenome-wide association studies for common human diseases. Nat Rev Genet 12: 529–541.
6. Okano M, Bell DW, Haber DA, Li E (1999) DNA Methyltransferases Dnmt3a and Dnmt3b Are Essential for De Novo Methylation and Mammalian Development. Cell 99: 247–257.
7. Bestor TH (2000) The DNA methyltransferases of mammals. Human Molecular Genetics 9: 2395–2402.
8. Wong CCY, Caspi A, Williams B, Craig IW, Houts R, et al. (2010) A longitudinal study of epigenetic variation in twins. Epigenetics 5: 516–526.

9. Bell JT, Pai AA, Pickrell JK, Gaffney DJ, Pique-Regi R, et al. (2011) DNA methylation patterns associate with genetic and gene expression variation in HapMap cell lines. Genome Biol 12: R10.

10. Bell JT, Spector TD (2011) A twin approach to unraveling epigenetics. Trends in Genetics 27: 116–125.

11. Bell JT, Tsai P-C, Yang T-P, Pidsley R, Nisbet J, et al. (2012) Epigenome-Wide Scans Identify Differentially Methylated Regions for Age and Age-Related Phenotypes in a Healthy Ageing Population. PLoS Genet 8: e1002629.

12. Dempster EL, Pidsley R, Schalkwyk LC, Owens S, Georgiades A, et al. (2011) Disease-associated epigenetic changes in monozygotic twins discordant for schizophrenia and bipolar disorder. Human Molecular Genetics 20: 4786–4796.

13. Rakyan VK, Down TA, Maslau S, Andrew T, Yang T-P, et al. (2010) Human aging-associated DNA hypermethylation occurs preferentially at bivalent chromatin domains. Genome Research 20: 434–439.

14. Cruickshanks KJ, Wiley TL, Tweed TS, Klein BE, Klein R, et al. (1998) Prevalence of hearing loss in older adults in Beaver Dam, Wisconsin. The Epidemiology of Hearing Loss Study. Am J Epidemiol 148: 879–886.

15. Provenzano MJ, Domann FE (2007) A role for epigenetics in hearing: Establishment and maintenance of auditory specific gene expression patterns. Hearing Research 233: 1–13.

16. Friedman L, Avraham K (2009) MicroRNAs and epigenetic regulation in the mammalian inner ear: implications for deafness. Mammalian Genome 20: 581–603.

17. Wilkin DJ, Liberfarb R, Davis J, Levy HP, Cole WG, et al. (2000) Rapid determination of COL2A1 mutations in individuals with Stickler syndrome: analysis of potential premature termination codons. American Journal of Medical Genetics 94: 141–148.

18. Donoso LA, Edwards AO, Frost AT, Ritter R, Ahmad N, et al. (2003) Clinical variability of Stickler syndrome: role of exon 2 of the collagen COL2A1 gene. Survey of ophthalmology 48: 191–203.

19. Buschdorf JP, Strätling WH (2004) A WW domain binding region in methyl-CpG-binding protein MeCP2: impact on Rett syndrome. Journal of Molecular Medicine 82: 135–143.

20. BSA (2011) Recommende Procedure Pure-tone air-conduction and bone-conduction threshold audiometry with and without masking. Reading: British Society of audiology.

21. Bibikova M, Le J, Barnes B, Saedinia-Melnyk S, Zhou L, et al. (2009) Genome-wide DNA methylation profiling using Infinium assay. Epigenomics 1: 177–200.

22. Bibikova M, Barnes B, Tsan C, Ho V, Klotzle B, et al. (2011) High density DNA methylation array with single CpG site resolution. Genomics 98: 288–295.

23. Willer CJ, Li Y, Abecasis GR (2010) METAL: fast and efficient meta-analysis of genomewide association scans. Bioinformatics 26: 2190–2191.

24. Bell JT, Loomis AK, Butcher LM, Gao F, Zhang B, et al. (2014) Differential methylation of the TRPA1 promoter in pain sensitivity. Nat Commun 5.

25. Horvath S, Zhang Y, Langfelder P, Kahn RS, Boks MP, et al. (2012) Aging effects on DNA methylation modules in human brain and blood tissue. Genome Biol 13: R97.

26. Grundberg E, Small KS, Hedman AK, Nica AC, Buil A, et al. (2012) Mapping cis- and trans-regulatory effects across multiple tissues in twins. Nat Genet 44: 1084–1089.

27. Huyghe JR, Van Laer L, Hendrickx JJ, Fransen E, Demeester K, et al. (2008) Genome-wide SNP-based linkage scan identifies a locus on 8q24 for an age-related hearing impairment trait. Am J Hum Genet 83: 401–407.

28. Wang SJ, Furusho M, D'Sa C, Kuwada S, Conti L, et al. (2009) Inactivation of fibroblast growth factor receptor signaling in myelinating glial cells results in significant loss of adult spiral ganglion neurons accompanied by age-related hearing impairment. Journal of Neuroscience Research 87: 3428–3437.

29. Olsson M, Durbeej M, Ekblom P, Hjalt T (2002) Nulp1, a novel basic helix-loop-helix protein expressed broadly during early embryonic organogenesis and prominently in developing dorsal root ganglia. Cell and Tissue Research 308: 361–370.

30. Steen H, Lindholm D (2008) Nuclear localized protein-1 (Nulp1) increases cell death of human osteosarcoma cells and binds the X-linked inhibitor of apoptosis protein. Biochemical and Biophysical Research Communications 366: 432–437.

31. Rosenbloom KR, Sloan CA, Malladi VS, Dreszer TR, Learned K, et al. (2013) ENCODE Data in the UCSC Genome Browser: year 5 update. Nucleic Acids Research 41: D56–D63.

32. Eppig JT, Blake JA, Bult CJ, Kadin JA, Richardson JE (2012) The Mouse Genome Database (MGD): comprehensive resource for genetics and genomics of the laboratory mouse. Nucleic Acids Research 40: D881–D886.

33. Pirvola U, Ylikoski J, Trokovic R, Hébert JM, McConnell SK, et al. (2002) FGFR1 Is Required for the Development of the Auditory Sensory Epithelium. Neuron 35: 671–680.

34. Byun H-M, Siegmund KD, Pan F, Weisenberger DJ, Kanel G, et al. (2009) Epigenetic profiling of somatic tissues from human autopsy specimens identifies tissue-and individual-specific DNA methylation patterns. Human Molecular Genetics 18: 4808–4817.

35. Ladd-Acosta C, Pevsner J, Sabunciyan S, Yolken RH, Webster MJ, et al. (2007) DNA methylation signatures within the human brain. The American Journal of Human Genetics 81: 1304–1315.

36. Sanchez-Calderon H, Rodriguez-de La Rosa L, Milo M, Pichel JG, Holley M, et al. (2010) RNA microarray analysis in prenatal mouse cochlea reveals novel IGF-I target genes: implication of MEF2 and FOXM1 transcription factors. PLoS One 5: e8699.

23

Induction of Enhanced Acoustic Startle Response by Noise Exposure: Dependence on Exposure Conditions and Testing Parameters and Possible Relevance to Hyperacusis

Rony H. Salloum[1], Christopher Yurosko[1], Lia Santiago[2], Sharon A. Sandridge[2], James A. Kaltenbach[1,2]*

1 Department of Neurosciences, The Cleveland Clinic, Cleveland, Ohio, United States of America, **2** Head and Neck Institute, The Cleveland Clinic, Cleveland, Ohio, United States of America

Abstract

There has been a recent surge of interest in the development of animal models of hyperacusis, a condition in which tolerance to sounds of moderate and high intensities is diminished. The reasons for this decreased tolerance are likely multifactorial, but some major factors that contribute to hyperacusis are increased loudness perception and heightened sensitivity and/or responsiveness to sound. Increased sound sensitivity is a symptom that sometimes develops in human subjects after acoustic insult and has recently been demonstrated in animals as evidenced by enhancement of the acoustic startle reflex following acoustic over-exposure. However, different laboratories have obtained conflicting results in this regard, with some studies reporting enhanced startle, others reporting weakened startle, and still others reporting little, if any, change in the amplitude of the acoustic startle reflex following noise exposure. In an effort to gain insight into these discrepancies, we conducted measures of acoustic startle responses (ASR) in animals exposed to different levels of sound, and repeated such measures on consecutive days using a range of different startle stimuli. Since many studies combine measures of acoustic startle with measures of gap detection, we also tested ASR in two different acoustic contexts, one in which the startle amplitudes were tested in isolation, the other in which startle amplitudes were measured in the context of the gap detection test. The results reveal that the emergence of chronic hyperacusis-like enhancements of startle following noise exposure is highly reproducible but is dependent on the post-exposure thresholds, the time when the measures are performed and the context in which the ASR measures are obtained. These findings could explain many of the discrepancies that exist across studies and suggest guidelines for inducing in animals enhancements of the startle reflex that may be related to hyperacusis.

Editor: Fan-Gang Zeng, University of California, Irvine, United States of America

Funding: This work was funded by National Institutes of Health Grant # DC R01-009097 to JK. The funders had no role in study design, data collection and analysis, decision to publish, or preparation of the manuscript.

Competing Interests: The authors have declared that no competing interests exist.

* Email: kaltenj@ccf.org

Introduction

Hyperacusis is a condition characterized by a heightened sensitivity to sounds and manifesting as diminished sound tolerance [1–4], but can include increased loudness perception or increased responsiveness to sound [5]. Hyperacusis is a common result of acoustic trauma and is frequently seen in association with tinnitus. The incidence of hyperacusis in the general population is unknown, but estimates range from 1 to 22% [6–8]. A large percentage (40–80%) of subjects with tinnitus also suffer from hyperacusis [1,3,9,10]. Like tinnitus, hyperacusis occurs in acute and chronic forms. Acute hyperacusis is experienced for short periods ranging from minutes to weeks, while chronic hyperacusis lasts many weeks, months or years. These different clinical features suggest that the mechanisms underlying hyperacusis may be complex and may share some characteristics with those underlying tinnitus. However, the ability

to test this hypothesis and separate those that are linked to tinnitus and those linked to hyperacusis requires the development of well-defined animal models of hyperacusis in its acute and chronic forms.

A growing number of studies have demonstrated induction of acute or chronic increases in responsiveness to sound that could be related to hyperacusis. Ison and colleagues found that mice show an augmentation of the acoustic startle reflex (ASR) with age [11]. Turner and Parrish [12] reported that the suppression of the ASR by a preceding pulse of sound (pre-pulse inhibition) was enhanced in rats treated with sodium salicylate, a finding which they interpreted as suggestive of hyperacusis. Two studies from the laboratory of Sun [13,14] found evidence for acute enhancements of the acoustic startle response (ASR) in rats treated with sodium salicylate. Subsequently, a transient strengthening of pre-pulse inhibition was also found in mice that had been exposed to intense noise [15]. Sun and colleagues [16] observed transient enhancements of the ASR in rats previously exposed to noise, while Dehmel et al. [17] found chronic enhancements of absolute startle amplitude and enhanced pre-pulse inhibition in noise-exposed guinea pigs. Thus, aging, salicylate treatment and noise exposure all appear to be factors that can trigger induction of heightened responsiveness to sound, although in most cases, the changes were found to be weak and very transient.

Recently, our laboratory showed that exposure to intense sound can lead to the induction of robust and long lasting enhancements of the ASR [18]. The enhancements were observed in the range of weeks to months following sound exposure and were associated with enhancements of noise-induced suppression of startle. Qualitatively similar chronic enhancements of the ASR and prepulse inhibition were observed in mice following moderate sound exposure [19], and such changes were found to be associated with cochlear neuropathy [20]. However, the results across studies have not always been consistent. While the study by Hickox and Liberman [19] showed enhancements of startle when the startle stimulus was immediately preceded by continuous background noise, only a slight suggestion of enhanced startle was observed when the startle stimulus was presented without background noise. Moreover, some studies have reported noise-induced changes in auditory responses that are not consistent with the above described enhancements of startle. Longenecker and Galazyuk [21] presented data showing little if any change in the ASR in noise exposed mice at or slightly above startle threshold, and startle amplitudes at moderate to high levels of startle stimulation were lower than control levels. Similarly, the data of Lobarinas et al. [22] showed a consistent weakening of startle amplitude at almost all startle stimulus levels above startle thresholds.

The different effects of noise exposure on the acoustic startle reflex across studies raise the question of what factors might be critical in determining whether a noise exposure condition or a condition of testing leads to enhancement of startle responses. In an effort to gain insight into these issues, we explored in depth how the acoustic startle response changes with variations in a number of different parameters. In particular, we sought to determine whether the induction of such enhancements is dependent on the intensity of exposure, and if so, what the optimal exposure condition might be to maximally induce enhanced startle responses. In order to understand the temporal nature of enhanced startle, we measured ASR at different post-exposure recovery times. Finally, we tested whether the changes in ASR might depend on the context of the measures. In particular, we examined the effect of performing ASR measures alone or in the context of the gap detection test. Our results suggest that all of these parameters are critical in determining whether enhancements of the ASR are induced and readily observable following sound exposure.

Methods

Ethical considerations

Animal work was performed using practices fully compliant with the NIH guidelines for the care and use of animals in research. Animals were lightly anesthetized by intramuscular injection of ketamine/xylazine (58 mg/kg- 9 mg/kg) for the measurements of Auditory Brainstem Responses. The animal handling protocol (#2013 1151) was approved by the Institutional Animal Care and Use Committee (IACUC) of the Cleveland Clinic.

Animal subjects

Adult hamsters (LVG strain), 60–70 days of age at the time of arrival were maintained on a 12:12-h day/night cycle by the animal housing facility of the Cleveland Clinic. After a 4-day quarantine period, they were divided into two groups, including an experimental group to be sound exposed, and a control group of unexposed animals. For each experiment, the exposed group was subdivided to allow testing of different variables. Exposures generally were conducted when the animals were between 2 and 3 months of age, except when noted otherwise. ASR tests were conducted beginning on each of the first three days after exposure, then every 2–3 days thereafter over an approximately 2 week period. ABRs were conducted upon completion of ASR tests.

Sound exposure

The animals were exposed to sounds inside a cylindrical chamber placed inside an Acoustic Systems sound attenuation booth. The chamber contained 4 compartments, allowing exposure of up to 4 animals simultaneously. Sound was introduced into the chamber through a Beyma CP-25 speaker mounted in the lid of the cylinder. The exposure sound was a 10 kHz continuous tone, calibrated using an Etymotic ER7C probe tube microphone whose tip was placed 2 cm above the chamber's floor to approximate the position where the animals ears would be located during the exposure. Since sound level varied when measurements were taken at different locations on the floor of the chamber, we chose a voltage input to the speaker that produced the desired sound level when averaged across those locations. Animals were allowed a few minutes of silence once placed inside the chamber to permit acclimatization to the exposure environment. The sound was then turned on and gradually increased in level over a 10 minute period before reaching the final exposure intensity. This approach was found to protect the animals from stress caused by sudden onset of intense sound. The exposure sound was delivered continuously for 4 hours. Behavior was monitored throughout the exposure period to ensure that the animals did not later develop behaviors indicative of stress. Exposures were performed in three different rounds, each differing in intensity level. Animals were exposed at 110 dB SPL in the first round, 115 dB SPL in the second, and at 120 dB SPL in the third. In each round, 5–8 animals were exposed to the tone, while 5–7 others were placed in the exposure chamber for a 4 hour period of silence and served as controls. Following the exposures the animals were returned to the animal facility. The acoustic startle reflex measurements began the following day in each trial.

Acoustic startle apparatus

Measures of acoustic startle were recorded as in our previous publication [18]. The testing apparatus consisted of a Kinder Scientific startle system (Model SM100) consisting of a small chamber measuring $28 \times 36 \times 50$ cm and containing a small animal housing designed for use with rats. The chamber was insulated with a 1 inch layer of dense foam material to reduce sound reflections [21]. Each animal was placed inside the housing on top of a plate that contained a pressure-sensitive piezoelectric transducer that converted sudden pressure changes caused by animal movement into voltages that were scaled to pressure units (Newtons, N). The plate sensitivity was adjusted to generate a 1 ± 0.05 N on the first positive peak of the pressure pulse waveform in response to a 1.0 N calibration wave. Calibration of the sound level at the level of the animals' ears was performed using a 1/4 in microphone and sound measurement system (B&K). Startle stimuli (and where applicable, stimuli used for the gap detection test) were introduced from speakers located in the ceiling of the test chamber. Inputs and measurements were controlled using Kinder software, with startle response collection windows spanning 100 ms from startle stimulus onset. Animals were weighed before ASR measurements to account for the potential contribution of weight differences to the startle amplitudes.

Acoustic stimuli

Testing was performed by quantifying the startle amplitude as a function of the startle stimulus level. For that purpose, each startle measuring session consisted of five sets of 15 trials, each having a battery of twelve 20-ms bursts of broad band noise varied in level from 57–120 dB SPL in steps of 3–6 dB, plus three no-stimulus trials. The order of these stimuli and the duration of inter-trial intervals were randomized. The same session was repeated daily for each of the animal subgroups, so that all exposed and control animals were alternately tested on the same day.

Because the ASR is known to be sensitive to the presence of background noise [23–26], we tested whether ASR amplitudes might differ significantly depending on the context in which the startle stimuli were presented. In this experiment, startle eliciting stimuli were presented in two different ways. In the first method, ASRs were tested using a stimulus battery that included only startle-eliciting noise bursts presented randomly at different levels (Fig. 1A). In the second, ASRs were measured using the same startle-eliciting noise bursts that were used in the first method, except that these stimuli were inserted randomly in a battery of stimuli used to measure gap detection ability; this stimulus battery thus included startle eliciting stimuli preceded by background noise (with or without gaps of silence) as well as startle eliciting noise bursts not preceded by background noise (Fig. 1B). This experiment design allowed us to address the question of whether the startle amplitude evoked by identical stimuli (noise bursts) differs depending on the acoustic context (i.e., the presence or absence of a recent history of background noise in the test battery).

Auditory brainstem responses (ABRs)

ABRs were recorded once behavioral testing was completed to assess the extent of hearing loss caused by sound exposure. This was generally a period of 3 to 5 weeks postexposure, but always

just after the last ASR measurement. Each animal was lightly anesthetized by intramuscular injection of ketamine/xylazine (58 mg/kg- 9 mg/kg). Temperature was maintained at 37°C throughout the period of ABR testing. Needle electrodes were placed subcutaneously, one in in the vertex (non-inverting), one each behind the ears (inverting), and one in the right hind limb (ground). Electrode signals were amplified 100,000X and bandpass filtered (30–3000 Hz). Stimuli were tone pips varied in frequency from 4 to 16 kHz and presented at a rate of 17.7/s. The pips were presented at the highest levels (80–100 dB SPL) first then lowered in 20 dB steps until no responses were visible. At each level, responses were averaged over 250 stimulus repetitions. Two responses were obtained at each stimulus level to confirm presence or absence of a response. Intensity was bracketed in 5 dB steps in the range of the lowest levels of stimulation to determine threshold. ABR waveforms displayed 5–6 biphasic responses, and thresholds were based on measures of P4 or P5, whichever gave the lower threshold.

Data analysis

Measures of startle amplitude were averaged for each animal, first across trials for each session then across sessions conducted on successive days. These were then averaged across animals for each of the stimulus levels tested. The result was a plot of startle amplitude vs. stimulus level for each animal. The mean startle amplitude vs. stimulus level (startle growth curve) was then obtained for each group by averaging across animals for each exposure or control group. Although control and exposed animals were age-matched, differences between growth curves in exposed and control animals could be due to group differences in mean weight. To control for this possibility, we averaged the weights across sessions to obtain a mean weight for each animal. Group weights were obtained by averaging the mean weights of all animals within each group. Group differences for all parameters of stimulation tested and for weights were tested using two-way ANOVAs or paired t-tests (one- or two-tailed), performed using Prism Graphpad. Differences between groups for each pairwise comparison were considered significant if $P \leq 0.05$.

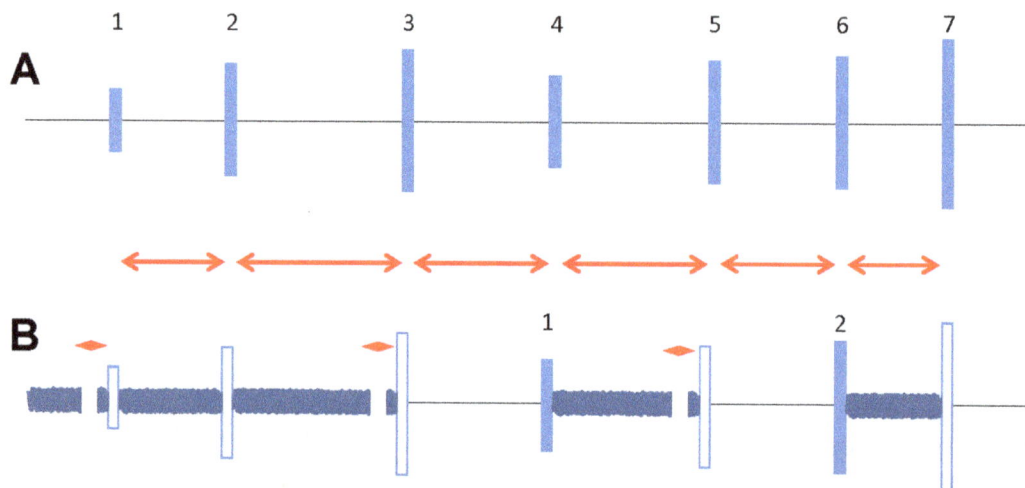

Figure 1. Stimulus sequences used to test the effect of acoustic context on ASR. Startle stimuli of different intensities (blue blocks) are presented as bursts separated by different time intervals (red double-headed arrows). In the first context (A), silence is maintained during the inter-stimulus interval (black lines) throughout the test battery. In the second context (B), a background noise, with or without an intervening gap of silence, fills some of the inter-stimulus intervals, but the startle stimulus only condition is identical to that in context 1. In either context, numbered solid blue block are those used to determine the ASR. Red diamond: time interval during which the background noise is interrupted by a gap.

Results

Effect of exposure intensity on response thresholds

In order to assess the impact of sound exposure on hearing function, we first compared mean ABR thresholds in animals exposed at each of the three levels of sound (110, 115 and 120 dB SPL) with those of control animals (Fig. 2A–C). Mean thresholds in control animals varied somewhat across frequencies but ranged between 18 and 33 dB SPL, which proved to be insignificant when comparing across the three control groups ($F_{2,55} = 2.32$, $P = 0.11$)(Fig. 2A–C, open circles). The mean threshold in exposed animals varied between 33 and 93 dB, increasing approximately linearly with the level of exposure at all frequencies ($R = 0.72$, $P = 0.0007$). The thresholds in exposed animals were significantly higher than those in their respective control groups in all three exposure level comparisons ($F_{1,31} = 53.64$, $P < 0.0001$ for the 110 dB SPL exposure group, $F_{1,35} = 50.08$, $P < 0.0001$ for the 115 dB SPL exposure group, and $F_{1,51} = 165.3$, $P < 0.001$ for the 120 dB SPL exposure group). Maximal threshold shifts in exposed animals were consistently at 8 and 12 kHz and measured 36–38 dB, 49–52 dB and 60–76 dB for the 110, 115 and 120 dB SPL exposure groups, respectively (Fig. 2D–F). The number of frequencies at which significant threshold shifts occurred, as well as the extent of the shift, also increased with exposure level: 8 and 12 kHz in the 110 dB SPL group ($P = 0.007$ and 0.04, respectively), 8 and 12 kHz in the 115 dB SPL exposure group ($P = 0.006$ for both), and all four test frequencies (4, 8, 12 and 16 kHz) in the 120 dB SPL group (P values, 0.003, 0.0006, 0.0004 and 0.01, respectively). Thus, both the degree of threshold shift and the spectral range of these shifts increased with the level of exposure.

Effect of post-exposure recovery time on ASR

Changes in the amplitudes of the ASR displayed considerable plasticity and rebound following tone exposure. The period of most dynamic change was the first few days following exposure, but additional quantitative changes continued through the remainder of the 3 or more weeks of measurements. The mean ASR growth curves for animals exposed at 115 dB SPL are shown in Fig. 3. Here, startle amplitudes can be seen to be either similar to or slightly diminished below control levels during the first 2 days following exposure (Fig. 3A–B). However, between 4 and 8 days post-exposure, a trend towards enhanced startle amplitudes were clearly evident at high levels of stimulation (Fig. 3C–D), and these enhancements continued to be apparent, albeit with some fluctuation, throughout the period of testing (Fig. 3E–G). The startle enhancements observed 1 week following exposure are similar to those described in our previous paper, which was based on a different set of animals [18], but the time series of Fig. 3 shows for the first time that the enhancement was a secondary effect that took several days to develop, suggesting the involvement of plastic mechanisms that are triggered by the initial insult.

ASR enhancements of the type shown in Fig. 3 were characteristic of most animals exposed at 115 dB SPL and some animals exposed at 110 dB SPL (Fig. 4, top and middle rows), although the precise details varied somewhat in the absolute amplitudes of startle and in the time course of the changes. When the data were averaged across animals on days 7–9 post-exposure, those exposed at 110 showed a trend suggestive of startle enhancements at high startle stimulus levels (≥ 105 dB SPL) ($F_{3,72} = 6.21$, $P = 0.01$), but the enhancement was significant only at a startle stimulus level of 110 dB SPL ($T_9 = 1.83$, $P = 0.05$) (Fig. 4B). However, in the animals exposed at 115 dB SPL, the increases in ASR amplitude were highly significant at all stimulus

levels from 105–120 dB SPL (Fig. 4D) ($F_{3,80} = 38.57$, $P < 0.0001$) and followed an initial period when startle responses were decreased below control levels (Fig. 4C). Post hoc t tests yielded P values no higher than 0.01 ($= 2.55$, $P < 0.01$ at 105 dB SPL, $T_9 = 2.63$, $P < 0.01$ at 110 dB SPL, $T_9 = 3.38$, $P < 0.005$ at 115 dB SPL and $T_9 = 4.83$, $P < 0.001$ at 120 dB SPL).

An altogether different pattern of change was observed in animals exposed at 120 dB SPL. In that group, both startle responses and the baseline level of activity below the startle threshold were below those of controls; moreover, the initial weakening of ASR amplitude observed above startle threshold on the first and second day after exposure (Fig. 4E) persisted and became even more pronounced when the same measures were performed 7–9 days after exposure (Fig. 4F). The decreases in ASR amplitude in this group of exposed animals were pronounced when tested by two-way ANOVA ($F_{12,364} = 45.66$, $P < 0.001$), with significant differences found at all startle stimulus levels from 70 to 110 dB SPL (P values for points represented by asterisks in Fig. 4F ranged from 0.000007 at 93 dB SPL to 0.02 at 110 dB SPL). Thus, our results show that the effect of exposure on ASR growth curves is dependent not only on the level of the exposure but also on the intensity of the startle-eliciting stimulus and the time after exposure when the measures are performed. None of the changes in ASR amplitude could be attributed to difference in weight of the animals. As shown in Fig. 5, there were no significant differences between mean weights in exposed and control animals at the beginning ($T_4 = 1.05$, $P = 0.35$ for the 110 dB SPL group, $T_5 = 1.81$, $P = 0.13$ for the 115 dB SPL group, and $T_6 = 0.99$, $P = 0.36$ for the 120 dB SPL group) and end ($T_4 = 1.02$, $P = 0.37$ for the 110 dB SPL group, $T_5 = 1.13$, $P = 0.31$ for the 115 dB SPL group, and $T_6 = 0.33$, $P = 0.75$ for the 120 dB SPL group) of the ASR testing periods (Fig. 5A–B). Moreover, there was no significant difference between mean weights in exposed and control animals when averaged over time through the period of ASR testing ($T_4 = 0.85$, $P = 0.44$ for the 110 dB SPL group, $T_5 = 1.17$, $P = 0.29$ for the 115 dB SPL group, and $T_6 = 0.99$, $P = 0.36$ for the 120 dB SPL group) (Fig. 5C).

ASR amplitude and threshold shift

The data in Fig. 4 suggests a link between the magnitude of change in the ASR and exposure level, but they obscure the more important relationship of how the change in ASR relates to the post-exposure thresholds. To examine this relationship, we plotted the maximal ASR amplitude as a function of average threshold, irrespective of the level of sound to which the animals were exposed. The results in Fig. 6 show that the enhancement of startle was highly dependent on the loss in sound sensitivity, being limited to a narrow range of thresholds between 50 and 70 dB SPL. Below this range (30–50 dB SPL), startle amplitudes were comparable to control levels, but above this range (80–100 dB SPL), ASR amplitudes declined toward sub-control values with further increases in threshold. Thus, moderate threshold elevation restricted to a narrow range resulted in ASR enhancements, whereas severe threshold elevation resulted in a weakening of ASR.

Effect of acoustic context

The results of this experiment are shown in Fig. 7. Control animals showed context-dependent differences in startle amplitudes at the low and high startle stimulus levels (Fig. 7A). The exposed animals showed even more pronounced context-dependent differences, startle amplitudes being consistently lower in the context of the gap suppression test (context 2) than in the context of the startle growth curve test (context 1) (Fig. 7B); also, exposed

110 dB SPL   115 dB SPL   120 dB SPL

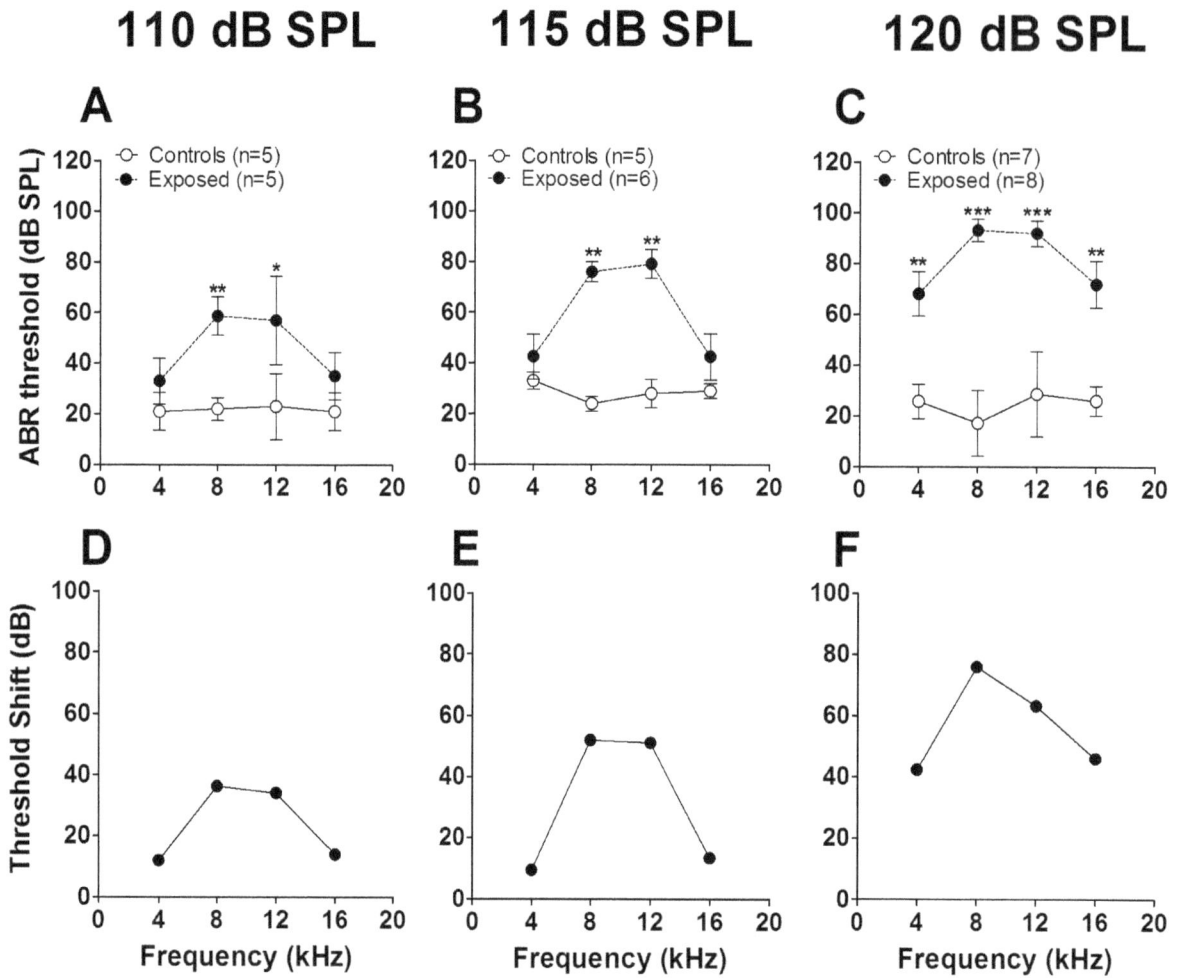

Figure 2. Effect of increasing the level of exposure on ABR thresholds. The exposure sound was a continuous 10 kHz tone presented for 4 hours at a level of 110 dB SPL (A), 115 dB SPL (B) or 120 dB SPL (C). Each point represents the mean (±S.E.M.) of ABR thresholds measured in 5–8 animals, upon completion of the ASR testing period. Results from A, B and C are represented as threshold shifts in D, E and F, respectively. *: p<0.05, **: p<0.01, ***: p<0.001.

animals showed a trend towards increasingly larger context-dependent differences with increases in stimulus level. Significantly weaker startle amplitudes were found in exposed animals at three of the four startle stimulus levels in context 2 than in context 1 ($F_{2,16} = 5.34$, P = 0.02 at 105 dB SPL, $F_{2,16} = 10.44$, P = 0.013 at

110 dB SPL and F = 13.03, P = 0.0004 at 115 dB SPL). Only in the condition where the startle stimulus level was 100 dB SPL were ASRs in exposed animals similar in the two contexts. Moreover, relative to controls, the significance of the enhancements of startle observed in exposed animals in context 1

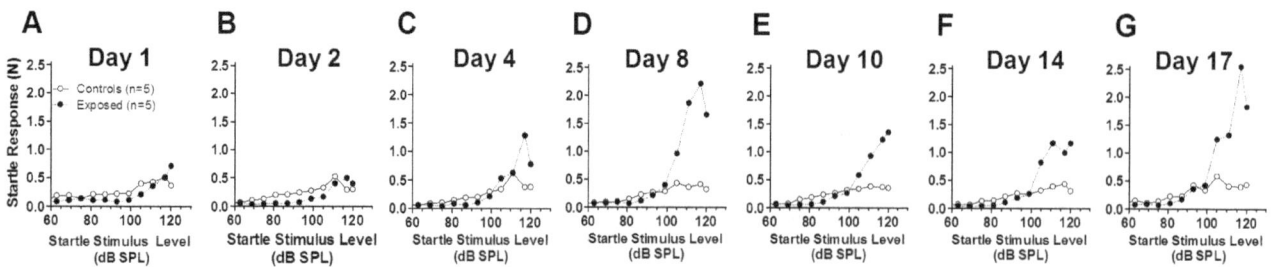

Figure 3. Comparison of the ASR growth curves from control (n = 5) and exposed animals (n = 6) at each of the 7 post-exposure times indicated at the top of each graph (panels A–G). The data shows decrements in ASR in exposed animals during the first two days post-exposure, but by the fourth day, there is a suggestion of enhanced ASR at the highest startle stimulus levels. This enhancement was better established by the 8th day at all stimulus levels above 100 dB SPL and continued through the remainder of the 2 weeks of measurements, although the degree of enhancement varied over time.

110 dB SPL Exposure level

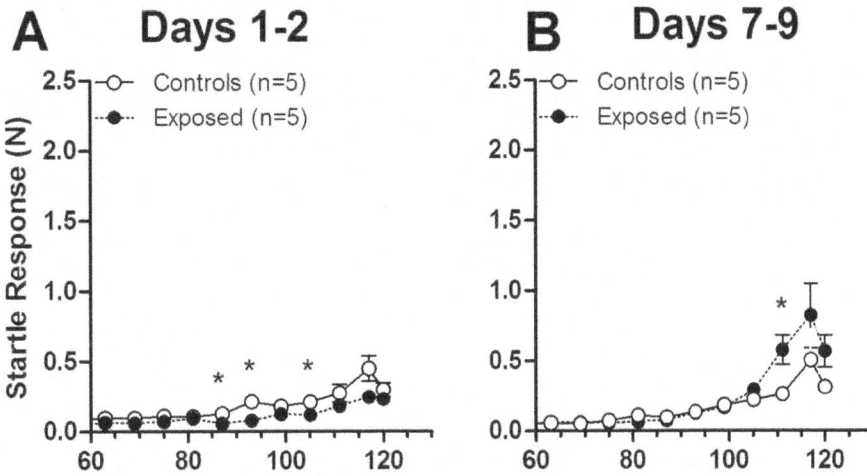

A   Days 1-2

Controls (n=5)
Exposed (n=5)

B   Days 7-9

Controls (n=5)
Exposed (n=5)

115 dB SPL Exposure level

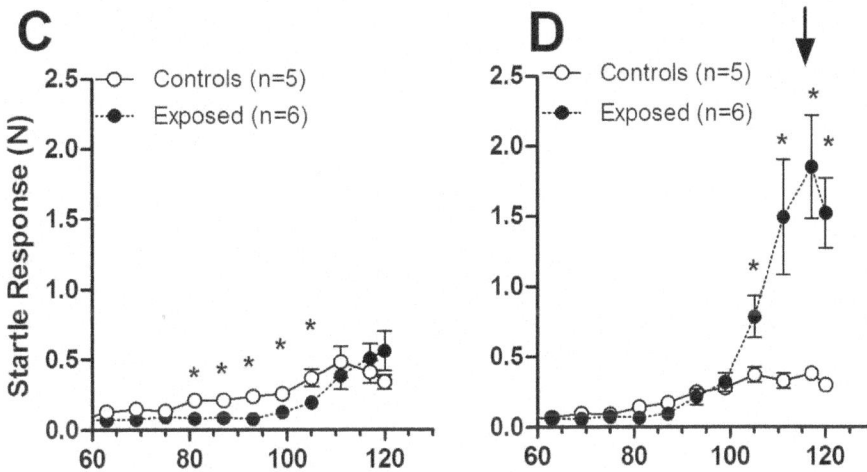

C

Controls (n=5)
Exposed (n=6)

D

Controls (n=5)
Exposed (n=6)

120 dB SPL Exposure level

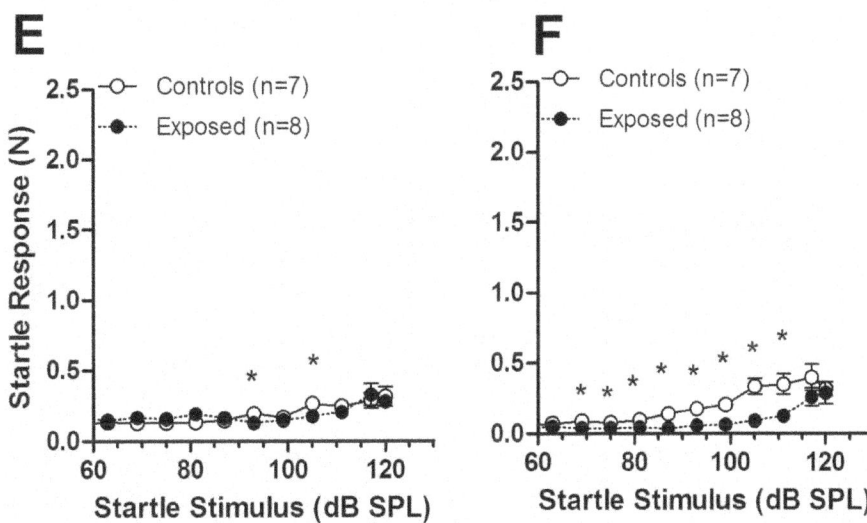

E

Controls (n=7)
Exposed (n=8)

F

Controls (n=7)
Exposed (n=8)

Figure 4. Effects of exposure level on ASR growth curves for early (1–2 days) and late (7–9 days) post-exposure time frames. A–B. Data for animals exposed at 110 dB SPL. C–D. Data for animals exposed at 115 dB SPL. E–F. Data for animals exposed at 120 dB SPL. Each point represents the mean (±S.E.M.). Group sizes are indicated in the graphs. Asterisks indicate points where differences between exposed and control animals were statistically significant (p<0.05).

$(F_{1,64} = 27.02, P<0.0001)$, was not observed in context 2 (Fig. 7C). In fact, the ASR obtained in context 2 were consistently lower than those obtained from control animals tested in context 1 $(F_{1,64} = 4.74, P<0.05)$. This indicates that the more complex stimulus battery of the gap detection test was suppressive of the ASR in both groups, although the suppression was more consistent and level dependent than in controls.

Discussion

Our results show that the direction and magnitude of change in the ASR is dependent on numerous factors, including the exposure level, the degree of threshold shift, the intensity of stimulation, the time after exposure when the ASR is measured, and on the context in which the startle stimuli are presented. We now discuss the possible underlying mechanisms of these changes and place our findings into a broader context by comparing them to those reported in other studies.

Enhanced startle responses were observed only in animals showing moderately elevated threshold

Animals with moderate thresholds (i.e., those in the range of 50–70 dB SPL) displayed robust enhancements of the ASR at stimulus intensities of 110–120 dB SPL. No enhancements were observed in animals with thresholds lower than 50 dB SPL or above 70 dB SPL. The enhanced startle responses observed in animals with thresholds in the range of 50–70 dB SPL emerged with a delayed onset of a few days and followed an initial period during which the ASR was either unchanged or slightly weakened.

One possible explanation of the enhanced ASR in sound exposed animals is that it was the result of Pavlovian conditioning or sensitization of the motor response caused by stress experienced during the initial sound exposure. Several of our observations argue against this explanation. First, we monitored the animals during the exposure periods and observed no evidence of a stressful response to the exposure sound. Animals moved about on the floor of their enclosures seemingly indifferent to the presence of

sound. The absence of any apparent stress response could be the result of a decrease in sensation level which the animals would experience as the hearing thresholds were shifted upward as the tone level was gradually stepped up in the beginning of the exposure period. Second, we observed no enhancement of ASR on the days immediately after the exposure, when the memory of the exposure would have been strongest. The enhanced startle responses observed in animals with thresholds in the range of 50–70 dB SPL emerged with a delayed onset of a few days and followed an initial period during which the ASR was either unchanged or slightly weakened. And third, ASR amplitudes were much weaker in the animals with the severest threshold losses, even after correcting for differences in sensation levels (see below). None of these observations seems consistent with the interpretation that animals exposed to intense sound developed enhanced ASRs because of a stress-associated conditioning. This conclusion is further supported by two other recent studies reporting chronically enhanced ASR in animals that were exposed while unconscious due to induction of anesthesia [17,27].

The enhanced ASR seems more likely to involve plastic mechanisms whereby the gain of the ASR at high stimulus levels is gradually readjusted in response to moderate hearing loss, as suggested in previous studies [13,18,28,29]. Although our data do not reveal mechanisms directly, we can offer some useful speculations concerning underlying mechanisms by considering knowledge based on previous studies. Those studies have shown that the main circuit that mediates the ASR includes cochlear root neurons (CRNs), which project to the caudal pontine reticular nucleus (cPRN), which, in turn, project to spinal motoneurons controlling body musculature [30–37]. A readjustment of gain of this startle circuit is likely to involve modulation by inputs to one or more of these nuclei from other sources. While such inputs come from multiple sources [30], the dorsal cochlear nucleus (DCN) is of special interest here because it has been shown to play a role in modulating the gain of the high intensity (110–115 dB SPL) component of the ASR [38], approximately the same range of intensities over which enhanced startle responses were observed

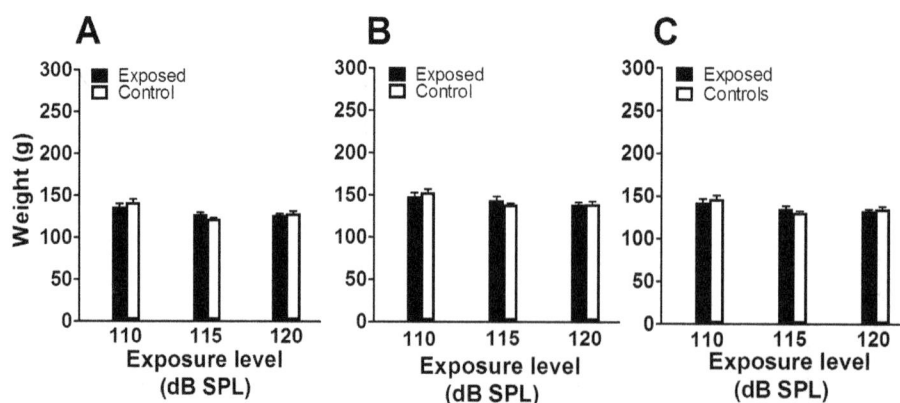

Figure 5. Representation of control and exposed animal weights, by group, from the beginning to the end of the ASR testing period. A. Weight averages on the first day of ASR testing, which is also the first day post-exposure. B. Weight averages on the last day of ASR testing. C. Weight averages over time through the entire ASR testing period. None of these measurements showed significant differences between exposed and control animals. (All P values >0.05, see text for exact values).

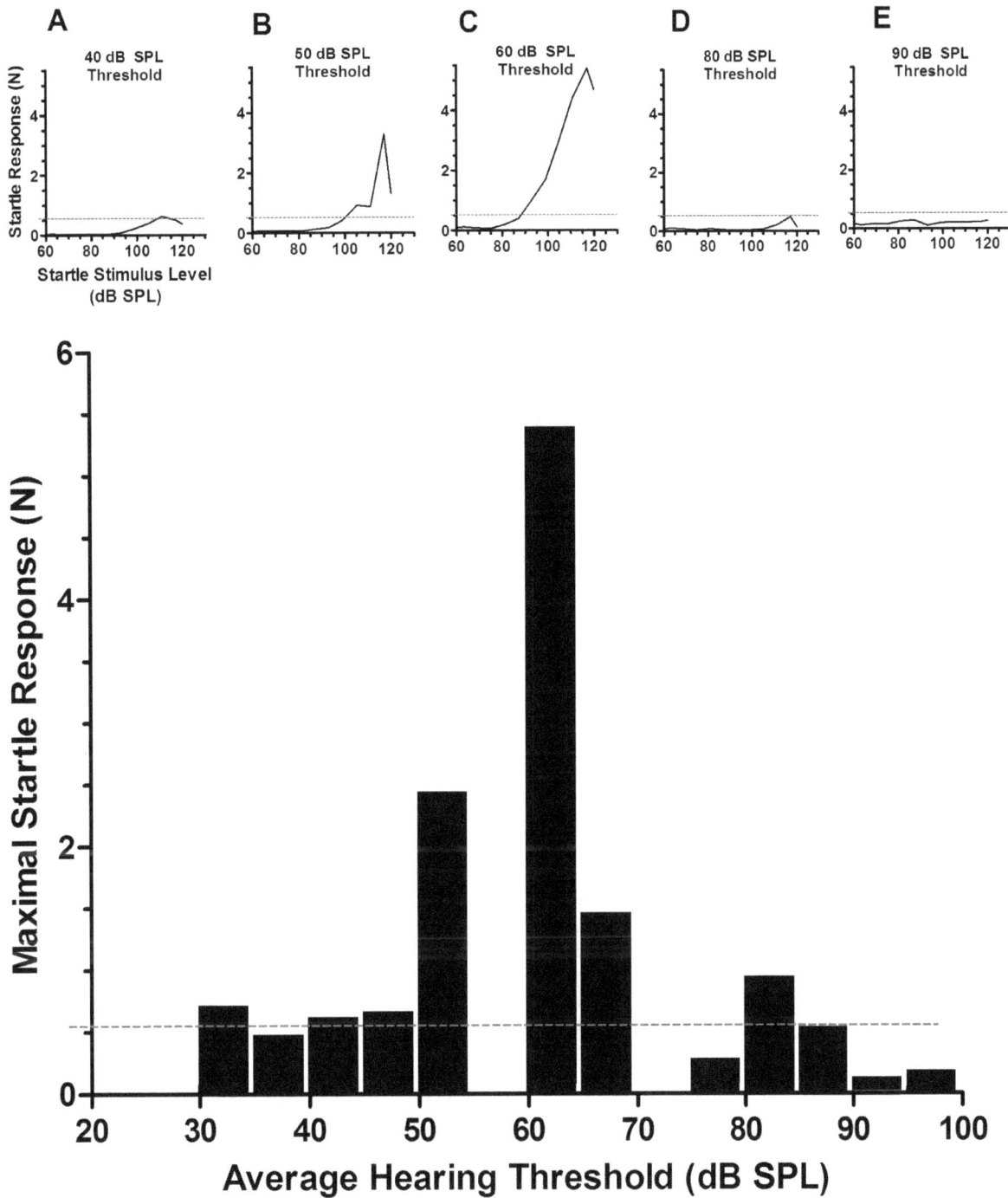

Figure 6. Dependence of enhancement of startle on threshold. The histogram depicts maximal ASR amplitudes with respect to thresholds for exposed animals. The dashed red line represents the mean maximal startle amplitude of control animals (thresholds for these animals ranged from 18 to 33 dB SPL). A–E: Representative ASR growth curves of exposed animals with different thresholds. When thresholds were less than 50 dB, startle amplitudes were similar to those of controls. For animals with thresholds of 50–70 dB, enhancements of startle were clearly apparent, but for animals with thresholds above 70 dB SPL, ASR amplitudes were in most cases reduced below control levels.

in the present study. Electrical stimulation of the DCN evokes large monosynaptic EPSPs in the giant neurons of the PRN [39], which activate the spinal motoneurons that recruit the muscles of the acoustic startle reflex [37]. Moreover, tracer injections into the giant cell regions of the PRN resulted in retrograde labeling of cochlear root neurons in the VCN and large neurons (probably fusiform and/or giant cells) in the DCN [35,37]. Thus, there are

both physiological and anatomical grounds on which to speculate that enhancements of startle might result from hyperactivity of output neurons in the DCN that synapse on the giant neurons of the PRN. Fusiform cells have been found to become hyperactive after intense sound exposure [40–43]. A number of studies suggest that noise exposure causes shifts in the balance of excitation and inhibition towards the side of excitation of DCN fusiform cells

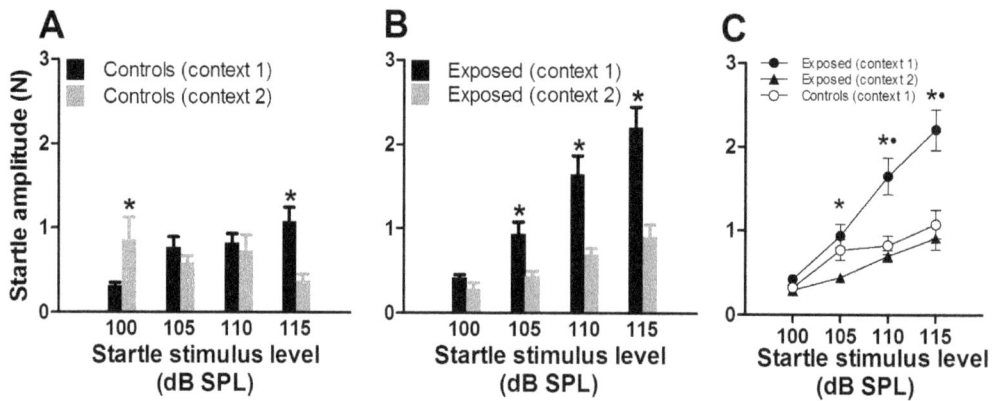

Figure 7. Effect of context on startle amplitudes. A. Data for control animals. B. Data for exposed animals. In each graph, data from animals tested in the context of startle stimuli alone (context 1) are compared with data from animals tested using startle stimuli alone presented randomly in the context of the gap detection test (context 2). Note that in control animals, ASR amplitudes were generally weaker in context 2 than in context 1, but for the most part, the decreases were not significant. In exposed animals, ASRs measured in context 2 were consistently weaker than those measured in context 1, indicating an effect of context on startle suppression. C. Comparison of startle amplitudes of exposed animals tested in contexts 1 and 2 with startle amplitudes of controls tested in context 1, showing the loss of hyperresponsiveness when animals were tested in context 2. *: P<0.05 for comparison between exposed animals tested in the two contexts. Dot represents P<0.05 for comparison between exposed and controls tested in context 1.

[44–46]. Increased activity of these cells would be expected to increase input to the giant cells of the PRN, thus increasing the amplitude of the ASR. Other sources of input to the acoustic startle circuit could also be involved, although thus far, none of these has been shown to play a role in adjusting the gain of the high intensity component of the acoustic startle reflex.

The ASR was weakened in animals with severe threshold shift

A fundamental question raised by our results is why, despite the induction of enhanced ASR with moderate thresholds (50–70 dB SPL), severely raised thresholds (those above 70 dB SPL) were associated with a persistent decrement of the ASR. Previous studies indicate that weakening of inhibition and strengthening of excitation can be induced in central auditory nuclei for different degrees (moderate and severe) of hearing loss [44,46]. Thus, to explain the decrement of the ASR observed in animals with the highest thresholds requires additional contributions via mechanisms that are not triggered by moderate hearing loss. The lack of enhancement of ASR in animals with thresholds greater than 70 dB SPL may be due in large part to the more severe hearing loss itself. Because sensation levels of high level startle stimuli would mostly be lower in animals with high thresholds than in those with moderate thresholds, the ASR would be expected to be correspondingly weaker. On the other hand, it seems unlikely that hearing loss can completely explain the lack of enhanced ASR in the highest threshold group. Weaker ASRs were found in this group even when comparing ASR amplitudes at startle stimulus levels evoking similar sensation levels. For example, using the highest ABR thresholds of Fig. 2B and 2C as benchmarks (80 dB SPL in animals exposed at 115 dB SPL and 93 dB SPL in the animals exposed at 120 dB SPL), startle stimuli at 25–30 dB SL would be in the range between 105 and 110 dB SPL for animals exposed at 115 dB SPL (Fig. 4D) and between 110 and 115 dB SPL for animals exposed at 120 dB SPL (Fig. 4F). Comparison of ASR amplitudes at these similar sensation levels still reveals a weaker response in the 120 dB group than those exposed at 115 dB group. Thus, other mechanisms would appear to contribute to the weakened ASR in the high threshold group.

One such mechanism may be the anatomical loss of primary afferent input to CRNs. Moderate levels of exposure (i.e., up to 110 dB SPL) typically causes loss of outer hair cells and injury to inner hair cells [47–49] as well as excitotoxic injury to the peripheral dendrites of spiral ganglion neurons [19,20,50]. This leaves surviving spiral ganglion cells and their centrally extending axons spontaneously inactive and unresponsive to sound [51,52], diminishing functional but not anatomical input to recipient CRN neurons. In contrast, higher levels of exposure cause more severe damage with widespread loss of outer and inner hair cells [47,53]. A secondary consequence of this type of injury is trans-neuronal degeneration of auditory nerve fibers which can spread to recipient neurons in the VCN [19,54–56]. Since CRNs receive direct input from primary afferents [57–60], this could lead to transneuronal degeneration of PRNs, irreversibly reducing the gain of the ASR, despite the survival of other cochlear nucleus cell types that may become hyperactive and also project to PRNs. Future studies examining the effects of severe acoustic insult on PRNs are needed to test this hypothesis more directly.

The present results may explain some of the differing effects of sound exposure on the ASR reported previously

One of the factors motivating our study was the puzzling discrepancies across studies describing the effects of sound exposure on the ASR. Whereas our previous study [18] and some others have shown chronic enhancement of the ASR in animals previously exposed to intense sound [19,27], the degrees and time courses of those enhancements as well as the types of stimulus batteries in which they have been observed have differed markedly across studies. Sun et al. [16] reported enhanced ASR immediately following noise exposure, but the enhancement was short lived, disappearing within the first 24 hours following exposure. The disappearance of enhanced ASR within the first 24 hours is not inconsistent with our results showing a lack of enhanced startle in animals tested 1–2 days post-exposure. Hickox and Liberman [19] found enhancements of ASR in animals tested with noise bursts against background noise, but only weak enhancements when tested with noise bursts in silence. This result is similar to the slight enhancement of startle observed in the present study in animals exposed at 110 dB SPL. The enhancement observed in silence by Hickox and Liberman might have been weak because the exposure level was only 100 dB SPL, inner hair cells were spared, and ABR thresholds were not permanently shifted. As our results from animals with near normal ABR thresholds show (Fig. 6), this would have been insufficient to cause robust enhancements of the ASR in the absence of background noise.

Two investigations have presented data showing reductions of ASRs after noise exposure. The reductions in these studies followed 1 hour exposures at levels between 115 and 120 [21] or between 120 and 126 dB SPL [22]. Although the amounts of threshold shift or injury to the ear were not reported, exposure sounds in both studies were presented to animals under anesthesia, a manipulation which could have increased injury to the inner ear by removing the protective effect of the middle ear muscles. Thus, the reductions in the latter two studies could have been a consequence of severely elevated thresholds (>70 dB), similar to the decrements of ASR which we observed in animals exposed at 120 dB SPL.

The response to a startle stimulus depends on the context

A surprising result of our experiments was the context dependency of the enhancement effect of exposure on ASR amplitude. We found that in exposed animals, when the ASR amplitudes were extracted from the startle-only stimulus conditions embedded in the gap detection test, the enhancement of startle was not observed. Context-dependent differences were also observed in control animals, but these were not as striking. These results are significant for at least two reasons. First, they underscore the importance of separating tests of startle growth functions from gap detection tests if enhancements of startle caused by noise exposure are the focus of investigation. As our results show, none of the startle amplitudes at any of the startle stimulus levels tested from 100–115 dB SPL, the range in which the startle amplitudes were enhanced when the startle stimuli were tested separately, was significantly elevated above control levels when such stimuli were presented in the context of the gap detection test. Second, they suggest that one consequence of sound exposure is a strengthening of suppressive mechanisms, which are either weak or absent in normal hearing animals. This is somewhat unexpected because generally, as discussed above, sound exposures are thought to cause weakening of inhibition and strengthening of excitation [61]. While the enhanced startle observed in our animals is consistent with this, the loss of that enhancement when the ASR is tested in the context of the gap detection test, suggests that the presence of the background noise or some other cue contained in the gap detection test battery elicits a suppression

of startle at high stimulus levels not seen in controls. These results may be related to two other forms of enhanced suppression observed in noise exposed animals, including enhanced prepulse inhibition [15,17] and increased suppression of the ASR by background noise [18]. The results in the present study suggest that noise exposure might increase the duration of the suppressive effect of background noise on the ASR. Whether these effects reflect an increase in the strength of inhibitory synapses [62] or changes in other non-synaptic mechanisms (e.g., adaptation, short term depression) is a topic for future investigation.

Are enhancements of the ASR related to hyperacusis?

Although the term 'hyperacusis' is most widely used in clinical audiology to refer to diminished sound tolerance [4,9], the underlying basis of diminished sound tolerance is unknown. One possibility is that it reflects a change in emotional sensitivity to sound, irrespective of a change in the sound sensation itself. Alternatively, diminished sound tolerance may result from heightened sense of loudness. Indeed, many clinicians measure hyperacusis either by assessing loudness discomfort level or by directly assessing loudness itself (magnitude estimation of loudness) or some emotional or behavioral quantity that increases with loudness, such as annoyance or fear [63]. As discussed recently in an in-depth review [5], many clinicians use the term 'hyperacusis' broadly to include any abnormally heightened percept evoked by sound, including not only loudness, but also increased responsiveness (hyperresponsiveness) to sound [3,29,64]. If indeed hyperacusis is a state of enhanced loudness, then one would expect that other quantities that vary with loudness, such as behavioral or physiological responses to sound, would also be enhanced. Evidence that this is true comes from functional imaging studies in humans with hyperacusis [2,65]. It follows that any circuit connected to the gain of the auditory system which underlies this increased responsiveness to sound, including the acoustic startle reflex circuit, might also show enhancement [28]. These are likely to be reasons why the terms hyperacusis or 'hyperacusis-like' are commonly used to refer to measures demonstrative of hyperresponsiveness to sound [11–14,17–19,28,63]. However, it should be acknowledged that until studies demonstrate that enhanced acoustic startle reflexes are a common characteristic of patients diagnosed with hyperacusis, the term 'hyperacusis' should be used with caution in seeking to establish animal models of this condition.

Author Contributions

Conceived and designed the experiments: JAK SAS. Performed the experiments: RHS CY LS. Analyzed the data: JAK RHS CY LS. Contributed reagents/materials/analysis tools: JAK SAS LS. Contributed to the writing of the manuscript: JAK RHS CY.

References

1. Fournier P, Hébert S (2013) Gap detection deficits in humans with tinnitus as assessed with the acoustic startle paradigm: Does tinnitus fill in the gap? Hear. Res. 295: 16–23.
2. Gu JW, Halpin CF, Nam EC, Levine RA, Melcher JR (2010) Tinnitus, diminished sound-level tolerance, and elevated auditory activity in humans with clinically normal hearing sensitivity. J. Neurophysiol. 104: 3361–3370.
3. Dauman R, Bouscau-Faure F (2005) Assessment and amelioration of hyperacusis in tinnitus patients. Acta Otolaryngol. 125: 503–509.
4. Baguley DM (2014) Hyperacusis: An Overview. Sem Hearing. 35: 4–83.
5. Tyler RS, Pienkowski M, Rojas Roncancio E, Jun HJ, Brozoski T, et al. (2014) Review of Hyperacusis and Future Directions: Part I. Definitions and Manifestations. Am J Audiol. Aug 7. AJA-14-0010.
6. Jastreboff PJ, Hazell JWP (2004) Tinnitus Retraining Therapy: Implementing the neurophysiological model. Cambridge University Press. 1–276.
7. Andersson G, Lindvall N, Hursti T, Carlbring P (2002) Hypersensitivity to sound (hyperacusis): a prevalence study conducted via the Internet and post. Int J Audiol. 41(8): 545–54.
8. Rubinstein B (1993) Tinnitus and craniomandibular disorders-is there a link? Swed Dent J Suppl. 95: 1–46.
9. Baguley DM (2003) Hyperacusis. J R Soc Med. 96(12): 582–5.
10. Schecklmann M, Landgrebe M, Langguth B, TRI Database Study Group (2014) Phenotypic characteristics of hyperacusis in tinnitus. PLoS One. 9(1): e86944.
11. Ison JR, Allen PD, O'Neill WE (2007) Age-related hearing loss in C57BL/6J mice has both frequency-specific and non-frequency-specific components that produce a hyperacusis-like exaggeration of the acoustic startle reflex. J. Assoc. Res. Otolaryngol. 8: 539–550.
12. Turner JG, Parrish J (2008) Gap detection methods for assessing salicylate-induced tinnitus and hyperacusis in rats. Am. J. Audiol. 17: S185–192.
13. Sun W, Lu J, Stolzberg D, Gray L, Deng A, et al. (2009) Salicylate increases the gain of the central auditory system. Neuroscience. 159(1): 325–34.

14. Lu J, Lobarinas E, Deng A, Goodey R, Stolzberg D, et al. (2011) GABAergic neural activity involved in salicylate-induced auditory cortex gain enhancement. Neuroscience. 189: 187–98.

15. Turner J, Larsen D, Hughes L, Moechars D, Shore S (2012) Time course of tinnitus development following noise exposure in mice. J Neurosci Res. 90(7): 1480–8.

16. Sun W, Deng A, Jayaram A, Gibson B (2012) Noise exposure enhances auditory cortex responses related to hyperacusis behavior. Brain Res. 1485: 108–16.

17. Dehmel S, Eisinger D, Shore SE (2012) Gap prepulse inhibition and auditory brainstem-evoked potentials as objective measures for tinnitus in guinea pigs. Front Syst Neurosci. 6: 42.

18. Chen G, Lee C, Sandridge SA, Butler HM, Manzoor NF, et al. (2013) Behavioral evidence for possible simultaneous induction of hyperacusis and tinnitus following intense sound exposure. J Assoc Res Otolaryngol. 14(3): 413–24.

19. Hickox AE, Liberman MC (2014) Is noise-induced cochlear neuropathy key to the generation of hyperacusis or tinnitus? J Neurophysiol. 111(3): 552–64.

20. Kujawa SG, Liberman MC (2009) Adding insult to injury: cochlear nerve degeneration after "temporary" noise-induced hearing loss. J Neurosci. 29(45): 14077–85.

21. Longenecker RJ, Galazyuk AV (2012) Methodological optimization of tinnitus assessment using prepulse inhibition of the acoustic startle reflex. Brain Res. 1485: 54–62.

22. Lobarinas E, Hayes SH, Allman BL (2013) The gap-startle paradigm for tinnitus screening in animal models: limitations and optimization. Hear Res. 295: 150–60.

23. Carlson S, Willott JF (2001) Modulation of the Acoustic Startle Response by Background Sound in C57BL/6J Mice. In: Willott JF, editor. Handbook of mouse auditory research: from behavior to molecular biology. CRC Press. Pp. 83–90.

24. Gerrard RL, Ison JR (1990) Spectral frequency and the modulation of the acoustic startle reflex by background noise. J Exp Psychol Anim Behav Process. 16(1): 106–12.

25. Ison JR, Hammond GR, Krauter EE (1973) Effects of experience on stimulus-produced reflex inhibition in the rat. J Comp Physiol Psychol. 83(2): 324–36.

26. Ison JR, Taylor MK, Bowen GP, Schwarzkopf SB (1997) Facilitation and inhibition of the acoustic startle reflex in the rat after a momentary increase in background noise level. Behav Neurosci. 111(6): 1335–52.

27. Pace E, Zhang J (2013) Noise-induced tinnitus using individualized gap detection analysis and its relationship with hyperacusis, anxiety, and spatial cognition. PLoS One. 8(9): e75011.

28. Zeng FG (2013) An active loudness model suggesting tinnitus as increased central noise and hyperacusis as increased nonlinear gain. Hear Res. 295: 172–9.

29. Hébert S, Fournier P, Noreña A (2013) The auditory sensitivity is increased in tinnitus ears. J Neurosci. 33: 2356–64.

30. Davis M, Gendelman DS, Tischler MD, Gendelman PM (1982) A primary acoustic startle circuit: lesion and stimulation studies. J Neurosci. 2(6): 791–805.

31. Davis M (1984) The mammalian startle response. In: Neural mechanisms of startle behavior. (Eaton RC, ed), 287–351. London: Plenum.

32. Pellet J (1990) Neural organization in the brainstem circuit mediating the primary acoustic head startle: an electrophysiological study in the rat. Physiol Behav. 48(5): 727–39.

33. Lee Y, López DE, Meloni EG, Davis M (1996) A primary acoustic startle pathway: obligatory role of cochlear root neurons and the nucleus reticularis pontis caudalis. J Neurosci. 16(11): 3775–89.

34. Kandler K, Herbert H (1991) Auditory projections from the cochlear nucleus to pontine and mesencephalic reticular nuclei in the rat. Brain Res. 562(2): 230–42.

35. Lingenhöhl K, Friauf E (1994) Giant neurons in the rat reticular formation: a sensorimotor interface in the elementary acoustic startle circuit? J Neurosci. 14(3 Pt 1): 1176–94.

36. López DE, Saldaña E, Nodal FR, Merchán MA, Warr WB (1999) Projections of cochlear root neurons, sentinels of the rat auditory pathway. J Comp Neurol. 415(2): 160–74.

37. Nodal FR, López DE (2003) Direct input from cochlear root neurons to pontine reticulospinal neurons in albino rat. J Comp Neurol. 460(1): 80–93.

38. Meloni EG, Davis M (1998) The dorsal cochlear nucleus contributes to a high intensity component of the acoustic startle reflex in rats. Hear Res. 119(1–2): 69–80.

39. Lingenhöhl K, Friauf E (1992) Giant neurons in the caudal pontine reticular formation receive short latency acoustic input: an intracellular recording and HRP-study in the rat. J Comp Neurol. 325(4): 473–92.

40. Brozoski TJ, Bauer CA, Caspary DM (2002) Elevated fusiform cell activity in the dorsal cochlear nucleus of chinchillas with psychophysical evidence of tinnitus. J Neurosci. 22(6): 2383–90.

41. Finlayson PG, Kaltenbach JA (2009) Alterations in the spontaneous discharge patterns of single units in the dorsal cochlear nucleus following intense sound exposure. Hear Res. 256(1–2): 104–17.

42. Li S, Choi V, Tzounopoulos T (2013) Pathogenic plasticity of Kv7.2/3 channel activity is essential for the induction of tinnitus. Proc Natl Acad Sci U S A. 110(24): 9980–5.

43. Shore SE, Koehler S, Oldakowski M, Hughes LF, Syed S (2008) Dorsal cochlear nucleus responses to somatosensory stimulation are enhanced after noise-induced hearing loss. Eur J Neurosci. 27(1): 155–68.

44. Asako M, Holt AG, Griffith RD, Buras ED, Altschuler RA (2005) Deafness-related decreases in glycine-immunoreactive labeling in the rat cochlear nucleus. J Neurosci Res. 81(1): 102–9.

45. Dong S, Mulders WH, Rodger J, Robertson D (2009) Changes in neuronal activity and gene expression in guinea-pig auditory brainstem after unilateral partial hearing loss. Neuroscience. 159(3): 1164–74.

46. Wang H, Brozoski TJ, Turner JG, Ling L, Parrish JL, et al. (2009) Plasticity at glycinergic synapses in dorsal cochlear nucleus of rats with behavioral evidence of tinnitus. Neuroscience. 164(2): 747–59.

47. Kaltenbach JA, Schmidt RN, Kaplan CR (1992) Tone-induced stereocilia lesions as a function of exposure level and duration in the hamster cochlea. Hear Res. 60(2): 205–15.

48. Fredelius L, Johansson B, Bagger-Sjöbäck D, Wersäll J (1987) Qualitative and quantitative changes in the guinea pig organ of Corti after pure tone acoustic overstimulation. Hear Res. 30(2–3): 157–67.

49. Emmerich E, Richter F, Linss V, Linss W (2005) Frequency-specific cochlear damage in guinea pig after exposure to different types of realistic industrial noise. Hear Res. 201(1–2): 90–8.

50. Puel JL, Ruel J, Gervais d'Aldin C, Pujol R (1998) Excitotoxicity and repair of cochlear synapses after noise-trauma induced hearing loss. Neuroreport. 9(9): 2109–14.

51. Liberman MC, Kiang NY (1978) Acoustic trauma in cats. Cochlear pathology and auditory-nerve activity. Acta Otolaryngol Suppl. 358: 1–63.

52. Liberman MC, Dodds LW (1984) Single-neuron labeling and chronic cochlear pathology. II. Stereocilia damage and alterations of spontaneous discharge rates. Hear Res. 16(1): 43–53.

53. Stebbins WC, Hawkins JE Jr, Johnson LG, Moody DB (1979) Hearing thresholds with outer and inner hair cell loss. Am J Otolaryngol. 1(1): 15–27.

54. Morest DK, Bohne BA (1983) Noise-induced degeneration in the brain and representation of inner and outer hair cells. Hear Res. 9(2): 145–51.

55. Morest DK, Kim J, Bohne BA (1997) Neuronal and transneuronal degeneration of auditory axons in the brainstem after cochlear lesions in the chinchilla: cochleotopic and non-cochleotopic patterns. Hear Res. 103(1–2): 151–68.

56. Kim J, Morest DK, Bohne BA (1997) Degeneration of axons in the brainstem of the chinchilla after auditory overstimulation. Hear Res. 103(1–2): 169–191.

57. Harrison JM, Warr WB, Irving R (1962) Second order neurons in the acoustic nerve. Science. 138: 893–895.

58. Merchan MA, Collia F, Lopez DE, Saldaña E (1988) Morphology of cochlear root neurons in the rat. J Neurocytol. 17(5): 711–25.

59. Gómez-Nieto R, Rubio ME, López DE (2008) Cholinergic input from the ventral nucleus of the trapezoid body to cochlear root neurons in rats. J Comp Neurol. 506(3): 452–68.

60. Sinex DG, López DE, Warr WB (2001) Electrophysiological responses of cochlear root neurons. Hear Res. 158(1–2): 28–38.

61. Roberts LE, Eggermont JJ, Caspary DM, Shore SE, Melcher JR, et al. (2010) Ringing ears: the neuroscience of tinnitus. J Neurosci. 30(45): 14972–9.

62. Dong S, Mulders WH, Rodger J, Woo S, Robertson D (2010) Acoustic trauma evokes hyperactivity and changes in gene expression in guinea-pig auditory brainstem. Eur J Neurosci. 31(9): 1616–28.

63. Tyler RS, Noble W, Coelho C, Haskell G, Bardia A (2009) Tinnitus and hyperacusis. In: Handbook of Clinical Audiology, Ed. Lippincott, Williams and Wilkins. New York, 726–738.

64. Song JJ, De Ridder D, Weisz N, Schlee W, Van de Heyning P, et al. (2014) Hyperacusis-associated pathological resting-state brain oscillations in the tinnitus brain: a hyperresponsiveness network with paradoxically inactive auditory cortex. Brain Struct Funct. 219: 1113–28.

65. Weber H, Pfadenhauer K, Stöhr M, Rösler A (2002) Central hyperacusis with phonophobia in multiple sclerosis. Mult Scler. 8: 505–9.

24

Predicting the Perceived Sound Quality of Frequency-Compressed Speech

Rainer Huber[1,2]*, **Vijay Parsa**[3], **Susan Scollie**[3]

1 Centre of Competence HörTech gGmbH, Oldenburg, Germany, **2** Cluster of Excellence Hearing4All, Oldenburg and Hannover, Germany, **3** National Centre for Audiology, Western University, London, Canada

Abstract

The performance of objective speech and audio quality measures for the prediction of the perceived quality of frequency-compressed speech in hearing aids is investigated in this paper. A number of existing quality measures have been applied to speech signals processed by a hearing aid, which compresses speech spectra along frequency in order to make information contained in higher frequencies audible for listeners with severe high-frequency hearing loss. Quality measures were compared with subjective ratings obtained from normal hearing and hearing impaired children and adults in an earlier study. High correlations were achieved with quality measures computed by quality models that are based on the auditory model of Dau et al., namely, the measure PSM, computed by the quality model PEMO-Q; the measure qc, computed by the quality model proposed by Hansen and Kollmeier; and the linear subcomponent of the HASQI. For the prediction of quality ratings by hearing impaired listeners, extensions of some models incorporating hearing loss were implemented and shown to achieve improved prediction accuracy. Results indicate that these objective quality measures can potentially serve as tools for assisting in initial setting of frequency compression parameters.

Editor: Bernd Sokolowski, University of South Florida, United States of America

Funding: The work was supported by the following: Deutsche Forschungsgemeinschaft (Research Unit "Individualized Hearing Acoustics"; For-1732) (to Dr. Huber), http://www.dfg.de/en/research_funding/programmes/coordinated_programmes/research_units/index.html; NSERC Discovery grant (to Dr. Vijay Parsa), http://www.nserc-crsng.gc.ca/professors-professeurs/grants-subs/dgigp-psigp_eng.asp; and NSERC Collaborative Health Research grant (to Dr. Scollie), http://www.nserc-crsng.gc.ca/Professors-Professeurs/grants-subs/CHRP-PRCS_eng.asp. The funders had no role in study design, data collection and analysis, decision to publish, or preparation of the manuscript.

Competing Interests: The authors have declared that no competing interests exist.

* Email: Rainer.Huber@HoerTech.de

Introduction

Nonlinear frequency compression

Frequency lowering techniques are now common in digital hearing aids as an alternative amplification strategy for hearing impaired listeners with severe to profound high frequency hearing loss. For this group of listeners, conventional amplification strategies may result in less than optimal performance due to a combination of inadequate gain at higher frequencies, limited bandwidth of the hearing instruments, and/or the potential presence of high frequency cochlear dead regions [1], [2], among other factors. Frequency lowering techniques aim to transfer high frequency information to lower frequency regions. These techniques can improve speech recognition, but may also affect perceived sound quality. In this paper, we investigate a broad range of objective indices of sound quality against a database of sound quality ratings for frequency-lowered speech. This work not only evaluates which models may be effective predictors of the impact of one form of frequency lowering on sound quality, but also develops insights as to the key features of a successful model by varying key modelling parameters and evaluating their impact on successful predictions.

Historically, frequency lowering has been achieved in many ways including slow playback, channel vocoding, frequency transposition, and frequency compression, as well as a combination of these alternative strategies [3]. As described in ([3] - Section 8.3), a frequency transposing hearing aid will shift a portion of high frequency spectrum to lower frequencies by a fixed amount (in Hz). Frequency compression can be linear or nonlinear; in linear frequency compression, all frequencies are proportionally reduced by the same factor (i.e., the output frequency is a fixed fraction of the input frequency), while in nonlinear frequency compression, only frequencies above a certain threshold are compressed.

Currently, frequency lowering is available as an option in commercial hearing aids as frequency transposition (termed "Audibility Extender") in Widex hearing aids [4], as nonlinear frequency compression (termed "SoundRecover") in Phonak and Unitron hearing aids and as "frequency compression" in Siemens hearing aids, as spectral warping (termed "SpectralIQ") in Starkey hearing aids, and as "Frequency Composition", another type of frequency transposition [5], in Bernafon hearing aids.

The differences in frequency lowering implementations can be expected to result in considerably different perceptual effects, even when they are fitted for the same audiometric configuration. For example, McDermott [6] conducted an electroacoustic comparison of Widex's Audibility Extender and Phonak's Sound Recover technologies. Spectrographic analyses with different speech and music samples showed that while both schemes were effective in lowering high frequency content, they also introduced distortion that may affect perception. It is therefore imperative to investigate the perceptual effects of frequency lowering technologies, and to develop electroacoustic tools and computational models that can predict these perceptual effects.

Since this paper focuses on a particular frequency lowering strategy, *viz.* the nonlinear frequency compression (NFC), a brief description of the NFC processing and the evidence surrounding its effectiveness is presented below.

The NFC processing in today's commercial hearing aids uses compression only for frequencies above a cutoff value. Mathematically, the relationship between input and output frequencies is given by

$$F_{out} = \begin{cases} F_{in}, & F_{in} < F_c \\ F_c^{1-p} \times F_{in}^p, & F_{in} \geq F_c \end{cases} \quad (1)$$

where F_{in} is the input frequency in Hz, F_{out} is the corresponding output frequency, F_c is the cutoff frequency, p is the compression exponent, and $1/p$ is the compression ratio (CR). Figure 1 illustrates the concept showing short time spectra of speech before and after nonlinear frequency compression.

The specification of the F_c ensures that the lower frequency information is unadulterated while the spectral content beyond the F_c is compressed into a narrower bandwidth. The NFC scheme has been evaluated with both adults and children. Simpson *et al.* [7] investigated the performance of prototype NFC with 17 hearing impaired adults with moderate to profound sensorineural hearing loss and found that the phoneme recognition scores for the group improved by 6%. Glista *et al.* [8] evaluated NFC processing with 13 adults and 11 children with moderately severe to profound sloping high-frequency hearing losses. On average, recognition scores for plurals and consonants improved significantly for the NFC scheme when compared with conventional amplification. Individual variability was present in the results and children derived greater plural recognition benefit from NFC as well as indicated preference for NFC over conventional amplification when compared to the adults [8]. Benefit was also related to audiogram: Those with greater high frequency hearing loss were most likely to demonstrate benefits. More recent studies have evaluated outcomes for those with moderate hearing losses [9], the time course of acclimatization [10] and effects on sound quality [11], [12]. Previous work indicated that sound quality is correlated with the strength of the frequency compressor, with stronger settings having poorer sound quality. This underscores the need for formal evaluation of sound quality of the NFC processor. In

particular, computational metrics which can effectively predict speech quality perception by hearing impaired listeners could be of use in determining an initial set of NFC parameters that have acceptable sound quality, potentially improving the acceptability of initial fittings.

Objective sound quality evaluation

The perceived quality of frequency-compressed sounds will depend on a number of variables, including the parameter settings, hearing loss, the type of sound, as well as highly individual, subjective factors like personal experiences, expectations and preferences. In order to estimate the expected sound quality for a given algorithm setting, sound, and listener, one could either follow a data-driven, i.e. statistical model approach (e.g, the E-model [13]), or a perception model approach (e.g. PESQ [14]). A data-driven approach would require a large base of empirical data containing subjective quality ratings of different types of sounds, processed with a variety of algorithm settings, obtained from many listeners with different hearing losses. A perception-model-driven approach would possibly require similar amounts of data if it was developed, trained or optimized, and validated particularly for this application.

Alternatively, existing quality models already validated for similar applications could be tested with a smaller amount of data. However, most of the existing quality models were designed, optimized and validated in the context of telecommunication applications and audio coding for normal-hearing listeners (see [15] for an overview). At present, very few sound quality models for hearing impaired listeners with application for hearing aid (algorithm) quality evaluations have been reported [16–19]. Most of the sound quality models, including current ITU standard methods for speech and audio quality, have in common that they follow the concept of comparing "internal representations", computed by a psychoacoustic model, of a test and a reference sound signal [20], [14]. Detected differences between internal representations are interpreted as quality degradations of the test signal with respect to the reference signal. Hence, these comparison-based models depend on the availability of a reference signal that represents the optimum, or desired, sound quality. This requirement is met in the evaluation of lossy signal processing systems, such as low-bitrate speech and audio codecs, where the unprocessed, original signal serves as a reference.

However, there is no known ideal reference for the evaluation of hearing aids (algorithms) in general. In contrast to audio codecs, whose aim is to produce output signals that are perceptually indistinguishable from the original input, hearing aids aim to alter the input sound in a way that it compensates for the listeners' hearing loss. This intentional alternation could result in the processed sound having higher sound quality than the original signal. Therefore, one would need a "perfect" hearing aid to produce the reference signal for sound quality evaluations. Unfortunately, the perfect hearing aid does not exist.

However, many hearing aid algorithms can be evaluated with comparison-based quality models. Examples include speech enhancement algorithms that operate on already distorted input signals, like noisy and/or reverberant speech. In these evaluations, the original, clean speech recording can serve as a reference signal, and comparison signals are generated by adding noise or reverberation. Such a comparison-based method may also be applicable in the case of frequency-lowering algorithms. Frequency-lowering will always degrade the naturalness of the input sounds. If subjective sound quality ratings are dominated by the perceived naturalness and not influenced by the possibly improved speech intelligibility or other positive effects of the frequency

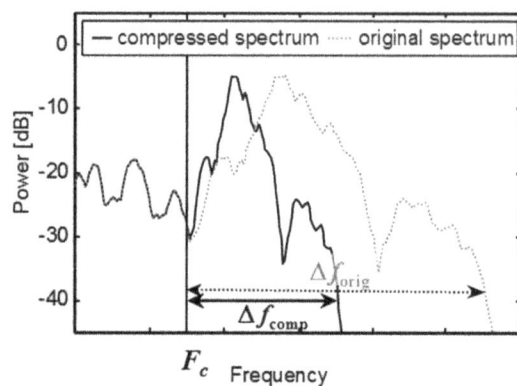

Figure 1. Illustration of nonlinear frequency compression. Dotted, grey line: Power spectrum of unprocessed speech. Solid, black line: spectrum after nonlinear frequency compression. Above a cutoff frequency F_c, the spectrum is compressed by a ratio CR = $\Delta f_{orig}/\Delta f_{comp}$.

compression, comparison-based quality models using the unprocessed input signal as a reference appear potentially qualified as predictors of sound quality also for this class of hearing aid algorithms.

Objective evaluation of frequency-compressed speech

NFC is a viable choice as an amplification solution for hearing impaired listeners with severe to profound high-frequency hearing loss. Since sound quality is one of the most important factors determining the overall satisfaction and acceptance of hearing aid users [21–24], the negative impact on sound quality by NFC must remain small enough to be overshadowed by the positive effects such as improved intelligibility in order to achieve acceptance and overall preference over conventional processing. Objective sound quality models are useful in this context as they can assist in the initial specification of NFC parameters that achieve a balance between intelligibility enhancement and quality degradation. In the present study, a number of established as well as rather new, mostly perceptual speech and audio quality models, including yet unpublished extended versions, have been applied to predict subjective sound quality ratings of nonlinear frequency-compressed speech [11]. It should be noted that none of the applied models was designed for the present application and some of them were particularly optimized for different experimental conditions, like (monaural) headphone presentation instead of loudspeaker presentation as used in the present study. In spite of this caveat, promising predictor candidates will be identified below.

Subjective Speech Quality Measurement

Speech signals and subjective quality ratings used to test the quality models were obtained from an earlier study [11] and shall be described only briefly here. See [11] for a more detailed description.

Speech quality ratings were obtained from a group of 12 normal hearing adults (ages 21–27 years, mean = 24 years), 12 normal hearing children (ages 8–18 years, mean = 12 years), 12 hearing impaired adults (ages 50–81 years, mean = 69 years), and 9 hearing impaired children (ages 8–17 years, mean = 12 years). The listeners with hearing impairment also participated in a field study with NFC hearing aids [8]. All normal hearing listeners had pure tone thresholds of 20 dB HL or better across the audiometric frequency range. Figure 2 depicts the mean and standard deviation of the pure tone thresholds for hearing impaired adults and children. While the children had higher absolute thresholds than adults, statistical analysis revealed there was no significant

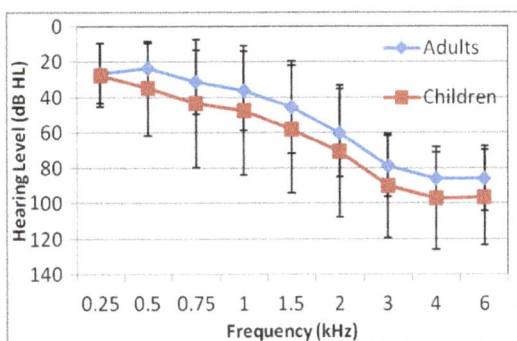

Figure 2. Mean and standard deviations of the pure-tone air conduction thresholds for hearing impaired adults and children.

interaction between frequency-specific thresholds and age [8], [11].

A database of frequency-compressed speech samples was created to obtain the subjective quality ratings. The database was constructed by first programming a prototype NFC hearing aid with specific cutoff frequency (F_c) and compression ratio (CR) parameters, placing this hearing aid in a Brüel and Kjær portable anechoic test box, and recording the output of the hearing aid separately in response to two male speech samples and two female speech samples. A total of five different NFC settings were investigated: (1) F_c = 4000 Hz, CR = 2:1; (2) F_c = 3000 Hz, CR = 2:1; (3) F_c = 3000 Hz, CR = 6:1; (4) F_c = 3000 Hz, CR = 10:1; and (5) F_c = 2000 Hz, CR = 2:1.

Hearing aid recordings were later played back to the bilaterally aided study participants in a sound booth through a loudspeaker positioned at 0° azimuth and at a distance of 1.5 m. The playback level was initially presented at 65 dB SPL and then individually adjusted, if needed, to the subject's most comfortable level (MCL) [11]. Calibration was performed using the Brüel & Kjær Sound Level Meter (SLM), Type 2270. Speech quality ratings were obtained using the ITU standard MUltiple Stimulus with Hidden Reference and Anchors (MUSHRA, [25]) protocol mediated by custom software. The MUSHRA protocol uses a numerical quality rating scale from 0 to 100 together with five verbal categories from "bad" to "excellent" as anchors for orientation. In this method, a "reference stimulus" was presented, which was the unprocessed male or female speech sample, while eight "test stimuli" were randomly associated with the five NFC-processed stimuli, the original signal itself ("hidden reference"), and a low-pass version and a peak-clipped version of the original signal, respectively. The low-pass version was obtained by passing the original signal through a 10th order Butterworth filter with a cutoff frequency of 2000 Hz, while the peak-clipped version was obtained through hard-clipping the original stimulus at 25% of its peak value. These stimuli served as "anchor" stimuli that represent sound with poor quality, as recommended by [25]. In the MUSHRA method, all stimuli are rated simultaneously using graphical slider buttons. Participants were instructed to listen to each of these stimuli in comparison to the reference, by clicking on the corresponding icons of the software's GUI and adjust the rating sliders such that a satisfactory quality rating of all eight stimuli was achieved. Participants were allowed to re-listen to any stimulus and re-adjust their quality ratings until they were satisfied with the final set of ratings.

Parsa et al. [11] have conducted a detailed statistical analysis of the subjective data collected through this procedure. A high degree of intra- and inter-rater reliability was observed with the speech quality ratings across both normal and hearing impaired groups. As such, this database was used to benchmark the performance of different objective speech quality estimators in predicting the quality of frequency-compressed speech.

Objective Speech Quality Measurement

This paper evaluated twenty-nine objective quality measures including sub-variants in order to benchmark model performance for prediction of sound quality with NFC processing. Table 1 provides a summary of the models/measures tested, and technical information on the nature of each model is provided below.

The objective models investigated in this paper are considered to be "double-ended" or "intrusive" in their operation. Double-ended models compare features extracted from the signal under test to those extracted from an undistorted reference version of the same signal. The comparisons quantify the degree of perceptual

Table 1. Quality models and measures used in this study.

Model/measure name	acronym	authors	ref.	measure(s)	HI?	no.
Hansen model		M. Hansen & Kollmeier	[37]	qc+W+B	–	M1
				qc+W-B	–	M2
				qc-W+B	–	M3
				qc-W-B	–	M4
Hansen model extended for hearing impaired		Huber	unpub.	qc+W+B (HI)	✓	M5
				qc+W-B (HI)	✓	M6
				qc-W+B (HI)	✓	M7
				qc-W-B (HI)	✓	M8
PEMO-Q	PEMO-Q	Huber & Kollmeier	[39]	PSM_fb+B	–	M9
				PSM_fb-B	–	M10
				PSM_lp+B	–	M11
				PSM_lp-B	–	M12
PEMO-Q extended for hearing impaired	PEMO-Q-HI	Huber	unpub.	PSM_fb+B (HI)	✓	M13
				PSM_fb-B (HI)	✓	M14
				PSM_lp+B (HI)	✓	M15
				PSM_lp-B (HI)	✓	M16
Hearing Aid Speech Quality Index	HASQI	Kates & Arehart	[19]	$HASQI_{lin}$	✓	M17
				$HASQI_{nonlin}$	✓	M18
				$HASQI_{comb}$	✓	M19
Perceptual Evaluation of Speech Quality (ITU-T Rec. P.862-2)	PESQ	ITU-T/Beerends et al.	[14], [31]	PESQ-LQO	–	M20
				PESQ-LQO (WB)	–	M21
Loudness Pattern Distortion	LPD	Guo & Parsa	[36]	LPD	–	M22
Moore quality model		Moore & Tan	[33–35]	D	–	M23
				R_{nonlin}	–	M24
				$S_{overall}$	–	M25
Itakura-Saito Distance	ISD	Itakura & Saito	[26]	ISD	–	M26
Log-Area Ratio	LAR	Quackenbush et al.	[28]	LAR	–	M27
Log-Likelihood Ratio	LLR	Itakura	[27]	LLR	–	M28
Weighted Spectral Slope Distance	WSSD	Klatt	[30]	WSSD	–	M29

("ref".: reference; "HI?": Does model account for hearing impairment? Yes: ✓; no: –) Quality measure suffixes: fb/lp: modulation filterbank/lowpass model version; +/– W: with/without frequency band weighting; +/–B: with/without asymmetric weighting of differences ("Beerends weighting").

overall difference or similarity. In contrast, single-ended models do not require a reference signal. The models in Table 1 can be broadly grouped into: (1) metrics based on speech production model parameters, and (2) metrics based on the comparison of "internal representations" obtained with computational models of auditory processing. Double-ended models were chosen for this work, because the subjective quality ratings were obtained using reference signals as well, according to the MUSHRA protocol.

Examples of objective models in the speech production model parameters include the Itakura-Saito Distance (ISD) [26] and the Log-Likelihood Ratio (LLR) [27], which calculate the weighted similarity between the linear prediction coefficients extracted from the distorted and reference speech signals, and the Log-Area Ratio (LAR) [28] measure, which computes the distance between the area ratio coefficients. Software implementations of ISD, LAR, and LLR were taken from a toolbox provided by Hansen and Pellom [29].

A basic objective measure that uses an auditory model is the Weighted Spectral Slope Distance (WSSD) [30] measure. It uses a psychoacoustically motivated bank of critical-band filters to decompose the speech signals, and weights the differences between the slopes of the log magnitudes in each band to produce the final quality measure. Again, the software implementation of the WSSD measure was taken from the Hansen and Pellom toolbox.

The method for the Perceptual Evaluation of Speech Quality (PESQ; ITU-T Recommendation P.862 [14]) and its wide band extension (PESQ-WB; ITU-T P.862.2 [31]) are perhaps the most popularly used objective quality assessment methods incorporating an auditory model. Conceptually, the PESQ technique computes the frame-by-frame internal representations of test and reference signals by first computing the power spectra, and then applying frequency and intensity warping functions based on Zwicker's loudness model [14].

Moore & Glasberg have developed a different loudness model [32], characterized by the computation of excitation patterns at the output of each auditory filter and the subsequent computation of the specific loudness pattern. Moore et al. [33–35] applied the Moore & Glasberg model and derived an objective quality metric based on comparisons of the excitation patterns of original and distorted signals. Two intermediate measures of linear (spectral) and nonlinear distortions (D and R_{nonlin}, respectively) are computed separately and combined to an overall subjective score predictor $S_{overall}$ in the end. For the Moore quality model, a custom software implementation was developed. Correlations between model output measures and mean subjective quality ratings will be reported for D, R_{nonlin} and $S_{overall}$.

Chen et al. [36] devised an objective measure based on the Moore & Glasberg loudness pattern differences between the reference and degraded speech samples. These differences were used to estimate sound quality in the degraded sample versus the reference sample. This measure was computed using custom software.

The speech quality model of Hansen & Kollmeier [37] (referred to as the "Hansen model" below) employs the auditory processing model of Dau et al. [38], "PEMO" (for "PErception MOdel"), for the computation of internal representations of test and reference signals. The bandwidth of the PEMO peripheral (gammatone) filterbank was adapted to telephone-bandpass-filtered speech. A "band importance weighting" function is applied to the frequency channels of the internal representations to emphasize higher frequency channels. The overall correlation between the weighted internal representations determines the quality measure qc.

The audio quality model PEMO-Q of Huber and Kollmeier [39] extends the Hansen model to include quality assessment of general, wideband audio signals (including speech) with low to very high audio qualities. By default, it uses the more recent version of the Dau model [40], with the option of selecting the earlier (much faster) version. The two model versions differ with respect to the processing of amplitude modulations: In [38], the final step of auditory preprocessing (i.e. before the decision stage) is an 8 Hz-lowpass filter, whereas in [40], this lowpass filter is replaced by a filter bank. The band importance weighting function used in the Hansen model was not adopted for PEMO-Q.

PEMO-Q outputs two quality measures: The Perceptual Similarity Measures PSM and PSM_t. The second variant evaluates the temporal course of the instantaneous audio quality, derived from a frame-wise correlation of internal representations, non-linearly mapped to the overall quality estimator PSM_t. In contrast, the PSM is the overall correlation of the complete internal representations. The PSM_t is more sensitive to small distortions and more independent of the type of input audio signal [39]. On the other hand, the "simpler" PSM seems to be more "robust" and more generally applicable, especially for low-to intermediate audio quality. For example, speech enhancement algorithms have been evaluated with this measure and showed good correlations with subjective quality ratings [41–43]. Since speech samples with rather strong quality differences are considered in this study, only the PSM was included here.

By default, PESQ and PEMO-Q apply an asymmetric weighting of differences between internal representations, putting more weight on "added" or increased elements of the internal representation of the distorted signal than on "missing" or attenuated ones [44]. This step is handled as an option for the Hansen model and PEMO-Q and has been switched on and off in this study. The second binary setting option of PEMO-Q that has been varied is the manner of amplitude processing in the auditory processing model (modulation lowpass vs. filterbank). This leads to four PEMO-Q output measure variants that have been tested in total. Since a benefit of the band importance function used in the Hansen model could only be found in the prediction of speech quality in the context of telecommunication, the Hansen model was also tested with the weighting function deactivated in this study. Hence, four versions of the Hansen model have been tested in total: with and without asymmetry weighting of internal

representations, and with and without applying the band importance weighting function.

Finally, the Hearing Aid Speech Quality Index (HASQI) by Kates and Arehart [19] was employed. In the computation of the HASQI, a relatively simple auditory processing model is applied to provide internal representations in terms of neural firing rates. Effects of possible sensorineural hearing losses are modeled by estimating the contributions of inner hair cell (IHC) and outer hair cell (OHC) losses to a total hearing loss given by the audiogram. Auditory filter bandwidths are increased and compression ratios are reduced depending on the OHC loss estimate. The effect of IHC loss is modeled by linear signal attenuation in each auditory filter before compression. From the comparison of internal representations of test and reference signals, two intermediate quality metrics are computed, quantifying the amount of linear and non-linear distortions, respectively. The final overall quality index is the product of the linear and the nonlinear distortion metrics. Again, correlations with subjective quality ratings will be reported for linear and nonlinear metrics and overall quality index, referred to as $HASQI_{lin}$, $HASQI_{nonlin}$ and $HASQI_{comb}$, respectively.

In summary, the models and measures for speech and audio quality listed in Table 1 have been applied to the signals of the database.

The versions of PEMO-Q and the Hansen model with extensions for hearing impaired data have not been published before and will therefore be discussed in the next section.

Extended versions of PEMO-Q and the Hansen model for hearing impaired

Modifications of the underlying auditory model of the audio quality prediction methods PEMO-Q and its predecessor, the speech quality model of Hansen and Kollmeier, for describing sensorineural hearing losses have been suggested by Derleth et al. [45]. One of their suggestions was to insert an instantaneous expansion and attenuation stage before the adaptation and compression stage in the PEMO (Figure 3), to account for a loss of sensitivity and reduced dynamic compression. This suggestion has been adopted and implemented in the extended version of PEMO-Q and the Hansen model. Given an audiogram as the input, the hearing thresholds in dB HL at audiometric frequencies are interpolated internally to the center frequencies of the model's peripheral filterbank. The inserted processing stage operates on the output of each of these filters, after envelope extraction. The total hearing loss in the respective channel is decomposed into contributions attributed to losses of inner (IHCL) and outer hair cells (OHCL), respectively, as shown in the equation below [32]:

$$OHCL = \begin{cases} \min\{65\,\mathrm{dB}, 0.8{\cdot}THL\}, f > 2000\,\mathrm{Hz} \\ \min\{55\,\mathrm{dB}, 0.8{\cdot}THL\}, f \leq 2000\,\mathrm{Hz} \end{cases} \quad (2)$$

$$IHCL = THL - OHCL$$

In the model stage, the signal amplitude is attenuated by the amount of IHCL. Then, it is raised to the power k, which itself is a function of the input signal amplitude I and OHCL. The attenuation and expansion operations are performed instanta-neously (i.e. sample-by-sample). For simulating normal hearing, k equals 1 for any I. For simulating impaired hearing, $k(I)$ becomes larger than 1 and increases with OHCL. The input/output

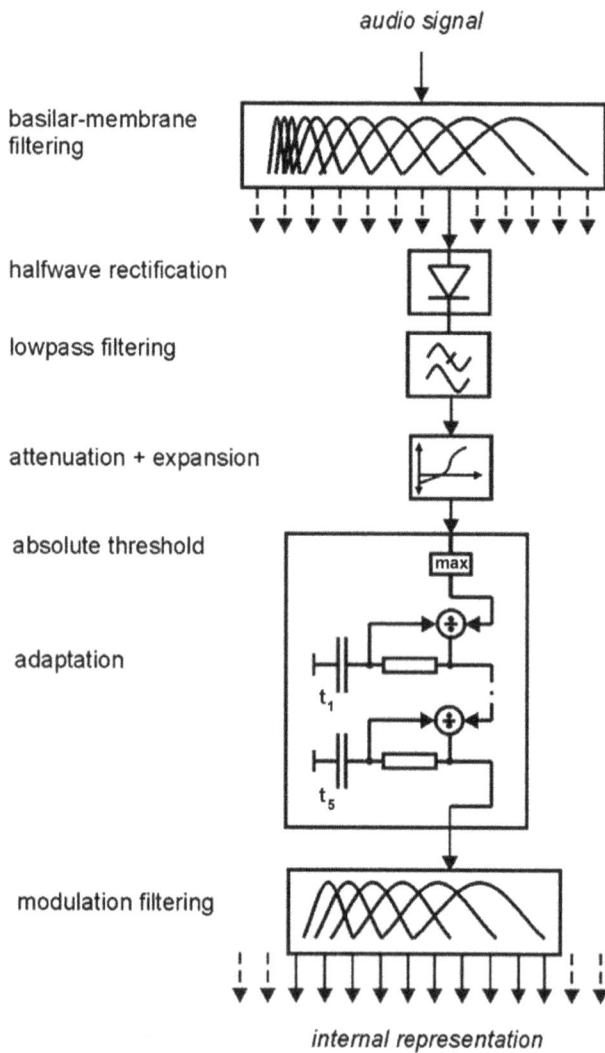

audio signal

basilar-membrane filtering

halfwave rectification

lowpass filtering

attenuation + expansion

absolute threshold

adaptation

modulation filtering

internal representation

Figure 3. Schematic plot of the auditory processing model PEMO, modified to simulate normal and impaired hearing (after [40] and [45]).

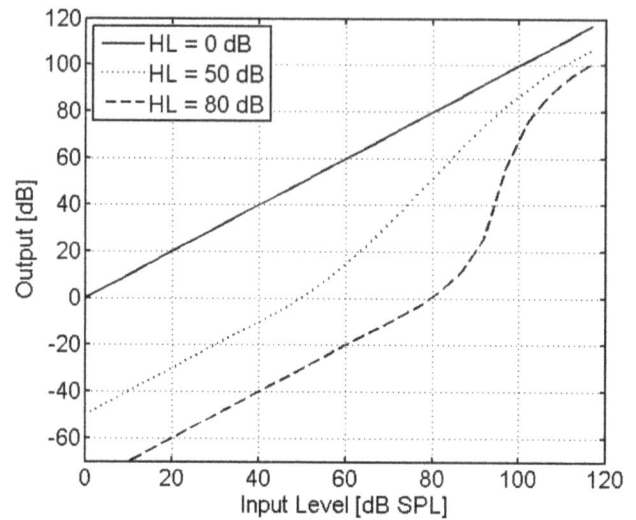

Figure 4. Input/output functions of the expansion and attenuation model stage for normal hearing (solid line) and impaired hearing with an assumed total hearing loss of 50 dB (dotted line) and 80 dB (dashed line).

impaired children, and (3) hearing impaired adults. In addition to averaging across subjects, quality ratings were also averaged across different talkers per processing condition. Results will be stated for both levels of averaging. For clarity, results per subject group will be presented separately in succession and only for a selection of measures. The complete results are reported in the Appendix S1. The relation between subjective ratings and corresponding model predictions will be illustrated by scatter plots for the best performing quality measures.

Results for normal hearing

Table 2 shows linear and rank correlations between selected model predictions and mean subjective ratings obtained from normal hearing subjects. (The complete correlation table is given in the Appendix S1) In this table, the suffixes of the PSM and qc measures have the following meaning: fb/lp indicate the modulation filterbank/lowpass version of PEMO-Q respectively, +/−W indicate the activation/deactivation of the frequency-band weighting, and +/−B denote activation/deactivation of the asymmetric weighting of internal representation differences ("Beerends weighting"). When frequency weighting is deactivated in the Hansen model, and the modulation lowpass version is used in PEMO-Q, these models become very similar. They mainly differ in the bandwidth of the peripheral filterbank. It must be noted that because the results obtained with the −B option tended to be better than with option +B, the latter are only reported in the complete set of results given in the Appendix S1.

It can be seen from Table 2 that the correlation coefficients are reasonable for several of the objective quality metrics, especially when averaged across different talkers per processing condition (right column "av.") Four of the five measures with highest correlations are PEMO-Q and related measures (PSM..., qc...), complemented by the LAR (M27 of Table 1) measure. The latter, however, shows only a rather poor rank correlation with the subjective ratings. Good correlations, especially rank correlations, are achieved when ratings are averaged across different talkers per processing condition because averaging reduces the statistical noise of the ratings and thus increases the reliability of the data. On the

function of this stage is shown in Figure 4 for normal hearing and two hearing losses. The parameters of the input/function were chosen such that its shape matches the inverse function of the assumed input/output function of the unimpaired cochlea proposed by Moore [46]. Again, model parameters were not adjusted in the present study.

Results

The performance of the objective measures was characterized by their correlations with averaged subjective quality ratings of all processing conditions (including hidden reference and anchors), quantified by Pearson's linear correlation coefficient r and Spearman's rank correlation coefficient rs. Quality measure values were taken directly as output by the models and not transformed by, e.g., nonlinear regression functions.

As there were no systematic differences between the quality ratings of normal hearing adults and children, quality ratings were averaged across the complete group of normal hearing subjects. Consequently, results are stated for three groups of subjects separately: (1) normal hearing (adults and children), (2) hearing

Table 2. Results of the quality predictions (including anchor conditions) for the normal hearing subjects, expressed by linear correlation coefficients and rank correlation coefficients (*italic*).

measure	ind.	av.
qc+W-B (M2)	0.84	0.86
	0.89	*0.93*
qc-W-B (M4)	0.84	0.87
	0.84	*0.95*
PSM_lp-B (M12)	0.85	0.88
	0.84	*0.91*
PSM_fb-B (M10)	0.88	0.89
	0.92	*0.98*
HASQ$_{comb}$ (M19)	*0.54*	*0.54*
	0.24	*0.19*
PESQ (M21)	0.64	0.64
	0.41	*0.45*
S$_{overall}$ (M25)$_l$	0.76	0.76
	0.63	*0.64*
LPD (M22)	−0.75	−0.77
	−0.64	*−0.62*
LAR (M27)	−0.83	−0.84
	−0.74	*−0.71*

Subjective ratings were averaged across subjects. Middle column: correlations based on ratings for individual talkers (ind.); right column: ratings averaged across talkers (av.). Quality measure suffixes: fb/lp: modulation filterbank/lowpass model version; +/−W: with/without frequency band weighting; +/−B: with/without asymmetric weighting of differences ("Beerends weighting").

other hand, the significance of the correlation coefficients gets lower as the number of data points is reduced to only eight.

Figure 5 shows a scatter plot of the results obtained with the measure PSM_fb-B (M10). It must be noted that the results for two of the four talkers processed by the NFC condition cr2_fc3k were not available due to a labelling error and a processing error of the concerned test files. It can be observed from this figure that the quality ratings for the NFC test conditions are bordered by the ratings of the high quality (hidden) reference and the low quality anchor stimuli (lowpass-filtered and clipped speech, respectively). The scatter plot reveals that the model underestimates the perceived quality of the clipped speech samples whose predicted quality was lower than that of the lowpass-filtered samples, whereas the subjects ranked the qualities of these conditions in an opposite manner. Another noteworthy difference between model predictions and the subjective ratings is the larger predicted quality difference between the reference condition and the processed conditions compared to the differences among processed conditions.

Both subjects and model rate the frequency-compressed signals with the lowest cutoff frequency 2 kHz (condition cr2-fc2k) very poorly compared to the other frequency compression conditions. A possible cause for this non-linear relation between compression cutoff frequency and perceptual effect could be the alteration of speech formant frequencies and/or the interference of down-shifted higher frequency contents with these formants. Vowel formants have significant energy in the second and third formants in approximately the 1000–4000 Hz region for female speech and approximately 750–3000 Hz for male speech, depending on the specific vowel and talker. Recalling that both male and female speech samples were used, it is reasonable to conclude that the cr2-fc2k setting was strong enough to lower significantly the upper

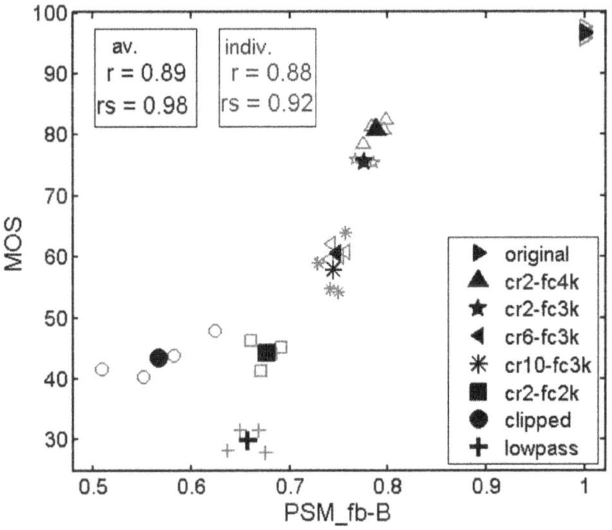

Figure 5. Scatter plot of the results obtained with the PEMO-Q measure PSM_fb-B for the normal hearing subjects. Subjective ratings (Mean Opinion Scores – MOS) are plotted versus corresponding model predictions. r: linear correlation, rs: rank correlation.

formants of many vowels for both male and female speech and was therefore much more noticeable than settings that likely did not disrupt the harmonic relationships within vowels, such as those that used a 4000 Hz cutoff frequency.

Figure 5 shows that in general, the influence of the talker on the measured and predicted quality ratings is very small, except for the clipping condition. Here, the influence of the talker is overestimated by the PSM measure.

Results for hearing impaired children

The results obtained for the hearing impaired children are shown in Table 3 and Figure 6. According to the correlations with subjective ratings (Table 3), the prediction accuracy of the models for hearing impaired listeners for separate talkers was very good (r up to 0.94), and even higher when averaged across talkers (r up to 0.99). The slightly better performance of the modulation filterbank version of PEMO-Q in the prediction of normal hearing subjects' ratings (Table 2) was not confirmed by the results obtained with hearing impaired children (Table 3).

Figure 6 depicts a scatter plot for PSM_lp-B, hearing impaired (HI) version (M16) and subjective ratings from hearing impaired children. In contrast to Figure 5, a greater variation of quality ratings and predictions for different talkers can be seen in this figure. Note that the predicted quality of the original, unprocessed condition is always maximal, since this condition is used as the reference by the comparison-based quality models. Hence, possible influences of different talkers cannot be modeled for this condition. Another difference from the normal hearing data concerns the rank order of the three processing conditions with the lowest ratings, i.e. lowpass filtering (LP), clipping (CL) and frequency compression with the lowest cutoff frequency, 2 kHz (cr2-fc2k). Normal hearing subjects ranked LP< CL ≈ cr2-fc2k. The model, in contrast, ranked CL<LP< cr2-fc2k. Hearing impaired children, however, ranked these conditions clearly differently: cr2-fc2k<CL<LP. This rank order was correctly predicted by the quality measure PSM_lp-B (HI) (M16). As a consequence, a very high linear correlation ($r = 0.99$) and a perfect

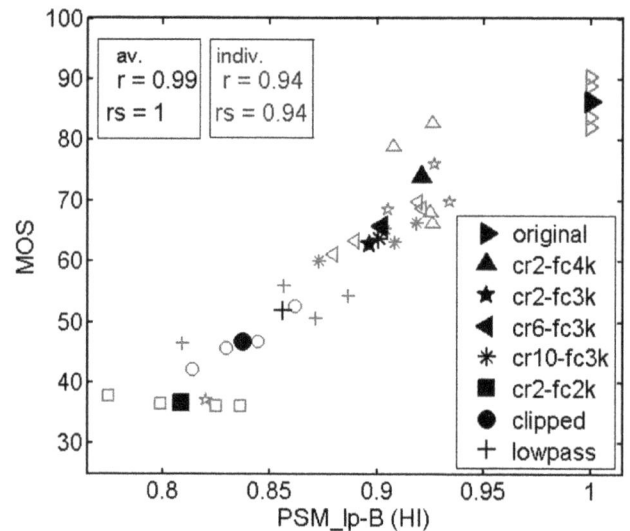

Figure 6. Same as Figure 5, but for hearing impaired children.

rank correlation ($rs = 1$) between PSM_lp-B and subjective ratings were achieved when averaged across talkers. Finally, the range of PSM_lp-B (HI) (M16) values is smaller compared to PSM_fb-B (M10) values used for normal hearing subjects, while the range of subjective ratings is about the same in both cases. This difference is due to the greater sensitivity of the modulation filterbank version of the auditory model PEMO used for the computation of

Table 3. Quality prediction results (linear and rank correlation (*italic*) coefficients) for the hearing impaired children group.

measure	NH models		HI models	
	ind.	**av.**	**ind.**	**av.**
qc+W-B (M2, M6)	0.58	0.59	0.87	0.90
	0.78	*0.88*	*0.89*	*0.93*
qc-W-B (M4, M8)	0.82	0.87	0.90	0.95
	0.80	*0.91*	*0.91*	*0.93*
PSM_lp-B (M12, M16)	0.87	0.91	0.94	0.99
	0.86	*0.95*	*0.94*	*1.00*
PSM_fb-B (M10, M14)	0.84	0.87	0.94	0.97
	0.87	*0.93*	*0.95*	*0.95*
HASQ_{comb} (M19)	*0.73*	*0.76*	*0.81*	*0.85*
	0.80	*0.69*	*0.87*	*0.88*
PESQ (M20)	0.90	0.92		
	0.90	*0.83*		
S_{overall} (M25)	0.83	0.85		
	0.90	*0.88*		
LPD (M22)	−0.51	−0.55		
	−0.53	*−0.57*		
LAR (M27)	−0.61	−0.63		
	−0.65	*−0.67*		

Results for the PEMO-Q measure PSM and the related measure qc are given for normal hearing (NH) and hearing impaired (HI) model versions. Quality measure suffixes: fb/lp: modulation filterbank/lowpass model version; +/−W: with/without frequency band weighting; +/−B: with/without asymmetric weighting of differences ("Beerends weighting").

PSM_fb-B (M10), compared to the modulation lowpass filter version used for computing PSM_lp-B (HI) (M16).

Results for hearing impaired adults

Hearing impaired adults exhibited a different rating behavior than hearing impaired children on average, although there were no significant differences between the distributions of hearing losses in these two groups (children's hearing losses were somewhat higher than adults' hearing losses on average). Adults rated NFC conditions generally higher, except for condition cr2-fc2k, whereas their ratings of the anchor condition (LP, CL) were similar to children's ratings (compare Figure 7 with Figure 6). As a result, adults' average ratings of cr2-fc2k, LP and CL conditions were very similar, whereas the quality measure PSM_lp-B (HI) (M16) clearly rated cr2-fc2k<LP< CL, which led to a lower correlation between measured and predicted mean quality ratings ($r = 0.88$) compared to the results obtained for the children ($r = 0.99$). In contrast, a very high correlation was achieved by the related quality measure qc-W-B (HI) (M8) ($r = 0.96$). As described earlier, qc-W-B (HI) (M4, M8) mainly differs from PSM_lp-B (HI) (M12, M16) in the lower cutoff frequency of the peripheral filterbank. Looking at Figure 8, the higher correlation obtained with qc-W-B (HI) (M8) is mainly due to a shift of quality ratings of NFC conditions towards higher values compared to the PSM_lp-B (HI) (M16) values, whereas ratings of the anchor conditions LP and CL basically correspond to the PSM_lp-B (HI) (M16) values. This agrees well with the observed difference in subjective ratings between hearing impaired children and adults. Table 4 summarizes the prediction performances of the different quality measures. Amongst others, it clearly shows the advantage of using models that account for hearing impairment, as evidenced by the higher

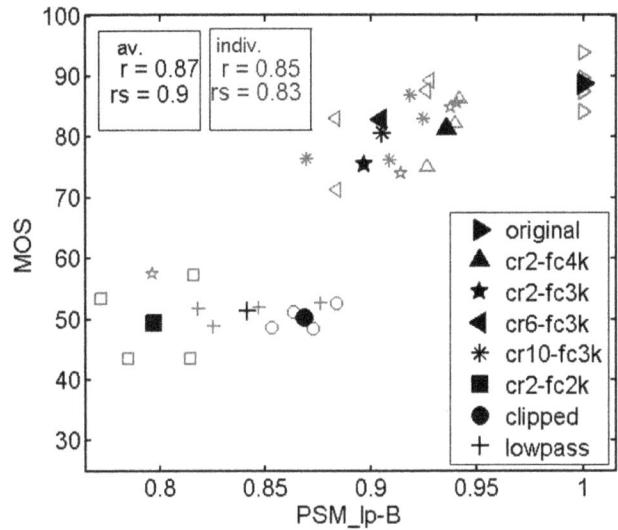

Figure 7. Same as Figure 5, but for hearing impaired adults.

correlations with subjective quality ratings for most of the evaluations.

Discussion

The obtained results show that predicting the perceived sound quality of nonlinearly frequency-compressed speech by means of objective, perceptual speech/audio quality models is possible. From the models tested, the PEMO-Q (related) measures, in

Table 4. Quality prediction results (linear and rank correlation (*italic*) coefficients) for the hearing impaired adults group.

measure	NH models		HI models	
	ind.	av.	ind.	av.
qc+W-B (M2, M6)	0.65	0.67	0.77	0.79
	0.68	*0.74*	*0.75*	*0.74*
qc-W-B (M4, M8)	0.85	0.88	0.91	0.96
	0.86	*0.76*	*0.87*	*0.81*
PSM_lp-B (M12, M16)	0.85	0.88	0.86	0.88
	0.86	*0.81*	*0.84*	*0.81*
PSM_fb-B (M10, M14)	0.78	0.81	0.82	0.85
	0.79	*0.81*	*0.79*	*0.86*
HASQ$_{comb}$ (M19)	*0.50*	*0.51*	0.78	0.79
	0.53	*0.62*	*0.86*	*0.95*
PESQ (M20)	0.62	0.63		
	0.79	*0.81*		
S$_{overall}$ (M25)	0.50	0.51		
	0.42	*0.48*		
LPD (M22)	−0.52	−0.57		
	−0.37	*−0.43*		
LAR (M27)	−0.62	−0.65		
	−0.49	*−0.48*		

Quality measure suffixes: fb/lp: modulation filterbank/lowpass model version; +/−W: with/without frequency band weighting; +/−B: with/without asymmetric weighting of differences ("Beerends weighting").

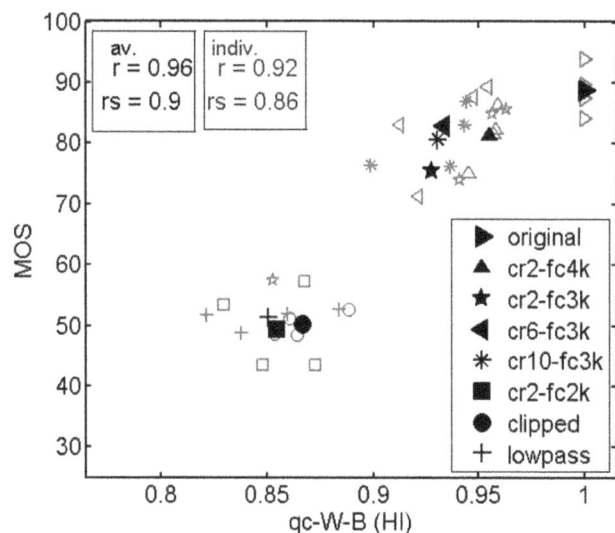

Figure 8. Quality prediction results for the hearing impaired adults group, obtained with quality measure qc-W-B (version for hearing impaired). r: linear correlation, rs: rank correlation.

particular, the Perceptual Similarity Measure (PSM) and the speech quality measure qc of the Hansen model (with deactivated frequency weighting function), showed the highest correlations with mean subjective ratings. These measures represent the most "basic" PEMO-based quality measures with the lowest degree of optimization for a specific task and hence the highest generality and robustness. This is in line with results of other studies where different quality measures have been applied for tasks other than those for which they were originally developed (e.g. [41–43]). Through the results of the present study, the generality of abovementioned measures is further proven given that the predicted quality degradations caused by very different kinds of distortions (i.e. frequency compression, amplitude clipping and lowpass filtering) correlated highly with subjective ratings.

A number of objective measures that were previously either applied to speech or audio quality estimation were evaluated in this paper. Of the objective measures based on speech production model parameters (viz. ISD (M26), LAR (M27), LLR (M28)), LAR (M27) performed the best. In the past, these metrics were primarily used for estimating narrowband (0–4 kHz bandwidth) speech quality (e.g. [28], [29]). Since some of the PEMO-based quality measures employed a wider bandwidth, experiments were conducted with implementations of ISD (M26), LAR (M27) and LLR (M28) metrics using an extended 8 kHz bandwidth. Results, however, showed a degradation in the correlation coefficients with subjective ratings for LAR (M27) and LLR (M28) metrics compared to the original versions with 4 kHz bandwidth. Similarly, the LPD (M22) metric was developed and validated for narrowband speech applications [36], and its performance with an extended bandwidth is not investigated in this work and is a worthwhile topic for future study.

Speech quality measures (M22, M25) based on the Moore & Glasberg model ([33–36]) performed decently with normal hearing data, but were inferior with the hearing impaired data. A revised model of loudness perception incorporating cochlear hearing loss was proposed by Moore and Glasberg [47], and further investigation would be interesting to determine whether the incorporation of this revised model would lead to an improvement in correlations with hearing impaired subjective data.

The Hearing Aid Speech Quality Index (HASQI, M17–M19) showed good rank correlations and moderate linear correlations with hearing impaired data, but only low correlations with normal hearing data. This is in clear contrast to the results reported in a recent publication on an updated version of the HASQI [48], which was also tested successfully on frequency-compressed speech. The main reason for the lower correlations observed in the present study was found to be a significant quality overestimation of the lowpass condition. The clipping condition was overestimated as well, although to a lesser extent. Without these anchor conditions, linear correlations of the HASQI_comb (M19) with subjective ratings increase to 0.83 for normal hearing data (0.85 when ratings are averaged across different talkers per condition), 0.75 (0.78) for hearing impaired adults' data, and 0.78 (0.82) for hearing impaired children's data. The HASQI submeasure for linear distortions (M17) achieves very high correlations in this case: 0.93 (0.95), 0.89 (0.95) and 0.95 (0.996) for normal hearing subjects', hearing impaired adults' and hearing impaired children's data, respectively.

In the present application, PESQ (M20, M21) surprisingly achieved poor correlations with subjective ratings from normal hearing listeners, but moderate and even high correlations with ratings from hearing impaired adults and children, respectively. The main reason for the poor results regarding normal hearing listeners was found to be a quality overestimation of the lowpass-filtered items by PESQ. Without this processing condition, the linear correlation obtained with the narrow-band version of PESQ increases to 0.89 (0.92) for normal hearing subjects. Correlations obtained with the wideband version of PESQ are lower in this case.

The successful "basic" PEMO-Q measures required minimal optimization during development, and use a very simple back-end of the underlying quality model. This result is interpreted as a reflection of the validity of the auditory model originally derived by Dau *et al.* [38], [40]. It represents a well-founded model of the "effective" signal processing in the auditory system and has been validated in a wide variety of psychoacoustical experiments [40], [49–55]. Its free parameters were adopted from psychoacoustical modeling and kept fixed in the development of the Hansen model and PEMO-Q as well as in the present study. When applied as a front-end for speech and audio quality prediction, only the bandwidth of the peripheral filterbank (i.e. the range of center frequencies) and the modulation filterbank were set appropriately. The bandwidth used in PEMO-Q appears to have been appropriate for use with the NFC data modeled in this study, too, although we did not evaluate impacts of any adjustments to these original settings. In the hearing-impaired adults group, however, better results were obtained with the quality measure qc with its smaller filterbank bandwidth compared to PSM. This suggests that the bandwidth could still be optimized for the present task and possibly lead to a further improvement of the quality prediction accuracy.

As already pointed out before, the higher correlation with the adults' quality ratings obtained with the measure qc-W-B (HI) (M8) compared to PSM_lp-B (HI) (M16) is mainly due to an upward shift of quality predictions for the 2 kHz-lowpass condition and the frequency-compressed condition with the lowest cutoff frequency of 2 kHz, which is in line with the adults' rating behavior. The upper cutoff frequency of the peripheral filterbank used in the computation of qc-W-B (HI) (M8) is 4 kHz, whereas it is 15.3 kHz for PSM. The two processing conditions of concern cancel (most of) the energy at frequencies higher than 4 kHz. The measure qc-W-B (HI) (M8) does not "notice" the missing energy above 4 kHz, in contrast to PSM_lp-B (HI) (M16). As a consequence, PSM_lp-B (HI) (M16) detects a larger overall difference between original and processed signals which leads to a lower quality estimate. A possible reason for the better correspondence between hearing impaired adults' ratings and the qc-W-B (HI) (M8) predictions could be a reduced sensitivity of these subjects for missing energy at frequencies above 4 kHz, or/and a lower perceptual weighting of this degradation component when rating the overall quality. Apparently, the hearing impaired children of this study were more sensitive or less tolerant towards the quality degrading effects of frequency compression than the hearing impaired adults. They rated the quality of frequency-compressed speech samples clearly lower than the adults did, although the distributions of hearing losses as described by audiograms are similar in these two groups; the children's hearing losses are in fact somewhat higher on average than the adults' hearing losses. There are two factors that may be related to this difference between age groups. First, age-related auditory and/or cognitive declines not revealed by the audiogram, but influencing quality perception might be factors related to this result. Moreover, age-dependent different experiences with and expectations on the quality of sound reproducing systems might play a role and have been speculated before [56]. However, to the knowledge of the authors, there is no data yet that would support such hypotheses, so these considerations remain speculative. Second, as is clinically typical, we provided the children with a higher level of gain and output in their hearing aids than was provided to adults [57]. For this reason, the children in this study may have had enhanced access to low-level effects in the processed signals and may have responded accordingly in their perceptual ratings. Again, this is a speculation and further study would be required to clarify whether this is a factor.

The fact that similar quality rating scores were obtained from normal hearing adults and children does not contradict the hypothesis of an age-related effect, because normal hearing adults in this study were much younger (mean = 24 years) than hearing impaired adults (mean = 69 years). However, in the present data, not all kinds of distortions were rated differently by older listeners, but mainly the frequency-compressed items. Lowpass-filtered and clipped samples received similar quality ratings from children and adults. The same is observed with the quality measure qc-W-B (HI) (M8), in contrast to PSM_lp-B (HI) (M16) for reasons explained above. As a result, qc-W-B (HI) (M8) correlates better with hearing impaired adults' quality rating scores, whereas PSM_lp-B (HI) (M16) is better suited to predict the hearing impaired children's ratings. However, the results obtained from hearing impaired adults and corresponding quality predictions obtained with the measure qc-W-B (HI) (M8) might represent a rather special data subset. In contrast, the measure PSM_lp-B (HI) (M16) appears to have a higher degree of generality and is thus recommended for general application.

Effect of PEMO-Q options

Modulation processing. A clear, consistent effect of the kind of modulation processing stage in PEMO-Q on the prediction accuracy could not be found in the results of the present study. Correlations achieved with the modulation lowpass and modulation filterbank versions of the PEMO-Q quality measure PSM, i.e. PSM_lp and PSM_fb, respectively, were mostly comparable and not consistently ranked with regard to subject group, individual vs. averaged talkers, and linear vs. rank correlation coefficients. Since the computational effort required for PSM_fb is about ten times

higher than for PSM_lp, the latter might be preferred for practical applications.

Asymmetric weighting of internal representation differences. The first application for which PEMO-Q was originally developed and optimized was the evaluation of audio codecs. For that purpose, a partial, asymmetric assimilation of internal representations of test and reference signals, equivalent to Beerends' asymmetry weighting of internal representation differences [44], was introduced into the quality model (option +B). In this procedure, negative deviations of the internal representation of the test signal from the reference are partially compensated (differences are halved), whereas positive deviations remain unchanged. This approach follows the hypothesis that "missing" components in a distorted signal are perceptually less disturbing than "additional" ones. This processing step was found to improve the quality prediction accuracy of PEMO-Q for audio codecs [58]. In the present application, however, better results were obtained without this processing step. The reason for this result is that the negative effect of strong frequency compression and lowpass filtering on sound quality by cancelling energy at medium to high frequencies (>3 kHz) is over-compensated by the assimilation procedure. Consequently, quality estimates are shifted towards higher values disproportionately with increasing frequency compression (i.e., increasing compression ratio and decreasing cutoff frequency) and for the 2 kHz-lowpass filter condition. Figure 9 illustrates this effect with the example of quality prediction results obtained with the quality measure PSM_fb (M9, M10) for the normal hearing subject group with and without assimilation of internal representations (+/−B).

Summary and Conclusions

In this paper, we presented results from a study on quality prediction of frequency-compressed speech in hearing aids by different objective speech and audio quality measures. Objective measures based on the audio quality model PEMO-Q and the related speech quality measure qc of the Hansen model achieved

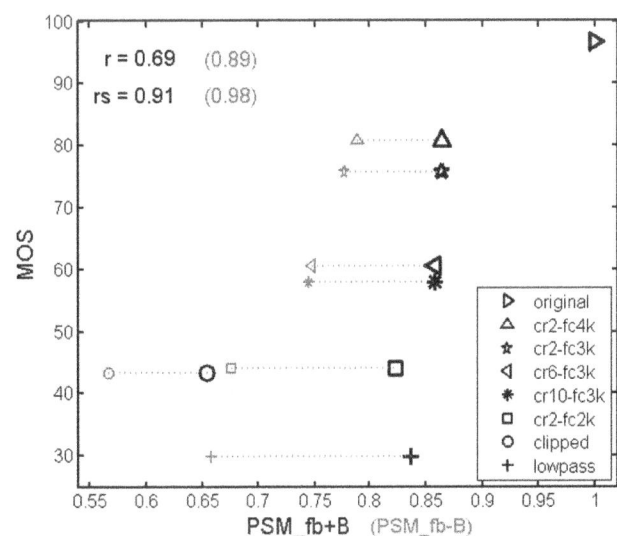

Figure 9. Effect of PEMO-Q model option +B (partial compensation of differences between test and reference internal representations) on quality estimates for the normal hearing subject group. Gray, small symbols: Results obtained with option −B (i.e. without partial compensation); black, large symbols: results obtained with option +B.

good correlations with averaged subjective ratings. The extension of these models incorporated hearing impairment, and improved prediction accuracy for quality ratings from hearing impaired subjects. Hearing impaired adults and children rated the quality of frequency-compressed speech differently. Best prediction results were achieved with different quality measures per subject group; adults' ratings were predicted better with a model that analyzes a smaller frequency bandwidth. Optimizations of bandwidth and possibly further model parameters were not carried out in the present study, but are considered to bear significant potential for further improvements. The HASQI model was also evaluated, and revealed consistently high results across subject groups for the linear submeasure of this index. Again, further evaluation could reveal optimization to the main HASQI model to further improve its performance.

In summary, the present study reports first-of-a-kind results on a broad range of objective sound quality evaluation models of frequency-compressed speech. Further studies are needed to validate the performance of the PEMO-Q quality measures for this application with a larger group of hearing impaired listeners and across more NFC parameter settings. Moreover, the predictability of perceived quality of other sound stimuli than speech, such as music, should be investigated. In addition, the objective modeling of sound quality for frequency lowering schemes other than the NFC scheme evaluated here would require further investigation. In addition, possible influences of age and acclimatization to frequency-compressed sound will have to be investigated and modeled. Research on this topic is driven by the fact that a successful objective speech quality model will have the potential to serve as a valuable supplemental tool for the fitting and evaluation of frequency lowering algorithms in hearing instruments.

Acknowledgments

We thank Andreas Seelisch and Danielle Glista for sharing their data and Prof. James Kates for sharing his HASQI code, and Phonak AG for providing hearing instruments for this work. We also thank four anonymous reviewers for their helpful comments on earlier versions of this article.

Author Contributions

Conceived and designed the experiments: RH VP SS. Performed the experiments: RH. Analyzed the data: RH VP SS. Contributed reagents/materials/analysis tools: RH VP SS. Wrote the paper: RH VP SS.

References

1. Moore BCJ (2010) Dead regions in the cochlea: conceptual foundations, diagnosis, and clinical applications. Ear and Hearing, 25(2): 98–116.

2. Stelmachowicz PG, Lewis DE, Choi S, Hoover B (2007) Effect of stimulus bandwidth on auditory skills in normal-hearing and hearing-impaired children. Ear and Hearing, 28: 483–494.

3. Dillon H (2012) Hearing Aids. Thieme Medical Publishers, 2nd edition.

4. Kuk P, Korhonen H, Peeters D, Keenan A, Jessen H et al. (2006) Linear frequency transposition: extending the audibility of high-frequency energy. Hearing Review, 13(10): 42–48.

5. www.bernafon.com/Professionals/Downloads/~/media/PDF/English/Global/Bernafon/WhitePaper/BF_WP_Frequency_Composition_UK.ashx.

6. McDermott HJ (2011) A Technical Comparison of Digital Frequency-Lowering Algorithms Available in Two Current Hearing Aids. PLoS ONE 6(7): e22358. doi:10.1371/journal.pone.0022358.

7. Simpson A, Hersbach AA, McDermott HJ (2005) Improvements in speech perception with an experimental nonlinear frequency compression hearing device. Int J Audiol, 44: 281–292.

8. Glista D, Scollie S, Bagatto M, Seewald R, Parsa V et al. (2009) Evaluation of nonlinear frequency compression: Clinical outcomes. Int J Audiol, 48: 632–644.

9. Wolfe J, John AB, Schafer E, Nyffeler M, Boretzki M et al. (2010) Evaluation of non-linear frequency compression for school-age children with moderate to moderately-severe hearing loss. J Amer Acad Audiol, 21(10), 618–628.

10. Glista D, Scollie S, Sulkers J (2012) Perceptual Acclimatization Post Nonlinear Frequency Compression Hearing Aid Fitting in Older Children. J Speech Lang Hear Res, 55(6): 1765–87. Doi: 10.1044/1092-4388(2012/11-0163).

11. Parsa V, Scollie S, Glista D, Seelisch A (2013) Nonlinear frequency compression: Effects on sound quality ratings of speech and music. Trends Amplif, 17(1): 54–88.

12. Souza PE, Arehart KH, Kates JM, Croghan NB, Gehani N. (2013) Exploring the limits of frequency lowering. J Speech Lang Hear Res., 56(5): 1349–63.

13. ITU-T Rec. G.107 (2002). The E-Model, a Computational Model for Use in Transmission Planning. International Telecommunication Union, CH-Geneva.

14. ITU-T (2001) Perceptual evaluation of speech quality (PESQ), an objective method for end-to-end speech quality assessment of narrow-band telephone networks and speech codecs. ITU-T Recommendation P.862, International Telecommunications Union, Geneva, Switzerland.

15. Rix AW, Beerends JG, Kim DS, Kroon P, Ghitza O (2006) Objective Assessment of Speech and Audio Quality - Technology and Applications. IEEE Trans Audio Speech Lang Processing, 14 (6): 1890–1901.

16. Beerends JG, Krebber J, Huber R, Eneman K, Luts H (2008) Speech quality measurement for the hearing impaired on the basis of PESQ. Proc. of the 124th AES Convention, Amsterdam, The Netherlands.

17. Nielsen LB (1993) Objective Scaling of Sound Quality for Normal-Hearing and Hearing-Impaired Listeners. The Acoustics Laboratory, Technical University of Denmark, Lyngby, Denmark.

18. Schmalfuß G (2004) Anwendung psychoakustischer Methoden und Modelle zur Feinanpassung von Hörgeräten mit natürlichen Schallen [Application of psychoacoustic methods and models for fine-fitting of hearing aids using natural sounds. Ph.D. thesis, Technical University of Munich, Germany, 2004.

19. Kates JM, Arehart KH (2010) The Hearing-Aid Speech Quality Index (HASQI). J Audio Eng Soc, 58(5): 363–381.

20. ITU-R (1998) Method for objective measurement of perceived audio quality. ITU-R Recommendation BS.1387, International Telecommunications Union, Geneva, Switzerland.

21. Hagerman B, Gabrielsson A (1985) Questionnaires on desirable properties of hearing aids. Scand Audiol, 14(2): 109–111.

22. Kochkin S (2002) Marketrak VI: 10-year customer satisfaction trends in the US hearing instrument market. Hearing Review, 9 (10): 14–25.

23. Ovegård A, Lundberg G, Hagerman B, Gabrielsson A, Bengtsson M et al. (1997) Sound quality judgment during acclimatization of hearing aid. Scand Audiol, 26: 43–51.

24. Wong LLN, Hickson L, McPherson B (2003) Hearing aid satisfaction: what does research from the past 20 years say? Trends Amplif, 7(4): 117–161.

25. ITU-R (2003) Method for the subjective assessment of intermediate quality levels of coding systems. ITU-R Recommendation BS.1534, International Telecommunications Union, Geneva, Switzerland.

26. Itakura F, Saito S (1997) A Statistical Method for Estimation of Speech Spectral Density and Formant Frequencies. In: Schafer RW, Markel, JD, editors. Speech Analysis. IEEE Press. New York.

27. Itakura F (1975) Minimum prediction residual principle applied to speech recognition. IEEE Trans Acoust, 23(1): 67–72.

28. Quackenbush S, Barnwell T, Clements M, (1998) Objective Measures of Speech Quality. Prentice Hall, Englewood Cliffs/New Jersey.

29. Hansen J, Pellom B (1998) An effective quality evaluation protocol for speech enhancement algorithms. Proc. ICSLP '98, Sydney, Australia.

30. Klatt D (1998) Prediction of perceived phonetic distance from critical-band spectra: A first step. Proc. IEEE ICASSP 1982: 1278–1281.

31. ITU-T (2005) Wideband extension to Recommendation P.862 for the assessment of wideband telephone networks and speech codecs. ITU-T Recommendation P.862.2 International Telecommunications Union. Geneva, Switzerland.

32. Moore BCJ, Glasberg BR (1997) A Model of Loudness Perception Applied to Cochlear Hearing Loss. Aud Neurosci, 3: 289–311.

33. Moore BCJ, Tan CT, Zacharov N, Matilla VV (2004) Measuring and predicting the perceived quality of music and speech subjected to combined linear and nonlinear distortion. J Audio Eng Soc, 52: 1228–1244.

34. Tan CT, Moore BCJ, Zacharov N, Matilla VV (2004) Predicting the perceived quality of nonlinearly distorted music and speech signals. J Audio Eng Soc, 52: 699–711.

35. Moore BCJ, Tan CT (2004) Development and Validation of a Method for Predicting the Perceived Naturalness of Sounds Subjected to Spectral Distortion. J Audio Eng Soc, 52: 900–914.

36. Chen G, Parsa V, Scollie S (2006) An ERB Loudness Pattern Based Objective Speech Quality Measure. Proc. Int. Conf. on Spoken Language Processing, Pittsburgh, USA, 2174–2177.

37. Hansen M, Kollmeier B (2000) Objective modelling of speech quality with a psychoacoustically validated auditory model. J Audio Eng Soc, 48: 395–409.
38. Dau T, Püschel D, Kohlrausch A (1996) A quantitative model of the 'effective' signal processing in the auditory system: I. Model structure. J Acoust Soc Am, 99: 3615–3622.
39. Huber R, Kollmeier B (2006) PEMO-Q - A New Method for Objective Audio Quality Assessment Using a Model of Auditory Perception. IEEE Trans Audio Speech Lang Processing, 14(6): 1902–1911.
40. Dau T, Kollmeier B, Kohlrausch A (1997) Modeling auditory processing of amplitude modulation: I. Modulation Detection and masking with narrowband carriers. J Acoust Soc Am, 102(5): 2892–2905.
41. Rohdenburg T, Hohmann V, Kollmeier B (2005) Objective Measures for the Evaluation of Noise Reduction Schemes. Proc. Int. Workshop on Acoustic Echo and Noise Control (IWAENC), Eindhoven, The Netherlands.
42. Goetze S, Albertin E, Kallinger M, Mertins A, Kammeyer KD (2010) Quality Assessment for Listening-Room Compensation Algorithms. Proc. ICASSP, Dallas, USA.
43. Huber R, Schulte M, Vormann M, Chalupper J (2010) Objective measures of speech quality in hearing aids: Prediction of listening effort reduction by noise reduction algorithms. Presented at the 2nd Workshop on Speech in Noise: Intelligibility and Quality, Amsterdam, The Netherlands Available: http://www.phon.ucl.ac.uk/events/quality2010/talks/RainerHuber.pdf.
44. Beerends JG (1994) Modelling cognitive effects that play a role in the perception of speech quality. Presented at the Workshop on Speech quality assessment at the Ruhr-Universität Bochum, Germany.
45. Derleth RP, Dau T, Kollmeier B (2001) Modelling temporal and compressive properties of the normal and impaired auditory system. Hearing Research, 159: 132–149.
46. Moore BCJ (1997) Psychoacoustic consequences of compression in the peripheral auditory system. In: Schick A, Klatte M, editors. Contributions to Psychological Acoustics. BIS Oldenburg, Germany.
47. Moore BCJ, Glasberg BR (2004) A revised model of loudness perception applied to cochlear hearing loss. Hearing Research, 188: 70–88.
48. Kates JM, Arehart KH (2014). The hearing-aid speech quality index (HASQI) version 2/J. Audio Eng. Soc. 62, 99–117.
49. Münkner S (1993) A psychoacoustical model for the perception of non-stationary sounds. In: Schick A, editor. Contributions to Psychological Acoustics. BIS Oldenburg, 121–134.
50. Fassel R (1994) Experimente und Simulationsrechnungen zur Wahrnehmung von Amplitudenmodulationen im menschlichen Gehör. [Experiments and simulations on the perception of amplitude modulations in the human auditory system.] PhD thesis, University of Göttingen, Germany.
51. Sander A (1994) Psychoakustische Aspekte der subjektiven Trennbarkeit von Klängen. [Psychoacoustic aspects of the subjective separability of sounds.] PhD thesis, University of Oldenburg, Germany.
52. Dau T, Püschel D, Kohlrausch A (1996) A quantitative model of the 'effective' signal processing in the auditory system: II. Simulations and measurements. J Acoust Soc Am, 99: 3623–3631.
53. Dau T, Kollmeier B, Kohlrausch A (1997) Modeling auditory processing of amplitude modulation. II. Spectral and temporal integration in modulation detection. J Acoust Soc Am, 102(5), 2906–2919.
54. Verhey JL (1998) Psychoacoustics of spectro-temporal effects in masking and loudness patterns. BIS, Oldenburg. ISBN 3-8142-0622-2.
55. Derleth RP, Dau T (2000) On the role of envelope fluctuation processing in spectral masking. J Acoust Soc Am, 108(1): 285–96.
56. Krebber J, Eneman K, Huber R (2007) Report on Experiments on the Performance of Normal and Non-normal-hearing Listeners for a Range of (Simulated) Transmission Conditions with Combined Technical Disturbances. HearCom Deliverable D-4-3 Available: http://hearcom.eu/about/DisseminationandExploitation/deliverables.html.
57. Scollie S, Seewald R, Cornelisse L, Moodie ST, Bagatto M et al., 2005. The desired sensation level multistage input/output algorithm. Trends Amplif, 9, 159–197.
58. Huber R (2003) Objective assessment of audio quality using an auditory processing model. PhD thesis, University of Oldenburg, Germany Available: http://docserver.bis.uni-oldenburg.de/publikationen/dissertation/2004/hubobj03/hubobj03.html.

Permissions

List of Contributors

Wilhelmina H. A. M. Mulders, Kristin M. Barry, Donald Robertson
The Auditory Laboratory, School of Anatomy, Physiology and Human Biology, The University of Western Australia, Crawley, Western Australia, Australia

Omar Akil, Jolie Chang and Lawrence R. Lustig
Department of Otolaryngology, Head & Neck Surgery, University of California San Francisco, San Francisco, California, United States of America

Faith Hall-Glenn and Tamara Alliston
Department of Orthopaedic Surgery, University of California San Francisco, San Francisco, California, United States of America

Alfred Li and Wenhan Chang
Endocrine Unit and Bone Imaging Core, San Francisco VA Medical Center, San Francisco, California, United States of America

Edward C. Hsiao
Division of Endocrinology and Metabolism, and the Institute for Human Genetics, Department of Medicine, University of California San Francisco, San Francisco, California, United States of America

Taro Yamaguchi, Reiko Nagashima, Masanori Yoneyama, Tatsuo Shiba and Kiyokazu Ogita
Laboratory of Pharmacology, Faculty of Pharmaceutical Sciences, Setsunan University, Hirakata, Osaka, Japan

Sherif F. Tadros and Mary D'Souza
International Center for Hearing & Speech Research, National Technical Institute for the Deaf, Rochester Institute of Technology, Rochester, New York, United States of America
Otolaryngology Dept., University of Rochester Medical School, Rochester, New York, United States of America

Xiaoxia Zhu and Robert D. Frisina
International Center for Hearing & Speech Research, National Technical Institute for the Deaf, Rochester Institute of Technology, Rochester, New York, United States of America
Otolaryngology Dept., University of Rochester Medical School, Rochester, New York, United States of America
Depts. Chemical & Biomedical Engineering, Communication Sciences & Disorders, and Global Center for Hearing & Speech Research, University of South Florida, Tampa, Florida, United States of America

Nicole Rosskothen-Kuhl and Robert-Benjamin Illing
Neurobiological Research Laboratory, Department of Otorhinolaryngology, University of Freiburg, Freiburg, Germany

Rui Deng, Ye Jiang and Bing Chen
Department of Otology and Skull Base Surgery, Eye Ear Nose and Throat Hospital, Fudan University, Shanghai, China

Duoduo Tao
Department of Otology and Skull Base Surgery, Eye Ear Nose and Throat Hospital, Fudan University, Shanghai, China
Division of Communication and Auditory Neuroscience, House Research Institute, Los Angeles, California, United States of America

Qian-Jie Fu
Department of Otology and Skull Base Surgery, Eye Ear Nose and Throat Hospital, Fudan University, Shanghai, China
Division of Communication and Auditory Neuroscience, House Research Institute, Los Angeles, California, United States of America
Department of Head and Neck Surgery, David Geffen School of Medicine, UCLA, Los Angeles, California, United States of America

John J. Galvin III
Division of Communication and Auditory Neuroscience, House Research Institute, Los Angeles, California, United States of America
Department of Head and Neck Surgery, David Geffen School of Medicine, UCLA, Los Angeles, California, United States of America

Dayong Wang, Liang Zong, Feifan Zhao, Wei Shi, Lan Lan, Hongyang Wang, Qian Li, Bing Han and Qiuju Wang
Chinese PLA Institute of Otolaryngology, Chinese PLA General Hospital, Beijing, China

Yali Zhao
Chinese PLA Institute of Otolaryngology, Chinese PLA General Hospital, Beijing, China
Beijing Institute of Otorhinolaryngology, Beijing Tongren Hospital, Capital Medical University, Beijing, China

Liping Guan, Peng Zhang, Jian Wang and Jun Wang
BGI-Shenzhen, Shenzhen, China

Xin Jin
BGI-Shenzhen, Shenzhen, China
School of Bioscience and Biotechnology, South China
University of Technology, Guangzhou, China

Ling Yang
BGI-Tianjin, Tianjin, China

Abhay Lodha and Reg Sauvé
Department of Pediatrics, Foothills Medical Centre,
Peter Lougheed Centre, Alberta Children's Hospital,
Calgary, Canada
Community Health Sciences, University of Calgary,
Calgary, Canada
Alberta Health Services, Calgary, Canada
Alberta Children's Hospital Institute of Child &
Maternal Health, Calgary, Canada

Harish Amin
Department of Pediatrics, Foothills Medical Centre,
Peter Lougheed Centre, Alberta Children's Hospital,
Calgary, Canada
Alberta Health Services, Calgary, Canada

Nalini Singhal
Department of Pediatrics, Foothills Medical Centre,
Peter Lougheed Centre, Alberta Children's Hospital,
Calgary, Canada
Alberta Health Services, Calgary, Canada
Alberta Children's Hospital Institute of Child &
Maternal Health, Calgary, Canada

Heather Christianson
Community Health Sciences, University of Calgary,
Calgary, Canada
Alberta Health Services, Calgary, Canada

Selphee Tang
Alberta Health Services, Calgary, Canada

Vineet Bhandari
Department of Pediatrics, Yale University School of
Medicine, New Haven, Connecticut, United States of
America

Anita Bhandari
Department of Pediatric Pulmonology, Connecticut
Children's Medical Center, Hartford, Connecticut,
United States of America

**Ann-Cathrine Lindblad, Åke Olofsson and Björn
Hagerman**
Department of Clinical Science, Intervention and
Technology, Division of Ear, Nose and Throat Diseases,
Unit of Technical and Experimental Audiology,
Karolinska Institutet, Stockholm, Sweden

Ulf Rosenhall
Department of Clinical Science, Intervention and
Technology, Division of Ear, Nose and Throat Diseases,
Karolinska Institutet; and Department of Audiology
and Neurotology, Karolinska University Hospital,
Stockholm, Sweden

Kaoru Ogawa
Department of Otolaryngology, Head and Neck
Surgery, Keio University, School of Medicine, Shinjuku,
Tokyo, Japan

Masato Fujioka
Department of Otolaryngology, Head and Neck
Surgery, Keio University, School of Medicine, Shinjuku,
Tokyo, Japan
Department of Physiology, School of Medicine, Keio
University, School of Medicine, Shinjuku, Tokyo, Japan

Hideyuki Okano
Department of Physiology, School of Medicine, Keio
University, School of Medicine, Shinjuku, Tokyo, Japan

Hirotaka James Okano
Department of Physiology, School of Medicine, Keio
University, School of Medicine, Shinjuku, Tokyo, Japan
Division of Regenerative Medicine, Jikei University
School of Medicine, Tokyo, Japan

Yasuhide Okamoto
Department of Otorhinolaryngology, Inagi Municipal
Hospital, Inagi, Tokyo, Japan
The Laboratory of Auditory Disorders and Division
of Hearing and Balance Research, National Institute
of Sensory Organs, National Tokyo Medical Center,
Meguro, Tokyo, Japan

Seiichi Shinden
Department of Otolaryngology, Saiseikai Utsunomiya
Hospital, Utsunomiya, Tochigi, Japan
The Laboratory of Auditory Disorders and Division
of Hearing and Balance Research, National Institute
of Sensory Organs, National Tokyo Medical Center,
Meguro, Tokyo, Japan

Tatsuo Matsunaga
The Laboratory of Auditory Disorders and Division
of Hearing and Balance Research, National Institute
of Sensory Organs, National Tokyo Medical Center,
Meguro, Tokyo, Japan

Alex Burdorf
Dept of Public Health, Erasmus MC University
Medical Center, Rotterdam, the Netherlands

Ineke Vogel
Dept of Public Health, Erasmus MC University Medical Center, Rotterdam, the Netherlands
Dept of Youth Policy, Municipal Public Health Service for Rotterdam Area, Rotterdam, the Netherlands

Petra M. van de Looij-Jansen, Cathelijne L. Mieloo and Frouwkje de Waart
Dept of Youth Policy, Municipal Public Health Service for Rotterdam Area, Rotterdam, the Netherlands

Yong-Yi Yuan, Feng Xin and Fei Yu
Department of Otolaryngology, Head and Neck Surgery, PLA General Hospital, Beijing, P. R. China

Guo-Jian Wang, Ming-Yu Han, Hui Zhao and Pu Dai
Department of Otolaryngology, Head and Neck Surgery, PLA General Hospital, Beijing, P. R. China
Department of Otolaryngology, Hainan Branch of PLA General Hospital, Sanya, P. R. China

Xue Gao
Department of Otolaryngology, Head and Neck Surgery, PLA General Hospital, Beijing, P. R. China
Department of Otolaryngology, Hainan Branch of PLA General Hospital, Sanya, P. R. China
Department of Otolaryngology, the Second Artillery General Hospital, Beijing, P. R. China

Jing-Qiao Lu and Xi Lin
Department of Otolaryngology, Emory University School of Medicine, Atlanta, Georgia, United States of America

Jin-Cao Xu and Mei-Guang Zhang
Department of Otolaryngology, the Second Artillery General Hospital, Beijing, P. R. China

Jiang Dong
Xi'an Research Institute of Hi_tech, Hongqing, Xi'an, Shaanxi, P. R. China

Alfred Ultsch
DataBionics Research Group, University of Marburg, Marburg, Germany

Jörn Lötsch
Institute of Clinical Pharmacology, Goethe - University, Frankfurt am Main, Germany
Fraunhofer Institute for Molecular Biology and Applied Ecology IME, Project Group Translational Medicine and Pharmacology TMP, Frankfurt am Main, Germany

Sandy Oba and Qian-Jie Fu
Division of Communication and Auditory Neuroscience, House Research Institute, Los Angeles, California, United States of America

Department of Head and Neck Surgery, David Geffen School of Medicine, University of California Los Angeles, Los Angeles, California, United States of America

John J. Galvin III
Division of Communication and Auditory Neuroscience, House Research Institute, Los Angeles, California, United States of America
Department of Head and Neck Surgery, David Geffen School of Medicine, University of California Los Angeles, Los Angeles, California, United States of America
Department of Otorhinolaryngology, Head and Neck Surgery, University Medical Center Groningen, University of Groningen, Groningen, The Netherlands
Research School of Behavioral and Cognitive Neurosciences, Graduate School of Medical Sciences, University of Groningen, Groningen, The Netherlands

Deniz Başkent
Department of Otorhinolaryngology, Head and Neck Surgery, University Medical Center Groningen, University of Groningen, Groningen, The Netherlands
Research School of Behavioral and Cognitive Neurosciences, Graduate School of Medical Sciences, University of Groningen, Groningen, The Netherlands

Stephanie C. P. M. Theunissen, Anouk P. Netten, Jeroen J. Briaire and Wim Soede
Department of Otorhinolaryngology and Head & Neck Surgery, Leiden University Medical Center, Leiden, The Netherlands

Johan H. M. Frijns
Department of Otorhinolaryngology and Head & Neck Surgery, Leiden University Medical Center, Leiden, The Netherlands
Leiden Institute for Brain and Cognition, Leiden, The Netherlands

Maartje Kouwenberg
Department of Developmental Psychology, Leiden University, Leiden, The Netherlands

Carolien Rieffe
Department of Developmental Psychology, Leiden University, Leiden, The Netherlands
Dutch Foundation for the Deaf and Hard of Hearing Child, Amsterdam, The Netherlands

Vera G. Pshennikova
Department of Molecular Genetics, Yakut Scientific Centre of Complex Medical Problems, Siberian Branch of the Russian Academy of Medical Sciences, Yakutsk, Russian Federation

Nikolay A. Barashkov
Department of Molecular Genetics, Yakut Scientific Centre of Complex Medical Problems, Siberian Branch of the Russian Academy of Medical Sciences, Yakutsk, Russian Federation
Laboratory of Molecular Biology, Institute of Natural Sciences, M.K. Ammosov North-Eastern Federal University, Yakutsk, Russian Federation

Aisen V. Solovyev
Laboratory of Molecular Biology, Institute of Natural Sciences, M.K. Ammosov North-Eastern Federal University, Yakutsk, Russian Federation

Maria V. Pak
Department of Pediatric, Medical Institute, M.K. Ammosov North-Eastern Federal University, Yakutsk, Russian Federation

Anatoliy N. Alexeev
Institute of Humanitarian Research and Indigenous Peoples of the North, Siberian Branch of the Russian Academy of Sciences, Yakutsk, Russian Federation

Lilya U. Dzhemileva
Department of Genomics, Institute of Biochemistry and Genetics, Ufa Scientific Centre, Russian Academy of Sciences, Ufa, Russian Federation

Thomas Lenarz
Department of Otolaryngology, Hannover School of Medicine, Hannover, Germany,

Mareike Hütten
Department of Otolaryngology, Hannover School of Medicine, Hannover, Germany,
University of Veterinary Medicine Hannover, Foundation, Institute of Zoology, Hannover, Germany

Verena Scheper
Department of Otolaryngology, Hannover School of Medicine, Hannover, Germany
Institute of Audioneurotechnology, Hannover School of Medicine, Hannover, Germany

Karl-Heinz Esser
University of Veterinary Medicine Hannover, Foundation, Institute of Zoology, Hannover, Germany

Roland Hessler and Claude Jolly
MED-EL Innsbruck, Research & Development, Innsbruck, Österreich

Anandhan Dhanasingh
MED-EL Innsbruck, Research & Development, Innsbruck, Österreich

Interactive Materials Research–DWI e.V. and Institute of Technical and Macromolecular Chemistry, RWTH Aachen University, Aachen, Germany

Martin Möller
Interactive Materials Research–DWI e.V. and Institute of Technical and Macromolecular Chemistry, RWTH Aachen University, Aachen, Germany

Jürgen Groll
Interactive Materials Research–DWI e.V. and Institute of Technical and Macromolecular Chemistry, RWTH Aachen University, Aachen, Germany
University of Würzburg, Department of Functional Materials in Medicine and Dentistry, Würzburg, Germany

Timo Stöver and J. W. Goethe
University Hospital and Faculty of Medicine, Department of Otolaryngology, Frankfurt am Main, Germany

Cornelis P. Lanting, Emile de Kleine and Pim van Dijk
Department of Otorhinolaryngology/Head and Neck Surgery, University Medical Center Groningen, University of Groningen, Groningen, Netherlands
Graduate School of Medical Sciences (Research School of Behavioural and Cognitive Neurosciences), University of Groningen, Groningen, Netherlands

Dave R. M. Langers
Department of Otorhinolaryngology/Head and Neck Surgery, University Medical Center Groningen, University of Groningen, Groningen, Netherlands
National Institute for Health Research, Nottingham Hearing Biomedical Research Unit, School of Clinical Sciences, University of Nottingham, Queen's Medical Centre, Nottingham, United Kingdom

Mark Edmondson-Jones, Heather Fortnum and Robert H. Pierzycki
NIHR Nottingham Hearing Biomedical Research Unit, Nottingham, United Kingdom
Otology and Hearing Group, Division of Clinical Neuroscience, School of Medicine, University of Nottingham, Nottingham, United Kingdom

David R. Moore
NIHR Nottingham Hearing Biomedical Research Unit, Nottingham, United Kingdom
MRC Institute of Hearing Research, University Park, Nottingham, United Kingdom
Cincinnati Children's Hospital Medical Center and Department of Otolaryngology, University of Cincinnati College of Medicine, Cincinnati, Ohio, United States of America

Abby McCormack
NIHR Nottingham Hearing Biomedical Research Unit, Nottingham, United Kingdom
MRC Institute of Hearing Research, University Park, Nottingham, United Kingdom
Otology and Hearing Group, Division of Clinical Neuroscience, School of Medicine, University of Nottingham, Nottingham, United Kingdom

Piers Dawes
School of Psychological Sciences, University of Manchester, Manchester, United Kingdom

Kevin J. Munro
School of Psychological Sciences, University of Manchester, Manchester, United Kingdom
Central Manchester University Hospitals NHS Foundation Trust, Manchester Academic Health Science Centre, Manchester, United Kingdom

Guanyin Chen, Zhi Liu, Yongzhu Sun and Pengcheng Cui
Department of Otolaryngology Head and Neck Surgery, Tangdu Hospital, the Fourth Military Medical University, Xi'an, China

Lining Feng
Department of Clinical Medicine, Faculty of Aerospace medicine, the Fourth Military Medical University, Xián, China

Haifeng Chang
Department of Radiology, Tangdu Hospital, the Fourth Military Medical University, Xi'an,China

Janaina Oliveira Bentivi Pulcherio
Department of Otolaryngology, Hospital Central da Polıćia Militar, Rio de Janeiro, Brazil

Aline Gomes Bittencourt, Patrick Rademaker Burke, Rubens de Brito, Robinson Koji Tsuji and Ricardo Ferreira Bento
Department of Otolaryngology, University of São Paulo School of Medicine, São Paulo, Brazil,

Rafael da Costa Monsanto
Department of Otolaryngology, Banco de Olhos de Sorocaba Hospital, São Paulo, Brazil

Lisa E. Wolber, Claire J. Steves, Pei-Chien Tsai, Tim D. Spector, Jordana T. Bell and Frances M. K. Williams
Department of Twin Research and Genetic Epidemiology, King's College London, London, United Kingdom

Panos Deloukas
William Harvey Research Institute, Barts and The London School of Medicine and Dentistry, Queen Mary University of London, London, United Kingdom
King Abdulaziz University, Jeddah, Saudi Arabia
Wellcome Trust Sanger Institute, Hinxton, Cambridge, United Kingdom

Rony H. Salloum and Christopher Yurosko
Department of Neurosciences, The Cleveland Clinic, Cleveland, Ohio, United States of America

James A. Kaltenbach
Department of Neurosciences, The Cleveland Clinic, Cleveland, Ohio, United States of America
Head and Neck Institute, The Cleveland Clinic, Cleveland, Ohio, United States of America

Lia Santiago and Sharon A. Sandridge
Head and Neck Institute, The Cleveland Clinic, Cleveland, Ohio, United States of America

Rainer Huber
Centre of Competence HörTech gGmbH, Oldenburg, Germany
Cluster of Excellence Hearing4All, Oldenburg and Hannover, Germany

Vijay Parsa and Susan Scollie
National Centre for Audiology, Western University, London, Canada

Index

R
Reduced Gpias, 1, 5, 8
Residual Hearing, 153, 160-161, 164, 201
Retinitis Pigmentosa, 113
Rna Extraction, 16, 33

S
Sensorineural Hearing Loss, 12, 19, 22, 67, 73, 75, 91, 99, 102, 105, 113, 144, 151, 177-178, 201, 204, 214
Signal-to-noise Ratio, 56, 168, 188
Single-channel Modulation, 128-129, 132
Speech Perception, 56-57, 59, 66, 128, 137, 153, 164, 179, 187-188
Speech-in-noise, 95-96, 179, 183, 185, 187-188
Spiral Ligament, 19, 21, 30, 99-101, 103, 105
Stria Vascularis, 8, 13, 17, 21, 104
Supplemental Oxygen, 76-77, 81, 84-85

T
Tartrate Resistant Acid Phosphatase, 11, 15
Temporal Amplitude Modulation, 128

Tinnitus, 1-3, 5-6, 8-10, 55, 69-70, 73, 88-90, 92-93, 95-98, 106-112, 114, 147, 166-171, 173-178, 182, 188-191, 193, 195-196, 202-203, 216, 225-226
Tinnitus Matching, 88, 92, 95, 167
Tmc1, 67, 70, 72-75, 122
Total Deafness, 42, 46, 51
Trabecular Bone Formation, 11, 19

U
Unilateral Eis, 46, 52-53
Unilateral Tinnitus, 166-167, 171, 173, 176, 178
Usher Syndrome, 113-114, 118-119

V
Vestibular Dysfunction, 19, 113

W
Working Memory Capacity, 56-57, 59, 63, 65, 188